An Introduction
to
Environmental
Toxicology

Third Edition

Michael H. Dong, MPH, DrPA, PhD

An Introduction to Environmental Toxicology
First (Student) Edition, 2011 (ISBN 978-0-578-09628-5)
Second Edition, 2012 (ISBN 978-1-477-66648-7)

CreateSpace Publishing
7290 Investment Drive
North Charleston, South Carolina, USA 29418
c/o ENVS130@gmail.com

ISBN-10: 1494324083
ISBN-13: 978-1-494-32408-7

Printed in the United States of America

Dedication

To my wife *Ivy* for her endurance, to my older daughter *Jennifer* for her appreciation, and to my younger daughter *Stephanie* for her inspiration, which together have made my writing of this book much easier as well as with greater enjoyment.

About the Author

Dr. Michael H. Dong (鄧振麟博士), born in Hong Kong, holds a Doctor of Public Administration (Dr.P.A.) degree in environmental health policy from the University of Southern California and a Doctor of Philosophy (Ph.D.) degree in environmental epidemiology from the University of Pittsburgh. Dr. Dong has also earned a Master of Public Health (M.P.H.) in environmental/nutritional sciences from the University of California at Los Angeles (UCLA), a B.Sc. in biochemistry from the University of California at Riverside, and a second B.Sc. in forensic science from the California State University at Sacramento (CSUS). Currently he is a full member of the American College of Nutrition, a full member of the (American) Society of Toxicology, a Certified Nutrition Specialist (CNS), and a Diplomate of the American Board of Toxicology (DABT).

Dr. Dong has been working for some 25 years as a regulatory toxicologist for the state of California. Prior to his state employment, for several years he was on military active duty as a U.S. Public Health Service Commissioned Corps officer serving at the U.S. Food and Drug Administration. He also served for several years as a U.S. Army Medical Service Corps officer with various assignments working as a nutritional, clinical, or research biochemist. Between the two U.S. military services, Michael worked for about a year as an occupational toxicologist as well as an environmental epidemiologist at the U.S. Occupational Safety and Health Administration.

For four years between 2005 and 2009, Michael served as one of the dozen board members of the American Board of Toxicology (ABT). From 2006 to 2008, he served as a voting member of the Scientific Advisory Committee on Alternative Toxicological Methods (SACATM) for the U.S. National Institute of Environmental Health Sciences. He is currently serving on the editorial board for the international journals *Environmental Geochemistry and Health* (since late December 2004) and *Human and Ecological Risk Assessment* (since January 2013). And since January 2008, he has been an adjunct lecturer teaching the environmental toxicology course for the Department of Environmental Studies at CSUS.

Michael's academic and professional trainings, his published work in such innovative concepts at the time as physiologically-based pharmacokinetic (PB-PK) modeling and aggregate exposure assessment through Monte Carlo (probabilistic) simulation, and the series of his online lectures on subjects such as toxicologic epidemiology, herbal medicine, and environmental endocrine disruption, all point to his continuing interest in and commitment to promoting environmental and global health. The Second Edition of this book was published in 2012. His most recent publication prior to this Third Edition was titled "Assessment of Field Reentry Exposure to Pesticides: Limitations, Uncertainties, and Alternatives" (*Hum. Ecol. Risk Assess.* 2013, 19:579-600).

Preface

This (Third) Edition continues to serve as an introduction to the basic principles, concepts, and issues for and of environmental toxicology intended for undergraduates majoring in environmental toxicology or a related field, as well as for graduate students taking a course in a related area as an elective. As with the earlier editions, this Edition is also intended to serve as supplementary reading for students whose instructors prefer to use their own lecture notes as class materials. This Edition remains as a primer covering lecture materials for a course of 3 to 6 semester units. As before, its 23 chapters have been arranged in a way that offers students the best flow and mode of comprehension, with each chapter including a set of review questions. Students using this book should already have completed a course in general biology and a course in general chemistry.

The content difference between the Second and this Edition is minimal. In addition to having corrected several typos found in the Second Edition, this Third Edition has made minor refinements and updated the status of several contemporary issues discussed in the text (e.g., H1N1 flu, SARS/MERS, persistent organic pollutants). In particular, Chapter 17 has now added the U.S. Code as a (legal) source for the definition of toxin. This Third Edition has also included in the back cover the encouraging book review conclusion given by Prof. Arthur L. Frank, M.D., Ph.D., chair of the Department of Environmental and Occupational Health, Drexel University School of Public Health.

It is expected that in the end, students can at least tell the commonality and difference between such two terms as *toxin* and *toxicant*, between *human health risk assessment* and *ecological risk assessment*, and between *environmental toxicology* and *ecotoxicology*. Students should also complete their course as well as the book with the appreciation that acute air pollution episodes such as London fog of 1952 and Meuse Valley of 1930 were environmental tragedies of the past. Nowadays, environmental toxicologists and health regulatory agencies around the world are more concerned with contemporary issues such as plastic marine pollution, melamine food poisoning, electronic waste problems in India or China, and Fukushima nuclear crisis in Japan. An undesired phenomenon happening today is that even some course instructors tend to forget that toxicology in general, and environmental toxicology in particular, should include those adverse effects caused by harmful biological and physical agents, not just by toxic chemicals.

As a book for a general course in environmental toxicology, it is written primarily *to* students who might not have heard much about the term *toxicology* or *environmental pollution*, and partly *for* those instructors who are overwhelmed by their research activities and other subspecialty interests but otherwise could have written a similar book. This textbook, or reference book to some, takes the position that a student who has completed the course should be familiar with not only the basic concepts of and the principles for environmental toxicology, but also the basic socioeconomic, environmental, regulatory, and global issues pertinent to the *practice* of environmental toxicology.

Toxicology is a study concerning the nature, the adverse effects, the biochemical actions, and the detection of all types and forms of toxicants in living systems and the ecosystem, as well as its applications to largely human health issues. Environmental toxicology is that branch of toxicology focusing on the sources and occurrence of (potential) biological, chemical, and physical contaminants in the environment, on their fate and transport in the environment, and on their adverse health effects on population dynamics of affected species. Siding with the belief or theory by some scholars that ecotoxicology is a branch of toxicology different from environmental toxicology, in this book the affected species of greater interest are humans and other mammalians, although some attention is given to other species such as plants and aquatic biota. Regardless, the toxic effects of concern in this book are not limited to the human health kind, but include also those pertaining to biological in origin and ecological in nature.

As reflected in its table of contents, the book's main objectives are for students and other readership to acquire an understanding on four general areas of knowledge in environmental toxicology: (1) the basic principles for/of environmental toxicology and the major contemporary issues relevant to human and ecosystem health; (2) the occurrence, fate, and transport of major or common pollutants in the environment; (3) the basic biological processes and physiochemical mechanisms through which toxicants (including toxins) exert their effects in humans and other species in the environment; and (4) the concepts and applications of both the ecological and the human health risk assessment, including those concepts relevant to health risk perception and communication as they concern the public's awareness pertaining to environmental pollution.

Two apologies are still due here; and they both have to do with the level at which the readership is targeted. While by certain professional standards this book may not have provided a fully comprehensive index, it has strived to index all the terms, concepts, events, names, and places that are deemed relevant, useful, or interesting to most readership. The end product of such an effort is the result of balancing the limited resources, intended readership, and professional judgment as well as personal bias. By personal bias it means that, for instance, in Table 17.2 the mycotoxin zearalenone is indexed whereas palutin is not. This is because the book takes the position that most readers are interested in the highly estrogenic effects (e.g., infertility, abortion) caused by zearalenone specifically in swine, more so than in the genotoxic effects caused by palutin in many animal species. In any event, Table 17.2 *per se* is indexed, which lists the major groups and subgroups of mycotoxins including zearalenone and palutin.

The other apology is for the bit of redundancy occurring throughout the book. Almost all the acronyms and some concepts have been re-decrypted or re-defined in a new chapter despite the fact that they have been introduced in (a) previous chapter(s). Such redundancy is considered necessary as the book takes the position that many of these acronyms and concepts are information still rather fresh to the majority of its readership.

Michael H. Dong
California, USA

Acknowledgments

I am deeply and truly grateful to Dudley Burton, Ph.D., professor and former chair of the Department of Environmental Studies, California State University at Sacramento (CSUS), for providing me with a great opportunity to teach as an adjunct lecturer the department's course in environmental toxicology.

Special thanks go to all the CSUS students who have taken the above course, which I have been teaching for several years since 2008. In fact, both the development of some of the lecture ideas and the mode of some of the lecture presentations owe much to many of these devoted students, from whose group presentations I have learned and continue to learn a great deal about environmental toxicology.

I am also indebted to many Wikipedia (largely anonymous) authors that have so effectively provided me with quick and relevant sources for many of the specifics presented in this book (this or the earlier editions). I would like to further acknowledge that if it had not been for some of the public domain images that I could use so freely, I would not have published the book so affordably and in such a timely and professional manner.

Last but not least, had I not been able to utilize the freeware version (12.01) of ACD's ChemSketch, I would not have been able to provide all the chemical structures in this book in such an effective, presentable, and affordable manner.

CONTENTS

I. TOXICOLOGIC CONCEPTS AND ENVIRONMENTAL CONCERNS

CHAPTER 1. Scope and Principles for Environmental Toxicology   **1**

1.1. Introduction   **1**

1.1.1. Some Basic Toxicology Terminology   2

1.1.2. Environmental Toxicology   3

1.2. Basic Principles for Environmental Toxicology   **3**

1.2.1. Knowledge on Toxic Dose/Environmental Exposure   4

1.2.2. Knowledge on Toxic or Undesired Effects   5

1.2.3. Knowledge on Dose-Response Relationship   5

1.2.4. Knowledge on Available Toxicity Testing Methods   6

1.2.5. Knowledge on Risk Assessment Framework   7

1.3. Setting the Proper Perspective   **7**

1.3.1. Professional Activities for Toxicologists   7

1.3.2. Environmental Toxicology *vs.* Ecotoxicology   8

1.3.3. Epidemiology as Another Very Close Ally   9

1.3.4. Importance and Scope of Environmental Toxicology   11

CHAPTER 2. Environmental Changes and Environmental Health   **15**

2.1. Introduction   **15**

2.1.1. Knowledge on the Changing World   15

2.1.2. Impacts of Global Environmental Changes   16

2.1.3. World's Perspective of Environmental Health   16

2.2. Major Specific Environmental Changes   **17**

2.2.1. Global Climate Changes   17

2.2.2. Air Pollution   17

2.2.3. Water Pollution   18

2.2.4. Soil Pollution   18

2.2.5. Red Tide Pollution   18

2.2.6. Electronic Waste Pollution   19

2.2.7. Deforestation   19

2.3. Incidence and Spectrum of Environmental Diseases   **20**

2.3.1. Incidence and Burden of Environmental Diseases   20

2.3.2. Spectrum and Nature of Environmental Diseases   21

2.4. Commonly Encountered Environmental Diseases   **22**

2.4.1. Cancer   23

2.4.2. Birth Defects   23

2.4.3. Reproductive Damage   23

2.4.4. Respiratory Diseases   24

2.4.5. Neurological Diseases   24

2.4.6. Skin Disorders   25

2.4.7. Diseases Induced by Specific Agents   25

CHAPTER 3. Environmental Pollution and Regulatory Agencies   **30**
  3.1. Introduction   **30**
    3.1.1. Impacts of Environmental Pollution   31
    3.1.2. Perception of Environmental Pollution   31
  3.2. Concerns with Environmental Pollution   **33**
    3.2.1. Regulatory Concerns in the United States   34
    3.2.2. Actions on Environmental Pollution Impacts   36
  3.3. Environmental Health Laws and Policies   **37**
    3.3.1. Regulatory Agencies in the United States   38
    3.3.2. Environmental Health Laws in the United States   39
    3.3.3. Foreign Environmental Health Laws and Agencies   41

CHAPTER 4. Occurrence and Types of Environmental Toxicants   **46**
  4.1. Introduction   **46**
    4.1.1. Contemporary Issues of Environmental Concern   46
    4.1.2. Grouping of Environmental Contaminants   47
  4.2. Contemporary Issues: 10 Select Cases   **48**
    4.2.1. Contaminants in Consumer Products   48
    4.2.2. Contaminants in Food Products   49
    4.2.3. Pollutants in the Open Environment   50
  4.3. Environmental Toxicants of Health Concern   **51**
    4.3.1. Group I: Individual, Specific Toxicants   52
    4.3.2. Group II: Specific Chemical/Biological Families   54
    4.3.3. Group III: per Use/Source or Toxic Effect   56

CHAPTER 5. Fate and Transport of Toxicants in the Environment   **62**
  5.1. Introduction   **62**
    5.1.1. Movement in the Environmental Media   62
    5.1.2. Distribution into the Living Organisms   63
  5.2. Fate and Transport of Air Pollutants   **63**
    5.2.1. Local and Long-Range Transport   63
    5.2.2. Direct and Indirect Deposition   65
    5.2.3. Changes in Chemical/Physical Form   65
  5.3. Fate and Transport of Water Contaminants   **68**
    5.3.1. Phase-Transfer and Transport Processes   69
    5.3.2. Chemical (Abiotic) Transformation   71
    5.3.3. Biological (Biotic) Transformation   71
  5.4. Fate and Transport of Soil Contaminants   **73**
    5.4.1. Volatilization from Soil   73
    5.4.2. Degradation in Soil   74
    5.4.3. Erosion and Runoff from Soil   74
    5.4.4. Leaching from Soil   75

II. BIOACCUMULATION AND BIODISPOSITION OF TOXICANTS

CHAPTER 6. Bioaccumulation of Persistent Environmental Toxicants   **78**
  6.1. Introduction   **78**
    6.1.1. Relevance of Food Chains   78
    6.1.2. Relevance to Exposure Assessment   79

6.2. Bioconcentration and Its Potential   **80**
6.2.1. Bioconcentration in the Aquatic Media   80
6.2.2. Bioconcentration Factor (BCF)   81
6.3. Bioaccumulation and Biomagnification   **82**
6.3.1. Toxic Equivalency (TEQ) in Bioaccumulation   83
6.3.2. Cases of Bioaccumulation and Biomagnification   83
6.3.3. Bioaccumulation of Organochlorine Compounds in Seafood   85
6.4. Factors Influencing Bioaccumulation   **87**
6.4.1. Lipophilicity and Bioavailability   87
6.4.2. Metabolic Potential   88
6.4.3. Environmental Mobility   88
6.4.4. A Dynamic Equilibrium Effect   89

CHAPTER 7. Uptake and Distribution of Toxicants   **94**
7.1. Introduction   **94**
7.1.1. Localized Effect of Non-Systemic Action   94
7.1.2. Disposition of Systemic/Internal Organ Toxicants   94
7.2. Mechanism of Entry   **95**
7.2.1. Structure of Cellular Membranes   95
7.2.2. Common Mechanisms of Entry   96
7.3. Uptake and Absorption of Toxicants   **97**
7.3.1. Uptake by Plants   97
7.3.2. Uptake and Absorption by Humans   99
7.4. Distribution and Excretion of Toxicants   **102**
7.4.1. Distribution via the Bloodstream   102
7.4.2. Excretion of Toxicants   103
7.5. Toxicokinetics of Toxicants   **106**
7.5.1. Principles and Models of Toxicokinetics   106
7.5.2. Basic Mathematical Concepts   107

CHAPTER 8. Metabolism/Biotransformation of Xenobiotics   **111**
8.1. Introduction   **111**
8.1.1. Metabolism *vs.* Biotransformation   111
8.1.2. Biotransforming Enzymes and Their Actions   112
8.2. General Sequence/Processes of Biotransformation   **112**
8.2.1. Phase I Enzymatic Reactions   114
8.2.2. Phase II Enzymatic Reactions   115
8.3. Other Sequences/Processes of Biotransformation   **116**
8.3.1. Bioactivation of Toxicants   116
8.3.2. Biotransformation of Endogenous Substances   116
8.4. Characteristics of Cytochrome P450 Enzymes   **117**
8.4.1. Families of Cytochrome P450   117
8.4.2. Catalytic Activities and Cellular Locations   117
8.5. Characteristics of Other Relevant Enzyme Groups   **118**
8.5.1. Enzymes in Phase II Reactions   118
8.5.2. Antioxidant Enzymes   119
8.5.3. EROD (7-Ethoxyresorufin *O*-Deethylase)   120
8.6. Factors Affecting Biotransformation   **121**
8.6.1. Genetic Polymorphism   121

8.6.2. Enzyme Inhibitors   122
8.6.3. Enzyme Inducers   122
8.6.4. Enzyme Cofactors and Coenzymes   124

CHAPTER 9. Adverse Action/Toxic Response   **129**
  9.1. Introduction   **129**
    9.1.1. Site and Mechanism of Action   129
    9.1.2. Basic Mechanisms of Action and Toxicodynamics   129
  9.2. Primary or Mediated Toxic Actions   **130**
    9.2.1. Direct Damage to Cellular Structure   130
    9.2.2. Reactions Mediated by Free Radicals   131
    9.2.3. Modulation of Receptor Functions   132
    9.2.4. Binding with a Cell Constituent   134
  9.3. Major Adverse Secondary or Indirect Actions   **135**
    9.3.1. Allergic Response   135
    9.3.2. Side Effects of Medications   135
    9.3.3. Complexation   135
    9.3.4. Microbic Invasion   136
  9.4. Disruption of Enzymatic Activities   **136**
    9.4.1. Inhibition of Cofactors or Coenzymes   137
    9.4.2. Inhibition/Inactivation of the Active Site   137
  9.5. Toxicodynamics of Toxicants   **139**
    9.5.1. Basic, Nonspecific Types of Adverse Effects   139
    9.5.2. Specific/Mechanism-Based Adverse Effects   141

CHAPTER 10. Factors and Conditions Affecting Toxicity   **149**
  10.1. Introduction   **149**
    10.1.1. Extrinsic Factors   149
    10.1.2. Intrinsic Cofactors   149
  10.2. Environmental Factors   **150**
    10.2.1. Level of Environmental Exposure   150
    10.2.2. Other Exposure-Related Factors   154
    10.2.3. Nonexposure-Related Factors   155
  10.3. Nutritional Factors   **157**
    10.3.1. Nutritional Status   157
    10.3.2. Macro- and Micro-Nutrients   158
  10.4. Physicochemical Factors   **160**
    10.4.1. Additivity of Toxic Effects   160
    10.4.2. Synergism of Toxic Effects   161
    10.4.3. Potentiation of Toxic Effects   161
    10.4.4. Antagonism of Toxic Effects   162
  10.5. Biological Factors   **162**
    10.5.1. Age, Gender, and Health Status   163
    10.5.2. Species, Strain, Race, and Genetics   164

III. NATURE AND EFFECTS OF ENVIRONMENTAL TOXICANTS

CHAPTER 11. Air Pollutants – I: Inorganic Gases   **172**
  11.1. Introduction   **172**

11.1.1. Hazardous Air Pollutants 172
11.1.2. Criteria Inorganic Gaseous Pollutants 172
11.2. Sulfur Dioxide 173
11.2.1. Sources of Pollution 173
11.2.2. Characteristics and Properties 174
11.2.3. Toxic Effects and Advisories 175
11.3. Nitrogen Oxides: Nitrogen Dioxide 177
11.3.1. Sources of Pollution 178
11.3.2. Characteristics and Properties 178
11.3.3. Toxic Effects and Advisories 179
11.4. Tropospheric Ozone 181
11.4.1. Sources of Pollution 181
11.4.2. Characteristics and Properties 181
11.4.3. Toxic Effects and Advisories 182
11.5. Carbon Monoxide 183
11.5.1. Sources of Pollution 184
11.5.2. Characteristics and Properties 184
11.5.3. Toxic Effects and Advisories 185

CHAPTER 12. Air Pollutants – II: Particulate Matter 191
12.1. Introduction 191
12.1.1. Composition of Airborne Particulates 191
12.1.2. Basic Characteristics of Airborne Particulates 192
12.2. Sizes of Particulate Matter 192
12.2.1. Sizes of Regulatory Importance 193
12.2.2. Non-Inhalable Coarse Particles (PM_{10+}) 194
12.2.3. Inhalable Coarse Particles ($PM_{2.5-10}$) 196
12.2.4. Fine Particles ($PM_{0.1-2.5}$) 196
12.2.5. Ultrafine or Nano Particles ($PM_{0.1}$) 197
12.3. Issues with Urban Airborne Particulate Pollution 197
12.3.1. Episodes of Particulate Pollution 198
12.3.2. Monitoring of Particulate Matter 199
12.3.3. Airborne Microbes 200
12.4. Toxic Effects of Airborne Particulates 202
12.4.1. Mechanisms and General Trends 203
12.4.2. Effects on the Respiratory Tract 203
12.4.3. Effects on the Cardiovascular System 204
12.4.4. Other Serious Health Effects 205
12.4.5. Effects on the Environment 206

CHAPTER 13. Volatile Organic Compounds 212
13.1. Introduction 212
13.1.1. As Precursors of Ozone and Particulate Matter 212
13.1.2. Sources of Pollution 213
13.2. Use Standards and Environmental Concerns 213
13.2.1. Standards for Consumer/Commercial Products 213
13.2.2. Select Compounds of Environmental Concern 214
13.3. Formaldehyde 215
13.3.1. Sources and Use 215

13.3.2. Exposures and Toxic Effects 216
13.4. Benzene **217**
13.4.1. Sources and Use 217
13.4.2. Exposures and Toxic Effects 218
13.5. Methyl *tert*-Butyl Ether **220**
13.5.1. Sources and Use 220
13.5.2. Exposures and Toxic Effects 221
13.6. Methylene Chloride **222**
13.6.1. Sources and Use 222
13.6.2. Exposures and Toxic Effects 222
13.7. Tetrachloroethylene **223**
13.7.1. Sources and Use 224
13.7.2. Exposures and Toxic Effects 224
13.8. Trichloroethylene **225**
13.8.1. Sources and Use 225
13.8.2. Exposures and Toxic Effects 226

CHAPTER 14. Toxic and Radioactive Metals **232**
14.1. Introduction **232**
14.1.1. Concepts of Minerals and Heavy Metals 233
14.1.2. Metals of Environmental Health Concern 233
14.2. The Three Heavy Metals **233**
14.2.1. Lead 234
14.2.2. Mercury 235
14.2.3. Cadmium 236
14.3. Select Secondary/Pseudo Heavy Metals **238**
14.3.1. Aluminum 239
14.3.2. Arsenic 240
14.3.3. Beryllium 241
14.4. Select Toxic Trace Metals **243**
14.4.1. Chromium 243
14.4.2. Nickel 244
14.4.3. Copper 246
14.5. Select Radioactive Metals **247**
14.5.1. Radium 248
14.5.2. Radon 249

CHAPTER 15. Pesticides and Pesticide Residues **255**
15.1. Introduction **255**
15.1.1. Health Impacts and Concerns 255
15.1.2. Pesticide Residues as Pollutants 256
15.2. Use and Classification of Pesticides **256**
15.2.1. Statistics on Pesticde Use 256
15.2.2. Classification of Pesticides 258
15.3. Organochlorine Pesticides **258**
15.3.1. The Dichlorodiphenylethane-Related 259
15.3.2. The Chlorinated Cyclodiene-Related 260
15.3.3. The Chlorinated Cyclohexane-Related 262
15.4. Organophosphate Pesticides **263**

15.4.1. Delayed Neurotoxic Agents 264
15.4.2. Acetylcholinesterase Inhibitors 264
15.5. Major Carbamate Pesticides **265**
15.5.1. Carbaryl 265
15.5.2. Propoxur and Several Others 266
15.6. Pyrethrin and Pyrethroid Pesticides **266**
15.6.1. Pyrethrins 266
15.6.2. Pyrethroids 267
15.7. Major Phenoxy Pesticides **268**
15.7.1. Dichlorophenoxyacetic Acid (2,4-D) 269
15.7.2. Trichlorophenoxyacetic Acid (2,4,5-T) 270
15.8. Major Triazine Pesticides **270**
15.8.1. Atrazine 270
15.8.2. Simazine and Propazine 271
15.9. Coumarin and Indandione Pesticides **271**
15.9.1. Coumarins 272
15.9.2. Indandiones 272
15.10. Select Novel/Specialty Pesticides **272**
15.10.1. Neonicotinoids 273
15.10.2. Glyphosate, Paraquat, and Compound 1080 274

CHAPTER 16. Persistent Toxic Substances **280**
16.1. Introduction **280**
16.1.1. Chemical *vs.* Environmental Persistence 280
16.1.2. Numerical Persistence Criteria 281
16.1.3. Relevance to Long-Range Transport 282
16.2. The Stockholm Convention of 2001 .... **282**
16.2.1. Persistent Pollutants of Global Concern 282
16.2.2. The Convention's Aims and Actions 283
16.3. Perfluorooctane Sulfonate **284**
16.3.1. Use and Pollution Sources 286
16.3.2. Environmental Health Concerns 286
16.4. Polybrominated Biphenyls **287**
16.4.1. Use and Pollution Sources 287
16.4.2. Environmental Health Concerns 289
16.5. Polybrominated Diphenyl Ethers **290**
16.5.1. Use and Pollution Sources 290
16.5.2. Environmental Health Concerns 291
16.6. Polychlorinated Biphenyls **292**
16.6.1. Use and Pollution Sources 292
16.6.2. Environmental Health Concerns 293
16.7. Polychlorinated Dibenzo-*p*-Dioxins/Dibenzofurans ... **294**
16.7.1. Use and Pollution Sources 294
16.7.2. Environmental Health Concerns 295
16.8. Toxic Equivalency Factors **296**
16.8.1. Concepts of Toxic Equivalency 296
16.8.2. Application of Toxic Equivalency Factor 296

CHAPTER 17. Biological and Physical Toxic Agents **303**

17.1. Introduction   **303**
17.1.1. Concepts of Biological Agents   303
17.1.2. Infection *vs.* Infectious Disease   304
17.2. Pathogenic Microbial Agents   **304**
17.2.1. Pathogenic Bacteria   305
17.2.2. Pathogenic Viruses   306
17.2.3. Pathogenic Fungi   307
17.2.4. Pathogenic Parasites   308
17.3. Toxins from Microorganisms   **309**
17.3.1. Toxins from Bacteria   310
17.3.2. Toxins from Fungi   310
17.4. Toxins from Fishes and Plants   **314**
17.4.1. Toxins from Fishes   315
17.4.2. Toxins from Plants   316
17.5. Venoms from Arthropods   **317**
17.5.1. Venoms from Arachnids   318
17.5.2. Venoms from Insects   319
17.6. Venoms from Reptiles and Amphibians   **319**
17.6.1. Venoms from Snakes   320
17.6.2. Venoms from Lizards   321
17.6.3. Venoms from Amphibians   321
17.7. Underrated Harmful Physical Agents   **322**
17.7.1. Traffic Congestion   322
17.7.2. Noise Pollution   323

IV. GENERAL CONSIDERATIONS AND SPECIAL FOCI

CHAPTER 18. Environmental Mutagenesis/Carcinogenesis   **328**
18.1. Introduction   **328**
18.1.1. DNA, RNA, Gene, and Chromosome   328
18.1.2. Characteristics of Cancer   330
18.2. Environmental Mutagenesis   **331**
18.2.1. Concepts of Mutagenesis   331
18.2.2. Point Mutation and Intragenic Mutation   332
18.2.3. Chromosome Aberration   332
18.2.4. Environmental Mutagens   333
18.3. Environmental Carcinogenesis   **336**
18.3.1. Concepts of Carcinogenesis   337
18.3.2. Mechanism of Carcinogenesis   337
18.3.3. Environmental Carcinogens   340
18.4. DNA Damage and Repair   **340**
18.4.1. DNA Damage   342
18.4.2. DNA Repair   343

CHAPTER 19. Reproductive Toxicity and Endocrine Disruption   **347**
19.1. Introduction   **347**
19.1.1. Impacts and Causes of Human Birth Defects   348
19.1.2. Concerns with Human Reproductive Disorders   348
19.1.3. Concepts of Endocrine Disruption in Humans   349

19.2. The Endocrine-Reproductive System   **350**
19.2.1. The Human Developmental-Reproductive Cycle   350
19.2.2. The Human Endocrine System   351
19.2.3. Hormones (The Chemical Messengers)   355
19.3. Endocrine/Hormonal Disruption   **357**
19.3.1. Modes of Endocrine Disruption   357
19.3.2. Types of Endocrine Disruptors   358
19.4. Developmental-Reproductive Effects in Humans   **359**
19.4.1. Birth Defects and Environmental Teratogens   361
19.4.2. Reproductive Effects and Environmental Toxicants   363

CHAPTER 20. Occupational Toxicology/Industrial Chemicals   **369**
20.1. Introduction   **369**
20.1.1. Classic Industrial Diseases   369
20.1.2. Uniqueness of Occupational Toxicology   370
20.1.3. Occupational Health Laws   370
20.2. U.S. Legislation for Occupational Health   **371**
20.2.1. U.S. Occupational Safety and Health Act   371
20.2.2. U.S. Occupational Safety and Health Administration   372
20.2.3. U.S. National Institute for Occupational Safety and Health   373
20.3. Relevant Concepts for Occupational Toxicology   **375**
20.3.1. Threshold Limit Values   375
20.3.2. Biological Exposure Indices   376
20.4. Occupational Toxic Agents/Industrial Chemicals   **377**
20.4.1. Pesticides   377
20.4.2. Metals   379
20.4.3. Organic Solvents   380
20.4.4. Fibers/Dusts   381
20.4.5. Other Groups of Toxic Agents   383

CHAPTER 21. Food Toxicants and Toxic Household Substances   **388**
21.1. Introduction   **388**
21.1.1. Concerns with Food Toxicants   388
21.1.2. Concerns with Toxic Household Substances   389
21.2. Toxic Substances in Food Products   **390**
21.2.1. Direct Food Additives   390
21.2.2. Indirect Food Additives   393
21.2.3. Food Contaminants   396
21.3. Toxic Substances in Household Products   **397**
21.3.1. Substances in Personal Care Products   398
21.3.2. Substances in Cleaning Agents   400
21.3.3. Substances in Over-the-Counter Medicines   401
21.3.4. Substances in Other Organic Compounds   402
21.4. Learning Lessons with Food and Household Products   **403**
21.4.1. Persistent Toxic Substances in Seafood   403
21.4.2. Lead on Children's Jewelry and Toys   403
21.4.3. Triclosan in Antibacterial Products   405
21.4.4. Self-Mitigation and Self-Prevention   405

CHAPTER 22. Human Health Aspects of Ecotoxicology   **411**

  22.1. Introduction   **411**
    22.1.1. Relevance of Aquatic Toxicology   411
    22.1.2. Relevance of Wildlife Toxicology   412
    22.1.3. Relevance of Hazardous Waste Pollution   412
  22.2. Aquatic Toxicology and Human Health   **413**
    22.2.1. The Basic Aquatic Environment   413
    22.2.2. Aquatic Toxicity Tests   414
    22.2.3. Regulatory Efforts for Water Quality   416
  22.3. Wildlife Toxicology and Human Health   **416**
    22.3.1. Scope and History of Wildlife Toxicology   417
    22.3.2. The Basic Wildlife Environment   418
    22.3.3. Ecological Risk Assessment   420
  22.4. Hazardous Wastes of Global/American Concern   **423**
    22.4.1. The RCRA Definition and Implications   424
    22.4.2. The Superfund Law and Program   425
    22.4.3. The United Heckathorn Site (A Case Study)   426

CHAPTER 23. Environmental Health Risk Assessment   **433**

  23.1. Introduction   **433**
    23.1.1. Health Risk Assessment Activities   433
    23.1.2. Subtleties of Health Risk Assessment   435
  23.2. Toxicity Assessment   **436**
    23.2.1. Hazard Identification   436
    23.2.2. Animal Toxicity Studies   437
    23.2.3. Dose-Response Assessment   438
  23.3. Human Exposure Assessment   **440**
    23.3.1. Past and Current Perspectives   441
    23.3.2. Direct and Indirect Measurements   442
    23.3.3. Aggregate and Cumulative Exposures   444
  23.4. Health Risk Characterization   **445**
    23.4.1. Health Risk Measures   445
    23.4.2. Uncertainty and Safety Factors   447
    23.4.3. Health Risk Perception   450
    23.4.4. Health Risk Communication   451

INDEX   **457**

An Introduction

to

Environmental Toxicology

Third Edition

CHAPTER 1

Scope and Principles for Environmental Toxicology

1.1. Introduction

The scope for environmental toxicology should begin with the definition of general toxicology, which in its simplest term is *the science of poisons*. The more descriptive definition of general toxicology is that it is *the science studying the nature, the adverse effects, the biochemical actions, and the detection of all types and all forms of poisons in living systems and the ecosystem, with a focus being more on human health issues.* Toxicology, much like medicine, is both a science and an art.

The historical development of toxicology dates back to the cave dwellers era, when prehistoric people utilized poisonous plants, animal venoms, and their extracts for execution, hunting, and warfare. By 1500 BC, when the metal mercury was discovered in an Egyptian tomb, medical documents such as the Egyptian *Papyrus Ebers* already revealed that *hemlock* (a herbal extract used to execute Socrates), certain *aconitum species* (as a Chinese arrow poison), and certain *metals* (lead, copper) were effective to poison foes. The Egyptian queen Cleopatra VII was suspected to have died of a venomous snakebite; and the Roman emperor Claudius reportedly was poisoned with mushrooms.

By the late Middle Age, poisons became widely applied in humankind with greater sophistication. During that time period, certain concepts fundamental to toxicology also emerged. Noteworthy in that movement were the work of Phillip von Hohenheim, otherwise known more commonly as Paracelsus (circa 1500 AD), and later the work of Mathieu J. B. Orfila (circa 1800 AD).

Paracelsus, a German-Swiss physician-alchemist known also as the father of (*classic*) toxicology, was the first person to focus on specific substances as *agents* responsible for the toxicity of a plant or an animal poison. He advanced the notion that the body's response to specific toxic agents depends on the dose received. That notion is now known as the dose-response relationship, one of the basic principles for toxicology. Paracelsus is frequently quoted for his famous assertion that *"All substances are poisons; there is none which (that) is not a poison. The right dose differentiates a poison and a remedy."*

Mathieu J. B. Orfila, a Spanish-born physician working in a French court, is generally regarded as the father of *modern* toxicology and the founder of clinical or forensic pathology. He was the first forensic toxicologist to apply autopsy materials and chemical analysis systematically as legal proof of poisoning, by way of demonstrating the *adverse effects* of poisons on *specific tissues* and *organs*.

1

Modern toxicology is the outgrowth of advances in many related scientific disciplines including analytical chemistry, biochemistry, ecology, epidemiology, medicine, molecular biology, nutritional science, pharmacology, physiology, public health, and many more. Since World War II, the production of synthetic fibers, drugs, pesticides, and industrial chemicals has increased markedly. So has people's knowledge on biochemical materials that sustain biological functions, including especially the hereditary material of life biochemically known as *deoxyribonucleic acid* (which nowadays is more commonly known by its acronym DNA). These developments have revolutionized toxicology (and many other life sciences as well) exponentially. Further discussion in this area has been given in numerous places in the literature including Gallo (2001), Lane and Borzelleca (2008), and the U.S. National Institutes of Health (NIH, 2008).

1.1.1. Some Basic Toxicology Terminology

Toxicology is an ever-evolving discipline, and so are the terms it uses in the literature. The terms that it uses for materials causing toxic effects are not always consistent. The most common terms used for these toxic materials include *toxicants*, *poisons*, *toxic substances, toxic agents, toxic chemicals, contaminants*, and *pollutants*. Although these terms are used interchangeably in some literature, by definition they differ from one another somewhat. The following are terms defined largely in accordance with two dictionaries of toxicology published in the 1990s (i.e., Hodgson *et al.*, 1998; Lewis, 1998).

Toxicants are natural or synthetic materials capable of causing adverse effects on or to living organisms. *Poisons* are toxicants that tend to cause *acute* death or *severe* illness even when exposed to in *trace* amounts. A *toxic substance* is simply any material having toxic properties, short of appreciating its ability to induce untoward effects. Note that gasoline should be referred to more appropriately as a toxic substance in that it contains a mixture of many chemicals, whereas something like cyanide is a discrete *toxic chemical*. Simply put, a *toxic agent*, like a toxic substance, refers to a toxicant using two words instead of one. In any event, a toxicant, a toxic substance, or a toxic agent can be *chemical* (e.g., mercury), *physical* (e.g., noise), or *biological* (e.g., snake venom) in nature.

Toxins are toxicants *produced* by *living cells* or *organisms*, and are capable of causing disease when present in the body tissue of a host organism (*see* Section 17.1). Most of them are protein-like materials. For example, botulinum toxin is a neurotoxin (i.e., that acting on the nerve cells) protein produced by the bacterium *Clostridium botulinum* and is perhaps the most potent biological substance known. Note that in toxicology, potency is defined as the ability or capacity to achieve or bring about the same toxic effect. By most potent, it means achieving the same lethal (or most severe) effect from the smallest amount of dose. Today, due to modern society's higher expectation for better life, the concern with a toxic substance's potency is no longer in terms of lethal dose or concentration at the 50th percentile (i.e., LD_{50} or LC_{50}, respectively, or more specifically the level required to kill half of the test population). Instead, today's concerns with the effect dose are down to the no observed effect level (NOEL), or the no observed *adverse* effect level (NOAEL) for non-cancer toxicity. These lower effect levels and other related risk measures, including those for cancer risk, are (further) discussed in Chapter 23.

Xenobiotic is the general term used for a *foreign* substance, usually a chemical, that is found in the body or has been taken into the body. The term is derived from the Greek word *xeno*, which means "foreigner". Xenobiotics may produce beneficial effects (e.g., pharmaceuticals) or may be toxic (e.g., arsenic, lead). They can be natural or synthetic materials, but must be exogenous in origin. A *contaminant* or *pollutant* is an undesired xenobiotic or agent (initially) present in a medium that contains a principal component, such as the case of a toxic chemical being the pollutant in the medium air, water, soil, foods, or other consumer products.

1.1.2. Environmental Toxicology

As generally accepted (e.g., Hodgson *et al.*, 1998; Lewis, 1998), *environmental toxicology* is that branch of toxicology focusing on three main aspects: (1) the sources of toxicants or potential toxicants in the environment; (2) their fate and transport under various environmental conditions and through food chains; and (3) their adverse effects on population dynamics of affected species. As such, and from a practical perspective, even a brief discussion of the scope and importance for or of environmental toxicology should start with those for or of general toxicology.

Environmental toxicology is best described as an interdisciplinary science currently at its adolescence. This branch of toxicology is an interdisciplinary science that continues to have a somewhat disputed core of knowledge for some time (and hence the urge for publication of this book). As Wright and Welbourn (2002) put it, "*There is still some controversy concerning the stage in a curriculum at which it should be introduced.*"

Siding with the theory advocated by a number of scholars (e.g., WHO, 1986; Wright and Welbourn, 2002) that ecological toxicology (or ecotoxicology for short) is a branch of toxicology different from environmental toxicology, in this book the affected species of greater concern are humans and other mammalians, although some attention is given to other species such as plants and aquatic biota. The toxic effects of concern in this book thereby are not limited to the human health kind, but also include those pertaining to biological or ecological in nature or origin. Even though ecotoxicology is perhaps the closest ally of environmental toxicology and hence to some people (e.g., WHO, 1986) the two should be considered together, they are two separate branches of toxicology. The distinction between the two branches is discussed in (Sub)Section 1.3.2 below.

1.2. Basic Principles for Environmental Toxicology

The basic principles for or of environmental toxicology are integral to the process what is now known as *health risk assessment* or *characterization,* where quantitative estimates are determined for the health risk associated with the (environmental) exposure of concern. As depicted in Figure 1.1, these principles involve (but are not limited to) the fundamentals, the concepts, and the understandings of five key subject matters: (1) *toxic dose/environmental exposure*; (2) *toxic or undesired effects*; (3) *dose-response relationship*; (4) *availability of toxicity testing methods*; and (5) *framework of health risk assessment*. Further discussion on these and related subject matters can be found in Eaton and Klaassen (2001), NIH (2008), and especially Chapter 23 of this book.

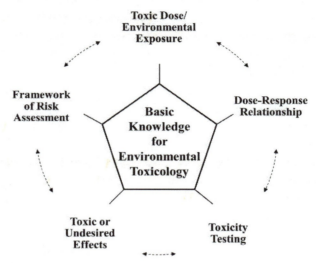

Figure 1.1. Basic Knowledge and Principles for Environmental Toxicology

1.2.1. Knowledge on Toxic Dose/Environmental Exposure

By definition, *toxic dose* is the amount of a toxicant applied to, or taken by, an organism during a specific time interval. *Exposure*, on the other hand, is the amount that the organism comes in contact with. There are, however, several variables that need to be considered in order to fully characterize the dosing with or exposure to a toxicant. The most critical are the magnitude, the frequency, and the duration of exposure or dosing. Toxic dose can be referred to by its type or form, such as *exposure* or *applied* dose, *absorbed* dose, and (total) *internal* dose. *Dosage* is a dose expressed as some function of the organism and time (e.g., mg of the toxicant per kg of body weight per day).

Dosage is a useful or more practical term in that the clinical and toxic effects of a dose are usually related to age and body size. This explains why there are adult Tylenol® (e.g., 350 mg each) *vs.* children Tylenol® (e.g., 80 mg each) tablets sold over the counter. Another important aspect is the *time* and *duration* over which a dose is given. This is particularly crucial for distinguishing doses that are required to induce a short-term *vs.* long-term (chronic) effect. For human exposure, the time unit commonly used is 24 hours and hence the usual dosage unit is *the amount (e.g., mg) per kg of body weight per day*.

The units for *environmental* exposure are usually expressed as the amount of a pollutant in a unit of an environmental medium (component). Examples of this type are mg/L (mg/liter) for pollutants in liquid or water, mg/g (mg/gram) for pollutants in solid or soil, and mg/m^3 (mg/cubic meter) for pollutants in the atmosphere. Smaller units are often encountered when expressing these environmental levels, such as µg/ml, or ppm (i.e., *parts of the substance per million* parts of the medium's principal component such as air, soil, water, or foods). Likewise, ppb (parts per billion) = µg/L or µg/kg.

1.2.2. Knowledge on Toxic or Undesired Effects

Toxicity is the degree or extent to which an agent can cause an adverse or undesired effect when an organism is exposed to it. The term can also be used as *such an adverse effect* on the organism's entire body or its substructures. In relation to *exposure* assessment, human adverse effects can be classified as follows: allergic reactions; idiosyncratic reactions (i.e., those peculiar to certain individuals); delayed *vs.* immediate toxicity; reversible *vs.* irreversible effects; and localized *vs.* systemic effects (Chapter 9).

Toxic effects are often influenced by the following factors: dosage; age; time and duration of dosing; route of exposure; species; gender; ability to be absorbed (into the host organism's body); nutrition; metabolism; disposition in the body; ability to be excreted (from the host organism's body); presence of other chemicals; and more. The biochemical mechanism in which an (adverse) effect is induced is complicated with many of these influencing factors, of which dosage is the most important or most relevant under normal circumstances (Chapter 10).

Some xenobiotics are themselves toxic. Others must be chemically biotransformed or otherwise broken down (i.e., metabolized) within the body before they can induce deleterious effects in a living organism (Chapter 8). Many xenobiotics available in the body of an organism affect only specific target organs. Others, however, can damage any of the organism's cells, tissues, or organs that they come in contact with. The target organs to be affected by these xenobiotics may vary depending on the dosage and route of exposure involved. For example, the site of toxic attack may be the central nervous system (CNS) for a toxicant after acute exposure at high levels. Yet the site may well be limited to the liver, the lungs, or the kidneys following chronic exposure to the same toxicant at lower doses or concentrations.

1.2.3. Knowledge on Dose-Response Relationship

Dose-response is defined as the (quantitative) relationship *between* the amount of a toxicant taken in or exposed to *and* the incidence or the extent of the toxic response (or of the toxic effect) induced. This relationship, when well founded, can strengthen the hypothesis that the toxicant is responsible for causing the observed effect(s). It can provide an estimate for the lowest dose that can induce the effect, which is the so-called threshold level or the lowest observed effect level (LOEL). By means of its slope, its curve, or the kind, it can also determine the dosage required to reach a certain level of toxic damage (or therapeutic effect). This type of quantitative inference has its limitations in that in most environmental settings, humans and other living organisms are exposed to multiple toxicants, rather than to a particular one for which the relationship is (to be) established.

Toxicants administered or taken in simultaneously may exert their toxic actions independently. Yet in many instances, the presence of one toxicant may drastically affect the host organism's response to another toxicant. The toxicity of a combination of toxicants may be less or more than that predicted from the known effect of each individual toxicant involved. The effect or influence that one toxicant has on the toxicity of another is known as a (bio- or physico-)chemical *interaction* which can fall into one of the following four joint effect patterns: *additivity* (additive effect); *antagonism* (reducing or inhibiting the target effect); *potentiation* (enhancing or promoting the effect which otherwise might not have occurred); and *synergism* (resulting in greater than additive effect). Further discussion on this topic is given in Chapter 10.

1.2.4. Knowledge on Available Toxicity Testing Methods

The investigation into chemical toxicity in general or into chemical interaction in particular is not without difficulty or limitations. Animal studies are rarely conducted to evaluate the toxicity of a chemical in a mixture, or to predict the combined effect of multiple toxicants in a mixture. One reason for not doing so as a common practice is that the toxic effect of the target toxicant could be easily confounded by those of the nontarget chemicals in the mixture. Another reason is logistic, as many more test animals and dosings would otherwise be required to sort out the various possible combined outcomes. The toxicity of a chemical is thus mostly determined by exposing test animals to the toxicant of concern only, amidst the reality that most humans and most other living organisms are exposed to multiple environmental pollutants at the same time.

Despite or amidst the limitations noted above, knowledge on toxicity continues to be derived mostly from studies in three categories: (1) epidemiological studies, including routine or clinical observations of people during their normal use of a substance or via accidental exposures; (2) controllable animal studies (i.e., *in vivo*); and (3) even more controllable test tube type assays (i.e., *in vitro*) at the molecular or cellular level using human, animal, or plant tissues. Of the three types, nowadays the last two are increasingly used for toxicity testing before most any new synthetic product is allowed to be on the market. This is especially the case for products such as food additives, pharmaceuticals, pesticides, medical devices, and industrial chemicals made since World War II.

The regulatory requirements of subjecting synthetic products to toxicity testing are crucial in terms of public health protection. In the past, a number of notable health tragedies had occurred, mostly in the United States, that were due to the populace's exposure to inadequately tested drugs and other substances: for example, the treatment of syphilis with arsenic (e.g., in pregnant women) until World War II, resulting in severe toxicity; the use of ethylene glycol as the first antibiotic (e.g., for treatment of Streptococcal infections), leading to over 100 American deaths in 15 states; and the use of thalidomide as an anti-nausea medicine, resulting in thousands of children born with severe birth defects worldwide. It was largely due to these health tragedies that in the United States, the following federal regulatory agencies were established or strengthened to (re)assure public health and safety: U.S. Food and Drug Administration (FDA: e.g., for pharmaceuticals, foods, cosmetics, medical devices, vaccines); U.S. Environmental Protection Agency (U.S. EPA: e.g., for agricultural and industrial chemicals released into the environment); U.S. Consumer Product Safety Commission (CPSC: e.g., for hazardous substances in consumer products, particularly those used in homes); and U.S. Occupational Safety and Health Administration (OSHA: e.g., for exposure to chemicals in workplaces). Further discussion on these agencies is given in Chapter 3.

1.2.5. Knowledge on Risk Assessment Framework

The assessment of environmental exposure and the evaluation of toxicity test results are all part of the so-called ecological or human health risk assessment activities. In the early years, the risk assessment activities performed by the various federal agencies in the United States were not always consistent or easy to follow. Accordingly, in 1983 the U.S. National Research Council (NRC) published standard terminology for *health* risk assessment and set out the basic framework for the process. There are four key analytical steps in NRC's initial risk assessment paradigm: *Hazard Identification*, *Dose-Response Assessment*, *Human Exposure Assessment*, and *Risk Characterization* (Chapter 23).

The (by-)products of regulatory risk assessments are generally exposure standards or guidelines that are set forth by government agencies to protect the public from harmful substances or activities that can cause serious health problems. These exposure standards and guidelines provide certain (perceived) acceptable exposure levels for various media (e.g., water, soil, air, foods, medicines, consumer products) that people come in contact with. In other cases, these standards or guidelines may be treated as preventive measures to reduce the exposures of concern (e.g., those pertaining to product labeling, personal protective equipment, and medical monitoring or surveillance). Exposure standards differ from exposure guidelines in that the former tend to be legally acceptable exposure limits or controls, whereas the latter are recommended or suggested maximum levels.

1.3. Setting the Proper Perspective

In what follows, brief accounts are given on four topics deemed to be especially relevant in setting a proper perspective for appreciating the role of toxicology in general, and of environmental toxicology in particular. These topics are: (1) professional activities for toxicologists; (2) environmental toxicology *vs.* ecotoxicology; (3) epidemiology as another very close ally; and (4) importance and scope of environmental toxicology. There are certainly more topics of this kind than the four discussed below. However, it is this book's position that these other topics are either considered as less relevant, or discussed more frequently in other forums (including in other chapters of this book).

1.3.1. Professional Activities for Toxicologists

There are three principal categories of professional activities for toxicologists, each of which interacts with or affects the other two (e.g., Eaton and Klaassen, 2001). These three activity categories are *descriptive*, *mechanistic*, and *regulatory*. Although the activities in these three categories have their own distinct characteristics, they each contribute to those in the other two. Mechanistic toxicologists have their focus on identifying and understanding the biochemical mechanisms by which chemical, physical, or biological agents exert their effects on living organisms. Descriptive toxicologists are largely analytical, clinical, or forensic scientists whose concerns include toxicity testing that directly or indirectly provides the needed information for safety evaluation and regulatory requirements. Their work may also provide significant clues to an agent's mechanism of toxicological action. A regulatory toxicologist's principal responsibility is to determine, through use of the data provided by descriptive and mechanistic toxicologists, whether the (environmental) exposure level is sufficiently safe or whether a product poses an acceptable low risk to be used for its intended purpose.

Toxicologists in each of the three categories may involve themselves in one or more of the numerous toxicology branches whose foci, interests, concerns, and functions are forever evolving and constantly shifting. The more prominent subspecialties of toxicology include environmental toxicology, occupational toxicology, analytical toxicology, pesticide toxicology, clinical toxicology, molecular and biochemical toxicology, regulatory toxicology, radiation toxicology, nutritional toxicology, epidemiologic toxicology, veterinary toxicology, ecotoxicology, inhalation toxicology, developmental toxicology, immunotoxicology, cardiotoxicology, neurotoxicology, and forensic toxicology.

1.3.2. Environmental Toxicology *vs.* Ecotoxicology

Much like ecology *vs.* environmental sciences, to this date a small number of scholars still do not care about or appreciate the distinction between ecotoxicology and environmental toxicology despite the fact that many others do. According to Truhaut (1977), ecotoxicology is defined as *"The branch of toxicology concerned with the study of toxic effects, caused by natural or synthetic pollutants, to the constituents of ecosystems, animal (including human), vegetable and microbial, in an integral context."*

Ecotoxicology is allegedly to have its main focus on the integration of toxicology and ecology or, as Chapman (2002) has suggested it, on *"ecology in the presence of toxicants"*. That branch of toxicology aims to understand, assess, and thereby reduce the adverse effects on natural populations, communities, or ecosystems, whether the stressors (e.g., toxic agents) are natural or anthropogenic in origin. It differs from environmental toxicology in that it integrates the effects of stressors across *all* levels of biological organization from the molecular to whole communities and ecosystems, whereas environmental toxicology has a stronger concern with the toxic effects on *individuals* living in a community (Maltby and Naylor, 1990), at least more so than on the ecosystem.

The publication of Rachel Carson's seminal volume *Silent Spring* in 1962 unquestionably catalyzed the separation of environmental toxicology, and later of ecotoxicology, from classical toxicology. The key revolutionary element in Carson's contribution was her extrapolation from effects on single organisms to effects at the whole ecosystem and the "balance of nature" (Bazerman *et al.*, 2005). Such a systematic study is distinct from the anthropocentric nature of classical toxicology. Overall, environmental toxicology is a discipline incorporating many aspects of analytical chemistry, biochemistry, environmental health, epidemiology, molecular biology, physiology, toxicology, and a wealth of other disciplines to study the adverse effects of xenobiotics in a community or population. The ultimate goal of this approach is to be able to *anticipate* the effects of environmental pollution so that, should such an incident occur, the most efficient or efficacious action to remediate the detrimental effects can be identified and implemented. As with ecotoxicology, there is a strong link *between* the legislative process on environmental pollution *and* the practice as well as the development of environmental toxicology.

1.3.3. Epidemiology as Another Very Close Ally

Epidemiology is the branch of medical or public health science concerned with the occurrence, transmission, and control of epidemic diseases in human populations. It also studies the factors that modify, or that are suspected to be capable of modifying, the distribution of a disease. The main purpose of studying disease distribution in a population is for one or both of the following two reasons: (1) to determine if there is a health crisis or risk with the disease; or (2) to use the disease distribution observed under some specific conditions as a measure of the association's strength between the disease and a suspected agent, hazard, or factor. Epidemiology students are thereby trained to measure incidence, prevalence, and their interrelation (e.g., Gordis, 1996; Lilienfeld and Stolley, 1994; Rothman and Sander, 1998; Szklo and Nieto, 2000).

Incidence and *prevalence* involve the number of *new* and *existing* cases, respectively, at a specific time point or during a time interval. These rates and other measures of morbidity and mortality are the main objectives of descriptive epidemiology, in which the attempt is to characterize the amount and distribution of disease within a population. Epidemiologists are also given training in analytical methods, in which several study designs are available as practical methodologies to measure associations between exposures and effects. These study designs include cohort study, clinical trial, case-control study, cross-sectional study, quasi-experimental study, and ecological study. All of these studies have human subjects or patients as the observational units (e.g., Gordis, 1996; Lilienfeld and Stolley, 1994; Rothman and Sander, 1998; Szklo and Nieto, 2000).

The selection of hazards or factors for epidemiologic investigation is rarely a random act. It is largely based on some physical or biological, but more typically, chemical and toxicological data and understandings. Although the assessment of this type of associations tends to be statistical in nature, the formulation of any of these associations is often based on some biological or toxicological speculation. For example, it might have been that by chance chimney sweeps were seen in the 1770s to associate with higher incidence of cancer of the scrotum. Yet it was largely due to the acceptance of the underlying biological process that more epidemiological studies were conducted to heighten this link.

Naturally, the most convincing evidence for supporting a causal relationship in humans is a well-conducted epidemiological study in which a strong link between exposure and disease in human subjects has been observed, as human data would offer most direct evidence. Yet well-conducted epidemiological studies are rather hard to come by, as it is unethical to deliberately subject humans to doses sufficient to cause them bodily harm. For somewhat different objectives, human exposure assessment is covered more fully and more frequently in epidemiology than in toxicology textbooks. In spite of this coverage preference, there are several reasons why some epidemiologists, like many toxicologists, do not find human exposure assessment appealing. These reasons are discussed in the final chapter (Chapter 23) on environmental health risk assessment.

Today's epidemiology is nevertheless found to play a greater role in health risk assessment than in early years. Recent advances in epidemiology that are pertinent to health risk assessment include several specialty areas into which general epidemiology at both the basic and the intermediate level have branched out. Coincidentally or not, these (sub)specialty areas parallel closely to those of toxicology, such as environmental epidemiology, occupational epidemiology, molecular epidemiology, cardiovascular epidemiology, nutritional epidemiology, reproductive epidemiology, genetic epidemiology, cancer epidemiology, pharmacoepidemiology, neuroepidemiology, and immunoepidemiology. The particular types of diseases that these individual specialties focus on also parallel closely to the various types of adverse effects that health risk assessors attempt to determine during the hazard identification phase; this phase is a key and usually the first component of the human health risk assessment process (Chapter 23).

In particular, environmental epidemiology and occupational epidemiology are the two branches oriented largely towards the study of causative exposures, rather than of disease outcomes. Occupational epidemiology is closely related to environmental epidemiology in that many of the environmental contaminants of concern are products or by-products initially present in a work setting. Accordingly, certain occupational groups are often subject to the same or similar types of contaminant insults as the general public are, even though the levels of exposure that each group encounters are likely different. Workers and users will receive the exposure during manufacturing or handling of the products. In contrast, the general public will be exposed to the (by-)products when these contaminants have been emitted, spread, or precipitated into the local environment.

The exposures to environmental and occupational health hazards are the domain of human health-based risk assessment because they are not only of great concern to the general public or workers, but are also thought to be highly preventable via regulatory intervention. It is under this premise that in many industrialized countries including notably the United States, many health statutes have been enacted to regulate the exposures to environmental health hazards. American health statutes in this category are summarized in Table 3.2 (in Chapter 3). Of all the branches of epidemiology, occupational epidemiology tends to use biomarkers the most for monitoring human exposures. This is because occupational groups are relatively easier to be identified, worked with, and followed up.

1.3.4. Importance and Scope of Environmental Toxicology

The importance of treating environmental toxicology as a distinct branch of toxicology is brought about in Section 1.3.2 concerning its distinction from ecotoxicology. Yet that section falls short of spelling out the subtle reasons why environmental toxicology is an important study subject on its own. In reality, there are at least three interrelated issues supporting the importance of environmental toxicology. One issue and perhaps the most crucial is that, as discussed further in Chapter 2, both the incidence and the spectrum of *environmental* diseases have been expanding markedly, particularly in the industrialized nations since World War II. Coincidentally or not, at about the same time, the use and the production of synthetic materials have increased at a similar rate. Another related issue is the enormous economic burden incurred from the widespread of environmental diseases that has been taking a substantial toll on human health and the ecosystem. The third closely related issue is that, owing to such huge economic burden, many governments begin to have insufficient resources to improve their people's quality of life, as they can no longer do more with other public health or welfare programs.

These issues are well reflected in the way in which the World Health Organization (WHO, 2003) looked at environmental health for children on the first year of the World Health Day. As WHO put it well, a child's world centers around the home, the school, and the local community. Yet in real life, these places are often so unhealthy that they underlie the majority of deaths as well as a huge burden of disease among children in the developing and underdeveloped regions. WHO went further to condemn and project that more than five million children under 15 years of age die every year from diseases linked to the environments in which they live, learn, and play.

Environmental toxicology is more than about the effects of chemical pollution. Its medical term covers not only the toxicity and toxicology of environmental pollutants in the air, dust, sediment, soil, water, foods, and other media, but also those of natural toxins in the environment. This definition reasserts the notion that the toxicants of concern are not limited to chemical, but include biological and physical agents (Chapter 17).

The reality is that, in the last decade or so between 2001 and 2013, there were at least four environmental pollution episodes reaching global concerns. Three of these concerns involved biological agents as the contaminants, whereas the fourth had to do with persistent toxic chemicals (Chapter 16). The three biological agents of global concern in the recent past were a mis-folded prion protein, a coronavirus which has a crown-like or halo appearance, and a subtype of influenza A virus named H1N1.

A mis-folded (i.e., mis-shaped) form of prion protein was implicated as the cause of a variety of diseases in mammals, including notably bovine spongiform encephalopathy (BSE). BSE is also known as mad-cow disease as it causes progressive neurological degeneration predominately in cattle. Similar to BSE in symptoms, Creutzfeldt-Jakob disease (CJD) is a rare brain disorder that occurs in humans. Neither the BSE nor the new variant of CJD (*v*CJD) cases were found in the United States until 2003. Yet between 1986 and 1992, over 180,000 BSE cases among cattle were confirmed in the United

Kingdom (WHO, 2011). And in more recent years, some BSE cases were also reported in other (predominately European) countries (e.g., Belgium, Denmark, France, Germany, Japan, Ireland, Italy, Spain). In addition, 129 cases of known vCJD (i.e., human) cases were reported between 1996 and 2002 mostly in the United Kingdom. As expected, the main concern with the BSE epidemic in the United Kingdom or other countries is that the infected animals would enter the human food chains. It was for such concerns that immediately following the first case of BSE reported in the United States on 23 December 2003, Japan stopped the $1.4 billion worth of beef imports from the United States until December 2005. A case of BSE found in the United States in April 2012 was the country's fourth and the world's most recently reported as of this writing. This 2012 case was discovered in a dairy cow brought to a transfer facility near Hanford, California.

A coronavirus was implicated as the agent responsible for the fatal *s*evere *a*cute *r*espiratory *s*yndrome (SARS) first reported in Asia in February 2003. Within a year, this infectious disease spread to more than two dozen countries in Europe, North America, South America, but predominately Asia before its global outbreak was contained. The 2003 outbreak involved 8,098 human victims worldwide, of which 774 died. What had made SARS a significant environmental disease was the observation that it tended to spread by close person-to-person contact. The virus was thought to be transmitted most readily and easily by respiratory droplets produced from an infected person's cough or sneeze. Some victims were found to have been exposed through foreign travel to other parts of the world with SARS. Air travel(er) thus can be an important transmission vehicle (vector), but is highly avoidable with effective traveling alerts or regulations. According to the U.S. Centers for Disease Control and Prevention (CDC, 2011a), the latest human cases of SARS were from laboratory-acquired infections reported in China in April 2004. However, recently over 100 SARS-*like* new cases have been confirmed by WHO (2013) since about a year after their first documentation in 2012. These new cases all involved a *novel* coronavirus, and were referred to by WHO as Middle East respiratory syndrome (MERS) as most of them occurred in the Middle East countries.

H1N1 is a new strain of influenza A virus. This strain is more specifically called 2009 H1N1 because it was first detected in the United States in April 2009, and was declared by WHO two months later as responsible for the flu pandemic initiated in Mexico. This disease was mistakenly and more commonly referred to as "swine flu" because many genes in the two proteins hemagglutinin (H) and neuraminidase (N) in the virus were thought to be very similar to those in influenza viruses commonly found in pigs. While showing some relief of a downward trend, human infections with H1N1 virus were still ongoing worldwide as of December 2013, such as in Alberta, Canada (CBCNews, 2013). H1N1 virus is highly contagious in humans, spreading in the same manner as a common seasonal flu transmits. According to CDC (2011b), the symptoms of H1N1 infection include fever, headaches, coughs, sneezes, sore throat, runny or stuffy nose, muscle or joint aches, chills, and fatigue. A considerable number of the infected individuals reportedly had diarrhea and vomiting. Hospitalization and death had occurred as a result of illness associated with this viral infection, primarily in children and adults under 60 years old and in those having one or more underlying medical conditions such as heart disease, diabetes, kidney disease, asthma, and pregnancy. A vaccine for this new virus strain has become available worldwide since October 2009.

Both the SARS/MERS and the H1N1 pandemic are agreeably more of a public health issue than one directly related to environmental toxicology or environmental pollution. Yet the laboratory confirmation of the viral pathogen in both cases and the development of a high-yield vaccine virus in the H1N1 case are indeed more related to toxicity testing, the role of a toxicologist with the proper training.

References

Bazerman C, De los Santos RA, 2005. Measuring Incommensurability: Are Toxicology and Ecotoxicology Bind to What the Other Sees? In *Rhetoric and Incommensurability* (Harris RA, Ed.). West Lafayette, Indiana, USA: Parlor Press, Chapter 10.

Carson R, 1962. *Silent Spring*. Boston, Massachusetts, USA: Houghton Mifflin.

CBCNews, 2013. Flu Clinics Reopened as H1N1 Cases Soar in Alberta. http://www.cbc.ca/news/canada/edmonton/flu-clinics-reopened-as-h1n1-cases-soar-in-alberta-1.2475970.

CDC (U.S. Centers for Disease Control and Prevention), 2011a. Severe Acute Respiratory Syndrome (SARS). http://www.cdc.gov/ncidod/sars/.

CDC (U.S. Centers for Disease Control and Prevention), 2011b. 2009 H1N1 Flu. http://www.cdc.gov/h1n1flu/.

Chapman PM, 2002. Integrating Toxicology and Ecology: Putting the "Eco" into Ecotoxicology. *Marine Pollut. Bull.* 44:7-15.

Eaton DL, Klaassen CD, 2001. Principles of Toxicology. In *Casarett and Doull's Toxicology: The Basic Science of Poisons* (Klaassen CD, Ed.). New York, New York, USA: McGraw-Hill, Chapter 2.

Gallo MA, 2001. History and Scope of Toxicology. In *Casarett and Doull's Toxicology: The Basic Science of Poisons* (Klaassen CD, Ed.). New York, New York, USA: McGraw-Hill, Chapter 1.

Gordis L, 1996. *Epidemiology*. Philadelphia, Pennsylvania, USA: Saunders.

Hodgson E, Mailman RB, Chambers JE (Eds.), 1998. *Dictionary of Toxicology*. New York, New York, USA: Grove's Dictionaries.

Lane RW, Borzelleca JF, 2008. Harming and Helping through Time: The History of Toxicology. In *Principles and Methods of Toxicology* (Hayes AW, Ed.). Boca Raton, Florida, USA: Taylor & Francis Group, Chapter 1.

Lewis RA (Ed.), 1998. *Lewis' Dictionary of Toxicology*. Boca Raton, Florida, USA: Lewis Publishers (CRC Press).

Lilienfeld DE, Stolley PD, 1994. *Foundations of Epidemiology*. New York, New York, USA: Oxford University Press.

Maltby L, Naylor C, 1990. Preliminary Observations on the Ecological Relevance of the Gammarus `Scope for Growth' Assay: Effect of Zinc on Reproduction. *Functional Ecol.* 4:393-397.

NIH (U.S. National Institutes of Health), 2008. *Toxicology Tutor I: Basic Principles Menu*. U.S. National Library of Medicine (Specialized Information Service), Environmental Health and Toxicology. http://sis.nlm.nih.gov/enviro/toxtutor/Tox1/amenu.htm.

NRC (U.S. National Research Council), 1983. *Risk Assessment in the Federal Government. Managing the Process.* Washington DC, USA: National Academy Press.

Rothman KJ, Sander G, 1998. *Modern Epidemiology.* Philadelphia, Pennsylvania, USA: Lipincott-Raven.

Szklo M, Nieto FJ, 2000. *Epidemiology – Beyond the Basics.* Gaithersburg, Maryland, USA: Aspen Publishers.

Truhaut R, 1977. Ecotoxicology: Objectives, Principles and Perspectives. *Ecotoxic. Environ. Safety* 1:151-173.

WHO (World Health Organization), 1986. Environmental Toxicology and Ecotoxicology: Proceedings of the Third International Course. WHO Regional Office for Europe, Copenhagen, Denmark.

WHO (World Health Organization), 2003. WHD (World Health Day) Brochure, Part II: Introduction. Geneva, Switzerland.

WHO (World Health Organization), 2011. Bovine Spongiform Encephalopathy. Fact Sheet No. 113. WHO Media Centre. http://www.who.int/mediacentre/factsheets/en/.

WHO (World Health Organization), 2013. Global Alert and Response (GAR) – Coronavirus infections. http://www.who.int/csr/don/archive/disease/coronavirus_infections/en/index.html.

Wright DA, Welbourn PA, 2002. *Environmental Toxicology.* Cambridge, UK: Cambridge University Press, Chapter 1.

Review Questions

1. What is environmental toxicology? And what is its relationship with general toxicology?

2. Who was Paracelsus? And what was his famous statement (assertion) frequently quoted by today's toxicologists?

3. Who was Mathieu Orfila? And what was his contribution to (classical) toxicology?

4. What are the subtle differences among the terms *toxicant, poison, contaminant, toxic agent, pollutant, toxic substance, toxic chemical, toxin,* and *xenobiotic*?

5. What are the three main categories of professional activities for or of (environmental) toxicologists?

6. Why is the term *dosage* a more practical concept than the term *dose*?

7. What are the more prominent factors affecting or influencing the (adverse) effects of an environmental toxicant?

8. What are the three main categories or types of studies from which knowledge on toxicity is constantly obtained?

9. How may chemical interaction affect a dose-response relationship?

10. Name the four basic steps (components) in the health risk assessment paradigm published by the U.S. National Research Council in 1983.

11. Name the five basic principles for and of environmental toxicology.

12. How is ecotoxicology different from environmental toxicology?

13. Why is epidemiology considered a very close ally of environmental toxicology?

14. What are the three issues underlying the importance of environmental toxicology?

CHAPTER 2

Environmental Changes and Environmental Health

2.1. Introduction

In addition to ecotoxicology (Section 1.3.2) and epidemiology (Section 1.3.3), two other key allies of environmental toxicology are environmental health (science) and environmental sciences, each of which is likewise an interdisciplinary science. Environmental health is the branch of public health that studies all aspects of exposures to pollutants in the environment that may affect human health. Environmental sciences, on the other hand, deals largely with the interaction of processes and systems that shapes the natural environment. This latter ally is built on a foundation of biological, chemical, physical, and socioeconomic sciences for the study of environmental processes and systems and for the solution of a wide range of environmental issues including pollution, natural resource, and global climate change. It is with such sense that the well-founded Society of Environmental Toxicology and Chemistry (SETAC) has its vision and mission to promote *"the advancement and application of scientific research related to contaminants and other stressors in the environment, the education in the environmental sciences, and the use of science in environmental policy and decision-making."*

Due to space limitation here, only global environmental changes and environmental diseases are discussed in this chapter. Both topics are among the three in the two ally disciplines deemed most relevant to environmental toxicology. The third topic is environmental pollution, which along with its regulatory burden is discussed in Chapter 3.

2.1.1. Knowledge on the Changing World

The world continues to bring forth significant global environmental changes every few years, due partly to nature's forces and partly to human activities including predominately industrialization and urbanization. As evident in subsequent chapters, knowledge on these changes is a prerequisite to studying environmental toxicology. There are at least three fundamental, interrelated aspects of environmental changes that are most relevant to environmental toxicology. One aspect involves a realization of the significant changes that have happened or are happening to the global and local environments. Another aspect necessitates an understanding of the impacts that these changes have on humankind and the natural environment. Still another need is for an appreciation of the actions that people, especially environmentalists and regulatory entities, undertake to cope with these environmental impacts. Whereas this third aspect is discussed as environmental and regulatory concerns in Chapter 3, the first two are the focal points of this chapter.

2.1.2. Impacts of Global Environmental Changes

It is important to note that not all the environmental changes discussed in this chapter or in this book are necessarily bad or health-related. Some of these can be positive, economic-related, or pertinent to advances in science and technology. For instance, certain food additives (Chapter 21) and almost all pest-killing chemicals known as pesticides (Chapter 15) are economic poisons, without which people would have less healthy foods to consume. The enormous volume of electronic waste (Section 2.2.6) which the world needs to cope with today simply reflects the trend that many people are living in a high-tech era. The outcome of deforestation is to have more land use. People also tend to improve their environmental conditions from the bad experiences that they encountered. In particular, pollution episodes such as the London fog of 1952 (Section 2.2.2) and the thousands of tons of chemical waste buried in Love Canal (Section 2.2.4) are things of the past, or things no longer occurring in a similar large order of magnitude.

Environmental changes nevertheless bring about dramatic changes in disease pattern as well. In the first half of 20th century, some infectious diseases such as tuberculosis and pneumonia were leading causes of death in the United States and most other countries. Yet since around the mid-1950s, cancer and cardiovascular diseases have become the two leading causes of death in the United States, and have accounted for much of the mortalities in many other countries including even those in the less developed regions. The upside of such a new disease pattern is that more chronic (i.e., long-term) diseases prevalent in a country means that overall its people live longer. This pattern also signifies a more sanitary place for people to live in now than before. The downside is that cancer and other chronic diseases (e.g., cardiovascular diseases) are more complex likely with multiple causes, of which many are considered as environmental in origin. It is this kind of concerns that has put environmental health into a world perspective.

2.1.3. World's Perspective of Environmental Health

Environmental health as considered by the World Health Organization (WHO, 2011) is that it: "*Addresses all the physical, chemical, and biological factors external to a person, and all the related factors impacting behaviours. It encompasses the assessment and control of those environmental factors that can potentially affect health. It is targeted towards preventing disease and creating health-supportive environments. This definition excludes behaviour not related to environment, as well as behaviour related to the social and cultural environment, and genetics.*"

Of all age groups, children are uniquely more vulnerable to environmental diseases. One reason for this is that as they grow and develop, there are periods in which the organs and systems in their body are particularly susceptible to the effects of many environmental threats. Another more important reason has to do with the environments that children are in. Again, as noted in Chapter 1, a child's world centers around the home, the school, and the local community. These should be healthy places where this youngster can thrive, while protected from diseases. Yet to the contrary, in most cases these places are found to be so unhealthy that they underlie the majority of deaths as well as a huge burden of diseases among children in the developing world (WHO, 2003).

Fortunately, the suffering of children and adults from most environmental diseases is not inevitable. Many of the environmental diseases and deaths can be prevented. Never before has there been such a wide range of tools and strategies to protect people from the hazards lurking in their environments. It is the advance of environmental toxicology that has been ultimately leading to the development of these strategies and tools.

2.2. Major Specific Environmental Changes

Amidst urbanization, industrialization, and advances in science or technology, many physical and material changes to the environment have occurred since World War II. The following are those regarded as more relevant to environmental toxicology: changes of global climate (particularly those leading to global warming); increased air and water pollutions; mounting quantities of solid and toxic wastes; destruction of the ozone (O_3) layer by pollutants; and presence of a growing number of environmental carcinogens and endocrine disruptors. Some of their more relevant, specific cases are highlighted below.

2.2.1. Global Climate Changes

This type of environmental changes, particularly those leading to global warming, has drawn much public attention in recent years. Studies reviewed by the Intergovernmental Panel on Climate Change (IPCC, 2007) showed that during the 20th century (i.e., 1901-2000), the global temperature at the lowest portion of the Earth's atmosphere (i.e., troposphere) increased about 0.5 to 1.0° C (1.0 to 1.7° F). IPCC concluded that most of the increases in the temperatures observed since the 1950s were caused by the increasing levels of greenhouse gases attributed to human activities such as fossil fuel burning and deforestation. Climate changes have reportedly affected the ocean's temperature as well as its productivity and ecosystems (Behrenfeld *et al.*, 2006; Sarmiento *et al.*, 2004). There has been suggestion that these changes can have serious implications for agricultural productivity resulting in food shortage (Lobell *et al.*, 2008). Ozone, water vapor (H_2O), carbon dioxide (CO_2), methane (CH_4), nitrous oxide (N_2O), and chlorofluorocarbons (CFCs) are the major greenhouse gases that help trap moderate level of atmospheric heat to sustain a habitable temperature of ~15.6° C (~60° F). Without the greenhouse effect (Chapter 5), the Earth would have an unlivable temperature of about −19° F (−2° F).

2.2.2. Air Pollution

Air pollution is the presence of contaminants in the atmosphere at such concentrations, durations, and frequencies that they can cause adverse effects on the health of living organisms or the ecosystem. The extent to which air pollution has affected public health can be illustrated by the numerous air pollution-related episodes occurring over the years, dating back earlier than December 1952 when the smoggy London experienced

4,000 excess deaths from respiratory and heart problems caused by acid rain and other air pollutants. Similar acute episodes, but less devastating and at times with different kinds of air pollutants, also occurred in other major cities around the world such as Beijing, Los Angeles, New York, and Osaka. Air pollutants of global concern include the following: sulfur oxides (SO_x); nitrogen oxides (NO_x); carbon monoxide (CO); ozone and other photochemical oxidants; different types and sizes of particulates; lead (Pb) and other toxic metals; and volatile organic compounds (known more commonly by its acronym VOCs). Major sources of air pollution are the combustion of fossil fuels for transportation, electricity, heating, cooking, as well as various industrial and combustion processes.

2.2.3. Water Pollution

Similarly, water pollution is the presence of contaminants in water at such concentrations, durations, and frequencies that they can cause undesired effects on the health of living organisms and the (aquatic) environment. In many developed countries including particularly the United States, many people generally regard water pollution not so much as a health issue, but more as an issue of conservation and preservation of natural beauty and resources. In either case, the major sources of water pollution include inorganic and organic wastes, petroleum compounds, municipal wastes, pesticide residues, agricultural wastes, and acid mine drainage. Many industrial processes have the potential to discharge various types of wastes that can cause significant water pollution problems. Water pollution can threaten not only aquatic life, particularly fish, but also human health. Evidence for this kind of human health threats includes the well-watched American film *Erin Brockovich*, which was released in 2000 publicizing specifically how human life was caused by water contamination with the toxic hexavalent metal chromium (Cr^{6+}).

2.2.4. Soil Pollution

For soil contamination, a major concern is the release of an increasing number or volume of toxic chemicals to the soil which is a relatively stationary medium. One noteworthy aspect is that the release of soil contaminants is not limited to areas adjacent to point sources (e.g., farmlands, industrial facilities). Rather, these contaminants can be transported to distant areas away from the point source. One widely known disaster related to land disposal of hazardous wastes in the American history is that of Love Canal, which initially was an abandoned area near Niagara Falls in the state of New York. The main issue with this environmental tragedy is that a neighborhood developed there in the late 1970s was discovered to have been sitting on top of some 20,000 tons of toxic waste buried more than two decades earlier. This pile of waste contained some 80 different harmful chemicals, of which about a dozen were suspected or known as human carcinogens.

2.2.5. Red Tide Pollution

Red tide, also known as *harmful algal bloom* (HAB), is a common name given to an environmental phenomenon when algae (e.g., phytoplankton) are present in water bodies in high enough concentrations that the water appears murky or discolored to green, brown, or mostly red (and hence the term *red tide pollution*). The most important environmental issue with red tides is their toxic and often lethal effects on the coastal species of birds, fish, and marine mammals. For the red tides occurring in the United States, particularly in the state of Florida, a potent neurotoxin named *brevetoxin* from algae is thought to be responsible for the much intoxication or killing of the coastal creatures. Red tide algae are also linked to skin irritation and burning in people who swim in nearby areas with high concentrations of the algae.

In certain regions, both the frequency and the severity of HAB have been linked to increased nutrient loading from human activities (Lam and Ho, 1989). In particular, the growth of marine phytoplankton has been linked to the availability of nitrates (NO_3^-) and phosphates (PO_4^{3-}), which can be abundant in and hence from agricultural runoff.

2.2.6. Electronic Waste Pollution

E-waste is the nickname for this type of waste, which is also known as waste electrical and electronic equipment. Technically, it includes the refuse from discarded or end-of-life electronic products that ends up in landfills or incinerators, instead of being reused or recycled. The environmental health concerns with e-waste may be justified with the statistics on electronics use. According to a somewhat outdated but still valid white paper report by Cairns (2005), waste electronic equipment has been one of the fastest growing categories of municipal solid waste. Both the rapid growth of the electronics sector and the swift changes in technology indicate that more consumers are replacing more electronic equipment more often than ever before. In that report, the then high-end estimates used were such that, the cumulative number of obsolete computers alone could well exceed 300 million, along with some four billion pounds of plastics, about one billion pounds of lead, two million pounds of cadmium (Cd), and four hundred pounds of mercury (Hg). These computer constituents are all considered toxic to human health and the ecosystem. Most electronic products, including computers, contain carcinogenic or highly toxic substances such as polychlorinated biphenyls (PCBs), which were once widely used as coolants and lubricants in transformers, capacitors, and other electrical equipment. It has been estimated that even though e-waste represents merely 2% of American trash in landfills, it amounts to 70% of the country's overall toxic waste (Slade, 2007).

2.2.7. Deforestation

For thousands of years, people have been using fire to clear land. Wildfires hence are a significant force for environmental change. Other means or causes of deforestation include logging, urbanization, mining and oil exploitation, and the conversion of forested lands for agricultural use and cattle-raising (TWI, 1999). The stability of a forest ecosystem is affected by changes of environmental conditions, such as by increasing temperatures, by increasing atmospheric carbon dioxide (CO_2), and by decreasing deposition rates of nutrients and acidity. Today, forest ecosystems are still threatened by nutrient depletion, soil acidification, and nutrient pollution or overload (Matzner, 2004). According to the United Nations Food and Agriculture Organization (FAO, 2001), during the ten-year period from 1990 to 2000 the global net annual rate of deforestation reached 36,000 sq. miles.

Forests are highly rich sources for foods, fuels, construction materials, fibers, and biological diversity, since much of the Earth's biomass and biodiversity above ground is held within its forests (UNEP, 2005). They are also important in water and air filtration, carbon (dioxide) sequestration, and soil stabilization (Williams, 1990, 1994). It has been estimated that roughly 3.7 acres of forestland are needed to supply each person on the planet with enough shelter and fuel (Lund and Iremonger, 1998).

2.3. Incidence and Spectrum of Environmental Diseases

In public health, environmental diseases are those caused by environmental factors that are not transmitted genetically or, to some scholars, not by infection either. This chapter however takes on a broader definition to include communicable diseases (i.e., those by infection). Pesticides, consumer products, food additives, cigarette smoke, radiation, air pollutants, water pollutants, and various types of toxic wastes are some of the major sources of environmental contaminants contributing to human diseases. Accordingly, there are many types of environmental diseases of health concern. Although environmental contaminants are found everywhere, the likelihood of people developing a specific environmental disease still depends on the type of contaminants present in their own environment and on their genetic susceptibility to such a hazard. Regardless, what seems certain is that environmental diseases thrive in conditions not conducive for better living (e.g., in where germs and disease-bearing insects tend to breed).

As a case in point, one of the Guyana government's national health concerns is their observation of a disproportionately high frequency of many communicable diseases including malaria, acute respiratory infections, acute diarrheal disorders, and worm infections (King, 2001). Their conclusion, that the causes of these diseases (including nervous disorders and hypertension) were largely environmental in nature, was nonetheless based on the fact that in their country, basic sanitation in most areas was (and still is) lacking or at best most rudimentary, amidst their ongoing problem of over-crowding.

2.3.1. Incidence and Burden of Environmental Diseases

High incidence of environmental diseases has been observed in many developed nations as well. Nearly four decades ago, *Time* (1975) magazine echoed the declaration made by Dr. Irving Selikoff of the New York Mount Sinai School of Medicine, likewise concluding that "*Environmental disease is becoming the disease of the century.*" Even then, they realized that industrialization along with expanding technology was changing the world radically and exposing humankind to growing amounts of harmful environmental pollutants, of which some were chemicals not available several decades ago.

In the industrialized countries, particularly the United States, the public's growing concern on environmental diseases dates back to the early 1960s, when Rachel Carson (1962) in her once widely read classic book *Silent Spring* asserted specifically that *"The economic costs of environmental disease and disabilities are very significant and they are largely preventable. By taking action to reduce or eliminate exposures to toxic chemicals, the US could save billions of dollars a year in health and related costs and significantly improve public health."*

According to a study (Landrigan *et al.*, 2002) published in the beginning of the 21st century, total annual health-related costs for the four categories of American pediatric diseases under investigation were estimated at over $50 billion, with $43.4 billion for lead poisoning, $9.2 billion for neurobehavioral disorders, $2.0 billion for asthma, and $0.3 billion for childhood cancer. These findings were not surprising at all, inasmuch as the U.S. National Health and Nutrition Examination Survey (also known commonly as NHANES) reported that during the years 1991-1994, 4.4% of American children aged 1 to 6 years had blood lead levels exceeding the critical level of 10 µg/dL (CDC, 1997). The study estimated that the total costs for the four categories came to about 2.8% of total U.S. health care costs. Another source (RDHN, 2006) suggested that the annual cost of environmental diseases in the United States might be as high as $165 billion.

Even at the state level, the total annual cost of asthma alone in California was estimated to be as much as $1.3 billion. This estimate was given in 2005 by a group of scientific staff who helped draft the California Senate Bill 600 in an effort to create a chemical monitoring program in the state. According to the bill, for individuals born in the late 1980s with one or more of the 18 most common and major birth defects (Section 2.4.2), the estimated lifetime costs for medical treatment and lost productivity would exceed $1 trillion. The bill's main point of argument was that approximately 85,000 chemicals were registered for use in the United States, with another some 2,000 chemicals being registered each year. Yet more than 90% of these chemicals had never been tested for their adverse effects on human health.

California is also known to have high incidences of cancer and birth defects. It was due to concerns over these high statistics that in 1986, its voters passed a law with the intent to keep their consumer products free of toxic substances that have the potential to cause illnesses in the two disease categories. This state law, officially entitled *"The Safe Drinking Water and Toxic Enforcement Act of 1986"*, is nicknamed *"Proposition 65"* or *"Prop 65"*. The law mandates that anyone in the state must be informed about the presence of any substance classified as a toxicant that may cause cancer or birth defect.

2.3.2. Spectrum and Nature of Environmental Diseases

Environmental toxicology is an important discipline mostly because there has been a growing concern on environmental diseases which now have been widely recognized and spreading, particularly in the developed countries and since World War II. These environmental diseases can be considered as the trade-offs for accelerating production of chemicals in the second half of last century. More bluntly, industrial society has since increased human exposure to thousands of chemicals present in the environment.

Again, environmental diseases and injuries are not caused by chemical agents alone. Some can be caused by biological or physical agents, such as those from venomous snakebites, from dermal contact with poisonous plants, from consumption of poisonous marine animals, from exposure to radiation, and those seen in foodborne outbreaks. Neither are humans the only victims of environmental diseases. For instance, corneal edema and ulcers can be seen in captive marine mammals (e.g., seals, walruses). According to the *Merck Veterinary Manual* (Kahn, 2008), the causes of these diseases are suspected to be lack of shade, excessive bright light, and nutritional deficiencies. The veterinary manual further points out specifically that for marine mammals, exposure to spills of petroleum hydrocarbons is a major health concern. Sea otters are particularly vulnerable to oil spills due to their natural grooming habits and their lack of an excessive fat layer. Kidneys, liver, and gastrointestinal tract are some of the body organs in the exposed marine mammals that can be seriously affected. In these mammals, the body organ affected the most is their respiratory tract, as petroleum hydrocarbons are fairly volatile.

The toxic effects of environmental exposure, in all settings and for all species (including humans), are greatly influenced by the route of exposure. Under normal circumstances, the primary sources (and hence routes) of exposure for most species (including humans) are air and water pollutions, followed by ingestion of contaminated foods and direct dermal contact. Plant diseases too can be caused from environmental exposure to biological agents. Many crops or plants are subject to pest infestation for which the treatment is with pesticides (Chapter 15).

In humans, many environmental diseases received first public attention during the late 18th and early 19th centuries when industrialized changes in agriculture, transportation, and manufacturing had profound socioeconomic and cultural impacts first in Britain and later in the rest of the world. Such public awareness reportedly stemmed from the recognition of occupational illnesses at the time, especially those associated with exposure to highly toxic chemicals. Supporting such a connection is the observation that chemical exposures generally are more intense in occupational settings than in the general environment, thereby readily yielding more noticeable illnesses in workplaces. Examples of these earlier occupational diseases included (as further discussed in Chapter 20): *cancer of the scrotal skin* (which in 1775 was linked to soot exposure in chimney sweeps); *silicosis* (a lung disease of miners, grinders, and potters from inhalation of silica dust, dating back to the 1700s); *neurological disorders* (found in workers exposed to lead glazes on pottery, dating back to the 1700s); and certain *bone diseases* (e.g., phossy jaw in workers exposed to white phosphorus in the manufacture of matches, dating back to the 1800s).

2.4. Commonly Encountered Environmental Diseases

In the (sub)sections that follow, brief overviews are presented for the various groups of environmental diseases that are not only more commonly encountered but also considered as having greater health concerns, with the specific aim of facilitating the appreciation of the materials covered in other chapters. For the more prominent specific environmental diseases emerging in recent years, they are discussed in the subsequent chapters that address specific causative agents or specific adverse health effects.

2.4.1. Cancer

This group of diseases begins when a cell or a small group of cells in the body multiply more rapidly than at the normal rate. As these cancer cells spread throughout the body, they eventually affect the normal functions of other healthy organs and tissues. It is thought that in most situations, several cancer-promoting factors may need to add up before a malignant growth can be developed in a person. Some of these promoting factors include short- or long-term exposure to certain (other) factors or toxic agents in the environment, such as cigarette smoke, radiation, natural or synthetic chemicals, alcohol, and sunlight. People therefore can reduce the risk of getting cancer by limiting their exposure to these harmful agents. More discussion on this group of diseases is given in Chapter 18.

2.4.2. Birth Defects

Diseases in this group are defined as abnormalities of structure, function, or body metabolism present in babies at birth. According to the U.S. Centers for Disease Control and Prevention (CDC, 2008), birth defects affect approximately 3% of babies born in the United States each year (i.e., affecting about 120,000 babies born annually). This group of diseases is one of the leading causes of infant deaths, accounting for more than 20% of all infant deaths in the United States. Babies born with birth defects tend to be more susceptible to illness and to long-term disability than those born healthy. There are 45 major types of birth defects identified by CDC (2006), of which 18 have been determined as more prevalent (e.g., cleft lip, neural tube defects; *see* Table 19.2). Birth defects can occur when pregnant women consume too much alcohol or when they are exposed to certain substances (e.g., the synthetic estrogen *diethylstilbestrol*, aspirin, contents in cigarette smoke, the drug *thalidomide* for morning sickness). These harmful substances can reach the fetus via the placenta. Ionizing radiation is also considered as a strong teratogen (i.e., an agent that causes birth defect). As a result of these maternal exposures, some babies are born with one or more organs, tissues, or body parts that have not developed in a normal way. Further discussion on this group of diseases is given in Chapter 19.

2.4.3. Reproductive Damage

Fertility is the ability to conceive and have children. It was estimated that about 10% of American couples had infertility problem (e.g., APA, 2013; CDC, 2013). Infertility occurs when a woman cannot produce an egg, or when a man cannot produce enough sperms. This condition can be caused by infections coming from sexual diseases, or from exposure to chemicals at work or elsewhere in the environment.

Some natural substances and synthetic pesticides are found structurally so similar to estrogen that they can actually "mimic" the action of this important (female) hormone (Chapter 19). As a result, these endocrine or hormone disruptors may interfere with the development of male and female reproductive organs or with their normal functions (Chapter 19). This type of interference can lead to increased risk of adverse reproductive conditions such as early puberty, low sperm counts, ovarian cysts, and cancer of the breast or the testicle. Certain solvents such as glycol ether can damage male reproductive health and a child's health. Other synthetic chemicals known as capable of inducing adverse reproductive effects in males include PCBs, lead compounds, and certain pesticides (e.g., dibromochloropropane, kepone, ethylene dibromide). Male adults therefore should avoid working with these chemicals for at least a few months prior to fathering a child.

2.4.4. Respiratory Diseases

Diseases in this group represent those affecting the respiratory tract which includes the lungs, bronchial tubes, trachea, and in some literature also the nose and the throat. These diseases can be broadly classified as the *obstructive* (that impeding the air flow; e.g., asthma, bronchiolitis) or the *restrictive* type (that characterized by a loss in lung volume; e.g., pulmonary fibrosis, lung cancer). Causes of these diseases range from infectious agents and environmental exposures, to allergens and genetic origin. It is suffice to say that the greatest interaction of humankind with the outside world is through their lungs which by nature need to constantly take in (and out) the omnipresent air.

According to the American Lung Association (ALA, 2010), about 3.7 million Americans have been diagnosed with a progressive, obstructive pulmonary condition termed *emphysema*. Emphysema is a subtype of chronic obstructive pulmonary disease (COPD) that limits the transfer of oxygen (O_2) and carbon dioxide (CO_2) in the lungs due to damage of the air sacs in the lung, with symptoms of chest tightness, shortness of breath, loss of appetite, and fatigue. Certain pollutants in the air and cigarette smoke can affect breathing by damaging sensitive tissues (e.g., the air sacs). Another subgroup of obstructive respiratory diseases is asthma, which affects some 235 million people worldwide (IUATLD, 2011). Some asthma attacks, including those leaving victims breathless and gasping for air, can be triggered by chemical pollutants in the air or in the home.

Some other airborne particles can be dangerous in the same way, but ending with different types of pulmonary damage. These include mineral (e.g., asbestos) or cellulosic (e.g., cotton) fibers and respirable dusts from silica, coal, or iron. These particles can cause scar tissue by damaging sensitive areas of the lungs. This black (as darkened with scars) lung condition is termed *pneumoconiosis*. Although the initial symptoms include only inflammation, fibrosis, chest pain, and shortness of breath, the condition often progresses to bronchitis, emphysema, or even death.

2.4.5. Neurological Diseases

Diseases in this group involve the nervous system, which is composed of the brain, the spinal cord, and billions of nerve cells. The brain and the spinal cord as a subsystem is generally referred to as the central nervous system (CNS), from which the nerve cells are responsible for carrying messages and instructions to other parts of the body. When the peripheral nerve cells or the cells in the CNS are damaged by toxicants, so is the neurological pathway or the neural signaling system. An impaired condition of this type can result in neurological disorders ranging from change in mood or memory to blindness, slurred speech, paralysis, and death. As noted in Chapter 15, certain pesticides are neurotoxic agents of environmental concern, particularly those of the organophosphate (OP) family such as parathion or malathion. Most organochlorine pesticides (e.g., dieldrin, lindane) and most in the pyrethroid (e.g., permethrin) family are also neurotoxic agents. So are certain metals (Chapter 14) and many organic solvents (e.g., Chapter 20).

2.4.6. Skin Disorders

One commonly encountered noncancerous disorder in this group is dermatitis, which is a fancy name for inflamed, irritated skin. This condition can be induced by contact with some pesticides (e.g., propargite) currently being used in farms. Many people also have experienced the oozing bumps and itching caused by poison ivy, poison oak, and poison sumac. Some chemicals found in paints, cosmetics, and detergents can cause skin rashes and blisters. Too much wind or sun can also make the skin dry and chapped. Certain medications, fabrics, and foods too can cause unusual skin reactions in some people.

2.4.7. Diseases Induced by Specific Agents

In addition to the environmental diseases categorized above by *effect* type, they and certain others can be characterized more effectively by concerning the specific (groups of) *agents* that induce them. Some examples for this type of disease concern or grouping are briefly discussed below. More examples along with more discussion can be found elsewhere in this book, mainly in Part III (i.e., Chapters 11 through 17).

Some environmental diseases are caused by *neurotoxins* found in seafood, such as *tetrodotoxin* in puffer fish and *ciguatoxin* in oysters and clams. *Mycotoxins* are toxins produced by microfungi which can be found harboring in a variety of plant foods. Among the various mycotoxins known, *aflatoxins* and especially *aflatoxin B_1* have been the subject of most intensive investigation worldwide owing to their acute toxic effects in humans and their potent hepatocarcinogenicity found in certain laboratory animals.

Many foreign substances in the body are metabolized (broken down) into harmless or less harmful compounds by the liver, a topic covered extensively in Chapter 8. Yet some xenobiotics are converted to *free radicals* which are highly reactive and unstable, as by definition they have an unpaired electron. In order to stabilize themselves, these free radicals each will take (steal) an electron from a nearby molecule which usually becomes another active free radical. This chain reaction may eventually disrupt the body's normal functions, including having radicals react constantly with lipoproteins in the blood to form plaque-like fatty deposits. These fatty plaques can clog blood vessels to block off blood supply to the heart, causing cardiac attacks. Examples of free radicals are *triphenylmethyl radical*, *superoxide radical*, and *hydroxyl radical*, of which the last two are referred to as *oxygen free radicals* as both are derived from the atom oxygen. Oxygen free radicals are also thought to play a key role in carcinogenesis.

Oftentimes adverse effects from environmental exposure to toxic metals are also conveniently considered as a special health concern. *Hexavalent chromium* (Cr^{6+}) is a metal used in electroplating, textile manufacturing, and paints, and has been found in some drinking water sources. There is mounting evidence that this compound can cause cancer in laboratory animals if they consume enough drinking water that contains it. The metal's harm to humans is publicized in the movie *Erin Brockovich* released in 2000. The toxic effects inducible by certain metals (e.g., Pb, Hg, Cd) are discussed in Chapter 14.

Some minerals and vitamins essential to human health can be harmful if they overload the body to beyond accommodation. Toxic effects from overdose of this group of chemicals too are sometimes regarded as a special group of environmental diseases for health concern purposes. *Zinc* (Zn), for example, is a mineral (or more correctly a metal) that the human body needs to function properly. However, in rare cases, some people can be poisoned if there is too much Zn in their body. Another example is *selenium* (Se), which is an essential trace element; yet at high enough doses it can cause abnormal nails, hair loss, peripheral neuropathy, irritability, dermatitis, and other disorders. *Vitamin A overdose* is more specifically termed *hypervitaminosis A*, which can cause birth defects, liver abnormalities, and osteoporosis; otherwise, it is an essential nutrient known for its role in maintaining good vision. Another example is *vitamin C overdose*, which can cause stomach aches and diarrhea. People in certain health conditions, such as with hemochromatosis or kidney stones, should avoid taking too much of this vitamin which otherwise is known as a highly effective antioxidant capable of reducing oxidative stress (as caused by free radicals).

Persistent organic pollutants (POPs) are hydrocarbon (hence by definition *organic*) compounds that persist in the environment likely for years. They are also capable of bioaccumulating and biomagnifying manifold in fatty tissues as they move up the food chains (Chapter 6). These environmental pollutants have been associated with many adverse health effects in humans and animals, including cancer, reproductive disorders, damage to the nervous system, interference with the immunological system, and disruption of the endocrine system. There is strong evidence showing long-range transport of certain POPs to remote regions where they have never been used or produced. It was partly due to such findings that in May 2001, at an international conference held in Stockholm, Sweden, over 150 nations including the United States signed a global treaty known as the *Stockholm Convention* (of 2001) *on POPs*. This treaty has its commitment to initially reduce or eliminate the global productions, uses, or releases of *twelve* POPs that are considered as having the most urgent concern to the global community.

These so-called "dirty dozen" POPs include: polychlorinated dibenzo-*p(ara)*-dioxins (PCDDs, also nicknamed *dioxins* for short); polychlorinated dibenzofurans (PCDFs, or *furans*); PCBs; and nine organochlorine pesticides (aldrin, chlordane, DDT, dieldrin, endrin, heptachlor, hexachlorobenzene, mirex, and toxaphene). The twelve POPs are also members of the chemical family known as persistent organochlorine compounds (POCs), as they all contain one or more chlorine atoms strongly bonded to their carbons. Most of these chemicals are known to be at least possible human carcinogens and fairly toxic to several body organs and systems including the liver, the kidneys, the immunological system, the reproductive system, the endocrine system, and the nervous system. As discussed in Chapter 16, ten more chemicals or chemical groups have been added to the Stockholm Convention's POPs action list since May 2011.

References

ALA (American Lung Association), 2010. Chronic Obstructive Pulmonary Disease (COPD) Fact Sheet. 1301 Pennsylvania Avenue NW, Suite 800, Washington DC, USA.

APA (American Pregnancy Association), 2013. Fertility FAQ. http://americanpregnancy.org/infertility/fertilityfaq.html.

Behrenfeld MJ, O'Malley RT, Siegel DA, McClain CR, Sarmiento JL, Feldman GC, Milligan AJ, Falkowski PG, Letelier RM, Boss ES, 2006. Climate-Driven Trends in Contemporary Ocean Productivity. *Nature* 444:752-755.

Cairns L, 2005. Electronic Waste: Finding Sustainable Solutions That Work Better for Consumers (A Consumers Union White Paper). Yonkers, New York, USA: Consumers Union.

Carlson R, 1962. *Silent Spring*. Boston, Massachusetts, USA: Houghton Mifflin.

CDC (U.S. Centers for Disease Control and Prevention), 1997. Update: Blood Lead Levels – United States, 1991-1994. *MMWR* (Morbidity and Mortality Weekly Report) 46:141-146.

CDC (U.S. Centers for Disease Control and Prevention), 2006. Improved National Prevalence Estimates for 18 Selected Major Birth Defects – United States, 1999-2001. *MMWR* 54:1301-1305.

CDC (U.S. Centers for Disease Control and Prevention), 2008. Update on Overall Prevalence of Major Birth Defects – Atlanta, Georgia, 1978-2005. *MMWR* 57:1-5.

CDC (U.S. Centers for Disease Control and Prevention), 2013. Infertility. http://www.cdc.gov/nchs/fastats/fertile.htm.

FAO (Food and Agriculture Organization of the United Nations), 2001. Forest Resources Assessment 2000. Main Report FAO Forestry Paper 140. FAO, Rome, Italy.

IPCC (Intergovernmental Panel on Climate Change), 2007. Summary for Policymakers. In *Climate Change 2007: The Physical Science Basis. Contribution of Working Group I to the Fourth Assessment Report of the Intergovernmental Panel on Climate Change* (Solomon S, Qin D, Manning M, Chen Z, Marquis M, Averyt KB, Tignor M, Miller HL, Eds.). New York, New York, USA: Cambridge University Press.

IUATLD (International Union Against Tuberculosis and Lung Disease), 2011. The Global Asthma Report, 2011. 68 Boulevard Saint Michel, 75006 Paris, France (in collaboration with the International Study of Asthma and Allergies in Childhood (ISAAC)).

Kahn CM (Ed.), 2008. *The Merck Veterinary Manual* (Exotic and Laboratory Animals – Marine Mammals: Environmental Diseases), Ninth Edition. Whitehouse Station, New Jersey, USA: Merck & Co.

King K, 2001. National Development Strategy − The Problems of the Health Sectors in Guyana. *Staboek News*, 23 September.

Lam CWY, Ho KC, 1989. Red Tides in Tolo Harbor, Hong Kong. In *Red Tides: Biology, Environmental Science and Toxicology* (Okaichi T, Anderson DM, Nemoto T, Eds.). New York, New York: Elsevier.

Landrigan PJ, Schechter CB, Lipton JM, Fahs MC, Schwartz J, 2002. Environmental Pollutants and Disease in American Children: Estimates of Morbidity, Mortality, and Costs for Lead Poisoning, Asthma, Cancer, and Developmental Disabilities. *Environ. Health Perspect.* 110:721-728.

Lobell DB, Burke MB, Tebaldi C, Mastrandrea MD, Falcon WP, Naylor RL, 2008. Prioritizing Climate Change Adaptation Needs for Food Security in 2030. *Science* 319:607-610.

Lund HG, Iremonger S, 1998. Omissions, Commissions, and Decisions − The Need for Integrated Resource Assessments. *Proceedings from First International Conference − Geospatial Information in Agriculture and Forestry − Decision Support, Technology, and Applications.* 1-3 June 1998, Lake Buena Vista, Florida, USA: ERIM International I:182-189.

Matzner E (Ed.), 2004. *Biogeochemistry of Forested Catchments in a Changing Environment − A German Case Study.* New York, New York, USA: Springer-Verlag.

RDHN (*Rachel's Democracy & Health News*), 2006. Environment, Health, Jobs and Justices − Who Gets to Decide? News #836, 5 January.

Sarmiento JL, Slater R, Barber R, Bopp L, Doney SC, Hirst AC, Kleypas J, Matear R, Mikolajewicz U, Monfray P, Soldatov V, Spall SA, Stouffer R, 2004. Response of Ocean Ecosystems to Climate Warming. *Global Biogeochem. Cycles* V18:GB3003.

Slade G, 2007. iWaste. *Mother Jones*, March/April Issue.

Time, 1975. Disease of the Century. 20 October.

TWI (Third World Institute; Instituto del Tercer Mundo − IteM), 1999. *The World Guide 1999/2000 − An Alternative Reference to the Countries of Our Planet* (1. The Earth and Its Peoples/Deforestation). PO Box 1539, Montevideo 11000, Uruguay.

UNEP (United Nations Environment Programme), 2005. *One Planet Many People: Atlas of Our Changing Environment.* United Nations Avenue, Gigiri, PO Box 30552-00100, Nairobi, Kenya.

WHO (World Health Organization), 2003. WHD (World Health Day) Brochure, Part II: Introduction. WHO, Geneva, Switzerland.

WHO (World Health Organization), 2011. Environmental Health (webpage). http://www.who.int/topics/environmental_health/en/.

Williams M, 1990. Forest. In *The Earth as Transformed by Human Action* (Turner BL II, Ed.). New York, New York, USA: Cambridge University Press.

Williams M, 1994. Forest and Tree Cover. In *Changes in Land Use and Land Cover. A Global Perspective* (Meyer WB, Turner BL, II, Eds.). New York, New York, USA: Cambridge University Press.

Review Questions

1. What are the three fundamental, interrelated aspects concerning environmental changes that deserve their consideration in studying environmental toxicology?
2. What is greenhouse effect? Name five major greenhouse gases that can induce this effect.

3. How can global warming affect human health, agricultural productivity, and/or the ocean eco-systems?

4. What may be defined as soil pollution?

5. What happened to London in December 1952 in relation to environmental health?

6. What was the main issue with the Love Canal tragedy?

7. Name a metal that was publicized in an American film in 2000 as a water pollutant threatening human health in the United States.

8. Name a neurotoxin found in algae that might have been responsible for the intoxication or killing of coastal birds, fish, and marine mammals.

9. Why is there a global environmental concern with e-waste?

10. What are some of the environmental concerns with deforestation?

11. Explain briefly why not all of the environmental changes should be regarded as undesirable.

12. Why are children uniquely more susceptible to environmental diseases?

13. Name two types of occupational diseases reported before the 1800s.

14. What are the four categories of pediatric diseases that appear to be responsible for nearly 3% of total health care costs in the United States?

15. List two or more environmental factors that may need to add up before a malignant growth can be developed in a person's body.

16. What are free radicals? Briefly explain why some of them can cause a cardiac attack.

17. Match each of the toxic agents in the left column to the disease or health effect in the right column that the agent can or tend to induce:

    (1) diethylstilbestrol   (a) reproductive effect
    (2) ethylene dibromide   (b) dermatitis
    (3) asbestos   (c) respiratory disease
    (4) DDT   (d) hepatocarcinogenicity
    (5) propargite   (e) birth defect
    (6) aflatoxin B_1 (f) stomach ache
    (7) hypervitaminosis C   (g) neurological effect

18. Briefly characterize the "dirty dozen" POPs (persistent organic pollutants) whose productions and uses are subjected to worldwide elimination or reduction under the global Stockholm Convention treaty.

CHAPTER 3

Environmental Pollution and Regulatory Agencies

3.1. Introduction

In line with the definitions of air pollution and water pollution given in Chapter 2, environmental pollution simply refers to the presence of one or more contaminants in the (or a certain) environment at such concentrations, durations, and frequencies that they can cause adverse effects on the health of living organisms or the environment. And urbanization and industrialization are human-based activities in modern time that represent just two of the major forces or phenomena driving environmental changes as well as pollution at the local, regional, or global level. For a quick overview, the reciprocal interrelationships (of uneven strength) among these forces or phenomena are summarized in the upper portion of Figure 3.1. Note that throughout this chapter as well as this book, the term *pollution* is synonymous with *contamination*.

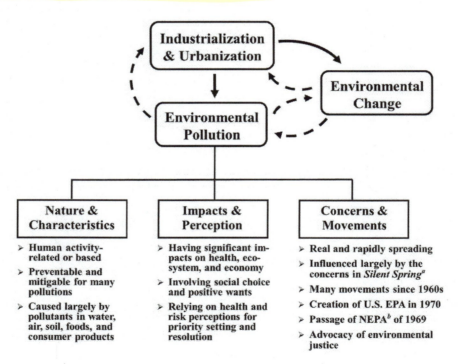

Figure 3.1. Major Characteristics, Impacts, and Concerns of Environmental Pollution in the United States (*Carson [1962]; *NEPA = U.S. National Environmental Policy Act)

Implicit in the reciprocal interrelationships depicted in Figure 3.1 is the general notion that most environmental pollutions are preventable or mitigable conditions, inasmuch as the underlying cause for each is almost always linked to one or more human activities. For example, motor vehicle emission is a human activity-based event that can lead to air pollution. And automobiles *per se* are the source contributing to as much as 90% of the noise pollution worldwide. Other major human activity-based sources include solid waste disposal facilities, incinerators, large farmlands, and industrial processes, as many common environmental contaminants involve toxic metals and chlorinated hydrocarbons. Environmental pollution can also be the consequence of a natural disaster, such as a hurricane which can lead to water pollution from sewage and can cause petrochemical spills from ruptured boats and automobiles. Even so, sewage is basically a human activity-related waste product whereas automobiles and boats are human-made conveyances.

3.1.1. Impacts of Environmental Pollution

The impacts of environmental pollution on human health and the ecosystem are real and profound. Environmental pollution along with environmental change has altered the disease pattern in many developed and developing countries over the past 50 or 60 years, largely from infectious diseases to chronic diseases being the major causes of death. The growing concern of the *health* impacts of environmental pollution is the focal point of Section 3.2. Yet another even more serious type of pollution impacts is the associated ultimate *economic* loss and burden. This type is far beyond the one incurred for health care alone, as readily reflected in the monetary example given in Table 3.1 below.

As shown in Table 3.1, China's total economic loss resulting from environmental pollution in 1992 alone was estimated at around US $13 billion (Xia, 1998). Of this total loss, about 59% and 36% were from air pollution and water pollution, respectively, with 40% being for or due to human health regardless of pollution type or source. In essence, the remaining 60% (of the US $13 billion) loss from air, water, and solid waste pollutions combined was for or due to causes other than health care-related.

In most instances, such huge economic and health impacts are considered preventable, though with the understanding that a total elimination of the source(s) is rarely a practical solution. Inasmuch as the causes of environmental pollution are related mostly to human activities, regulatory actions that reflect or involve some form of public decision are generally needed in order to maintain a balance between a community's positive wants and negative impacts. And it is the need for such a balance that sets a place for ecological (Chapter 22) or human health (Chapter 23) risk assessment, a scientific paradigm as well as a socioeconomic ideology that has preoccupied, if not masterminded, the field of environmental toxicology since the 1980s.

3.1.2. Perception of Environmental Pollution

In addition to scientific concerns, the decision for the balance between the community's positive wants and negative impacts involves cultural, ethical, socioeconomic, and legal considerations. Given the limited resources that most governments have, there is a further need to determine whether one pollution source has more or less impacts on human health or the ecosystem than another source has. Regulatory bodies in the position to make such decisions often need to share the complex information on their risk assessment with their stakeholders (i.e., those with an interest in or a concern with the matter). Such sharing is considered highly desirable, if not inevitable, since public health activity is a subset of social choice. This subset is a systematic process through which collective goals are pursued and appropriate decisions are resolved. In reality, the public's support for any of such decisions comes down to a matter of local and individual perception of health risk, since many citizens lack much of the required technical background.

Table 3.1. Estimated Economic Losses Resulting from Pollutions in China in 1992[a]

Impact Factor/Cause Category	Economic Loss (US $ Billion)	Percentage of Total Loss
Water Pollution	4.95	36.1
human health	2.68	(19.5)
industry	1.92	
crop yields	0.19	
livestock	0.10	
fisheries	0.06	
Air Pollution	8.05	58.7
human health	2.80	(20.4)
agriculture	1.00	
household upkeep	1.87	
clothing	0.15	
vehicles	0.15	
buildings	0.13	
acid rain	1.95	
Solid Waste	0.71	5.2
Total	*13.72*	*100.0*

[a]adapted from Xia (1998); 1 US $ ≈ 7.2 Chinese *Yuan* (around the year 1992).

The concept that (health) risk perception is a subjective judgmental behavior may be best illustrated starting with the example given by Neely (1994) on traffic accidents. From the 1980s to the 1990s, each year there were roughly 20,000 to 30,000 deaths reported in the United States as from traffic accidents caused by drunk driving. Statistics of this kind were accepted by most Americans with little reactions, at least on prevention and regulatory action. In contrast, the tampon-toxic shock scare in the early 1980s had received far more public attention, even though the total number of victims did not amount to one weekend's traffic fatalities. The contrast made here bears no accusation that public concerns on drunk driving were lacking in those days. Rather, people's dread over a situation is what has just been contrasted. To many people, dread is a main factor responsible for the development of a person's health risk perception (e.g., Tversky and Kahneman, 1974; U.S. EPA, 2007), as so evident in the tampon-toxic shock story.

Toxic shock syndrome (TSS) was not officially recognized as an illness by the U.S. Centers for Disease Control and Prevention (CDC) until the early months of 1980, when the institute received the first 55 cases characterized by a sudden onset of fever, sunburn-like rash, hypotension, desquamation (i.e., skin shedding), and abnormalities in three or more major body organs (CDC, 1990). This disease, occurring predominately in women, was soon determined to be caused by the bacterium *Streptococcus aureus* and highly correlated to the use of super-absorbent synthetic tampons. The panic over TSS then started creeping quickly into the minds of many American women in that year which had reportedly the highest as well as the only significant annual incidence of 852 cases and 38 deaths (CDC, 1990). *Streptococcus aureus*, a species commonly colonized in the vagina as well as the nasal and throat passages, is harmless to about 95% of the American population as these people have antibodies to the bacterium's toxin responsible for the toxic shock. For the 5% lacking the antibodies, they are highly susceptible to the fatal disease; yet they would have a much higher risk when using super-absorbent synthetic tampons, since this type of material provides an ideal breeding ground for the bacteria.

The fear for TSS among American women, which lingered over to the next couple of years long after the successful recall of the super-absorbent tampons, was apparently not due to the low morbidity and small death toll experienced. Rather, it was largely due to the *dread* that at the time TSS was conceived as a highly uncontrollable epidemic sweeping across the nation. That situation was in many ways similar to the more recent situation involving the H1N1 flu pandemic in 2009, where CDC released a novel harmless virus for vaccine production (CIDRAP, 2009) even two weeks ahead of the pandemic declaration on 11 June 2009. Such an urgency for the vaccine development was based more on the public's concern over the virus being a new strain with unpredictable epidemic virulence, than on the unimpressive statistic toll experienced at the time.

The H1N1 pandemic is used as another example here not so much that it fits well the common definition of environmental pollution. It is included here because the urgency for the vaccine development and production was based on some form of environmental health risk assessment. Again, as noted in Chapter 1, any laboratory confirmation of the viral pathogen or any laboratory development of a high-yield vaccine virus is highly related to toxicity testing, the role of a toxicologist with the appropriate training.

3.2. Concerns with Environmental Pollution

In the United States and many other countries, the public's concerns of environmental pollution are real and rapidly spreading. It was back in the 1960s that most scholars and organizations proclaimed the work in *Silent Spring* by Rachel Carson (1962) the starting point of the modern environmental movement. In Carson's book, numerous case studies (or anecdotes as so treated by some people) are included to describe the environmental problems associated with the use of hazardous pesticides and other chemicals in the United States and worldwide. In particular, the book cites several experimental observations purporting to show the link between the spraying of the organochlorine pesticide DDT and the survival or the reproductive failure of several bird species. That book also describes in detail the toxic effects that chemical control had placed on all key components of the environment, including air, water, land, wildlife, and humans.

Carson's book was not without serious criticism, as there were enough people appreciating the vital role in which DDT played in controlling malaria transmission by killing the mosquitoes that carried the disease. Yet in numerous places in her book, Carson's concerns and arguments should still be regarded as fair, objective, and valid. At the least, she did point out explicitly that *"No responsible person contends that insect-borne disease should be ignored. The question that has now urgently presented itself is whether it is either wise or responsible to attack the problem by methods that are rapidly making it worse. The world has heard much of the triumphant war against disease through the control of insect vectors of infection, but it has heard little of the other side of the story."*

3.2.1. Regulatory Concerns in the United States

The relatively modern environmental concerns reflected in *Silent Spring* were more than just welcome by the environmental movement community. These concerns were regarded by many sectors as the driving forces behind the creation of both a powerful regulatory agency and the most significant piece of environmental legislation in American history. It was in late 1969, less than 10 years since the publication of *Silent Spring*, that U.S. Congress presented to the Executive Branch a landmark bill known as the National Environmental Policy Act (NEPA), which was signed into law by then President Richard Nixon on New Year's Day in 1970. NEPA's stated purpose was (and still is) threefold as follows:

- ◆ To declare a national policy which will encourage productive and enjoyable harmony between man and his environment.

- ◆ To promote efforts which will prevent or eliminate damage to the environment and biosphere and stimulate the health and welfare of man.

- ◆ To enrich our (the) understanding of the ecological systems and natural resources important to the Nation.

Initially and quickly, the U.S. Council of Environmental Quality (CEQ) was formed to fulfill NEPA's statutory intents. Yet the environmental concerns at the time were so intensified by the influence of Rachel Carson's work that, before the year 1970 was over, President Nixon was compelled to form a strong, independent agency by piecing together various programs from other federal agencies. That strong, independent body was named the U.S. Environmental Protection Agency, a federal agency now known commonly by its acronym (U.S.) EPA (and henceforth so used in this book). The intense concern for environmental issues at the time was best evident from the first Earth Day celebration held on 22 April 1970, which brought about 20 million Americans out into the spring sunshine for peaceful grassroots type demonstrations in favor of environmental reform (Lewis, 1985). Coincidentally or not, the notion for Earth Day evolved over a period of seven years beginning in 1962, the year *Silent Spring* was first published.

As Jack Lewis (1985) of U.S. EPA put it well in his article *The Birth of EPA*, "Silent Spring *played in the history of environmentalism roughly the same role that* Uncle Tom's Cabin *played in the abolitionist movement. In fact, EPA today may be said without exaggeration to be the extended shadow of Rachel Carson. The influence of her book has brought together over 14,000 scientists, lawyers, managers, and other employees across the country to fight the good fight for environmental protection.*" At the time of its formation, President Nixon wanted U.S. EPA to be a powerful regulatory agency with the specific responsibility to:

- ◆ Establish and enforce environmental protection standards.

- ◆ Conduct environmental research.

- ◆ Provide assistance to others combating environmental pollution.

- ◆ Assist the CEQ in developing and recommending to the President new policies for environmental protection.

Many of U.S. EPA's early efforts, including the enforcement of Federal Insecticide, Fungicide, and Rodenticide Act (FIFRA) which underwent a significant revision in 1972, are thought to have been related to Carson's work (Hynes, 1989). Some such early efforts are summarized in *The Birth of EPA*, in which Rachel Carson is specifically described as a person who "*derived her missionary zeal from her fear that fewer species of birds would be singing each spring unless pesticide poisoning was curtailed.*"

It is not surprising that today the concerns with environmental pollution are far more in scope than dealing with such fundamentals as the creation of U.S. EPA or the passage of NEPA. Nowadays, the concerns and movements on environmental pollution have much to do with, among other things, *environmental justice*. Environmental justice is an idealism centering on the principle that no one sector of the community, including racial, ethnic, national origin, or socioeconomic groups, should be disproportionately impacted by pesticides or other toxic substances. It asserts that anyone whose health or environment may be affected by any chemical exposure shall hold a stake in the regulatory process at any level of government. In essence, this idealism or ideology is upheld seriously by U.S. EPA and many state agencies including the California Environmental Protection Agency. This kind of concerns, along with other aspects of environmental pollution discussed earlier, is summarized schematically in the lower portion of Figure 3.1.

3.2.2. Actions on Environmental Pollution Impacts

Many regulatory and organizational actions have been implemented in the modern past to cope with the health and economic impacts of environmental pollution. Such actions are evident from several environmental legislations enacted and several environmental movements advocated in recent years in the United States and worldwide. Examples of these include: the U.S. Clean Air Act; the U.S. Clean Water Act; the Stockholm Convention on POPs (Persistent Organic Pollutants); the aforesaid FIFRA; the reforestation movement; the anti-red tide movement; and the United Nations' (UN's) formation of the Intergovernmental Panel on Climate Change (IPCC). Some of these environmental movements and regulatory actions have caused significant changes to local and global environments or have led to new perspectives on environmental regulation, such as the Superfund (law) of 1980 (which was passed under public pressure to provide funding initially for the cleanup of toxic waste buried in Love Canal, *see* Chapter 2 or 22).

In brief but more specifically, the U.S. Clean Air Act was amended once again in 1990 to curb three major threats to the nation's environment and the health of millions of Americans. The three threats of main concern are acid rain, urban air pollution, and toxic air emissions (e.g., U.S. EPA, 2008a). Similar clean air acts have been passed in some states and some other countries.

As proclaimed by U.S. EPA (2008b), the U.S. Clean Water Act amended in 1977 is regarded as "*The cornerstone of surface water quality protection in the United States.*" This federal statute employs a variety of regulatory and non-regulatory tools to limit direct contaminant discharges into waterways, to finance the municipal wastewater treatment systems, and to manage non-point pollution (e.g., polluted runoff).

The main focus of FIFRA of 1972 was to provide federal control of pesticide distribution, sale, and use in the United States (U.S. EPA, 2008c). The act gives U.S. EPA the authority not only to assess the consequences of pesticide usage, but also to require certain users (e.g., farmers) to register their pesticides at time of purchase.

Under the global Stockholm Convention treaty on POPs, participating parties need to commit to both the development and the implementation of a plan to fulfill their obligations of eliminating or reducing the releases of certain POPs into the environment. It has been projected at an international scientific conference (Dong, 2006), and there is now evidence (Chapter 16), that their share of the commitment and the number of POPs under consideration continue to expand.

Reforestation movement appeared to have gained serious public attention beginning in the early 1920s (e.g., *The New York Times*, 1922). Yet in recent years, the American *movement* of reforestation is somewhat slow compared to those occurring in some developing regions. For instance, it was estimated that between 1990 and 2010, the United States *gained* slightly over 900,000 acres of forest each year (FAO, 2010). In contrast, close to 80 million trees (roughly 20,000 acres) were planted in Indonesia as part of the country's 2007 National Reforestation Movement, all completed just within one week of November with its people from all walks of life (Pathoni, 2007).

One prominent American organization with a mission to control and mitigate red tide pollution is Solutions to Avoid Red Tide (also known by its acronym START), which is a member of the Red Tide Alliance. The alliance, which is a partnership located in the state of Florida, consists of the Florida Department of Health in Tallahassee, the Mote Marine Laboratory in Sarasota, and the Florida Fish & Wildlife Research Institute in Saint Petersburg. A similar organization also founded in the United States is the Gulf Coast Preservation Society, with a mission to restore, preserve, and protect the rich marine habitat of the Gulf of Mexico. On the other side of the globe, Japan and South Korea have been in the forefront in dispersing clays on a large scale as flocculants to protect fish from red tide pollution (Sengco and Andersen, 2004).

For actions on global climate change, former U.S. Vice-President Al Gore and the UN panel IPCC were awarded the 2007 Nobel Peace Prize for their work on global warming. This award can be regarded as a recognition signifying their many years of efforts in building up and disseminating greater knowledge about human-made climate changes. Al Gore also won an Oscar in 2007 for his documentary film on global warming. The film, distributed by Paramount Pictures in 2006, was entitled *"An Inconvenient Truth"*. Yet despite these high levels of recognition, neither IPCC's work nor Al Gore's on global warming is without merit challenge. There are enough skeptics not convinced that global warming is an environmental issue, especially in light of the e-mail controversy on climate change. In 2009, hundreds of private e-mail messages and documents were hacked from a computer server at the University of East Anglia in England. The hacked climate e-mails, some of which were sent as far back as in the late 1990s, reportedly caused a stir among skeptics who argued that climate scholars had conspired to deliberately overstate the case for a *human* influence on global warming (Revkin, 2009).

3.3. Environmental Health Laws and Policies

In general, treaties, legislations, regulations, and policies for environmental health are enacted or adopted as a result of certain environmental health concerns or movements. Yet the extent to which the entities are concerned with a particular environmental health issue is influenced greatly by their appreciation and perception of environmental health. As noted in Chapter 2, the World Health Organization (WHO, 2011) considers environmental health as the realm of concern that *"Addresses all the physical, chemical, and biological factors external to a person, and all the related factors impacting behaviours. It encompasses the assessment and control of those environmental factors that can potentially affect health."* Environmental health laws or legislations thereby refer to the rules of conduct adopted specifically to address the various key aspects of this realm. It should be noted that all laws, including those pertaining to environmental health, are with binding legal force and are enforced by appropriate government authorities at the local, national, or international level. Laws are found in treaties, statutes, constitutional provisions, regulations, and court decisions.

More often than not, there are chaos and disorder over the interpretation of certain key legal jargon among toxicologists, particularly among those not working in a regulatory agency. Therefore, an understanding of certain legal terms may become necessary or advantageous for health scientists working in a regulatory agency. For instance, it is important to note that *statute* is a law created by a legislative body, whether at the regional, federal, state, or local level. It may mean a single or a collection of acts. *Regulation*, on the other hand, is an official rule or order promulgated by government authority. Regulations too have the force of law and are intended to implement a specific statute, oftentimes to direct the conduct of those regulated by the regulating authority.

Another term subject to confusion likewise requiring clarification is *(agency) policy*, which refers to a deliberate program or course of action intended to guide, influence, or determine certain (agency) decisions, actions, or outcomes. It can also be defined as a statement or an agendum set forth by an (a public) organization to relate its goals and intents to the overall performance of its action or activity. And the term *order* is an authoritative direction given by a court, another adjudicative entity, or an authority intended to be obeyed. In contrast, the terms *guidelines, guidance,* and in some cases *standard* are advisory in nature and do not have the full force of law. At most, they represent rules or a series of steps to be carried out to implement a policy more efficaciously.

3.3.1. Regulatory Agencies in the United States

In the United States, environmental health laws at the national level are regulated and enforced by certain federal agencies, which have the added duties to establish and implement their own agency policies and standards relevant to these statutes. The more prominent of these U.S. federal agencies include: U.S. Environmental Protection Agency (U.S. EPA); U.S. Food and Drug Administration (FDA); U.S. Occupational Safety and Health Administration (OSHA); U.S. Consumer Product Safety Commission (CPSC); and U.S. Department of Transportation (DOT).

Briefly, U.S. EPA is a non-cabinet regulatory agency charged with protecting human health and with safeguarding as well as improving the nation's natural environment. Its areas of environmental health and regulatory concerns include, but are not limited to: air pollution; water pollution; hazardous substances; ecosystems and natural resources; solid and toxic wastes; pesticides; ocean dumping; indoor air; drinking water; and oil pollution. The agency began operation on 2 December 1970, less than a year since the passage of NEPA (U.S. National Environmental Policy Act).

FDA is part of the U.S. Department of Health and Human Services. It is responsible for the safety (and health) regulation of most types of foods, drugs, cosmetics, food additives, dietary supplements, veterinary products, radiation-emitting devices, medical devices, vaccines, and blood products. The agency's current name was officialized in 1930, with its root dating back to the early 1900s or earlier.

CPSC is an independent agency of the U.S. federal government, and was established in 1972 under the federal Consumer Product Safety Act. This federal agency is charged with safeguarding consumers (especially children in families) against unreasonable risks of illnesses or injuries associated with products that pose a fire, electrical, chemical, or mechanical hazard or that can cause injury specifically to children.

OSHA is an agency of the U.S. Department of Labor. It was created by U.S. Congress under the federal Occupational Safety and Health Act of 1970. The agency's mission is to prevent work-related injuries, illnesses, and deaths by promulgating and enforcing standards for workplace safety and health.

Beginning operation on 1 April 1967, DOT was established by U.S. Congress as a cabinet department of the Executive Branch. It has a mission to ensure a fast, safe, efficient, accessible, and convenient transportation system for the nation. In terms of environmental health, its areas of regulatory concern include: water shipment of toxic materials (sharing responsibility with U.S. Coast Guard); oil pollution (with U.S. Coast Guard and U.S. EPA); and transport of hazardous materials in general.

3.3.2. Environmental Health Laws in the United States

Table 3.2 provides an overview of the more prominent federal laws dealing with environmental exposures. Also listed in the table are both the areas of environmental health and regulatory concerns that each statute covers, and the principal federal agency(ies) that is (are) charged with regulating and enforcing that specific statute.

For the most part, the connection should become clear between each federal statute listed in Table 3.2 and the principal federal agency(ies) charged with enforcing it, once the areas of concern covered by that law have become transparent. One exception is the connection for the Food Quality Protection Act (FQPA) of 1996, as the law involves the responsibilities of both FDA and U.S. EPA. FQPA was enacted as an amendment to both FIFRA and the Federal Food, Drug, and Cosmetic Act (FD&C Act). This amendment calls for stricter safety standards for pesticide residues in foods, particularly for young children under the presumption that this age group tends to be more susceptible to environmental exposure. FQPA requires a complete health risk re-assessment of all existing tolerances (i.e., limits) set on the amount of pesticide residues being allowed to remain in or on foods marketed in the United States.

Another connection lacking transparency to some people is that for the Oil Pollution Act (OPA) of 1990, which involves not only U.S. Coast Guard and DOT but also U.S. EPA. The OPA was enacted in response to the pollution problem caused by the oil tanker *Exxon Valdez*, which on 24 March 1989 spilled over 10 million gallons of crude oil into the water of Prince William Sound. The law amended the U.S. Clean Water Act and addressed the wide range of problems associated with the prevention of, response to, and cleanup payment for oil pollution incidents in navigable U.S. waters. Three other statutes are likewise noteworthy here. These are the Federal Hazardous Substances Act (FHSA) of 1960, the Comprehensive Environmental Response, Compensation, & Liability Act (CERCLA) of 1980, and the Bioterrorism Act of 2002. From its title, FHSA might not be thought of as primarily for household products and hence not for CPSC alone to regulate

Table 3.2. The More Prominent Federal Environmental Health Laws and Regulatory Concerns in the United States[a]

Federal Statute[b]	Areas of Regulatory and Environmental Health Concerns	Agency[c,d]
Food, Drug, & Cosmetic Act (FD&C Act, 1906; amended 2007)	Safety regulation on foods, drugs, cosmetics, vaccines, medical devices, blood products, dietary supplements, color additives, veterinary products, radiation-emitting devices, and more.	FDA
Federal Insecticide, Fungicide & Rodenticide Act (FIFRA, 1947; amended 2007)	Safety regulation on use, sale, and distribution of pesticides	EPA
Federal Hazardous Substances Act (1960; amended 2011)	Safety regulation on household products (especially on labeling)	CPSC
National Environmental Policy Act (1969; amended 1982)	Promotion of harmony between the people and the environment	EPA
Occupational Safety and Health Act (1970; amended 2004)	Safety standards for toxic agents in (nongovernment) workplaces	OSHA
Poison Prevention Packaging Act (1970; amended 2008)	Child-resistant packaging for toxic household products	CPSC
(U.S.) Clean Air Act (1970; amended 1990)	Regulation and improvement of nation's air quality	EPA
(U.S.) Clean Water Act (1972; amended 2011)	Regulation and improvement of nation's water quality	EPA
Consumer Product Safety Act (1972; amended 2011)	Safety regulation on hazardous consumer products	CPSC
Safe Drinking Water Act (1974; amended 1996)	Protection and improvement of nation's drinking water quality	EPA
Hazardous Materials Transportation Act (1975; amended 1990)	Safety regulation on transportation of hazardous and toxic materials in commerce	DOT
Resource Conservation & Recovery Act (1976; amended 1984)	Safety regulation on solid waste disposal, including disposal of hazardous wastes, on *active* sites	EPA
Toxic Substances Control Act (1976; amended 1992)	Safety regulation on hazardous substances not covered by other statutes, including pre-market review/approval	EPA
Comprehensive Environmental Response, Compensation, & Liability Act (1980; amended 1986; a.k.a. Superfund)	Safety regulation on *inactive* sites contaminated with hazardous wastes	EPA
Oil Pollution Act (1990; amended 2000)	Mitigation and prevention of oil pollution and oil spills	DOT, USCG
Pollution Prevention Act (1990)	Reduction of pollution at and through the source	EPA
Food Quality Protection Act (FQPA, 1996; amended versions of FIFRA and the FD&C Act)	Safety regulation on pesticide residues in food, with a focus on children's exposure	EPA, FDA

[a] *see, e.g.,* Beck *et al.* (2008) for further discussion, which is the primary source for this table; [b] in parentheses are year of the act's passage and, if any, year of its (key or latest) amendment; [c] primary or sole agency(ies); [d] FDA = U.S. Food and Drug Administration, EPA = U.S. Environmental Protection Agency, CPSC = U.S. Consumer Product Safety Commission, OSHA = U.S. Occupational Safety and Health Administration, DOT = U.S. Department of Transportation, and USCG = U.S. Coast Guard.

and enforce. Yet it is narrower in scope than its title might suggest. The statute is intended primarily for regulation of children's toys and household goods.

As further discussed in Chapter 22, CERCLA is known more commonly as Superfund (law). The law was enacted initially in response to the threat of hazardous waste buried and released at the Love Canal toxic site (Section 2.2.4). It allows the federal government to tax on the chemical and petroleum industries for compensation and liability purposes, as reflected in the law's title. Over the first five years after the law's passage, $1.6 billion was collected into a trust fund for use to clean up abandoned or uncontrolled hazardous waste sites. The accumulated trust fund is now known as Superfund, which now also becomes CERCLA's nickname. Despite the fact that Superfund created the U.S. Agency for Toxic Substances and Disease Registry (ATSDR), it empowers U.S. EPA alone to compel the responsible parties to clean up sites that they have contaminated.

Note that the Bioterrorism Act of 2002 (or more formally, the Public Health Security & Bioterrorism Preparedness and Response Act of 2002) is not listed in Table 3.2, since it is treated as having less pertinence to factors that are generally addressed under the realm of environmental health. It is nonetheless regarded by some people as the more recent U.S. federal statute on issues relevant to some form of environmental health.

3.3.3. Foreign Environmental Health Laws and Agencies

There are likewise many environmental health laws and regulatory agencies abroad that are equally influential, whether at the global, regional, or national level, in protecting human health from exposure to environmental contaminants. A case in point is, again, the global treaty *Stockholm Convention on POPs*, that adopted in 2001 (and put into force in 2004) by more than 150 nations. The aims of this treaty are to schedule and implement worldwide reduction or elimination of all POP uses, by starting with the twelve that are considered as the worst (and hence the term *dirty dozen*).

Another case is the *Basel Convention on the Control of Transboundary Movements of Hazardous Wastes and Their Disposal*, or Basel Convention for short. This global treaty is regarded as the most comprehensive global environmental agreement on hazardous and other wastes. It represents more than 170 parties with the aims of protecting human health and the environment against the harmful effects that may result from improper handling of hazardous and other wastes, including their disposal, generation, and transboundary movements. The Basel Convention came into force in 1992.

A third example for treaties at the global level is the *Montreal Protocol on Substances That Deplete the Ozone Layer*, or Montreal Protocol for short. This international treaty was adopted to protect ozone (O_3) in the air zone second closest to the Earth (i.e., the stratosphere layer) by phasing out the production of a number of substances (e.g., freons, halons) determined to be responsible for ozone depletion. The treaty was opened for signature on 16 September 1987, and put into force on 1 January 1989.

For international health agencies with a regulatory role, among the first that comes to the mind of many people is WHO. Yet legally or technically, WHO may assume only a *coordinating* authority for all public health matters within the United Nations system. While the organization's stated mission is "*the attainment by all peoples of the highest possible level of health*", its main activities include: providing leadership on environmental health and other global health matters; shaping health research agenda; setting public health norms and standards; monitoring and assessing health trends; and offering technical support to countries in the world.

Another equally relevant, equally prominent international organization is the United Nations Environment Programme (UNEP). It serves as the *designated* authority of the United Nations system in tackling and resolving environmental issues at the global and regional levels. As with WHO, UNEP is not truly a health *regulatory* agency. Regardless, its influential activities indeed cover a broad range of environmental issues concerning the atmospheric, oceanic, and terrestrial ecosystems, as well as human health.

There are also many regulatory agencies abroad at the national or regional level that are as influential and active as those in the United States. These foreign agencies include: the Commission for Environmental Cooperation (CEC); the European Environmental Agency (EEA); the Environment Canada (EC); Japan's Ministry of the Environment (JMOE); China's Ministry of Environmental Protection (CMEP); the Brazilian Institute of Environmental and Renewable Natural Resources (IBAMA, as from the institute's name in Portuguese); and Germany's Federal Environment(al) Agency (UBA, as from the agency's name in German). The visions and missions of these foreign agencies are similar, all aiming to control and prevent environmental pollution as well as to safeguard public health and preserve the natural environment. As with those in the United States (e.g., U.S. EPA, FDA, CPSC, OSHA), many of these foreign agencies are charged with a similar responsibility of enforcing their own regional or national laws, regulations, and policies that are highly pertinent to environmental health.

More specifically, CEC was established by Canada, Mexico, and the United States in 1994 through the North American Agreement on Environmental Cooperation, with the aims to address the region's environmental concerns. The commission was created to foster conservation, protection, and enhancement of the North American environment for the benefit of present and future generations, in the context of increasing economic, trade, and social links among the three nations.

EEA is a research arm as well as a monitoring unit of the European Union. Its task is to provide sound, independent information concerning the quality of the natural environment. The agency serves as a major information source for the general public as well as for those entities that are involved in developing, adopting, implementing, and evaluating environmental policy. Currently, EEA has 32 countries as its members.

EC is a federal level agency accountable to Canada's Minister of the Environment. Its mandate includes preserving as well as conserving the nation's natural environment and water resources. In addition, the agency is required to perform the following agenda for the people of Canada: forecast weather conditions and warnings; provide detailed meteorological data; and coordinate all federal environmental policies and programs.

CMEP (or China's MEP) is a new cabinet-level ministry established in 2008 to take over the responsibility of China's State Environmental Protection Administration (SEPA) for the nation's environmental governance. The ministry's regulatory role includes efforts to control and prevent environmental pollution, preserve the nation's natural environment, ensure nuclear safety, and protect public health. Many of these national agenda were those of the SEPA that survived for 20 years.

JMOE is a cabinet-level ministry in Japan. It was upgraded in 2001 from its sub-cabinet level Environmental Agency established in 1971. The then sub-cabinet agency, as well as now JMOE, had many regulatory agenda similar to those of U.S. EPA.

IBAMA is an environmental enforcement agency in Brazil affiliated with the country's Ministry of Environment. Its regulatory role includes environmental protection, environmental licensing, environmental quality, sustainable use of forest management, and animal resources.

UBA is Germany's central federal authority on all environmental issues. It has two key statutory mandates: (1) the provision of scientific support to the various federal government bodies (e.g., Federal Ministry for the Environment, Federal Ministry of Health); and (2) the implementation of environmental laws (e.g., those pertaining to emissions trading and to authorization of chemicals, pharmaceuticals, and plant protection agents). The agency also has the responsibility to provide the public with information concerning environmental protection.

References

Beck BD, Calabrese EJ, Slayton TM, Rudel R, 2008. The Use of Toxicology in the Regulatory Process. In *Principles and Methods of Toxicology* (Hayes AW, Ed.), Fifth Edition. Boca Raton, Florida, USA: Taylor & Francis Group, Chapter 2.

Carlson R, 1962. *Silent Spring*. Boston, Massachusetts, USA: Houghton Mifflin.

CDC (U.S. Centers for Disease Control and Prevention), 1990. Historical Perspectives Reduced Incidence of Menstrual Toxic-Shock Syndrome – United States, 1980-1990. *MMWR* (Morbidity and Mortality Weekly Report) 39:421-423.

CIDRAP (University of Minnesota Center of Infectious Disease Research & Policy), 2009. CDC Releases Viruses for Novel H1N1 Vaccine Development. *CIDRAP News*, 7 May (by Robert Roos, its News Editor).

Dong MH, 2006. Human Health Risk from Consumption of Fish Contaminated with Persistent Organochlorine Compounds (POCs). Planetary lecture presented at the *International Conference on Environmental and Public Health Management: Aquaculture and Environment*, 7-9 December, 2006, Croucher Institute for Environmental Sciences, Hong Kong Baptist University, Hong Kong.

FAO (Food and Agriculture Organization of the United Nations), 2010. Global Forest Resources Assessment 2010. FAO Forestry Paper 163. Rome, Italy.

Hynes HP, 1989. *The Recurring Silent Spring*. New York, New York, USA: Pergamon Press.

Lewis J, 1985. The Birth of EPA. *EPA Journal*, November Issue. http://www.epagov/history/topics/epa/15c.htm.

Neely WB, 1994. *Introduction to Chemical Exposure and Risk Assessment*. Boca Raton, Florida, USA: CRC Press.

Pathoni A, 2007. Indonesia Starts Planting 79 Million Trees. *Reuters.com*, 28 November.

Revkin AC, 2009. Hacked E-Mail Is New Fodder for Climate Dispute. *The New York Times*, 20 November.

Sengco MR, Andersen DM, 2004. Controlling Harmful Algal Blooms through Clay Flocculation. *J. Eukaryol. Microbiol.* 5:169-172.

The New York Times (nytimes.com), 1922. Reforestation Spreading; Conservation Commission Reports 31,994,000 Plantings since 1908, published 29 January.

Tversky A, Kahneman D, 1974. Judgment under Uncertainty: Heuristics and Biases. *Science* 185: 1124-1131.

U.S. EPA (U.S. Environmental Protection Agency), 2007. Risk Communication in Action: The Risk Communication Workbook. EPA/625/R-05/003. Office of Research and Development, Cincinnati, Ohio, USA.

U.S. EPA (U.S. Environmental Protection Agency), 2008a. Clean Air Act. http://www.epa.gov/air/caa/index.html.

U.S. EPA (U.S. Environmental Protection Agency), 2008b. Clean Water Act. http://www.epa.gov/r5water/cwa.htm.

U.S. EPA (U.S. Environmental Protection Agency), 2008c. Federal Insecticide, Fungicide, and Rodenticide Act (FIFRA) Enforcement. http://www.epa.gov/compliance/civil/fifra/index.html.

WHO (World Health Organization), 2011. Environmental Health (webpage). http://www.who.int/topics/environmental_health/en/.

Xia G, 1998. II. An Estimate of the Economic Consequences of Environmental Pollution in China. In *The Economic Costs of China's Environmental Degradation* (Smil V, Yushi M, Eds.). Cambridge, Massachusetts, USA: American Academy of Arts and Sciences.

Review Questions

1. Briefly describe the nature, characteristics, impacts, and concerns of environmental pollution.

2. What was (and still is) U.S. NEPA's stated purpose?

3. On what date did the *first* Earth Day celebration take place in the United States? And roughly how many Americans participated on that day?

4. From *air* pollution in China in the early 1990s, what impact factor or cause category was responsible for the *second* most economic loss in that nation?

5. What were the three major threats to the nation's environment that the U.S. Clean Air Act has aimed to curb through its amendment in 1990?

6. What was the major environmental concern that U.S. Vice-President Al Gore's documentary film *An Inconvenient Truth* attempted to publicize as a worldwide health problem?

7. What was the main focus of the U.S. FIFRA amended in 1972?

8. Name the principal U.S. federal agency(ies) responsible for regulating and enforcing the following statutes: a) *Poison Prevention Packaging Act;* b) *Federal Hazardous Substances Act;* c) *Toxic Substances Control Act;* d) *Oil Pollution Act.*

9. What is the basic legal distinction between *law* and *order*, and between *guidance* and *regulation*?

10. Which federal statute in the United States is known as *Superfund (law)*? And how is it related to the missions or functions of U.S. EPA and ATSDR?

11. Name the U.S. federal agency(ies) that is (are) primarily responsible for the health and safety regulations concerning the following: a) blood products; b) radiation-emitting devices; c) oil pollution; d) pesticide residues in food.

12. Name the treaty that is regarded as the most comprehensive global environmental agreement concerning the treatment of hazardous and other wastes.

13. What is the global treaty concerned with the worldwide depletion of ozone layer?

14. Name four regulatory agencies abroad that are as influential and active as those in the United States.

CHAPTER 4

Occurrence and Types of Environmental Toxicants

4.1. Introduction

In this chapter, brief accounts of 10 environmental contamination cases are given to illustrate of two points deemed crucial to the practice of environmental toxicology. First, this short list is intended to offer a sense of what the current sensitivity is regarding public and regulatory concerns with environmental health. Second, the list also aims to assure that the *occurrence* of today's environmental health issues rests more on social values than on the severity of the health effect involved. For example, trans fats are chemically known as unsaturated fatty acids with at least one double bond in the *trans* position. The ban of trans fats for use in restaurants in the state of California (Section 4.2.2.C below) signifies a new perspective from at least some sectors in the United States concerning environmental health. After all, it is not as if the harmful cardiovascular effects of trans fats were unbeknown to many people until in recent years.

From the first three chapters (notably Section 2.3.1), it becomes clear that there appear to be countless environmental toxicants of concern regarding their effects on human health and the ecosystem. Many of these toxicants are systematically characterized in groups in Part III of this book (Chapters 11 through 17) for a fuller appreciation of their environmental nature and effects. In the second half of this chapter, many of these toxicants are revisited in groups in a different manner for yet two other reasons. The first reason is that, much like the adverse effects that they can cause (Chapter 2), further discussion on topics covered in Part II (Chapters 5 through 10) cannot be as productive without some knowledge on the general nature and effects of these toxicants. A subtle issue here, if not a dilemma, is that neither is it practical to have a fair understanding of the environmental nature and effects of these toxicants unless there is some appreciation of the topics covered in Part II. The other reason is more subtle. The toxicants discussed in this chapter represent those that appear to be of greater concern to the general public, such as parents and news media, than to other sectors, thus re-signifying to some extent what the public's *current* sensitivities or concerns are with environmental health.

4.1.1. Contemporary Issues of Environmental Concern

In addition to the three biological agents (i.e., those causing mad-cow disease, severe acute respiratory syndrome, and H1N1 flu) and the one notorious group of persistent organic pollutants briefly discussed in Chapters 1 and 2, respectively, there are many environmental contaminants (re)emerging within the past decade or so. Despite the fact that to certain people these other toxicants may not deserve as much national or global attention, some can indeed cause a considerable level of harm or threat to human health or the environment. For the reasons given earlier, overviews for 10 select contemporary cases are given in Section 4.2 one by one. This short list is selected among the many that are currently considered as having a public health problem or to cause some significant issues on safety regulation in the context of environmental health and toxicology.

4.1.2. Grouping of Environmental Contaminants

Inasmuch as there are seemingly countless contaminants present in the environment, there are bound to be numerous schemes in which these toxicants can or should be grouped for better consideration or analysis. For example, toxicants in the environment can be grouped according to *site of exposure.* To that end, there are indoor air pollutants, outdoor air pollutants, drinking water contaminants, pesticide residues in foods, food contaminants, soil contaminants, and so forth. Another way is to classify environmental pollutants based on the *type* of health or ecological *effects* that they tend to cause, such as environmental carcinogens, environmental teratogens, environmental endocrine disruptors, and environmental stressors (e.g., air pollutants, soil contaminants, traffic congestion, noise pollution). Still another scheme is to group them according to their chemical structure, their chemical family or subfamily, or their physicochemical state, such as toxic metals, pesticides (or their subfamilies insecticides, fungicides), persistent organochlorine compounds (POCs), and volatile organic compounds (VOCs).

There is simply no definitive or correct way to place environmental contaminants into certain types, groups, or classes. After all, residues of many pesticides that belong to a certain subfamily (e.g., organochlorines, organophosphates, herbicides) are commonly present in the air, water, soil, or foods. Many pesticides also can cause multiple toxic effects in humans or test animals. Still some pesticides are metals, while some others can be both an endocrine disruptor (Chapter 19) and a persistent organic pollutant.

In this chapter, the way in which environmental contaminants are grouped for a brief overview below is based partly on some of the above example schemes and partly on the ease of their referral or referencing in the literature, but more on their availability for environmental exposure and the perceived or confirmed importance of their health or ecological implications. As a result, a few of the contaminants included below have a specific place all by themselves. Regardless, the list presented below is by no means exhaustive and is subject to change from time to time, but does include most of those currently being considered by U.S. EPA (2008a) as having a great deal of interest or concern to parents, news media, and other public sectors. Note that throughout this book, the term *contaminant* or *environmental contaminant* is used as defined by the U.S. Agency for Toxic Substances and Disease Registry (ATSDR, 2008): "*A substance (or an agent) that is either present in an environment where it does not belong or is present at levels that might cause harmful health effects.*" Moreover, here the words *environment* and *contamination* are defined in their broadest scope as can be.

4.2. Contemporary Issues: 10 Select Cases

Note that the 10 cases discussed below are not meant to represent those current issues highly debatable in nature (e.g., gun control, marijuana cultivation). They are simply specific contemporary issues, events, or otherwise cases relevant to environmental toxicology or pollution that have occurred within the past decade or so. These select cases tend to have more regional than global ramifications as they all reflect the social, economic, or cultural concerns at the national or community level. More specifically, for the cases discussed below, all but one mean more to American people than to those living in other countries. The tenth case is an issue more to people living in some other countries, particularly those residing around an e-waste (electronic waste) recycling site.

4.2.1. Contaminants in Consumer Products

Three cases have been specifically selected to represent the contemporary issues for this group. The toxicants of environmental health concern representing this group are triclosan ($C_{12}H_7Cl_3O_2$), lead (Pb), and bisphenol A ($C_{15}H_{16}O_2$).

A. The Ubiquitous Antibacterial Ingredient

Triclosan is a disinfectant showing up in hundreds of consumer products used every day (especially in the United States), such as soaps, toothpastes, deodorants, cosmetics, kitchenware, toys, and clothing (Cone, 2006). Despite the fact that this chemical has been used since the 1970s, environmental health concerns with its overuse have come up only in recent years, when its efficacy in soaps has since become questionable for preventing infectious illness symptoms and for reducing bacterial levels on the hands (Aiello *et al.*, 2007). There have been many studies linking triclosan to a variety of health and environmental effects ranging from destruction of aquatic ecosystems to skin irritation, antibiotic resistance, and contamination with the carcinogenic dioxins (Glaser, 2004). In particular, a Swedish study detected high levels of triclosan in 3 out of 5 human breast milk samples (Adolfsson-Erici *et al.*, 2002), implicating that this antibacterial agent can be absorbed into the human body and that newborns can easily be exposed to it.

B. Lead on Toys

According to the U.S. news media (e.g., Hartman, 2007), in the summer of 2007 as many as 1.5 million railway toys manufactured for Thomas & Friends Wooden Railway in the United States joined the growing list of Chinese-made products to be pulled out of the American store shelves for children safety reasons. The surface paint of these toys reportedly contained an unacceptable level of lead (Chapter 14), a metal that is highly toxic to the human body if swallowed (e.g., through licking).

C. Baby's Toxic Bottle

Bisphenol A (BPA) is the building block of hard polycarbonate plastics and epoxy resins used in a wide variety of consumer products including baby bottles. This chemical, first synthesized in 1895 and discovered in 1936 as a synthetic hormone, is now shown to be capable of mimicking the sex hormone estrogen to interfere with healthy growth and normal body functions. Animal studies have consistently demonstrated that BPA can cause damage to the reproductive, neurological, and immunological systems during critical stages of development, such as during infancy and in the womb (WGFSM, 2008). The one critical health concern with BPA is apparently the finding that, when heating the bottles to 80° C or higher, the chemical was shown to leach out of six major brands of baby bottles available in Canada and the United States (WGFSM, 2008). In those studies, the synthetic hormone in the leachates was measured at 4.7 to 8.3 ppb (parts per billion).

4.2.2. Contaminants in Food Products

Three cases have been specifically selected to represent the contemporary issues for this group. The food toxicants of concern in these three cases are mercury (Hg), melamine ($C_3H_6N_6$), and trans fats (*trans*-isomer fatty acids).

A. Mercury Level in Tuna

According to a national survey conducted in the United States by an ocean conservation organization named Oceana (Burros, 2008), both store-bought tuna and those sold to customers in sushi restaurants were found to have mercury concentrations almost twice as much as the action level recommended by FDA (U.S. Food and Drug Administration) as unsafe. Mercury is a metal that can be highly toxic to humans when available in soluble form in high doses (Chapter 14). In 2004, both FDA and U.S. EPA formally advised women of childbearing age to limit their consumption of certain canned tuna to 6 ounces per week or less, due to the metal's toxic effects on the developing fetus.

B. Melamine Poisoning

As reported by MSNBC.com (2009), on 22 January 2009 a court in China "*sentenced two men to death for their role in the production and sale of melamine-tainted milk that killed at least six children and made nearly 300,000 ill.*" Melamine is an organic base with the molecular formula $C_3H_6N_6$ and hence highly rich in nitrogen (N). According to the court case, the organic base was illegally added to milk formulas by the two men to falsify the milk's protein content which is typically measured in terms of N content. Melamine *per se* has low acute toxicity. Yet the organic base can form crystals to give rise to kidney stones when reacting with cyanuric acid ($C_3H_3N_3O_3$), a weak organic acid commonly present in melamine powder. In 2007, it was found that pet food manufactured in the United States using wheat gluten imported from China had led to the death of a large number of dogs and cats due to kidney failure. Further investigation indicated that the wheat gluten was contaminated with melamine.

C. Trans Fat Ban in California

Effective New Year's Day 2010, all restaurants in California (the most populous state in the United States) can no longer cook foods with trans fats (McGreevy, 2008). The state law was signed in July 2008 but did not take effect until 2010. Trans fats are made from vegetable oil by adding hydrogen to saturate the unsaturated plant oil, in order to increase the shelf life and the flavor stability of foods containing this type of fats. Trans fatty acids can be found commercially in vegetable shortenings and some margarines. Overwhelming scientific evidence has indicated that the consumption of trans fats can raise the LDL (low-density lipoprotein) "bad" cholesterol levels in the blood, thereby increasing the risk of coronary heart disease (FNB, 2005).

4.2.3. Pollutants in the Open Environment

Four cases have been specifically selected to represent the contemporary issues for this group. Here the environmental contaminants of concern are nonchemical-specific. They include plastics, pharmaceuticals, pesticides, and organochlorine compounds.

A. Plastic Marine Pollution

On 27 March 2007, San Francisco became the first city in the United States to approve a groundbreaking ordinance banning petroleum-based plastic bags at checkouts of large supermarkets and pharmacy stores. One key argument supporting the ban was that *"Plastic bags are blamed for gumming up recycling machines taking up space in landfills and killing or sickening marine mammals* (Goodyear, 2007)." According to a Greenpeace report (Allsopp *et al.*, 2006), hundreds of thousands of marine creatures (e.g., whales, dolphins, fish, whales, sea turtles, seabirds) die each year from entanglement or ingestion of plastic debris present ubiquitously in the seabed, particularly near the coastal regions where large volumes of plastic bags are used and left behind as litter (e.g., Galgani *et al.*, 1995; Thiel *et al.*, 2003).

B. Pharmaceutical Wastes

On 2 December 2008, U.S. EPA (2008b) filed a proposal in the *Federal Register* to add hazardous pharmaceutical wastes to the federal Universal Waste Rule (UWR), which at the time included only batteries, pesticides, lamps, and mercury-containing equipment all in the *used* form. The agency has not set a date for the finalization of this long process rulemaking (but with spring 2013 tentatively scheduled for public comment). The proposed amendment applies to all facilities that generate hazardous pharmaceutical wastes, including hospitals, pharmacies, medical offices, dental offices, and veterinary clinics. Although pharmaceuticals are crucial to the maintenance of human health, they can pollute the environment. A study by the U.S. Geological Survey (USGS, 2002) found that, between 1999 and 2000, many personal care products (e.g., fragrances) and pharmaceuticals (e.g., prescription drugs, over-the-counter medicines, steroids, hormones) were detected in water samples collected from 139 streams in 30 states, though at low concentrations. It is important to note that fish and other aquatic animals residing near the contamination sites are likely to be exposed to the wastes throughout their entire life cycle even prior to birth. Some pharmaceutical wastes can be endocrine disruptors, as they have been shown to cause reproductive effects in fish (Palace *et al.*, 2006; Schultz *et al.*, 2003). At least one study has implicated that antidepressants could accumulate in fish living in streams that received a high level of treated urban effluent (Brooks *et al.*, 2005).

C. The United Heckathorn Superfund Site

The U.S. Comprehensive Environmental Response, Compensation, & Liability Act (CERCLA), or known commonly as Superfund (law), was enacted by U.S. Congress on 11 December 1980 initially in response to the appalling tragedy of Love Canal (Sections 2.2.4 and 3.3.2). This act authorizes U.S. EPA to compel responsible parties to clean up toxic waste sites and, where a responsible party cannot be found, to clean up the site on the agency's own effort using a special trust fund nowadays known as Superfund. In 2001, U.S. EPA issued a summary of the first five-year review of its cleanup efforts for the United Heckathorn (U.H.) site located in Richmond Harbor in Contra Costa County, California. From 1947 to 1966, the U.H. Superfund toxic site was a place for formulating and packaging pesticides. It now becomes a major source of DDT and other persistent pesticides polluting the nearby San Francisco Bay. As authorized under CERCLA, in March 1990 U.S. EPA took over from the state of California the investigation and clean-up of this toxic site. In October 2008, U.S. EPA launched and completed its first fish survey since the dredging to assess the lingering pollution. The objective of the fish sample collection was to update the baseline information for the human health and ecological risks involved. Further elaboration on this case is given in Chapter 22 (Section 22.3.2).

D. Electronic Waste (E-Waste) Problems in China

As noted in Chapter 2, e-waste is an emerging major environmental health issue. This is particularly true in China. There are as many as 50 million tons of e-waste generated worldwide each year, of which more than 50% is legally or illegally imported to Asia, mainly to China (Puckett *et al.*, 2002; UNEP, 2005). Most of this e-waste flowing into China ends up in families residing around the recycling sites, where many of these families have members as laborers working to disassemble the waste electronics manually for reclaimable materials. Wearing little protective gear, these workers (and their families) are exposed to a host of toxic chemicals including acids, PCBs (polychlorinated biphenyls), polybrominated diphenyl ethers (PBDEs), and toxic metals (e.g., lead, cadmium).

4.3. Environmental Toxicants of Health Concern

Highlighted in this section are the toxicological issues with environmental toxicants that are considered as having great concerns to the public sectors as well as having great relevance to environmental toxicology. The toxicological issues discussed are comparable to those given in Hodgson *et al.* (1998), at the U.S. EPA website, or at the ATSDR website. Serving as further references, where applicable the one or more chapters in this book that provide specific elaboration on the toxicant are listed in parentheses in the subject heading given for the toxicant under discussion.

4.3.1. Group I: Individual, Specific Toxicants

This group includes 11 chemicals that each appear to have a specific place by themselves in terms of their public health impacts. Of these, three are inorganic gases (carbon dioxide, carbon monoxide, ozone), two are volatile organic compounds (benzene, formaldehyde), and the remaining six are chemical elements with metallic properties (arsenic, cadmium, chromium, lead, mercury, radon).

A. Arsenic (As; Chapter 14)

This contaminant is best characterized as a group of arsenic compounds (commonly called arsenicals), not as a single metalloid element. One concern with these compounds is that they can come from drinking water and are used in pesticides. Epidemiological studies revealed that the *tri*valent form As^{3+} could cause skin carcinogen. Chromated copper arsenate (CCA) is a wood preservative pesticide containing chromium (Cr), copper (Cu), and As. Since the 1970s, CCA-pressure treated wood has been part of the majority of the outdoor residential structures, even though it is no longer being produced (but not yet completely eliminated) for use in decks or playsets in the United States.

B. Benzene (C_6H_6; Chapter 13)

It is a volatile organic compound (VOC) widely used as a constituent of motor fuels and as an intermediate to make other chemicals that in turn are used to make plastics, resins, nylons, and other chemical materials. This VOC has been listed by U.S. EPA as both a human carcinogen and a priority toxic pollutant.

C. Cadmium (Cd; Chapter 14)

This metal was used for a long time as a pigment and for corrosion resistant plating on steel, with its compounds being used mainly to stabilize plastics. In recent years, over 85% of all the cadmium has been used in batteries, especially in the rechargeable nickel-cadmium kind. Like lead, it has no known useful role in higher order animals. The most dangerous form of occupational exposure to cadmium is inhalation of its fine dusts and fumes, or ingestion of its soluble compounds. Severe chronic cadmium poisoning can result in renal abnormalities, or in the ill-known *itai-itai* (ouch, ouch) disease (Chapter 14).

D. Carbon Dioxide (CO_2)

It is one of the gases readily found in the atmosphere. This gas can be an asphyxiant by replacing an excessive portion of the oxygen in the breathing zone. At high blood concentrations, it can cause unconsciousness or death. When fossil fuels such as gasoline and propane (containing mostly carbon) react with oxygen, they produce carbon dioxide. Deforestation can increase the atmospheric level of this gas since forests will otherwise break down the compound during photosynthesis. It has been speculated that too much carbon dioxide in the air can overwhelm the greenhouse effect to cause global warming.

E. Carbon Monoxide (CO; Chapter 11)

This is a highly acute toxic gas responsible for the most common type of fatal human poisoning in many parts of the world including the United States. The gas is readily produced by the incomplete burning of many common types of fuels (e.g., charcoal, coal, kerosene, natural gas, oil, wood), and by many common types of equipment powered by internal combustion engines (e.g., automobiles, lawn mowers, portable generators). Carbon monoxide is considered as one of the criteria air pollutants in the United States. The gas is also known as a silent killer owing to the fact that it is not only an acutely fatal but also a completely colorless, odorless, and tasteless compound.

F. Chromium (Cr; Chapter 14).

This metal is commonly used in electroplating, paints, and textile manufacturing. It has been found in some drinking water sources. Studies showed that the metal caused cancer in laboratory animals when they consumed enough water containing it in the hexavalent form (Cr^{6+}). In contrast, its trivalent form (Cr^{3+}) in low doses is an essential human nutrient, as Cr^{3+} shortage can cause heart conditions and disruptions of metabolism.

how diff forms have diff. effects

G. Formaldehyde (CH_2O; Chapter 13)

This is a colorless, strong-smelling gas used widely by industry to manufacture building materials and many household products (e.g., as an adhesive resin in pressed wood products). Accordingly, it can be found in substantial levels in the indoor and outdoor air. This VOC gas is a by-product of combustion and some other natural processes. It is a designated carcinogen in the United States and may trigger an asthma attack.

H. Lead (Pb; Chapter 14)

This is a highly toxic metal used for many years in products found around homes. The metal can cause a wide range of health effects from behavioral problems and learning disabilities to seizures and death. Young children are most at risk, largely due to their naïve nature and the fact that many defensive mechanisms in their body are still being developed. The following are major sources of lead exposure for children: lead contaminated dust; deteriorating lead-based paint (from chewing the paint chips); and lead contaminated residential soil. Lead is one of the six criteria air pollutants in the United States.

I. Mercury (Hg; Chapter 14)

As with lead, mercury is a highly toxic metal found in the air, water, and soil. The metal exists in several forms: elemental or metallic mercury (Hg^0), inorganic mercury compounds (e.g., $HgCl_2$), and organic mercury compounds (e.g., $[CH_3Hg]^+$). At high levels, exposure to mercury can harm the brain, heart, kidneys, lungs, and immunological system of people at all ages. Exposure to certain forms of the metal at high levels can cause similar biological effects in many animals, especially those that consume fish (which as a group tend to be a rich reservoir for mercury). Severe chronic mercury poisoning can result in the ill-known Minamata disease (Chapter 14).

J. Ozone (O_3; Chapter 11)

This gas is an allotrope (i.e., a certain form) of oxygen occurring both near the ground level (troposphere) and in the Earth's next upper air layer (stratosphere). Depending on its location in the atmosphere, ozone can be "good" or "bad" to human health and the ecosystem. Tropospheric ozone is a gas pollutant posing a significant health threat, especially to children with asthma. At high levels, it will damage trees, crops, and other vegetation. It is a main component of urban smog. In the stratosphere, the gas plays a key role in keeping the sun's harmful ultraviolet radiation from striking the Earth's surface.

K. Radon (Rn; Chapter 14)

This is a cancer-causing natural radioactive gas that reportedly claims some 20,000 American lives each year. It is formed from mostly the radioactive decay of the metal uranium (U) which is available in small amounts in most rocks and soils. Radon itself undergoes radioactive decay to yield yet another unstable radioactive daughter. The daughter then also divides herself into radiation and still another radioactive daughter. Although radon is no longer used in the treatment of various human diseases (e.g., diabetes, cancer, arthritis, ulcers), it is still being used to predict earthquakes, in the study of atmospheric transport, and in exploration for petroleum and uranium.

4.3.2. Group II: Specific Chemical/Biological Families

This group consists of one biological and five chemical families. Entities in this group include: asbestos; nitrogen oxides (NO_x); persistent organochlorine compounds (POCs); polybrominated diphenyl ethers (PBDEs); sulfur oxides (SO_x); and the one family of biological organisms termed *fungi* (or known loosely as molds to most people).

A. Asbestos (Chapter 20)

This is a name given to a family of six naturally occurring fibrous silicate minerals in two kinds: the one in serpentine named chrysotile; and the five in amphibole named actinolite, amosite, anthophyllite, crocidolite, and tremolite. Collectively these minerals are used in a variety of building materials for acoustic and thermal insulation and as a fire retardant. Higher incidences of lung cancer and mesotheliomas have been linked to occupational exposure to asbestos (e.g., to those entering the air and water from the breakdown of manufactured goods), especially when in combination with cigarette smoking.

B. Molds (Chapter 17)

These microbes are the dominate group of fungi that are found indoors and outdoors in many places. Common fungal genera include *Alternaria, Aspergillus, Cladosporium,* and *Penicillium.* Certain exposed individuals with chronic pulmonary illnesses (e.g., obstructive lung disease) could develop mold infections in their lungs. These microbes may trigger asthma attacks. Areas causing high mold exposures are typically moist or damp surfaces, such as in antique shops, farms, saunas, greenhouses, mills, and constructions.

C. Nitrogen Oxides (NO$_x$; Chapter 11)

This is the generic term given to a family of highly reactive gases containing the nitrogen (N) and a varying number x of oxygen (O) atoms. The common anthropogenic sources of NO$_x$ include automobile exhausts, electric utilities, and facilities that burn fuels. Nitrogen oxides and sulfur dioxide (SO$_2$) are known to react with certain atmospheric substances to form acids which fall onto the ground as acid rain, fog, snow, or dry particles. Acid rain has harmful effects on aquatic animals, plants, and infrastructures (Section 5.2.3.C). Nitrogen dioxide (NO$_2$) and nitric oxide (NO) are the two principal members of NO$_x$. The health effects of nitrogen dioxide include: eye, nose, and throat irritation; impaired lung function; and increased respiratory infections in young children.

D. Persistent Organochlorine Compounds (POCs; Chapter 16)

These are hydrocarbon (hence *organic*) compounds that each have substituted one or more of their hydrogen (H) atoms for chlorines (Cl). As the carbon-chlorine (C-Cl) bond is highly stable, organochlorines (OCs) are by structure highly persistent in the environment. The two most prominent POC families *not* used as pesticides are discussed below.

Dioxins. This is the general name given to two classes of highly toxic and environmentally persistent OCs with chemical structures very similar to one another: polychlorinated dibenzo-*p(ara)*-dioxins (PCDDs); and polychlorinated dibenzofurans (PCDFs). Of the some 200 dioxin congeners (i.e., members), 2,3,7,8-TCDD is the most potent and hence uniquely referred to as *the dioxin.* Most, if not all, dioxin congeners are not intentionally produced but are by-products from industrial or chemical processes such as the chlorine bleaching process at pulp mills and the chlorination by waste or drinking water treatment plants. Many of these compounds are hormone disruptors (Chapter 19). Their acceptable levels in human fat are typically set at the range of parts per *trillion* (ppt).

Polychlorinated Biphenyls (PCBs). These are some 130 congeners (i.e., structurally similar chemicals) that were once manufactured in the United States for a variety of industrial and commercial applications, such as coolants and insulating fluids for electronic transformers and capacitors. (As explained in Table 16.2, up to 209 congeners of PCBs are *theoretically* possible for the PCB family.) As with PCDDs and PCDFs, the most commonly observed health effects of these PCB congeners in humans are skin conditions such as (chlor)acne and rashes. Studies in exposed workers showed changes in blood and urine that might lead to liver damage. Several other occupational studies also implicated that PCBs could cause cancer of the liver in humans.

E. Polybrominated Diphenyl Ethers (PBDEs; Chapter 16)

These congeners are part of the brominated flame retardant family. Many are components of flame retardants used in furniture foam (e.g., *penta*BDE congeners), plastics for TV cabinets (*deca*BDE congeners), and plastics for small appliances and computers (*octa*BDE congeners). Many PBDE congeners are highly persistent, bioaccumulative, and toxic to humans, with an array of adverse health effects including thyroid hormone disruption, fetal malformations, delayed puberty onset, and permanent learning impairment.

F. Sulfur Oxides (SO$_x$; Chapter 11)

Inhaled sulfur dioxide (SO$_2$), which is the principal member of sulfur oxides, readily reacts with the moisture of mucous membranes (e.g., in the respiratory tract) to form the more severe irritant sulfurous acid (H$_2$SO$_3$). Sulfur dioxide is produced from the burning of fossil fuels and the smelting of mineral ores that contain sulfur (S). Erupting volcanoes is a significant natural source of sulfur dioxide emissions. When sulfur dioxide combines with water (e.g., with atmospheric water vapor), it forms sulfuric acid (H$_2$SO$_4$) which is the principal component of acid rain that can seriously irritate the respiratory tract as well as the eyes and can cause serious damage to plants, aquatic animals, and infrastructures.

4.3.3. Group III: per Use/Source or Toxic Effect

Thirteen entities are included in this group. Each entity is a collection of toxicants or toxins grouped together because they are recognized by the general public as having similar use (household chemicals, pesticides), similar toxic effect (asthma triggers, environmental endocrine disruptors, free radicals), or similar exposure source (diesel fuel, drinking water contaminants, food contaminants and additives, particulate matter, plant toxicants, radioactive wastes, terrestrial venoms and poisons, volatile organic compounds).

A. Asthma Triggers

Asthma attack can be a fatal or very serious respiratory illness. The agents that can trigger this attack are usually allergenic in nature, including cockroaches, molds, paints, dust mites, secondhand smoke, warm-blooded pets, perfumes, and many more.

B. Diesel Fuel (Chapter 12)

In many cities, the exhausts from this type of fuel can take on a significant toll of the urban particulate load, insomuch as diesel fuel is currently used widely to power delivery trucks, farm rigs, boats, and the kind. The exhaust particulates from such engines burning diesel fuel are usually of nano size. These particulates are a complex mixture containing over 40 toxic pollutants including benzene, arsenic, nitrogen oxides, and formaldehyde.

C. Drinking Water Contaminants

Drinking water, including bottled water, almost always contains at least some small amounts of contaminants. U.S. EPA has set standards for approximately 90 contaminants in drinking water. In addition to the fuel additive methyl *tert(iary)*-butyl ether (MTBE) being a single chemical entity, the major subfamilies of water contaminants on U.S. EPA's list currently include: microbes (e.g., *E. coli*); radionuclides (e.g., radium^{226}, radon); organic chemicals (e.g., dioxins, PCBs, pesticides, benzene); inorganics (e.g., Pb, Cr, As); disinfectants (e.g., chlorine); and disinfection by-products (e.g., chlorite).

D. Environmental Endocrine Disruptors (Chapter 19)

These disruptors are generally defined as exogenous substances that may interfere with the synthesis, secretion, metabolism, distribution, elimination, and normal function of natural hormones in the body, leading to adverse developmental, reproductive, neurological, immunological, or carcinogenic effects in humans and wildlife. They include a large number of pesticides, toxic metals, industrial chemical pollutants, foods, fluoride, cosmetics, toys, and more. As specifically defined in Chapter 19, hormones are chemical messengers that a body uses to regulate or influence its many crucial day-to-day functions including those pertaining to its development, reproduction, and behavior.

E. Food Contaminants and Additives (Chapter 21)

Contaminants in foods are substances inadvertently placed in cooked, processed, or raw foods. These substances include: bacterial toxins (e.g., exotoxin of *Clostridium botulinum*); mycotoxins (e.g., aflatoxins from *Aspergillus flavus*); animal toxins; pesticide residues; animal drug residues (e.g., diethylstilbestrol, antibiotics); plant alkaloids; and a variety of industrial chemicals (e.g., PBDEs, PCBs). Substances (mostly antimicrobials and antioxidants) that are *purposely* added to foods as preservatives are termed *direct additives* (e.g., butylated hydroxyanisole [BHA], butylated hydroxytoluene [BHT]). Food additives can also be used to change the physical characteristics for processing, or to change the taste or odor (e.g., nitrate). Due to the recent concerns by some sectors, the adverse health effects of many of these additives are subjected to further investigation.

F. Free Radicals (Chapters 2, 8, and 9)

As noted in Chapter 2 and further discussed in Chapters 8 and 9, these are strong oxidants that can damage other molecules nearby and the cell structures. Some free radicals will react with lipoproteins in the blood to form plaque-like fatty deposits which can end up clogging blood vessels to block off blood supply to the heart, leading to cardiac attacks. Those derived from the atom oxygen, and thus referred to as reactive oxygen species (ROS) or oxygen free radicals, are thought to also play a key role in carcinogenesis.

G. Household Chemicals (Chapter 21)

In the 1980s, the U.S. National Institute for Occupational Safety and Health (NIOSH) analyzed 2,983 chemicals contained in personal care products and found 884 of them (30%) toxic (e.g., Berns, 1989; Miller, 1990; Douillard, 2003). A five-year report by U.S. EPA (1989) also concluded that the toxic substances in household cleaners were three times more likely to cause cancer than outdoor air pollution. Moreover, according to the U.S. Consumer Product Safety Commission (CPSC, 2009), more than 90% of suspected poison exposures that occurred at homes generally involved the use of household products. CPSC (2009) estimated that each year, some 80,000 American children visited hospital emergency rooms due to unintentional poisonings, of which many involved exposures to products commonly found in the home.

H. Particulate Matter (Chapter 12)

This matter is also known as particle or particulate pollution which is a complex mixture of extremely small solid particles and liquid droplets. Particulate matter is made up of hundreds to thousands of tiny components, including acids (e.g., nitrates and sulfates), metals (e.g., Pb, Cd), organic chemicals, and soil or dust particles. This type of particulates has been linked to a range of serious respiratory and cardiovascular disorders. As a single entity, it is one of the six designated criteria air pollutants in the United States.

I. Pesticides (Chapter 15)

Most of the pesticides available today are compounds that are specifically synthesized for use to prevent, destroy, repel, or mitigate one or more types of agricultural and public health pests which include insects, rodents, weeds, fungi, bacteria, and viruses. Oftentimes, pesticides that are used specifically on insects are referred to as insecticides; those used specifically on rodents (and some other nuisance animals) are referred to as rodenticides; those used on weeds are referred to as herbicides; and so forth. Many of these chemicals are acutely highly toxic, carcinogenic, or capable of disrupting the endocrine system. Pesticides of the organochlorine group (e.g., DDT, aldrin, dieldrin, chlordane, lindane, toxaphene, mirex) are particularly persistent in the environment; and many are members of POPs (persistent organic pollutants), of which many are POCs (persistent organochlorine compounds). Some naturally occurring compounds such as certain metals (e.g., As, Cu, Hg) and certain plant extracts (e.g., pyrethrum, citronella, rotenone) have been used as pesticides.

J. Plant Toxicants (Chapter 17)

These include many types of chemical substances, such as sulfur compounds, alkaloids, cardiac glycosides, phenols, lipids, and some of the drugs of abuse (e.g., nicotine, cocaine, morphine). These toxicants collectively can cause a wide array of health effects including allergic or contact dermatitis, gastrointestinal disturbance, cardiac arrhythmias, hepatocyte (i.e., liver cell) damage, kidney tubular degeneration, seizures, soft tissue calcification, birth defects, abortion, and more.

K. Radioactive Wastes (Chapters 14 and 22)

Toxic wastes in this group are generated by processes that produce or use radioactive materials, such as those used for or in national defense, scientific research, nuclear power generation, medicine, and industrial applications. These radioactive wastes can be in a gas, liquid, or solid form. The radioactivity in these waste products can remain for a few days (e.g., the radioactive isotope iodine-135) or for as long as thousands of years (e.g., spent or used nuclear fuel). The adverse effects of radiation can be mild (e.g., reddening of the skin) or with severe consequence (e.g., cancer or early death).

L. Terrestrial Animal Venoms/Poisons (Chapter 17)

These are mostly protein-like toxins produced by animals specifically for the poisoning of other species through a mechanism designed to deliver the toxin to their prey. Examples of this kind include the venoms of bees and wasps (delivered by a sting) and the venoms of snakes (delivered by fangs).

M. Volatile Organic Compounds (VOCs; Chapter 13)

These compounds are readily emitted as gases from thousands of volatile solid and liquid chemicals: paints; lacquers; paint strippers; cleaning supplies; household products; cosmetics; pesticides; and many more. Collectively, they can cause a wide array of health effects: irritation of the skin, eyes, nose, throat, and/or lungs; nausea; loss of coordination; headaches; and damage to the liver, kidney, and/or central nervous system. Some VOCs are found to cause cancer in animals, whereas some others are known (e.g., benzene) to cause cancer in humans.

References

Adolfsson-Erici M, Pettersson M, Parkkonen J, Sturve J, 2002. Triclosan, A Commonly Used Bactericide Found in Human Milk and in the Aquatic Environment in Sweden. *Chemosphere* 46: 1485-1489.

Aiello AE, Larson EL, Levy SB, 2007. Consumer Antibacterial Soaps: Effective or Just Risky? *Clin. Infect. Dis.* 45:S137-S147.

Allsopp M, Walters A, Santillo D, Johnston P, 2006. *Plastic Debris in the World's Oceans.* Greenpeace International, Ottho Heldringstraat 5, 1066 AZ Amsterdam, The Netherlands.

ATSDR (U.S. Agency for Toxic Substances and Disease Registry), 2008. ATSDR Glossary of Terms. http://www.atsdr.cdc.gov/glossary.html.

Berns J, 1989. The Cosmetic Cover-up. *The Human Ecologist*, 43 (Fall Issue).

Brooks BW, Chambliss CK, Stanley JK, Ramirez A, Banks KE, Johnson RD, Lewis RJ, 2005. Determination of Select Antidepressants in Fish from an Effluent-Dominated Stream. *Environ. Toxicol. Chem.* 24:464-469.

Burros M, 2008. National Study Finds High Levels of Mercury in Tuna. *The New York Times*, 24 January.

Cone M, 2006. Threat Seen from Antibacterial Soap Chemicals: The Compounds End Up in Sewage Sludge That Is Spread on Farm Fields Across the Country. *Los Angeles Times*, 10 May.

CPSC (U.S. Consumer Product Safety Commission), 2009. *CPSC Warns That 9 Out of 10 Unintentional Child Poisonings Occur in the Home.* Release #09159 (dated 18 March). Washington DC, USA.

Douillard J, 2003. *Perfect Health for Kids: Ten Ayurvedic Health Secrets Every Parent Must Know.* Berkeley, California, USA: North Atlantic Books.

FNB (Food and Nutrition Board), 2005. *Dietary Reference Intakes for Energy, Carbohydrate, Fiber, Fat, Fatty Acids, Cholesterol, Protein, and Amino Acids (Macronutrients).* Washington DC, USA: The National Academies Press.

Galgani F, Jaunet S, Campillo A, Guenegen X, His E, 1995. Distribution and Abundance of Debris on the Continental Shelf of the North-Western Mediterranean. *Marine Poll. Bull.* 30:713-717.

Glaser A, 2004. The Ubiquitous Triclosan, a Common Antibacterial Agent Exposed. *Pesticides and You* 24(3):12-17.

Goodyear C, 2007. SF Supes Vote to Ban Plastic Bags in Stores, March 27. *San Francisco Chronicle*, 27 March.

Hartman B, 2007. Thomas & Friends Wooden Railway Toys Recalled: Chinese Manufacturer Used Lead Paint on 1.5 Million Toys, as Nation's Recall Rate Troubles Safety Experts. *ABC News*, 13 June.

Hodgson E, Mailman RB, Chambers JE (Eds.), 1998. *Dictionary of Toxicology.* New York, New York, USA: Grove's Dictionaries Inc.

McGreevy P, 2008. State Bans Trans Fats: Restaurants in California Must Stop Cooking with the Substances, Except in Tiny Amounts, by 2010. *Los Angeles Times*, 28 July.

Miller, GT, 1990. *Living in the Environment: An Introduction to Environmental Science.* Belmont, California, USA: Wadsworth Publishing.

MSNBC.com (MSNBC.com News Services), 2009. 2 Face Execution Over China Poison Milk Scandal: Relatives Express Outrage after Tainted Product Killed 6 Kids, Left 300,000 Ill. Updated 22 January.

Palace VP, Wautier KG, Evans RE, Blanchfield PJ, Mills KH, Chalanchuk SM, Godard D, McMaster ME, Tetreault GR, Peters LE, Vandenbyllaardt L, Kidd KA, 2006. Biochemical and Histopathological Effects in Pearl Dace (*Margariscus margarita*) Chronically Exposed to a Synthetic Estrogen in a Whole Lake Experiment. *Environ. Toxicol. Chem.* 25:1114-1125.

Puckett J, Byster L, Westervelt S, Gutierrez R, Davis S, Hussain A, Dutta M, 2002. *Exporting Harms: The High-Tech Trashing of Asia.* The Basel Action Network, c/o Asia Pacific Environmental Exchange, 1305 Fourth Avenue, Suite 606, Seattle, Washington, USA.

Schultz IR, Skillman A, Nicolas J-M, Cyr DG, Nagler JJ, 2003. Short-Term Exposure to 17α-Ethynylestradiol Decreases the Fertility of Sexually Maturing Male Rainbow Trout (*Oncorhynchus mykiss*). *Environ. Toxicol. Chem.* 22:1272-1280.

Thiel M, Hinojosa I, Vásquez N, Macaya E, 2003. Floating Marine Debris in Coastal Waters of the SE-Pacific (Chile). *Marine Poll. Bull.* 46:224-231.

UNEP (United Nations Environment Programme), 2005. *E-Waste, the Hidden Side of IT Equipment's Manufacturing and Use: Environmental Alert Bulletin No. 5.* UNEP, P.O. Box 30552, Nairobi, Kenya.

U.S. EPA (U.S. Environmental Protection Agency), 1989. Report to Congress on Indoor Air Quality, Volume II: Assessment and Control of Indoor Air Pollution. EPA 400-1-89-001C. Office of Air and Radiation, Washington DC, USA.

U.S. EPA (U.S. Environmental Protection Agency), 2008a. Search Potential Environmental Hazards. http://yosemite.epa.gov/ochp/ochpweb.nsf/frmchemicals.

U.S. EPA (U.S. Environmental Protection Agency), 2008b. Amendment to the Universal Waste Rule: Addition of Pharmaceuticals. *Federal Register* 73:73520-73544.

USGS (U.S. Geological Survey), 2002. Pharmaceuticals, Hormones, and Other Organic Wastewater Contaminants in U.S. Streams. Fact Sheet FS-027-02. Toxic Substances Hydrology Program, Reston, Virginia, USA.

WGFSM (Work Group for Safe Markets), 2008. Baby's Toxic Bottle: Bisphenol A Leaching from Popular Baby Bottles. WGFSM-Clean Water Fund, 262 Washington Street, No. 301, Boston, Massachusetts, USA.

Review Questions

1. Name an antibacterial ingredient used in hundreds of consumer products (e.g., soaps, shampoos, toothpastes, cosmetics) every day in the United States. And briefly describe its potential adverse health effects to humans.

2. Name one type of debris from entanglement and ingestion of which hundreds of thousands of marine creatures die each year.

3. Name the endocrine-disrupting chemical that was shown in a 2008 report to leach out of popular brands of baby bottles sold in Canada and the United States.

4. What was U.S. EPA's regulatory intent to add pharmaceutical wastes to the federal Universal Waste Rule?

5. How does cyanuric acid affect melamine's toxicity in dogs, cats, and humans?

6. How do trans fats biochemically increase the risk of coronary heart disease?

7. Briefly describe three ways in which environmental toxicants may be grouped or classified.

8. Name five environmental agents that may trigger an asthma attack.

9. Which gas is commonly nicknamed the silent killer?

10. Briefly describe the characteristics of free radicals and their biochemical actions in the human body.

11. What is airborne particulate matter?

12. Name three classes of chemicals that are often referred to as POCs (persistent organochlorine compounds).

13. What are some of the adverse health effects that plant toxicants can cause?

14. Which chemical family is commonly used as flame retardants in furniture foam and in plastics for TV cabinets?

15. How is radon formed, and what is (are) its major adverse health effect(s)?

16. What are VOCs? And what are some of the adverse health effects that they can induce?

CHAPTER 5

Fate and Transport of Toxicants in the Environment

5.1. Introduction

Exposures of humans and other organisms to environmental toxicants are regarded by most scholastic and regulatory entities as highly preventable and mitigable, a point also made explicitly in Chapters 2 and 3. This notion is supported by the argument that there is sufficient knowledge on how toxicants generally move and behave in the environment. In general, when a toxicant is released into the environment, it may move from the point of source into different environmental media (e.g., air, water, soil, sediment, foods, living organisms) at various locations. The toxicant may move as the original, parent compound or as different degradates (i.e., breakdown products). More specifically, the contaminants or their degradates may move within or across various environmental media and undergo biological (biotic) or chemical (abiotic) transformation. These numerous various transport and transformation processes are the subject matters of this chapter.

Of note here is that apparently there has been a lack of general consensus on some of the terms used in describing the behavior and movement of toxicants in the environment. For instance, the word *dispersion* usually means the spread, diffusion, or distribution of materials. Yet in air pollution modeling, it is a technical term referring to specifically the process of spreading out pollution emission over a large area resulting in a lower concentration in the emission source. Regardless of how some of the terms may be used differently in different fields, there are fundamentals about the behavior and movement of materials in the environment that are not subject to much dispute among scholars.

5.1.1. Movement in the Environmental Media

For the most part, a toxicant in the atmosphere or water may move from one location to another by the two common transport processes termed *advection* and *diffusion*. Advection refers to the process in which a substance in the environment is moved *horizontally* by the mass motion of the medium (e.g., mostly air or water). Therefore, unsurprisingly, the variables that have strong impacts on atmospheric or oceanic advection include predominately the strength and direction of the wind in effect or the characteristics of the eddies in place. Diffusion on the other hand refers to the *spontaneous* movement of a substance from an area of high concentration to one of low concentration. The two transport processes can occur at the same time. There have been rather sophisticated advection-diffusion equations developed to simulate the concurrent occurrence of these two processes (e.g., Buske *et al.*, 2007; Lee *et al.*, 2007).

Animal migration, or the so-termed *biotransport* process, is also known to be capable of transporting environmental toxicants to a different location far away (Chapter 6). Surface runoff, leaching, and volatilization are the more prominent phase-transfer processes responsible for transporting soil contaminants from one location to another.

5.1.2. Distribution into the Living Organisms

Pollutants moving in the environment enter terrestrial (or aquatic) plants largely via one of two processes. They can be deposited onto foliage via air (or water) movement, or be taken up by roots in contaminated soil. Following uptake by plants, a toxicant can be distributed into the various organs and tissues in these non-mobile organisms.

In humans and other mammalians, the main portals of entry for environmental toxicants are skin, eyes, lungs, and gastrointestinal tract. Upon absorption, these toxicants may be bound to proteins in the blood. Their rapid transport via the bloodstream or the lymphatic system then follows (Chapter 7). Certain chemicals (particularly those that are persistent in the environment) may undergo bioconcentration and bioaccumulation upon contact with the body of a biological system. These two biotransfer phenomena, along with biomagnification in a food web, are the topics discussed extensively in Chapter 6.

ex?

5.2. Fate and Transport of Air Pollutants

Air pollutants are toxic substances (e.g., chemicals, particulate matter, biological materials) that are introduced into the atmosphere where they can be in the form of solid particles, liquid droplets, or gases. They may be emitted directly from a natural source such as the ashes from volcanic eruptions, or from an anthropogenic source such as nitrogen dioxide (NO_2) from automobile exhausts or sulfur dioxide (SO_2) discharged from factories. Many air pollutants are not emitted directly, however. Instead, they are formed in the atmosphere when other primary pollutants react or interact and thereby are termed *secondary* (i.e., second-generation) pollutants. An example of important secondary air pollutants is ozone (O_3) formed in the troposphere (i.e., the air layer closest to the Earth). This type of ozone is one of the secondary air pollutants that make up photochemical smog. Smog is fog that has become polluted with smoke. In photochemical smog, the smoke usually comes from such air pollution as motor vehicle exhausts which usually contain high contents of NO_2 and nitric oxide (NO). Not surprisingly, some air pollutants may occur with one portion coming from direct emission and the other portion coming from reactions or interactions of other primary pollutants. The general sources of air pollutants and their movement schemes are outlined graphically in Figure 5.1.

5.2.1. Local and Long-Range Transport

Many air pollutants, owing to their physicochemical properties, tend to travel short distances within a confined area especially where meteorological conditions are not as conducive. Yet even for a short distance, the travel could still mean hundreds of miles away, particularly if they travel with the aid of strong wind. In some cases, these air pollutants are so vulnerable to chemical or physical transformation (Section 5.2.3) that they will not be in the air for long. For example, even though elemental mercury (Hg^0) emitted from coal-fired utilities can be transported in the atmosphere for long distances (e.g., thousands of miles), it can be oxidized quickly to divalent mercury (Hg^{2+}). The divalent form of Hg in the gas phase is then removed from the atmosphere within a short distance from the emission source. In general, air pollutants can be removed from the atmosphere by falling onto the ground in precipitation or dust, or simply due to gravity. This type of removal of atmospheric substances is termed *air (atmospheric) deposition*.

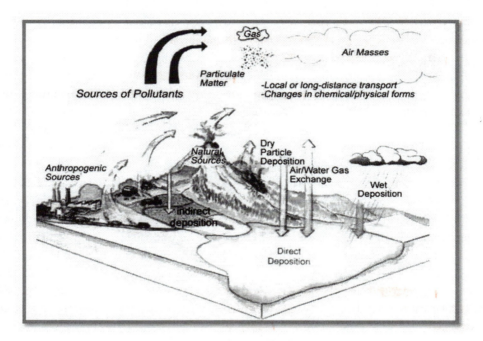

Figure 5.1. A Schematic of the Fate and Transport of Air Pollutants
(from public domain source: U.S. EPA, 2001)

Some pollutants from air deposition do not remain deposited on soil or in water for long. These are usually the persistent kind, such as PCBs, dioxins, organochlorine pesticides, and certain forms of mercury. Due to their chemical stability along with a set of conducive meteorological variables, these substances can be *re-emitted* from contaminated soil or water. This then can lead to a pattern known as *the grasshopper effect*, whereby a pollutant is emitted from an original source, transported for some short distance, deposited, and followed by a portion of the deposited residues being re-emitted, being re-transported further, and being re-deposited. The pattern may be repeated almost indefinitely until the pollutant residues reach high elevations or northern climates where cold condensation can and will take effect to retard their hopping (e.g., U.S. EPA, 2001).

5.2.2. Direct and Indirect Deposition

Pollutants from the atmosphere can reach a water body in one of two modes. They can be deposited directly onto water surface (i.e., direct deposition) or onto land and later be carried away to water bodies through runoff (i.e., indirect deposition). Once these pollutant residues are deposited in the water, they can pose certain undesirable health and environmental threats, such as contaminated seafood and unsafe drinking water.

Direct atmospheric deposition can be divided into two subprocesses: *dry* and *wet* deposition. Dry deposition can be caused by or due to one of several common phenomena in the absence of precipitation. For instance, airborne particles can fall down simply by gravitation or be transported to a surface by another physical force such as random air turbulent motions. A familiar physical phenomenon for this type of deposition is when particles flow too close to a branch of a tree, such as by advection, they may collide and thus be intercepted. Dry deposition is affected by a multiplicity of factors that usually interact in complex ways. The most important variables are the characteristics of the atmosphere (e.g., temperature, wind speed), the nature of the landing surface (e.g., porosity, pH, aerodynamic roughness), and properties of the depositing species (e.g., diameter, shape, surface charge). Transport of gases through the atmosphere depends on turbulent and molecular diffusion. The chemical's solubility and reactivity are additional factors that can affect the capture of gases by the landing surface.

Wet deposition occurs when any form of precipitation (e.g., rain, snow, sleet, cloud, fog) removes the atmospheric particles and delivers them to the Earth's surface. Precipitation occurs when the atmosphere, which basically is a huge volume of gaseous solution, becomes saturated with water vapor to the point that the water molecules condense, causing them to precipitate out of this huge tank of gaseous solution and down to the Earth's surface. The water vapor that precipitates out may contain the air pollutant particles. A well-known example is acid rain which is caused by the emissions of mostly sulfur, nitrogen, or carbon compounds that can react with water molecules in the atmosphere to produce acids. The more accurate term for acid rain is thus *acid deposition*.

5.2.3. Changes in Chemical/Physical Form

Depending on its physicochemical properties, an air pollutant may be subject to one or more chemical or physical transformations in the atmosphere. Those crucial reactions or phenomena involving the more prominent air pollutants are highlighted below.

A. Absorption and Release of Solar Radiation

There are gases such as water vapor (H_2O) and carbon dioxide (CO_2) in the atmosphere with their atoms being held together loosely enough that they wobble when they absorb heat from the sun. Eventually, the trembling molecules release the absorbed heat in the form of radiant energy which is likely to be absorbed by nearby molecules with similar structural vulnerabilities. This process, which traps heat to near the Earth's surface, leads to the *greenhouse effect* in the same sense that a greenhouse works by keeping heat from the sun. The gaseous molecules responsible for the trapping effect are naturally termed *greenhouse gases*. Without these gases, heat would escape back into space above the troposphere; and the Earth's average temperature would then be below the habitable level. In addition to water vapor and carbon dioxide, the major greenhouse gases are methane (CH_4), nitrous oxide (N_2O), ozone, and chlorofluorocarbons (CFCs). The principal uses of CFCs are as refrigerants (e.g., freons) in refrigeration units and as propellants in air conditioners, at least in the recent past. Although CFCs in the atmosphere can induce greenhouse effect, they have been found to cause serious depletion of the Earth's ozone shield. It has been said that too much greenhouse effect can lead to global warming.

B. Photochemical Reaction

Photolysis (a.k.a. photodissociation or photodecomposition) is a photochemical reaction occurring frequently in the atmosphere. It is a photoreaction whereby a chemical compound is broken down by a photon (*hv*), which is an elementary particle as well as the basic unit of all forms of electromagnetic radiation including light. Two of the most important photolysis reactions in the troposphere are:

$$O_3 + hv \rightarrow O_2 + O^\bullet \tag{5.1}$$

$$NO_2 + hv \rightarrow NO + O^\bullet \tag{5.2}$$

In Reaction 5.1, the excited oxygen atom ($O^\bullet$) may react with H_2O vapor to produce the hydroxyl radical ($HO^\bullet$). This radical is central to atmospheric chemistry in that it acts as an atmospheric detergent to cleanse many hydrocarbon (HC) pollutants by initiating their oxidation in the atmosphere. The oxygen atom produced from Reaction 5.2 (or even from Reaction 5.1), on the other hand, can react with oxygen molecules (O_2) to form O_3; and the other co-product nitric oxide (NO) from Reaction 5.2 can remove O_3 by reacting with the latter to form NO_2 and O_2. These three subsequent or secondary reactions are shown below as Reactions 5.3 through 5.5, respectively:

$$O^\bullet + H_2O \rightarrow O_2 + HO^\bullet \tag{5.3}$$

$$O^\bullet + O_2 \rightarrow O_3 \tag{5.4}$$

$$NO + O_3 \rightarrow NO_2 + O_2 \tag{5.5}$$

In the presence of sunlight, NO_2 can react with O_2 and some HCs, but more notably as well as more commonly with O_2 and acetaldehyde (CH_3CHO) to produce *peroxyacetyl-nitrate* (PAN; $CH_3CO\text{-}OO\text{-}NO_2$) by first yielding the radical $CH_3CO\text{-}OO^\bullet$:

$$NO_2 + O_2 + CH_3CHO + hv \rightarrow CH_3CO\text{-}OO\text{-}NO_2 \tag{5.6}$$

Nitrogen dioxide, nitric oxide, ozone, and PAN are considered as the principal substances in photochemical smog. Both ozone and PAN in this type of pollution are secondary (i.e., second-generation), harmful pollutants which can cause breathing difficulties, eye and nose irritation, fatigue, headaches, and can aggravate respiratory problems.

C. Formation of Acid Rain

In addition to being one of the major ingredients in photochemical smog, atmospheric NO_2 can produce nitric acid (HNO_3) when it is oxidized by the hydroxyl radical ($HO^{\bullet}$) which is easily available (e.g., Reaction 5.3). HNO_3, as produced from NO_2 in Reaction 5.7 below, is one of the acidic components frequently found in acid rain.

$$NO_2 + HO^{\bullet} \rightarrow HNO_3 \tag{5.7}$$

Another acidic component even more commonly found in acid deposition is sulfuric acid (H_2SO_4). The common route of sulfuric acid formation, as shown in Reactions 5.8 through 5.10, involves the primary ingredient SO_2 and the intermediate ingredients $HO^{\bullet}$, bisulfite radical ($HOSO_2^{\bullet}$), and sulfur trioxide (SO_3).

$$SO_2 + HO^{\bullet} \rightarrow HOSO_2^{\bullet} \tag{5.8}$$

$$HOSO_2^{\bullet} + O_2 \rightarrow SO_3 + HO_2^{\bullet} \text{ (perhydroxyl radical)} \tag{5.9}$$

$$SO_3 + H_2O \rightarrow H_2SO_4 \tag{5.10}$$

When the precipitation that falls onto the Earth's surface is acidic, it has harmful effects on plants, aquatic animals, and infrastructures. When reacting with H_2O vapor molecules in the atmosphere, CO_2 (carbon dioxide) too can produce an acidic component of acid rain. This acidic component is carbonic acid (H_2CO_3), which is considerably less acidic than H_2SO_4 or HNO_3.

D. Lightning and Photosynthesis

Motor vehicle exhaust is not the only source of atmospheric NO and NO_2. These nitrogenous oxides can be formed when atmospheric N_2 reacts with atmospheric O_2 in the presence of high temperatures and pressures polarized by lightning strikes. It is the enormous and powerful electric current of lightning that can break N_2 into N atoms which can then react with O_2 to form NO_2 in the air (of which ~80% is N_2 gas).

Carbon dioxide can lower its atmospheric level when pulled for use by plants nearby. Through photosynthesis (Reaction 5.11), plants can use sunlight to convert the captured atmospheric CO_2 into the sugar *carbohydrate* ($C_6H_{12}O_6$) molecules to sustain their life.

$$6CO_2 + 6H_2O + \text{sunlight } (hv) \rightarrow C_6H_{12}O_6 + 6O_2 \tag{5.11}$$

5.3. Fate and Transport of Water Contaminants

For organic and inorganic compounds, separate discussions on their general physico-chemical behaviors in water can be found in the chapter by Lyman (1995). Those discussions provide the foundation for much of the overview given in this section. A modified version of Lyman's discussion on organic compounds is outlined graphically below in Figure 5.2, only now with a focus on POCs (persistent organochlorine compounds). Here the focus on POCs is more by preference, as some other organic compounds (e.g., those also included in Chapter 16) and some inorganics (e.g., arsenic, cadmium, mercury) are equally persistent in the aquatic environment as well as highly toxic to human health. The main reason for the POC preference is that although much of what follows applies to these other chemicals as well, certain physicochemical properties discussed below (e.g., lipophilicity) are more unique to or better known for POCs.

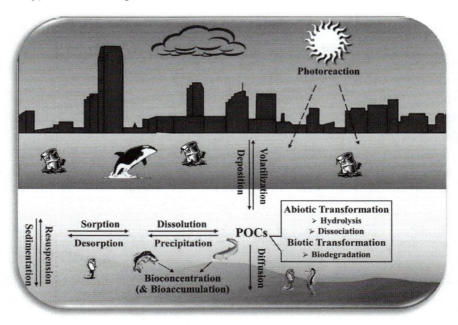

Figure 5.2. A Schematic of the Fate and Transport of Water Pollutants
(POCs = persistent organochlorine compounds)

In most instances, whenever a chemical manages to get onto or into a water body, initially it will undergo one or more transport or physicochemical phase-transfer processes. For POCs as a group, *dissolution*, *volatilization*, and *(ad)sorption* appear to be the better-known processes for phase-transfer, whereas *sedimentation* and *diffusion* are the more common processes for transport. Within an aquatic system, POCs can likewise be transformed into a different chemical form or species via one or more of the common abiotic or biotic processes. These transformation processes include, but are not limited to: *dissociation*, *hydrolysis*, *oxidation*, *photolysis*, and *biodegradation*. Each of these transport, phase-transfer, and transformation processes is strongly governed or influenced by both the substance's physicochemical properties and the properties as well as the conditions of the aquatic system in which the chemical is present. The properties considered important to the fate and transport of POCs in aquatic systems are listed below in Table 5.1.

Table 5.1. Physicochemical and Water Properties Relevant to the Fate and Transport of Persistent Organochlorine Compounds in the Aquatic Environment[a]

Physicochemical Variable	Environmental Variable(s)
Molecular structure	Surface area and depth
Molecular weight	Flow; extent of mixing; bottom scouring
Water solubility	Sedimentation rate
Vapor pressure	Solar irradiation; presence of sensitizer
Henry's law constant (air-water partition)	Population and activity of microbes
Octanol-water partition coefficient (K_{ow})	Concentrations of nutrients and minerals
Light absorption spectrum	Temperature; pH
Quantum yield	Nature of suspended particles
Diffusion coefficient	Concentration of suspended particles
Sorption constant for sediments (K_{oc})	Hardness; salinity; ionic strength
Bioconcentration factor	Level of dissolved organic matter
Biodegradation constant	Nature of bottom sediments

[a] *see*, e.g., Lyman (1995) for further reading, which is also the primary source for this table.

5.3.1. Phase-Transfer and Transport Processes

For POCs in water, one of the key phase-transfer processes is *dissolution*, which involves a solute (e.g., a POC) getting dissolved in a solvent (e.g., water). POCs are extremely hydro*phobic* (i.e., lipo*philic*). Therefore, dissolution is most relevant to POCs in water only when bulk quantities of these organic compounds are discharged into the water, such as from a chemical spill or an improper waste disposal.

POCs are nonetheless not totally insoluble in water. In spite of the fact that the water solubility of most any POC is extremely low, thus making the chemical to behave rather hydrophobically, the total quantity of this chemical that is eventually dissolved in the water could still be tremendous. This is because in many aquatic systems, water is present in a huge volume compared to the POC content in the same volume, thus making the ratio of (local) water to chemical volume abnormally high (which in turn offers an aquatic system where a chemical with very low solubility can still be treated as highly soluble). Another reason is that in the presence of suspended particles acting like a sponge constantly taking up the dissolved POC (a reaction as well as a process called sorption), the organic compound's quantity in the water can easily exceed what would be expected from its water solubility. In addition, a POC's water solubility will be enhanced by decayed materials or dissolved organic carbon being present in the same water body.

In accordance with Lyman (1995), the actual rate of dissolution for any POC will depend on a number of factors including but not limited to:

- Ratio of the local water volume to POC volume.
- Degree of mixing in the water.
- Water's temperature (and in some cases its pH as well).
- Solubility of the POC in water.
- Presence of other organic materials affecting the POC's water solubility.

One easy and perhaps the most practical approach to estimating a POC's water solubility is through use of its *octanol-water* partition coefficient (K_{ow}) as the predictor. This coefficient is measured as the ratio of a chemical's concentration in octanol to its concentration in water at equilibrium and at a specified temperature, with the fatty alcohol octanol being used as a surrogate for fatty tissue and other natural organic matters.

Another crucial phase-transfer for certain POCs is *volatilization* (a.k.a. evaporation) whereby the chemical can be transported out of a water surface, across the air-water interface, and into the air directly above the aquatic system, all happening without breaking down the chemical into degradates. As to all other chemical groups, volatilization will be most relevant to POCs when the water body in which the organics are present is shallow and clear, and when there is sufficient air movement over the water surface. For this phase-transfer process, it is important for the POC to have a sufficiently high air-water partition coefficient commonly known as Henry's law constant. This constant can be estimated from the chemical's vapor pressure, molecular weight, and water solubility.

The third crucial phase-transfer process for POCs in water is *sorption*, known also as *adsorption*, a process involving the transfer of a chemical from the dissolved state to one in which the chemical is attached (i.e., sorbed) to a solid, such as to soil or in this case often to a sediment. In other words, once the POC is dissolved in an aqueous solution and is relatively nonvolatile, it can be (*ad*)sorbed to a sediment. The sediment can be treated as acting like a sponge or magnet constantly taking up and harboring the dissolved particles in the water.

The physicochemical basis for sorption of most chemicals, including POCs, can vary greatly depending on the chemical's properties and the nature of the adsorbent (e.g., the sediment). The general rule is that for low organic carbon sediments, physical adsorption dominates. If the adsorbent has high organic carbon, then chemical adsorption dominates. By chemical adsorption, it means that the binding or interaction responsible for sorption is of chemical nature, rather than physical.

For sediments or other adsorbents with high *o*rganic *c*arbon, a practical value used to describe the sorption potential of a chemical (e.g., POC) is its chemical-specific sorption constant K*oc*. This constant can be approximated with some accuracy through correlation with the chemical's K*ow* (e.g., Karickhoff, 1981; Winegardner, 1996).

Once the POC molecules are sorbed to solids suspended in the water column, they will be deposited onto the bottom of the water body when the suspended solids eventually settle onto the bottom, even simply by gravitation. This entire process is termed *sedimentation*. It is not uncommon for bottom sediments to move away horizontally (e.g., via advection) at some appreciable rates. On the other hand, a POC in its undissolved state may be diffused into a sediment directly under the influence of concentration gradient; that is, by moving from areas of high concentration to areas of low concentration. Although *diffusion* is a slow process for most POCs in water, it occurs continuously.

It is important to note that, in the three phase-transfer processes discussed above, the chemical movements are bidirectional or reversible. That is, for chemical dissolution in water there is *precipitation*, which results in a solute forming a solid phase composed of the solute itself after the chemical has exceeded its solubility limit. For volatilization from water, there is *atmospheric deposition*. And for chemical sorption to a sediment, there is *desorption*, which results in the release of the chemical from the sediment.

5.3.2. Chemical (Abiotic) Transformation

In many cases, a POC in water (or in any medium) is not only subject to transport or phase-transfer. It can be *transformed* into another chemical form or species when reacting with water or other materials in or around the aquatic system. For some POCs with low volatility when they are in clear water, sunlight *photolysis* may be a dominant degradation process. This type of transformation forms oxidation products that are more water-soluble while less volatile, typically resulting in reductive dechlorination through cleavage of the carbon-chlorine bond. The process is specific to the wavelength and the sensitizer factors present around the aquatic system. The final end results of photolysis often involve a variety of reactions of the secondary kind such as dissociation, isomerization, and photoionization (e.g., Lyman, 1995). The aqueous half-lives for photolysis of POCs are usually shortened when the process is induced with decayed materials in the aquatic system. This may explain why the potent persistent dioxin 2,3,7,8-TCDD at water surface reportedly had a very short half-life of 24 hours in the summer to about 5 days in the winter (Podoll *et al.*, 1986; ATSDR, 1998).

One insignificant abiotic transformation process for most POCs but not for the pesticide heptachlor is *hydrolysis*, which involves replacing a chlorine atom by the OH group from a water molecule. Moreover, if a POC acts as an acid or a base, it can undergo *dissociation*. Although this reaction does not apply much to most POCs, a few including the wood preservative pentachlorophenol (PCP) are highly susceptible to it.

5.3.3. Biological (Biotic) Transformation

As for most other chemical groups, the other type of transformation for POCs within an aquatic environment is *biotic*. This type of transformation is commonly referred to as microbiologically-induced degradation, or biodegradation for short. This process is induced largely by microbes with great physiological versatility in sediments that tend to provide a good habitat for benthic biota. More specifically and biochemically, biodegradation is a process of electron transfer (that moving an electron from one atom or molecule to another) catalyzed by microbial enzymes. Since many specific enzymes (a group of complex proteins whose general characteristics and functions are given in Chapter 8) are not released outside of microbial cells, water contaminants subject to biodegradation must be brought into these cells first. Oftentimes when a specific hydrocarbon compound cannot be (readily) utilized as a carbon or energy source by the indigenous microorganisms, it can still be degraded by similar or the same types of enzymes released by the microbes from metabolizing (breaking down) other coexisting compounds for energy. This type of biodegradation is termed *co-metabolism*.

Biodegradation is considered as one of the few crucial processes for many POCs in water, in spite of the fact that it involves a series of slowly occurring metabolic activities with half-lives typically in years. The process is usually slower for more complex structures such as dioxins and PCBs, than for relatively simpler structures such as certain OC (organochlorine) pesticides. This kind of structural effect is expected given that a more complex POC structure would involve the cleavage of more carbon-chlorine bonds (with the resultant carbon being used as an energy substrate for microbial growth).

Biodegradation of POCs may be induced in water under *aerobic* (i.e., oxygen-rich) or *anaerobic* (i.e., oxygen-depleted) conditions. In aerobic biodegradation, the microbes use oxygen as the ultimate electron acceptor in breaking down the organic chemical whereas in anaerobic biodegradation, they utilize electrophilic substrates such as sulfate and nitrate instead. Still some microbes can use both oxygen and inorganic salts as oxidants. The typical end result of biodegradation, regardless of the type of oxidants used, is either the conversion of the chemical into another form or the degradation of the chemical into more or less toxic degradates. Rarely would there be a thorough biodegradation leading to the same compound with minor changes in structure.

For POCs, historically aerobic biodegradation was thought to be the more important biotic transformation process compared to anaerobic biodegradation. This notion was based on the general observation that more chemicals are degraded at a higher rate with aerobic microbes, and thus on the misconception that larger volumes take place under aerobic conditions. Yet many sediments are now known to be good habitats for many more anaerobic than aerobic microbes, and are the places where many POCs can be adsorbed onto. For instance, an extensive collaboration study (Lin *et al.*, 2006) confirmed the existence of a large community of anaerobic bacteria living on rocks about two miles below the Earth's surface, somewhere in a South Africa gold mine. These microbes were found to have been sustained solely by geologically-produced sulfate and hydrogen, with no apparent reliance on substrates (e.g., oxygen) derived from photosynthesis.

For many PCBs and dioxins, the parent compounds can be metabolized aerobically with carbon as an energy substrate for microbial growth. These compounds can be degraded by co-metabolism as well; that is, they can be broken down in the presence of one or more other chemicals serving as the needed substrates for microbial growth. Another way in which these parent compounds can be metabolized is with anaerobic microbes by reductive dechlorination through cleavage of the carbon-chlorine bond. In all cases, for the rationale given earlier, the rate of biodegradation decreases with increasing chlorination; and the process on the whole is very slow, with half-lives typically in years. For example, the half-lives of 2,3,7,8-TCDD in *deep* water range from 2 to 6 years, depending on the aquatic conditions (e.g., aerobic, anaerobic, pH, temperature, in groundwater, in sediment) in which the organic is present (Chiao *et al.*, 1994; Segstro and Muir, 1995). Yet in spite of such slowness, biodegradation is the ultimate and, in most cases, the only pathway for complete destruction (degradation) of many POCs.

Because biodegradation of PCP (pentachlorophenol) is relatively rapid and extensive (especially when this wood preservative is present at low aqueous concentrations), certain indigenous microbes have been utilized on many occasions to bioremediate (i.e., to clean up) this POC contaminant in various groundwater systems (e.g., Frick *et al.*, 1988; DoD, 2002). Studies have also shown that with the addition of oxygen and within a month's time, certain indigenous microbes could remove PCP at the low water level of <10 mg/L to near or below the drinking water standard of 1 μg/L (Schmidt *et al.*, 1999).

5.4. Fate and Transport of Soil Contaminants

Compared to air and water contaminants, there appear to be fewer health issues and less direct discussion in the environmental toxicology literature concerning soil contaminants or other non-aquatic surface deposits. One reason is that this type of surface contaminants is housed in a much more stationary environment and hence is often assumed to be less accessible to other ecosystems or to people. It is also for this very reason that this section's focus is on soil contaminants, not on other non-aquatic surface deposits, as the terrestrial pollutants of environmental health concern. Overall, the fate and transport mechanisms or processes for soil contaminants in a terrestrial environment involve predominately the following:

♦ Volatilization from soil

♦ Degradation in soil

♦ Erosion and runoff from soil

♦ Leaching from soil

5.4.1. Volatilization from Soil

Volatilization can significantly affect the dissipation of soil (and other non-aquatic surface) contaminants, as this process can discharge them into the atmosphere in considerable quantities. As with water pollutants, volatilization reactions are most significant to contaminants in surface soils that are in (nearly) direct contact with the atmosphere and are contingent mostly on a chemical's volatility.

Precipitation events (e.g., rain, irrigation) are found to increase volatilization of certain soil contaminants only. For example, a study showed that volatilization of mercury in soil after a series of rain events was five orders of magnitude greater than that measured prior to those events (Lindberg *et al.*, 1999). However, this does not appear to be the case for some organic compounds, such as propargyl bromide (C_3H_3Br) which has been used as a soil fumigant and a pharmaceutical intermediate. This organic was found to evaporate three times less from irrigated than non-irrigated soil (Allaire *et al.*, 2004).

5.4.2. Degradation in Soil

In some situations, soil tends to provide a more conducive environment for biodegradation of organic compounds than an aquatic system would. For one thing, it is comparatively easier to artificially stimulate the number and activity of indigenous microbes in contaminated soil than in contaminated water. This type of microbial enhancement has been used for the cleanup of organic contaminants in soil, such as the case with the wood preservative PCP noted earlier in relation to its groundwater contamination. Many factors affecting biodegradation of water pollutants apply here as well. More specifically, for biodegradation of soil contaminants to be efficacious, elements or factors comparable to those listed in Table 5.1 should also be considered. These elements or factors include, but are not limited to: soil condition (e.g., moisture, pH); suitability of microbes; availability of nutrients; and availability of oxygen and other electron acceptors.

In addition, soil contaminants can be degraded via several common abiotic reactions, including photolysis and hydrolysis. For photolysis, the degradation is again most effective when the chemical is close to the soil surface where it is exposed to sunlight. Likewise, for hydrolysis requiring reaction with water, the degradation is most efficacious when the chemical is in the zone of saturation (i.e., the area just below the water table).

5.4.3. Erosion and Runoff from Soil

Erosion is the process in which the rocks, soils, or the deposits on their surfaces are being worn away by action of water, ice, wind, or the kind. For example, high winds can scrub fine contaminant particles bound to soils and discharge them downwind. Water erosion and surface runoff from heavy precipitation events can scrub these fine particles from surface soils as well. Runoff is the water flow that arises when the soil is infiltrated to beyond capacity thereby allowing the excess water to flow over and through the soil. When runoff flows along the ground, it can pick up soil contaminants such as toxic metal or herbicide residues. Surface runoff can be generated by rainfall, by the melting of snow glaciers, or by frequent heavy irrigation on a large farmland.

With soil contaminants dissolved or suspended in runoff, there likely comes water pollution since the contaminant load can reach various receiving aquatic systems (e.g., estuaries, lakes, rivers, streams, oceans). One study showed a strong positive correlation between the mercury levels measured in surface runoff and those measured in the catchment water (Eckley and Branfireun, 2008).

5.4.4. Leaching from Soil

In addition to surface runoff, another major source of water pollution by soil contaminants is leaching. Chemicals in the soil have the potential or tendency to migrate downward to greater depths with infiltrating water, even down to the groundwater layer. When the (soluble) contaminant residues are lost (extracted) from a layer of the soil by percolating precipitation, they are carried downward (eluviated) and generally re-deposited (illuviated) in the lower layer. This transport process may eventually allow the contaminant residues to reach beyond the water table down to the groundwater layer. The extent to which a contaminant is leached is strongly influenced by hydraulic loading (e.g., amount of rainfall), water table conditions (e.g., temperature, pH), soil permeability, the chemical's tendency to partition to the solid *vs.* aqueous phase (which is primarily a function of the chemical's solubility as well as its sorption potential binding to organic matters and clay in the soil). Many chemical fertilizers (e.g., ammonium nitrate), pesticides (e.g., atrazine, simazine), and metals (e.g., arsenic, cadmium) are highly subject to leaching.

References

Allaire SE, Yates SR, Ernst FF, 2004. Effect of Soil Moisture and Irrigation on Propargyl Bromide Volatilization and Movement in Soil. *Vadose Zone J.* 3:656-667.

ATSDR (U.S. Agency for Toxic Substances and Disease Registry), 1998. Toxicological Profile for Chlorinated Dibenzo-*p*-Dioxins. U.S. Department of Health and Human Services, Atlanta, Georgia, USA.

Buske D, Vilhena MT, Moreira D, Tirabassi T, 2007. Two-Dimensional Steady State Advection-Diffusion Equation – An Analytical Solution. In *Developments in Environmental Science Series 6: Air Pollution Modeling and Its Application XVIII* (Borrego C, Renner E, Eds.). Oxford, UK: Elsevier, Poster 22 (pp.802-804).

Chiao FF, Currie RC, McKone TE, 1994. Final Draft Report: Intermedia Transfer Factors for Contaminants Found at Hazardous Waste Sites: 2,3,7,8-Tetrachloro-Dibenzo-*p*-Dioxin (TCDD). Risk Science Program, Department of Environmental Toxicology, University of California, Davis, California, USA.

DoD (U. S. Department of Defense), 2002. Building on Cleanup Success, FY02 DERP (Defense Environmental Restoration Program) Annual Report to Congress. Washington DC, USA.

Eckley CS, Branfireun B, 2008. Mercury Mobilization in Urban Stormwater Runoff. *Sci. Total Environ.* 403:164-177.

Frick TD, Crawford RL, Martinson M, Chresand T, Bateson G, 1988. Microbiological Cleanup of Groundwater Contaminated by Pentachlorophenol. *Basic Life Sci.* 45:173-191.

Karickhoff SW, 1981. Semi-Empirical Estimation of Sorption of Hydrophobic Pollutants on Natural Sediments and Soil. *Chemosphere* 10:833-846.

Lee M-M, Nurser AJG, Coward AC, de Cuevas BA, 2007. Eddy Advective and Diffusive Transports of Heat and Salt in the Southern Ocean. *J. Phys. Oceanogr.* 37:1376-1393.

Lin L-H, Wang P-L, Rumble D, Lippmann-Pipke J, Boice E, Pratt LM, Lollar BS, Broide EL, Hazen TC, Andersen GL, DeSantis TZ, Moser DP, Kershaw D, Onstott TC, 2006. Long-Term Sustainability of a High-Energy, Low-Diversity Crustal Biome. *Science* 314:479-482.

Lindberg SE, Zhang H, Gustin M, Vette A, Marsik F, Owens J, Casimir A, Ebinghaus R, Edwards G, Fitzgerald C, Kemp J, Kock HH, London J, Majewski M, Poissant L, Pilote M, Rasmussen P, Schaedlich F, Schneeberger D, Sommar J, Turner R, Wallschläger D, Xiao Z, 1999. Increases in Mercury Emissions from Desert Soils in Response to Rainfall and Irrigation. *J. Geophys. Res.* 104:21879-21888.

Lyman WJ, 1995. Transport and Transformation Processes. In *Fundamentals of Aquatic Toxicology: Effects, Environmental Fate, and Risk Assessment* (Rand GM, Ed.), Second Edition. Washington DC, USA: Taylor & Francis, Chapter 15.

Podoll RT, Jaber HM, Mill T, 1986. Tetrachlorodibenzodioxin: Rates of Volatilization and Photolysis in the Environment. *Environ. Sci. Technol.* 20:490-492.

Schmidt LM, Delfino JJ, Preston JF 3rd, St. Laurent G 3rd, 1999. Biodegradation of Low Aqueous Concentration Pentachlorophenol (PCP) Contaminated Groundwater. *Chemosphere* 38:2897-2912.

Segstro MD, Muir DCG, 1995. Long-Term Fate and Bioavailability of Sediment-Associated Polychlorinated Dibenzo-p-Dioxins in Aquatic Mesocosms. *Environ. Toxicol. Chem.* 14:1799-1807.

U.S. EPA (U.S. Environmental Protection Agency), 2001. Frequently Asked Questions About Atmospheric Deposition – A Handbook for Watershed Managers. EPA-453/R-01-009. Office of Wetlands, Oceans & Watersheds and Office of Air Quality Planning & Standards, Washington DC, USA.

Winegardner DL, 1996. *An Introduction to Soils for Environmental Professionals*. Boca Raton, Florida, USA: CRC Press.

Review Questions

1. Briefly describe the two basic transport processes whereby a water or an air contaminant generally travels from one location to another in the environment.

2. Name two secondary (i.e., second-generation) air pollutants and describe in general terms how they can occur in the environment.

3. Briefly describe the grasshopper effect in relation to atmospheric deposition.

4. Briefly describe the main differences between dry and wet deposition of air pollutants.

5. Briefly explain how acid deposition can be formed.

6. Briefly describe how some air pollutants can cause a greenhouse effect.

7. Give an example to illustrate how hydroxyl radical ($HO^{\cdot}$) can be formed. And briefly explain why this radical is central to atmospheric chemistry.

8. What is a photon? And why does it play a key role in photochemical smog?

9. Name four principal chemical components in photochemical smog.

10. Name two most toxic acidic components that are likely to be found in acid rain.

11. Name three phase-transfer processes and two transport processes that are common to most water contaminants.

12. Why is it true that dissolution could still lead to a potential water pollution with POCs even though most (if not all) of these organic compounds have very low water solubility?

13. With respect to (ad)sorption of a POC onto sediments with high organic carbon, how is its sorption constant K_{oc} related to its octanol-water partition coefficient K_{ow}?

14. What may be a common abiotic transformation process for pollutants present near a clear water surface?

15. Briefly explain the processes *biodegradation* and *co-metabolism* used in characterizing the biotic transformation of water or soil contaminants. Why is biodegradation not as practical a transformation process for air pollutants?

16. Briefly explain why biodegradation is typically slower for dioxins and PCBs than for many organochlorine pesticides.

17. Name a POC that may serve as an exception to the rule (or notion) that biodegradation is a very slow process for many POCs.

18. Name the four key processes for transporting soil contaminants in the environment.

19. Name two abiotic reactions through which soil contaminants can be greatly degraded.

20. What may be a reason that there appear to be less immediate environmental health concerns with soil contaminants, when compared to air and water pollutants?

21. Briefly describe two transport processes whereby soil contaminants can pollute groundwater.

CHAPTER 6

Bioaccumulation of Persistent Environmental Toxicants

6.1. Introduction

In its broadest term, *bioaccumulation* is a construct concerning the accumulation of substances in a living organism. It involves primarily three interrelated quantitation processes termed *bioconcentration*, *bioaccumulation*, and *biomagnification*. The three processes are highly relevant to both the ecological and the human health risk assessment covered extensively and respectively in Chapters 22 and 23, especially to their exposure analysis component. In this chapter, POCs (persistent organochlorine compounds) in aquatic systems are used to illustrate the dynamics and relevance of bioaccumulation of persistent environmental toxicants. Aquatic systems and POCs are used in this chapter as the bioaccumulation setting because most POCs have high lipophilicity and the water environment is conducive to bioaccumulation. The significance of lipophilicity to bioaccumulation, along with other crucial factors, is discussed in Section 6.4.

It should be noted that bioaccumulation is not limited to organochlorine (OC) compounds. For example, in addition to elemental mercury (Hg^0), the main forms of mercury commonly found in the aquatic environment are ionic Hg (e.g., those binding to chloride, organic acids) and organic Hg (e.g., notably the monomethyl mercuric cation). The organic monomethyl mercuric cation CH_3Hg^+ (a.k.a. methylmercury) is highly bioaccumulative, at least much more so than inorganic Hg. This is because its organic methyl (CH_3) group is lipophilic and as such, the cation is better retained by organisms in a food chain.

6.1.1. Relevance of Food Chains

The conception of bioaccumulation cannot be fully appreciated without a basic understanding of the dynamic construct of a food web, inasmuch as the two constructs are closely interrelated. In human health or ecological risk assessment, the bioaccumulation construct that is abstracted into a model is commonly used to simulate chemical accumulation in a food web in order to give a fuller account of the dietary exposure to the chemical at issue. A food web model on the other hand offers a practical means to validate the abstracted bioaccumulation construct, in that the former model can be applied to systematically characterize the latter and can relate causality to the interconnections observed between the biota and their ecosystem, ecoregion, or ecozone.

Food webs are each a representation of the feeding relationships between species within an ecosystem, an ecoregion, or as high up as an ecozone. They can be treated as systematic, graphic descriptions of the prey-predator relationships among species in an ecological community. A food web is a series of related food chains which each show a simpler, linear link of prey-predator relationship. Each food web thereby attempts to outline a more complex but more complete interconnected system of the feeding relationships (i.e., of the related food chains) occurring within a given community.

Organisms in a food chain are grouped into hierarchic positions known as trophic levels. The trophic level of an organism is its position in a food chain or, more specifically, its position in the sequence of feedings and food energy transfer within a community. A simple and yet relatively complete food chain is often illustrated by the four basic trophic levels as follows: plants → herbivores → carnivores → omnivores. Plants or phytoplankton are *auto*trophs as they produce their own food. As such, they are the primary producers and are on the first (i.e., base) trophic level. Herbivores are their primary consumers and as such are on the second trophic level. Carnivores that consume these herbivores are considered as secondary consumers to the plants and are placed on the third trophic level. There are omnivores such as humans that consume both the herbivores and carnivores. These organisms are thereby called tertiary consumers and are put on the fourth trophic level. Figure 6.1 shows a simplified food chain (or even a simplified food web) that can be used to characterize the bioaccumulation of POCs involving human exposure.

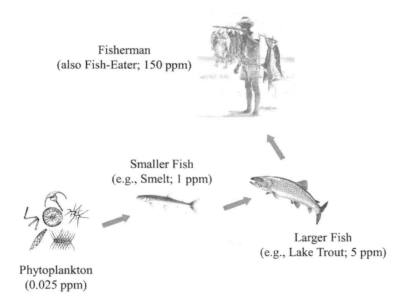

Fisherman
(also Fish-Eater; 150 ppm)

Smaller Fish
(e.g., Smelt; 1 ppm)

Larger Fish
(e.g., Lake Trout; 5 ppm)

Phytoplankton
(0.025 ppm)

Figure 6.1. A Simplified Aquatic Food Chain for Persistent Bioaccumulative Toxic Substances *(e.g., for polychlorinated biphenyls in ppm [parts per million])*

6.1.2. Relevance to Exposure Assessment

Bioaccumulation is a crucial component of exposure hazard assessment (and hence of health and ecological risk assessments as well) for POCs and other groups of persistent chemical substances. The capability of predicting accurately the bioaccumulation of substances in aquatic systems, which typically involve fish, has become a key element in assessing human health and ecological impacts of chemical pollutants. This notion is based on the argument that the assessment of a more realistic, fuller dietary exposure of humans or piscivorous wildlife to a chemical needs to account for the chemical's bioaccumulation in the environment (which includes likely an aquatic system).

For non-bioaccumulative substances, human health or ecological risk is related more directly to their external (e.g., environmental) concentrations. In contrast, the risk of bioaccumulative substances (as defined in Section 6.2 below) is related more to their levels in the body tissues of the target organism. This complicates the older, conventional approach to health or ecological risk assessment for bioaccumulative substances, as there is a need to account for the bioaccumulation of these substances in a food web.

Substances that are lipophilic tend to build up to higher concentrations in humans or other higher order animals since their bodies have relatively more fatty tissues, a point being made explicitly in the sections that follow. Persistent, bioaccumulative, toxic substances (PBTs) released into the aquatic environment thus have the potential to bioaccumulate to the point where these contaminants can adversely affect the health of the aquatic biota (e.g., fish, marine animals) or of humans and animals that consume them.

6.2. Bioconcentration and Its Potential

When contaminants are not already degraded in the environment, they are subject to *bioconcentration*. From a health risk assessment perspective, bioconcentration is one of the few most crucial biotransfer processes in the overall fate and transport of persistent toxicants in the environment. This process refers to *both* the uptake *and* the retention of a toxicant in an organism's tissue, typically to the extent that its concentration in the tissue can eventually be much higher than its concentration in the surrounding medium.

6.2.1. Bioconcentration in the Aquatic Media

Toxicants such as the lipophilic POCs can be accumulated in fish tissue through direct uptake, with concentrations up to *million* times greater than their concentrations in the surrounding water (i.e., the source). The extent of this type of chemical concentration is commonly measured as an index known as *bioconcentration factor* (BCF). This index is expressed as the ratio of the chemical's concentration in an organism's tissue (e.g., in mg kg^{-1} wet or lipid weight) to the chemical's concentration in the surrounding medium (typically in water in mg L^{-1}) at equilibrium. Many BCF estimations have been based on aquatic measurements because fish and other aquatic creatures typically provide a rich lipophilic microenvironment conducive to bioconcentration.

In the United States, substances are considered to have an alarming potential for bioconcentration if they have a degradation half-life >30 days, a BCF >1,000, or a $\log_{10} K_{ow}$ (*o*ctanol-*w*ater partition coefficient, as briefly described in Chapter 5) value >4.2 (Corl,

2001; U.S. EPA, 1999, 2000). These criterion values are below those adopted by Canada (CEPA, 1999) and some other western countries.

6.2.2. Bioconcentration Factor (BCF)

For POCs in fish, their BCFs can be approximated from the log of their K_{ow}, using the log-linear regression $log_{10} (BCF) = [(0.79) \times log_{10} (K_{ow}) - 0.40]$ given by van Gestel *et al.* (1985). Similar equations by others (e.g., Veith *et al.*, 1980) may be used, though expectedly ending with somewhat different results. As shown in Table 6.1, using the van Gestel equation, a BCF value of over one million has been estimated for the PCB 209 and the *octa*CDD congener (*see* Chapter 16 for their definitions and congener nomenclature).

Table 6.1. Bioconcentration Factors (BCFs) Estimated for Select
Persistent Organochlorine Compounds (POCs) [a]

Select POC	$log_{10} K_{ow}$ [b]	BCF
p,p'-DDT	5.90 (a)	18,239
Heptachlor	4.95 (a)	3,240
HCB (Hexachlorobenzene)	5.18 (a)	4,923
Lindane	3.55 (a)	254
Aldrin	6.29 (a)	37,077
Dieldrin	4.95 (a)	3,240
PCP (Pentachlorophenol)	4.59 (a)	1,683
PCB 28	5.80 (b)	15,205
PCB 138	6.97 (c)	127,732
PCB 209	8.27 (d)	1,359,252
2,3,7,8-TCDD	6.80 (b)	93,756
*hexa*CDD (1,2,3,4,7,8-)	7.80 (b)	578,096
*octa*CDD (1,2,3,4,6,7,8,9-)	8.20 (b),(e)	1,196,741
2,3,7,8-TCDF	6.10 (b)	26,242

[a] from correlation with $log_{10} K_{ow}$ based on the equation log_{10} (BCF) = [0.79 x log_{10} (K_{ow}) – 0.40] (van Gestel *et al.*, 1985), using where applicable the midrange of the $log_{10} K_{ow}$ calculated or measured within $20° – 25° C$, with the majority at $25° C$; K_{ow} = *o*ctane-*w*ater partition coefficient (*see* text); *see* Table 16.2 for numbering of PCB, PCDD, and PCDF congeners.

[b] (a) Montgomery (1993); (b) MacKay *et al.* (1992); (c) ATSDR (2000); (d) Hawker and Connell (1988); (e) Shiu *et al.* (1988).

Another quantitative approach widely used for approximating BCFs from K_{ow} is through application of the log-log *q*uantitative *s*tructure-*a*ctivity *r*elationship (QSAR) framework. Several regulatory agencies including especially U.S. EPA have used the K_{ow}-based QSAR model to approximate BCFs for hundreds of chemicals including many POCs. An extensive review (Cronin *et al.*, 2002) was published relating the application of the QSAR framework for BCF approximation.

A BCF value can also be estimated directly from a site-specific field study, which must show that the chemical's concentration in water remained constant over the range of the organism's inhabitation and for a time interval not less than 4 weeks (to ensure an equilibrium state). Another condition is that the chemical's bioavailability must not be affected by its removal from the solution through competing mechanisms. The third, final condition is that the chemical's concentration which the test organism was exposed to must be below the lowest that would cause an adverse effect on the organism.

For BCFs measured in a laboratory setting instead, a total of five conditions should be met. First, the BCF should be calculated from the chemical's concentrations measured in a test solution. Second, the test should be either of sufficient duration to reach steady state or, alternatively, lasting 4 weeks or longer. Third, as for the site-specific field data, the chemical's concentration which the test organism was exposed to must be below the lowest that would cause harm to the organism. Fourth, the BCF should be calculated on a wet tissue weight basis. Fifth and lastly, the (geometric) mean should be used if more than one BCF estimate for the same species is available.

In many western and European countries, it is recommended that the laboratory studies be conducted using a method consistent with the one specified in the Organization for Economic Cooperation and Development (OECD, 2002) Test Guidelines 305. In certain aspects, the OECD guidelines are similar to those given by U.S. EPA (2003). Overall, most regulatory entities have agreed that compared to those from laboratory studies, field data generally provide more accurate or realistic BCF estimates.

6.3. Bioaccumulation and Biomagnification

Bioaccumulation as a technical phenomenon refers to *a single* organism's uptake *and* retention of a toxicant from *all sources*, including all sites and routes, not just from one medium (e.g., water, soil) as in the bioconcentration case. When this organism is eaten up by its predator, *biomagnification* occurs. This is because the toxicant is now bioaccumulated in the predator, with its concentration magnifying in a food chain, in that the predator is likely to consume more than one similar prey. Bioaccumulation is most relevant to POC type toxicants because they tend to concentrate in fatty tissues, particularly in species at the top of the food chain. The reality is that in species on higher trophic levels, the fatty tissues tend to be more abundant and more lipophilic.

In short, aquatic systems can be contaminated easily and substantially by OCs (organochlorines) which are mostly highly persistent substances. These POCs subsequently can be concentrated and accumulated inside small aquatic biota in the same aquatic environment. As these contaminated creatures fall prey to carnivorous fish, birds, and large terrestrial or amphibian species nearby, a contaminant's concentrations are progressively magnified in each of this chain of predators. Therefore, human fish eaters too may suffer adverse health effects from bioaccumulation and biomagnification of POCs and other POPs (persistent organic pollutants). Similarly, many ecosystems (e.g., plants, soil, or any of their combinations with or without water) can provide a conducive environment for bioconcentration, bioaccumulation, and biomagnification of these substances.

6.3.1. Toxic Equivalency (TEQ) in Bioaccumulation

One reality about bioaccumulation is that an organism can be exposed to the same toxicant multiple times. An axiom to this notion is that insofar as the organism's health is the endpoint at stake, two structurally similar or even two different chemicals can be treated as the same one if, for all practical purposes, both exert the same kind of adverse effects of concern in (nearly) all aspects. It is based on this axiom that in the literature, the concentrations of DDT and its two equally persistent metabolites DDD and DDE (Chapter 15) in a sample were usually combined and reported as one; that is, simply as the concentration of the sum of all DDT-related compounds (often denoted by ΣDDTs) found in the sample. This approach is also frequently applied for reporting the concentrations of all PCB congeners measured in environmental samples.

The above approach is not used across the board, however. For reporting the concentrations of all dioxin congeners in a sample, a modification of the approach is used. This deviation owes to the fact that the dioxin member 2,3,7,8-TCDD (or TCDD for short) is regarded as the most potent of all congeners in the dioxin family. Therefore, for all other congeners in a mixture, their measured amounts usually are each adjusted downward for their potency relative to that of TCDD. For example, suppose a sample was measured to have 1 unit of TCDD and 5 units of 2,3,7,8-TCDF (or TCDF for short), then the *total* TCDD-equivalent amount of the two dioxins in the sample would be reported as 1.5 units since the TCDF potency was determined by the World Health Organization (WHO) to be *one-tenth* of the potency of TCDD (as published by van den Berg *et al.*, 2006). That is, TCDF has been given a (mammalian) toxic equivalency factor (TEF) of 0.1.

There are theoretically 75 possible congeners of PCDDs (polychlorinated dibenzo-*p*-dioxins) and 135 possible congeners of PCDFs (polychlorinated dibenzofurans) in the environment simply due to the various positions that the chlorine atoms can be structurally bonded to the carbon atoms. Nonetheless, when based on just the *number* of chlorine atoms present, there are only 29 members subject to TEF consideration. These include: 7 congeners of PCDDs; 10 congeners of PCDFs; and 12 dioxin-like congeners from the PCB family. These various POC congeners, along with the 29 (mammalian) TEFs assigned and utilized by WHO, are discussed more extensively in Chapter 16.

6.3.2. Cases of Bioaccumulation and Biomagnification

Bioaccumulations of PCBs and certain other OCs are real phenomena. These POCs have been found in some remote areas where these chemicals have never been produced or used (Matthies and Scheringer, 2001; Cone, 2005). For instance, the Inuit living in the Canadian arctic have never used PCBs or other OCs. Yet a study on these people living in northern Quebec showed that their whole blood samples had levels of PCBs and PCB metabolites (e.g., OH-PCBs) up to 70 times higher than the whole blood sample pooled from the non-arctic southern part of Canada (Sandau *et al.*, 2000). One possible source of the Inuit's elevated exposure to these chemicals was likely from consuming contaminated marine mammals and fish, which are part of their regular high-protein, high-fat diet.

Coincidentally, detectable to high levels of PCBs, DDTs, and some other OCs were found in marine mammal samples collected around that time from California (Kajiwara *et al.*, 2001), Finland (Koistinen *et al.*, 1997; Kostamo *et al.*, 2002), and Russia (Muir *et al.*, 2003). These data showed support of the bioaccumulative nature of many of these pollutants, as evident from some of the study results elaborated on briefly below.

The American study by Kajiwara *et al.* (2001) was conducted to analyze the contents of PCBs, DDTs, and other persistent substances in the blubber and livers of 31 marine mammals. These mammals included 15 California sea lions, 6 northern elephant seals, and 10 harbor seals that were found stranded along the Pacific coasts off California between 1991 and 1997. Among the substances analyzed, DDTs were found predominant, followed by PCBs. The highest levels were found in the blubber of sea lions, with the highest DDT and PCB levels being 2.9 and 1.3 mg/g, lipid weight, respectively.

In the Finnish study by Koistinen *et al.* (1997), the contents of several OCs were measured in seal samples from the Gulf of Finland and in sediments from the gulf or near Gotland, all collected around 1991. The OCs under analysis included PCBs, their structurally related cousins polychlorinated diphenyl ethers (PCDEs), and dioxins. The sediment samples included one surface core per sampling site. The seal specimens consisted of 14 ringed seals and 6 grey seals that were found dead and examined for pathology in late 1991. For all the 50 *tetra-* through *deca*-CDE congeners analyzed (i.e., those with 4 to 10 chlorines, as per congener nomenclature described in Chapter 16), their levels in seal blubber ranged from <0.3 to 62 ng/g, lipid weight. In ringed seals with good nutritional status, the levels of most PCDE congeners were found higher in the two adult females than in the young. In the sediments, the levels of dioxin congeners expressed as TCDD-equivalents were found higher than those of the dioxin-like PCBs.

The other Finnish study by Kostamo *et al.* (2002) was conducted to assess in part the biomagnification potential for OCs and mercury (Hg) from the main prey fish to Saimaa ringed seals that died between 1981 and 2000 at Lake Haukivesi, Finland. The study found a considerably higher biomagnification from prey fish to the ringed seal than to the pike. Its finding as well as conclusion was based on the higher feeding rate and the metabolism differences observed in the ringed seals.

In the Russian study by Muir at al. (2003), the contents of PCBs, DDTs, and several other OCs were analyzed in the blubber of harp seals, ringed seals, and bearded seals, as well as in several fishes and invertebrates, all from the White Sea in northwest Russia. Highest concentrations of ΣPCBs and ΣDDTs were found in specimens from two male bearded seals (with mean concentrations of 4.2 ng/kg and 4.0 ng/kg, lipid weight, respectively). Female harp seals had mean ΣPCB and ΣDDT concentrations of 1.1 ± 0.5 ng/kg and 0.6 ± 0.3 ng/kg, lipid weight, respectively. The male and female adult ringed seals had similar mean concentrations of ΣPCBs found in the harp seals. The blubber concentrations were considerably lower for all other OCs analyzed in all the seal specimens. The predominant OCs found in the fish samples were PCBs and DDT-related compounds, ranging from approximately 16 to 41 ng/kg, wet weight.

6.3.3. Bioaccumulation of Organochlorine Compounds in Seafood

Bioaccumulation of POCs in seafood is an important concern to human health for a good reason. Seafood is a global commodity of great value to humans. According to the Food and Agriculture Organization of the United Nations (FAO, 2012), global supply of food fish from capture fisheries and aquaculture reached 130 million tons in 2011, which is sufficient to provide an apparent consumption of over 18 kg (live weight equivalent) per capita for the world population of over 7 billion people. Fish is a good commodity not simply due to its availability in relatively huge quantities. It is also an important part of a healthy diet. Fishes contain little "bad" (saturated) fats, which are commonly found in red meat; yet at the same time, they provide high quantities of complete proteins, "good" (e.g., polyunsaturated) fats, and other high quality nutrients (e.g., minerals). Proteins are the main component of human muscles, organs, and glands. These highly complex organic macromolecules, which are each made of chains of amino acids, are in every part of the human body except the bile and urine.

The good fats rich in fish include *Omega*-3 fatty acids, such as ALA (alpha-linolenic acid), EPA (eicosapentaenoic acid), DHA (docosahexaenoic acid), and DPA (docosapentaenoic acid). These unsaturated fatty acids provide humans with great health benefits. They were found to reduce mortality rates of coronary heart disease (Kris-Etherton *et al.*, 2002) and were linked to lower risks for Alzheimer's disease (Morris *et al.*, 2003) and stroke (Friedland, 2003). In particular, DHA is a critical component for building brain tissue, nerve growth, and retina function (Horrocks and Yeo, 1999). This 22-carbon *Omega*-3 fatty acid is thereby considered essential for infant development. It is also an important nutrient for normal brain function in adults.

Despite their high nutritious values, fishes in many localities are often contaminated with persistent toxic (organic) compounds. As shown in Table 6.2, some POCs were reportedly found to have bioaccumulated in fish (and shellfish) tissue from localities inside and outside the tropical Southeast Asia and Oceania. The data included in this table were compiled and reported in the 1990s. They all showed that for all localities under study, the residue levels monitored in fish tissue far exceeded U.S. EPA's screening values for at least one of the POCs included in the analysis. The worst case appeared to have been in the Lake Michigan area in the United States, where the residue levels of PCBs in fish tissue reportedly exceeded even the action level of 2.0 ppm set forth by the United States (FDA, 2001) and Canada (CIFA, 2005).

Levels of POC residues in fish tissue from studies conducted in the early 2000s are listed in Table 6.3. From a public health perspective, these residue levels appeared to fare better compared to the values reported in the 1990s, except in India where the upper-end DDT levels were extremely high. The levels from India exceeded even Australia's *legal* standard of 1.0 ppm (as footnoted in Table 6.2). While the residue data shown in Table 6.3 are limited to what had been gathered to the early 2000s, what has become certain is that fish contamination by POCs is a global phenomenon. In fact, in the early 2000s, a rather extensive collaboration study (Hites *et al.*, 2004) was conducted to monitor the POC residue levels in salmon. That study revealed that for many of the POCs analyzed, the residue levels monitored in farmed salmon whether purchased or imported from worldwide greatly exceeded U.S. EPA's screening values (Table 6.3).

Table 6.2. Mean Tissue Residue Concentrations of Select Persistent Organochlorine Compounds in Fishes from Select Localities, around the Years 1990s[a]

Locality	ΣPCBs	ΣDDTs	Aldrin/ Dieldrin	Chlordane	HCB
Screening Value[b]	*2.5 ppb*	*14.4 ppb*	*0.3 ppb*	*14.0 ppb*	*3.1 ppb*
Tropical Southeast Asia and Oceania[c]					
India	3.5	15.0	3.1	2.4	0.07
Thailand	1.6	6.2	3.7	2.6	0.24
Vietnam	10.0	26.0	0.29	0.11	0.05
Indonesia	2.6	28.0	1.2	0.45	0.05
Papua, New Guinea	7.5	0.4	1.3	0.37	0.03
Solomon Islands	3.6	4.8	0.3	0.57	0.02
Australia	55.0	22.0	10.0	51.0	4.2
Outside of Southeast Asia and Oceania[d]					
Canada (Baffin Island)	165	129	24.4	127	–
Canada (Banks Island)	202	128	24.4	115	–
Morocco (Mediterranean)	–	17.4	2.8	–	0.6
Egypt (Maryut Lake)[e]	21.9	39.6	7.8	–	–
Finland (Teno River)[e]	15.3	8.4	–	4.5	1.3
Finland (Simo River)[e]	241.1	299.2	–	17.0	7.8
Russia (Ob River)[e]	2.5	0.9	–	0.7	–
Spain (Catalonia rivers)[e]	181	81	–	–	–
USA (Lake Michigan)[e]	2,440	1,830	130	320	–

[a]in ppb (parts per billion) = ng/g, wet weight; ΣPCBs = all polychlorinated biphenyl congeners; ΣDDTs = all isomers of DDT and its metabolites; HCB = hexachlorobenzene; except PCBs (Chapter 16), the other four are organochlorine pesticides (Chapter 15).

[b]concentrations exceeding the screening values (from U.S. EPA, 2000) are considered as having a potential public health concern.

[c]extracted from values compiled by Allsopp and Johnston (2000) for studies conducted by other investigators mostly in the 1990s.

[d]extracted from values compiled by Allsopp *et al.* (2000) for studies conducted by other investigators mostly in the 1990s.

[e]in freshwater fish; all others in marine fish.

Overall, the fish residue data in Table 6.2 and Table 6.3 together reveal that a sufficient number of monitoring sites had residue levels greater than U.S. EPA's screening values by more than 30-fold. For those localities, no more than one or two fishmeals per month thus may become necessary, particularly for children and pregnant women, so that their intake of POCs can be kept below the screening levels which are considered by some authorities to be of potential public health concern. However, it is well taken that such a health advisory may not be practical to people who rely on fish as their main diet.

Table 6.3. Tissue Residue Concentrations of Select Persistent Organochlorine Compounds in Fishes from Select Localities, around the Early 2000s[a,b]

Locality	ΣPCDDs/Fs	ΣPCBs	ΣDDTs	Aldrin/ Dieldrin
Screening Value[c]	*0.03 ppt*	*2.5 ppb*	*14.4 ppb*	*0.3 ppb*
China (Pearl River Delta) (a)	–	–	1.5-62	–
China (Shanghai, Tianjin) (b)		0.8-11.4	28.9	–
China (Taihu Lake) (c)	0.5-3.8	1.5-27.6		
Egypt (Demietta) (d)	–	–	20-211	
India (River Ganges) (e)	–	–	13.6-1,666	3.1-86.1
Italy (central Adriatic Sea) (f)	–	51.4-177.2	5.2-65.6	–
Korea (coastal waters) (g)	–	3.0-96.6	0.8-27.0	–
Portugal (h)	–	–	30.1-109.9	–
Spain (Atlantic SW Coast) (i)	0.04-0.19	0.86-23.8	–	–
Sweden (Baltic sea) (j)	0.5-33.4	–	–	–
USA (salmon worldwide) (k)	65	73	28	6.3

[a]all residue concentrations are in ppb = parts per billion (ng/g) wet weight, except for ΣPCDDs (including PCDFs); ppt = TEQ-based parts per trillion (ng/kg), *see* Section 6.3.1 for concept of TEQ.

[b](a) Kong *et al.* (2005); (b) Yang *et al.* (2006); (c) Zhang and Jiang (2005); (d) El Nemr and Abd-Allah (2004); (e) Kumari *et al.* (2001); (f) Perugini *et al.* (2006), converted from values given on fat basis assuming a fat content of 10% for Atlantic mackerel (Gall, 2004); (g) Yim *et al.* (2005); (h) Campos *et al.* (2005); (i) Bordajandi *et al.* (2006); (j) SNFA (2004); (k) Hites *et al.* (2004).

[c]concentrations exceeding the screening values (from U.S. EPA, 2000) are considered as having a potential public health concern.

6.4. Factors Influencing Bioaccumulation

Both bioaccumulation and bioconcentration begin as soon as a contaminant enters an organism from the environment where both the chemical and the organism co-exist. This first phase is referred to as the uptake of the toxicant, which by and in itself is a complex process. Within the scientific sector, it is a widely accepted concept that chemicals tend to diffuse passively from an area of high concentration to one of low concentration. The driving force for this passive transport is the natural tendency of molecules proceeding from order (e.g., highly packed places) to chaos (e.g., loosely packed places). However, as discussed below, a number of factors can facilitate or hinder this passive process.

6.4.1. Lipophilicity and Bioavailability

Certain chemicals such as POCs do not mix well with water, as they are lipophilic.

Lipophilic substances tend to move out of water and into the cells of a living organism that they come in contact with, as the latter (particularly their membranes) offer a less lipid-resistant microenvironment. The same factors facilitating the uptake of a toxicant by an organism continue to operate inside that organism, thereby minimizing the toxicant's opportunity of returning to the outer microenvironment. Once inside a mammalian organism, toxicants travel rapidly to its body organs and tissues via the bloodstream and the lymphatic system. At any given time, these chemicals inside the organism are present either as bound or unbound to plasma proteins present in the various tissues. It is the unbound fraction of the chemical that is generally considered more biologically active or available, leading to the important concept of chemical bioavailability.

Different POCs have different unique binding interactions with different plasma proteins. Therefore, the type of plasma proteins, their concentrations, the plasma flow rate, and the binding kinetics between a POC and the plasma proteins involved all affect the amount of the POC in the bioactive form. Some toxicants are attracted to certain cellular sites and are temporarily if not permanently stored there upon distribution. If uptake proceeds slowly or is discontinued, or if the protein binding is weak enough, the chemical can eventually be excreted from the body. The uptake and the storage of chemicals are also influenced by their water solubility. Chemicals that are highly water-soluble generally do not readily enter the cells of an organism. Therefore, even when water-soluble toxicants somehow find their ways into an organism (e.g., by oral), they are easily removed unless the cells inside have specific biochemical processes for retaining them.

6.4.2. Metabolic Potential

Another factor affecting bioaccumulation of toxicants is whether or not an organism's body can break down the chemical that has entered its cell or tissue. The process as well as the ability for such a biological breakdown is termed *metabolism*, or more specifically *biotransformation* (Chapter 8). This ability varies among species of living organisms and depends largely on a chemical's physicochemical properties. For example, natural pyrethrins are insecticides derived from plants of the chrysanthemum species (Chapter 15). They are highly fat-soluble (lipophilic) but are easily degraded. As such, they do not accumulate in an organism. This is one reason why this chapter has its focus on toxicants that are *persistent* in the (aquatic or any micro-) environment.

6.4.3. Environmental Mobility

Still another crucial factor that influences bioaccumulation is a chemical's mobility in the environment. As discussed in Section 6.3.2, it is evident that PCBs and other OCs can reach remote regions of the Earth. This type of long-range transport is thought to be generally via atmospheric, oceanic, or terrestrial transport. Of the three, terrestrial transport appears less likely as a major mode for long-range mobility, insomuch as soil, plants, surface runoff, leaching, and the kind are fairly stationary objects or processes. Regardless, in the late 1990s a fourth mode for long-range transport was identified and analyzed rather extensively (e.g., Ewald *et al.*, 1998; UNEP, 1998; Wania, 1998). This transport mode was via animal migration, or technically known as *biotransport*.

In particular, in the study by Ewald *et al.* (1998), pacific salmon were noted to deposit eggs in freshwater and then migrate downstream to the ocean to spend the majority of their lifecycle there. Prior to migration back upstream to freshwater for spawning, they accumulated lipids for the energy required for migration as well as for gonadal development. The lipids that the salmon accumulated in their body were found to have been contaminated by lipophilic pollutants, such as PCBs and DDT, present in the ocean.

The salmon study concluded that biotransport of environmental pollutants was more significant than other modes of transport for two reasons. First, lakes that were within reach of salmon migration are quantitatively a larger contributor to *local* contaminant loads compared to an ocean, as the latter is a much larger aquatic system. Second, contaminants via biotransport tend to be more biologically active and less vulnerable to environmental degradation, as they are all within an organism's lipid stores and thereby protected from various oxidation processes (e.g., via ultraviolet radiation).

Pacific salmon is not the only species known as capable of transporting POCs to remote areas. Wania (1998) had used whales and seabirds to exemplify the ability of migratory animals in transporting POPs, of which many were POCs, to the arctic. According to his analysis, the annual amount ranged from grams to kilograms for POPs (particularly PCBs and DDT) transported by seabirds in and out of the arctic. With whales, the estimate for the annual amount transported was in the order of several tons. These estimates all suggested that the quantities of some POPs transported by migratory animals, especially whales, might be in a similar order of magnitude as the gross rates estimated for atmospheric and oceanic transports.

In an earlier analysis performed by Comba *et al.* (1993), an effort was made to quantify the transport of the pesticide mirex ($C_{10}Cl_{12}$, an OC uniquely with no hydrogen atoms) from Lake Ontario to the St. Lawrence river system. That study estimated that, for the years 1950 to 1990, nearly 300 kg of mirex was transported downstream with water and sediments, and another 60 kg by migrating eels. Those estimates suggested that biotransport was of a similar order of magnitude as the transports in abiotic media. In another yet earlier study, Lum *et al.* (1987) determined that eels transported more mirex out of Lake Ontario than what these aquatic creatures did to suspended particulate matter (Chapter 12). As still one more example, according to the United Nations Environment Programme (UNEP, 1998), each year many migrating birds die in their winter quarters in the warmer (southern) regions. These birds were seen to frequently leave behind in their winter quarters a considerable amount of POCs that their bodies had accumulated from their (northern) summer quarters prior to migration.

6.4.4. A Dynamic Equilibrium Effect

As a recap and in essence, when a POP enters the cells of an organism, it is subject to distribution and then to storage, metabolism (biotransformation), and elimination within that organism (Chapter 7). Bioaccumulation thereby results from a dynamic equilibrium between an organism's exposure to a chemical and its uptake, storage, and degradation inside the organism. As expected, persistent lipophilic toxicants such as POCs are the ones posing a great threat of bioaccumulation within an ecosystem. Posing even a greater threat are those toxicants resistant to biotransformation once inside an organism. Due to their high lipophilicity, many POCs can be stored in fat deposits for years inside an organism. In general, those POCs that tend to move more freely within an organism's body, or to be excreted rapidly from its body, are less likely to be bioaccumulated. All these may explain why the accumulation of POCs was found to be much more in an old trout than in a young yellow perch from the same lake, since by comparison the older fish is a larger, fatter, and longer-lived creature with a lower rate of chemical excretion.

References

Allsopp M, Johnston P, 2000. Unseen Poisons in Asia: A Review of Persistent Organic Pollutant Levels in South and Southeast Asia and Oceania. Greenpeace Research Laboratories, Department of Biological Sciences, University of Exeter, Exeter, UK.

Allsopp M, Erry B, Stringer R, Johnston P, Santillo D, 2000. Recipe for Disaster: A Review of Persistent Organic Pollutants in Food. Greenpeace Research Laboratories, Department of Biological Sciences, University of Exeter, Exeter, UK.

ATSDR (U.S. Agency for Toxic Substances and Disease Registry), 2000. Toxicological Profile for Polychlorinated Biphenyls (PCBs). U.S. Department of Health and Human Services, Atlanta, Georgia, USA.

Bordajandi LR, Martin I, Abad E, Rivera J, Gonzalez MJ, 2006. Organochlorine Compounds (PCBs, PCDDs and PCDFs) in Seafish and Seafood from the Spanish Atlantic Southwest Coast. *Chemosphere* 64:1450-1457.

Campos A, Lino CM, Cardoso SM, Silveira MIN, 2005. Organochlorine Pesticide Residues in European Sardine, Horse Mackerel and Atlantic Mackerel from Portugal. *Food Addit. Contamin.* 22: 642-646.

CEPA (Canadian Environmental Protection Act), 1999. Persistence and Bioaccumulation Regulations (SOR/2000-107; 23/3/2000). *Canada Gazette* Part II, 134 (7):607-612.

CFIA (Canadian Food Inspection Agency), 2005. Canadian Shellfish Sanitation Program – Manual of Operations. Ontario, Canada.

Comba ME, Norstrom RJ, MacDonald CR, Kaiser KLE, 1993. A Lake Ontario-Gulf of St. Lawrence Dynamic Mass Budget for Mirex. *Environ. Sci. Technol.* 27:2198-2206.

Cone M, 2005. *Silent Snow: The Slow Poisoning of the Arctic.* New York, New York, USA: Grove Press.

Corl E, 2001. Bioaccumulation in the Ecological Risk Assessment (ERA) Process (Issue Papers, dated 7 August). Technical Support, Atlantic Division, Naval Facilities Engineering Command, Norfolk, Virginia, USA.

Cronin MTD, Walker JD, Jaworska JS, Comber MHI, Watts CD, Worth AP, 2002. Use of QSARs in International Decision-Making Frameworks to Predict Ecologic Effects and Environmental Fate of Chemical Substances. *Environ. Health Perspect.* 111:1376-1390.

El Nemr A, Abd-Allah AMA, 2004. Organochlorine Contamination in Some Marketable Fish in Egypt. *Chemosphere* 54:1401-1406.

Ewald G, Larsson P, Linge H, Okla L, Szarzi N, 1998. Biotransport of Organic Pollutants to an Inland Alaska Lake by Migrating Sockeye Salmon (*Onchorhynchus nerka*). *Arctic* 51:478-485.

FAO (Food and Agriculture Organization of the United Nations), 2012. The State of World Fisheries and Aquaculture: Part 1. World Review of Fisheries and Aquaculture. FAO Fisheries Department, Rome, Italy.

FDA (U.S. Food and Drug Administration), 2001. Fish and Fisheries Products: Hazards and Control Guidance –Third Edition (Chapter 9). U.S. Department of Health and Human Services, College Park, Maryland, USA.

Friedland RP, 2003. *Editorial*: Fish Consumption and the Risk of Alzheimer Disease: Is It Time to Make Dietary Recommendations? *Arch. Neurol.* 60:923-924.

Gall K, 2004. Seafood Nutrition and Health. New York Seafood Council, 23 Bay Avenue, Hampton Bays, New York, USA.

Hawker DW, Connell DW, 1988. Octanol-Water Partition Coefficients of Polychlorinated Biphenyl Congeners. *Environ. Sci. Technol.* 22:382-387.

Hites RA, Foran JA, Carpenter DO, Hamilton MC, Knuth BA, Schwager SJ, 2004. Global Assessment of Organic Contaminants in Farmed Salmon. *Science* 303:226-229.

Horrocks LA, Yeo YK, 1999. Health Benefits of Docosahexaenoic Acid (DHA). *Pharmacol. Res.* 40:211-225.

Kajiwara N, Kannan K, Muraoka M, Watanabe M, Takahashi S, Gulland F, Olsen H, Blankenship AL, Jones PD, Tanabe S, Giesy JP, 2001. Organochlorine Pesticides, Polychlorinated Biphenyls, and Butyltin Compounds in Blubber and Livers of Stranded California Sea Lions, Elephant Seals, and Harbor Seals from Coastal California, USA. *Arch. Environ. Contamin. Toxicol.* 41: 90-99.

Koistinen J, Stenman O, Haahti H, Suonpera M, Paasivirta J, 1997. Polychlorinated Diphenyl Ethers, Dibenzo-p-Dioxins, Dibenzofurans and Biphenyls in Seals and Sediment from the Gulf of Finland. *Chemosphere* 35:1249-1269.

Kong KY, Cheung KC, Wong CK, Wong MH, 2005. The Residual Dynamic of Polycyclic Aromatic Hydrocarbons and Organochlorine Pesticides in Fishponds of the Pearl River Delta, South China. *Water Res.* 39:1831-1843.

Kostamo A, Hyvarinen H, Pellinen J, Kukkonen JVK, 2002. Organochlorine Concentrations in the Saimaa Ringed Seal (*Phoca hispida saimensis*) from Lake Haukivesi, Finland, 1981 to 2000, and in Its Diet Today. *Environ. Toxicol. Chem.* 21:1368-1375.

Kris-Etherton PM, Harris WS, Appel LJ, 2002. Fish Consumption, Fish Oil, Omega-3 Fatty Acids, and Cardiovascular Disease. *Circulation* 106:2747-2757.

Kumari A, Sinha RK, Gopal K, 2001. Organochlorine Contamination in the Fish of the River Ganges, India. *Aquatic Ecosys. Health & Magnt.* 4:505-510.

Lum KR, Kaiser KLE, Comba ME, 1987. Export of Mirex from Lake Ontario to the St. Lawrence Estuary. *Sci. Total Environ.* 67:41-51.

MacKay D, Shiu WY, Ma KC, 1992. *Illustrated Handbook of Physical-Chemical Properties and Environmental Fate of Organic Chemicals*. Boca Raton, Florida, USA: Lewis Publishers, Volumes I and II.

Matthies M, Scheringer M, 2001. *Editorial*: Long-Range Transport in the Environment. *Environ. Sci. Pollut. Res.* 8:149.

Montgomery JH, 1993. *Agrochemical Desk Reference: Environmental Data*. Chelsea, Michigan, USA: Lewis Publishers.

Morris MC, Evans DA, Bienias JL, Tangney CC, Bennett DA, Wilson RS, Aggarwal N, Schneider J, 2003. Consumption of Fish and n-3 Fatty Acids and Risk of Incident Alzheimer Disease. *Arch. Neurol.* 60:940-946.

Muir D, Savinova T, Savinov V, Alexeeva L, Potelov V, Svetochev V, 2003. Bioaccumulation of PCBs and Chlorinated Pesticides in Seals, Fishes and Invertebrates from the White Sea, Russia. *Sci. Total Environ.* 306:111-131.

OECD (Organization for Economic Cooperation and Development), 2002. Test No. 305: Bioconcentration – Flow-Through Fish Test. OECD Guidelines for the Testing of Chemicals (Vol. 1, pp.1-23). Paris, France.

Perugini M, Giammarino A, Olivieri V, Di Nardo W, Amorena M, 2006. Assessment of Edible Marine Species in the Adriatic Sea for Contamination from Polychlorinated Biphenyls and Organochlorine Insecticides. *J. Food Protect.* 69:1144-1149.

Sandau CD, Ayotte P, Dewailly E, Duffe J, Norstrom RJ, 2000. Analysis of Hydroxylated Metabolites of PCBs (OH-PCBs) and Other Chlorinated Phenolic Compounds in Whole Blood from Canadian Inuit. *Environ. Health Perspect.* 108:611-616.

Shiu WY, Doucette W, Gobas FAPC, Andren A, MacKay D, 1988. Physical-Chemical Properties of Chlorinated Dibenzo-p-Dioxins. *Environ. Sci. Technol.* 22:651-658.

SNFA (Swedish National Food Administration), 2004. Persistent Organic Pollutants in Fatty Fish in Sweden 2000-2003 (Interim Report 5: Study of Dioxin-like PCBs in Fatty Fish from Sweden 2000-2002). Swedish National Food Administration (Toxicology Division), Box 622, SE-751 26, Uppsala, Sweden.

UNEP (United Nations Environment Programme), 1998. Preparation of an International Legally Binding Instrument for Implementing International Action on Certain Persistent Organic Pollutants. UNEP/POPS/INC. 1/6 (dated 30 April), Geneva, Switzerland.

U.S. EPA (U.S. Environmental Protection Agency), 1999. Category for Persistent, Bioaccumulative, and Toxic New Chemical Substances. *Federal Register* 64:60194-60204.

U.S. EPA (U.S. Environmental Protection Agency), 2000. Bioaccumulation Testing and Interpretation for the Purpose of Sediment Quality Assessment: Status and Needs. Bioaccumulation Analysis Workgroup. EPA/823/R-00/001. Washington DC, USA.

U.S. EPA (U.S. Environmental Protection Agency), 2003. Water Quality Guidance for The Great Lakes System, USA. *Code of Federal Regulations* Title 40, Part 132.

van den Berg M, Birnbaum LS, Denison M, De Vito M, Farland W, Feeley M, Fiedler H, Hakansson H, Hanberg A, Haws L, Rose M, Safe S, Schrenk D, Tohyama C, Tritscher A, Tuomisto J, Tysklind M, Walker N, Richard E, Peterson RE, 2006. The 2005 World Health Organization Re-evaluation of Human and Mammalian Toxic Equivalency Factors for Dioxins and Dioxin-like Compounds. *Toxicol. Sci.* 93:223-241.

van Gestel CAM, Otermann K, Canton JH, 1985. Relation Between Water Solubility, Octanol/Water Partition Coefficients, and Bioconcentration of Organic Chemicals in Fish: A Review. *Regul. Toxicol. Pharmacol.* 5:422-431.

Veith GD, Macek KJ, Petrocelli SR, Carroll J, 1980. An Evaluation of Using Partition Coefficients and Water Solubility to Estimate Bioconcentration Factors for Organic Chemicals in Fish. In *Aquatic Toxicology* (Eaton JG, Parrish PR, Hendricks AC, Eds.). ASTM STP 707. American Society for Testing and Materials (ASTM), Philadelphia, Pennsylvania, USA.

Wania F, 1998. The Significance of Long Range Transport of Persistent Organic Pollutants by Migratory Animals. WECC Report 3/98. WECC Wania Environmental Chemists Corp, 289 Simcoe Street, Suite 404, Toronto, Ontario, Canada.

Yang N, Matsuda M, Kawano M, Wakimoto T, 2006. PCBs and Organochlorine Pesticides (OCPs) in Edible Fish and Shellfish from China. *Chemosphere* 63:1342-1352.

Yim UH, Hong SH, Shim WJ, Oh JR, 2005. Levels of Persistent Organochlorine Contaminants in Fish from Korea and Their Potential Health Risk. *Arch. Environ. Contamin. Toxicol.* 48:358-366.

Zhang G, Jiang G, 2005. Polychlorinated Dibenzo-p-Dioxins/Furans and Polychlorinated Biphenyls in Sediments and Aquatic Organisms from the Taihu Lake, China. *Chemosphere* 61:314-322.

Review Questions

1. Give both the broader and the more specific definition for *bioaccumulation*.

2. How are the dynamic construct of bioaccumulation and that of food web related to each other in terms of exposure assessment?

3. What is the definition of *bioconcentration* as a technical phenomenon? And how are the biological events involved in this phenomenon typically assessed quantitatively?

4. What are some of the general methods or techniques used to measure bioconcentration factors for persistent toxic chemicals?

5. Why does bioconcentration or bioaccumulation appear to be better studied for toxicants in an aquatic environment than in an atmospheric or a terrestrial environment?

6. How are the technical processes *biomagnification* and *bioaccumulation* related to each other?

7. What is a toxic equivalency factor (TEF)? And how is it generally used in estimating the total TCDD-equivalent concentration of all the dioxin congeners in a mixture?

8. Why is it important to study the bioaccumulation of environmental contaminants in seafood?

9. Which locality inside or outside of the tropical Southwest Asia and Oceania appeared to have the worst case (i.e., the highest levels) of fish contamination by POCs in the 1990s?

10. Which locality appeared to have the worst case (i.e., the highest level) of fish contamination by DDT(s) in the early 2000s?

11. Briefly describe three basic factors that can strongly affect or influence bioaccumulation of environmental toxicants.

12. How is bioaccumulation relevant to long-range transport of PBTs?

13. Give two reasons why migration of contaminated Pacific salmon may be a significant mode for transport of environmental contaminants.

14. Besides salmon, name three species of migratory animals that were studied in the late 1980s through the late 1990s for the biotransport load of POCs.

15. Briefly explain why the accumulation of a PBT is expected to be more in an old trout than in a young yellow perch from the same aquatic environment.

CHAPTER 7

Uptake and Distribution of Toxicants

7.1. Introduction

In this and the three chapters that follow, the focus is on the fate and transport of environmental toxicants that are entering or have entered the body of an organism, particularly that of a human or a physiologically similar mammalian. Within a biological system being the microenvironment, the fate and the transport of toxicants are generally about their uptake by and disposition in the organism's body. The preference in species here is due to the notion that unlike ecotoxicology, this is where the emphasis lies with environmental toxicology. The foci of these four chapters are on *systemic* effects which are those occurring at sites distant from the toxicant's point of entry.

7.1.1. Localized Effect of Non-Systemic Action

Systemic effect (more on this topic in Chapter 9) tend to be more a concern to environmental toxicologists in that, in many environmental settings, the levels of most toxicants are not alarming enough to call for immediate public health or regulatory action. Yet when toxicants are present in sufficiently high levels within the microenvironment outside of an organism, their (acute) toxic effects exerted on the organism can be localized on its outer structure (e.g., skin, surface of respiratory tract, surface of gastrointestinal tract), not necessarily systemic. For example, serious localized rash or irritation of the skin (Section 2.4.6) can be induced by contact with certain pesticide residues, such as with those of propargite left on treated foliage upon a fieldworker's reentry.

Another example of non-systemic effect is with ozone (O_3) which at atmospheric levels above 0.1 ppm (parts per million) can irritate the eyes and upper respiratory tract of people exposed to it. As with sulfur dioxide (SO_2), nitrogen dioxide (NO_2), and hydrogen fluoride (HF), ozone is a major and highly phytotoxic air pollutant capable of causing acute, direct damage to a leaf's structural components without entering its stomata (i.e., air spaces each between guard cells on a leaf's surface tissue, *see* Figure 7.3). This type of damage frequently results in leaf chlorosis (yellowing) or necrosis (browning and death), largely due to direct oxidative stress (and thereby oxidative damage) to the leaf's cellular membrane (e.g., Schraudner *et al.*, 1998).

7.1.2. Disposition of Systemic/Internal Organ Toxicants

Following environmental exposure, the disposition of a xenobiotic inside a biological system may be broadly divided into a series of biochemical events or phases outlined in

Figure 7.1. This series of events also applies to plants which can excrete certain wastes (e.g., minerals) via their roots, shoots, or leaves (Larcher, 2003). In some plants, certain wastes can be transported to the cytoplasmic sacs called vacuoles on the leaves which are destined to shed. In some other plants, certain wastes can be actively secreted through the roots into the soil.

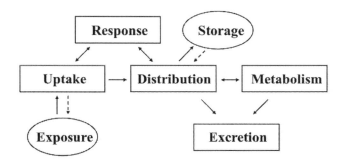

Figure 7.1. Disposition of Xenobiotics inside a Biological System

In Figure 7.1, those disposition phases in a box are the ones each involving enormous complex and more dynamic biochemical reactions, whereas those in an eclipse are each requiring relatively fewer, simpler, more static biochemical events. The *uptake*, *distribution*, and *excretion* phases, along with exposure and storage, are discussed in this chapter. Due to their complexities, *metabolism* (largely *biotransformation*) of toxicants and toxic *response* are covered separately in Chapters 8 and 9, respectively. Note that the phase *response* by the organism's body includes the *adverse action* induced by the toxicant.

7.2. Mechanism of Entry

As alluded to in Figure 7.1, upon exposure all systemic effects begin with the uptake or absorption of the xenobiotic by the organism's body. In many instances, the term *uptake* or *intake* is more appropriate than *absorption* when discussing the entry of a xenobiotic into a biological organism, in that absorption also connotes the specific process whereby a xenobiotic *actively penetrates* a cellular membrane on the host organism's outer structure. Cellular membranes are commonly referred to as biological membranes or, in this book, biomembranes for short.

7.2.1. Structure of Cellular Membranes

Biomembranes, such as those of plasma, tissues, cells, and cell organelles, are vital to an organism's life. They are those that either protect a cell from the outside environment, or separate the compartments inside a cell in order to safeguard important biological processes and specific events. These biomembranes, especially those in a mammalian body, are composed of predominately proteins and phospholipids, with the lipid portions being arranged as bilayer leaflets embedded with the proteins (Figure 7.2). Each phospholipid in each (e.g., outer) layer has a polar (i.e., water-soluble) head and two much longer non-polar fatty acid hydrocarbon tails. The two tails are packed together as well as with one or more of those in the opposite (e.g., inner) layer. With such a structural arrangement, biomembranes are generally permeable to certain toxicants only, depending on the particular physicochemical properties of the intruders, such as their molecular size, lipid solubility, polarity, and structural similarity to endogenous molecules.

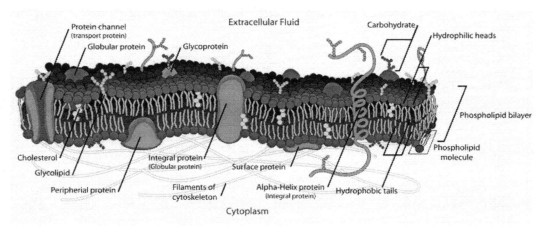

Figure 7.2. General Structure of a Mammalian Biomembrane
(public domain image from www.freeclipartnow.com)

The membrane proteins generally fall into two types termed *peripheral proteins* and *integral* (a.k.a. *transmembrane*) *proteins*. The main function of an integral protein is to transport substances such as ions and macromolecules across the phospholipid bilayer. A peripheral protein, on the other hand, does not interact with the hydrophobic (i.e., nonpolar) core of the bilayer. Instead, it is there to safeguard the membrane surface, regulate cell signaling, and participate in some other crucial cellular events.

Two major secondary lipids found in a typical biomembrane are glycolipids and steroids. Glycolipids are those that have one or more carbohydrate groups attached. Sphingolipids are the main glycolipids found in many biomembranes and, due to their backbone molecule sphingosine, play a key role in signal transmission and cell recognition. The majority of steroids found in a biomembrane are cholesterols which, due to their alcoholic hydroxyl (OH) group, can interact with water and thereby can act as important spacers in the bilayer's hydrophobic core. They are there to prevent crystallization of the fatty acids and to give rigidity or stability to the biomembrane.

7.2.2. Common Mechanisms of Entry

There are broadly five common mechanisms of entry enabling or aiding xenobiotics to get inside an organism's body or to cross its cellular membranes. These include:

♦ *Passive diffusion* (a.k.a. *passive transport*) – This is the movement of molecules across a cell membrane *without* any expenditure of energy by the cell.

♦ *Active transport* – This is the movement of molecules *against* a concentration gradient or an electrical potential in the direction opposite to passive diffusion, thereby *requiring* certain expenditure of energy by the cell.

♦ *Filtration* – This is the movement of molecules across a cell membrane due to hydrostatic pressure (e.g., that generated by the cardiovascular system).

♦ *Facilitated diffusion* – This is the movement of molecules across a cell membrane using *special transport proteins* (primarily integral proteins) as carriers that are embedded within the cellular membrane.

♦ *Endocytosis* – This is the process whereby cells absorb molecules from outside the cell by engulfing these molecules with their membranes. Where the ingested molecules are solids, the process is specifically termed *phagocytosis*; and when liquids are taken in instead, the process is termed *pinocytosis*.

For many xenobiotics, passive transport is the predominant entry mechanism. For a system at constant temperature and for diffusion over unit distance, the rate of passive transport of nonpolar, nonionized lipid-soluble molecules is generally thought to follow closely Fick's law of diffusion as follows:

$$Rate\ of\ diffusion = K \times A \times (C_1 - C_2) \tag{7.1}$$

where K is a rate constant specific to the intruder, A is the surface area in which the diffusion takes place, C_1 is the intruder's concentration outside the membrane, and C_2 is its concentration inside. When C_2 is negligible relative to C_1, $(C_1 - C_2)$ is treated as C_1.

7.3. Uptake and Absorption of Toxicants

The routes and processes involved in the uptake and absorption of toxicants vary considerably across the plant and animal kingdoms. This variation is largely due to the differences in their body structures but to some extent also to the ways in which they are exposed to the toxicants. Plants are more dependent on local habitat conditions for their survival, as they are stationary structures. They are included here for discussion not only because this provides a further appreciation of the numerous and various ways in which toxicants can enter an organism, but also because the damage on plants, especially on the consumable kind, has a considerable effect on the health of humans and wildlife.

7.3.1. Uptake by Plants

Plants each consist of two main organ systems for uptake of nutrients and other foreign substances: the shoot and the root. The shoot system includes all parts of a plant above ground, such as leaves, buds, stems, flowers (if any), and fruits (if any). The root system includes those parts below ground, such as roots, tubers, and rhizomes. Plant cells are formed with undifferentiated cells termed *meristems* and then develop into various cell types, which can be broadly grouped into three tissue categories as follows: *dermal*, *ground*, and *vascular* (e.g., Purves *et al.*, 1995; Taiz and Zeiger, 2006) .

The *dermal* tissues comprise epidermal cells closely packed to shield the outer surface of herbaceous plants (Figure 7.3). These cells secrete a waxy cuticle atop to help reduce water loss from the leaf. Most of the leaf interior between the upper and the lower epidermis are the palisade and the spongy parenchyma (both together also called mesophyll) cells. The parenchyma cells in these *ground* tissues are most functional, as they are rich in chloroplast and are actively involved in photosynthesis, storage, and support. The xylem and phloem tubes, along with some other kinds of parenchyma cells, are included in the *vascular* bundles. The vascular bundles (not specifically shown in Figure 7.3) are located among the spongy mesophyll and are the units responsible for transporting food, water, minerals, hormones, and other materials within a plant.

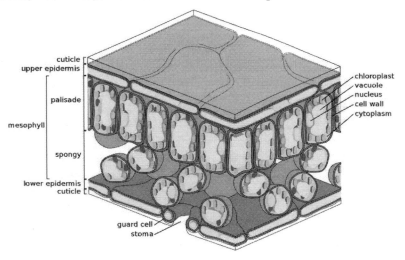

Figure 7.3. Internal Anatomy of a Typical Leaf *(permission directly from author Zephyris [Richard Wheeler]; http://en.wikipedia.org/wiki/file:leaf_tissue_structure.svg)*

Uptake of environmental toxicants by most terrestrial plants occurs in two common pathways. One is from exposure of their roots to soil contaminants and the other, from exposure of their foliage to pollutants in the air (Kvesitadze *et al.*, 2006). Indirect damage retarding plant growth can occur when the pollutants cause disturbance of water or nutrient uptake. In particular, when the contaminated soil is acidified by decayed material or acid rain, the metallic ions (e.g., Pb^{2+}, Cd^{2+}) in the soil become more mobile toward the plant roots. These ions may damage the plant's roots and then its leaves by disrupting its uptake of water and nutrients. Soil acidification can also cause leaching of nutrients, leading to an unhealthy plant suffering from nutrient deficiency or growth disturbance.

A. Uptake via Plant Leaves

Inasmuch as the amount of a contaminant that enters a plant is what matters the most in terms of plant damage, the stomata on the plant's leaf cells are the most significant structural component. This is because they are the ones mainly responsible for regulating the passage of pollutants into the leaf cells. The extent of such uptake depends on the environmental setting as well as the physicochemical properties of a pollutant along the leaf surface. For example, the flow of a pollutant may be hindered by the leaf's morphology, by the reactions of chemical scavengers occurring within the leaf, or by air movement across the leaf. These factors can affect the polluted air's flux to the leaf surface.

Again, of all the determinants considered, stomatal opening is by far the most crucial in that little or no uptake will occur when the stomata are closed. This surface opening is regulated by a number of factors including meteorological variables (e.g., temperature, light), physicochemical conditions in the guard cells, starch content in the guard cells, and amount of potassium (K^+) ions accumulated in the guard cells (Humble and Raschke, 1971; Jinno and Kuraishi, 1982; Kim and Lee, 2007).

Many toxic substances that enter the leaves of a plant are in solution (e.g., pesticide spray, liquid aerosol), rather than in gas. The permeability of liquids on a leaf surface depends on the moistening of the leaf surface, surface tension of liquid, and morphology of stomata (Kvesitadze *et al.*, 2009). Once inside the leaf cells, toxicants are subject to biochemical reactions that are similar in kind to those observed in a mammalian body (e.g., Kvesitadze *et al.*, 2006).

B. Uptake via Plant Roots

Like their leaves, the roots of many plants also have stomata serving as crucial passages for soil contaminants. These air spaces on roots have been found open in all cases to this date (e.g., Christodoulakis *et al.*, 2002; Tarkowska and Wacowska, 1987). As water can enter the root via the epidermis, minerals in their inorganic forms can enter the root by being dissolved in water, or by entering on their own as free molecules through predominately the root hairs. Minerals can enter the root against their concentration gradient (i.e., via active transport). However, most if not all soil contaminants can enter the root only through cuticle-free unsuberized cells (Kvesitadze *et al.*, 2009). The ability of plant roots to absorb or extract soil contaminants is most evident from their application for phytoremediation (Kvesitadze *et al.*, 2006; McCutcheon and Schnoor, 2003; Tsao, 2003), a biotechnology relying on the ability of plant roots to remove contaminants such as toxic metals in soil.

7.3.2. Uptake and Absorption by Humans

Like the above overview for plants, the one for humans here is likewise necessarily succinct due to space limitation. In general, the main portals for entry of xenobiotics into a human (or another mammalian) body are dermal, respiratory, and gastrointestinal (GI). Secondary routes include the eyes, injection, sexual, anal, and wound.

Materials that have just been taken in (or up, depending on one's perspective) via inhalation or ingestion are still treated as outside the body until they penetrate the cellular barriers of the respiratory or GI tract, respectively. More so than the uptake or intake process, absorption varies greatly with the chemical and the portal of entry involved.

A. Skin Penetration

Figure 7.4 provides a simplified schematic overview of the penetration and distribution of xenobiotics via the human skin which is a complex, multilayered structure comprising about 2 m^2 of surface in an average adult. This skin is a biomembrane relatively impermeable to most ions and aqueous solutions. This inability is due to the fact that the human skin's outermost layer, termed *epidermis*, has an outermost surface layer of dead, keratinized cells called *stratum corneum* serving as a physical barrier to most chemical penetration. Yet despite such a structural advantage, many toxicants can still find their ways deep into the human skin (e.g., organophosphate pesticides in agricultural workers). This is particularly the case when the xenobiotic is a lipid-soluble compound given that biomembranes are composed of largely phospholipids which are highly lipophilic (*see* Section 7.2).

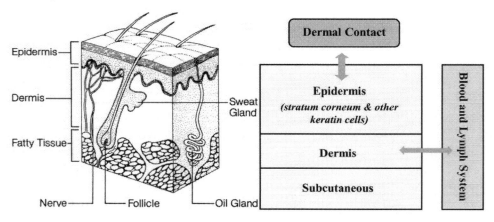

Figure 7.4. Penetration of Xenobiotics through the Human Skin
(skin image from public domain at www.freeclipartnow.com)

B. Respiratory Uptake

Figure 7.5 provides a simplified schematic overview of the uptake and distribution pathways of toxicants in the human respiratory tract. The main function of this respiratory system is to exchange gases between the bloodstream and the air present in the air sacs termed *alveoli* (located in the lowest region of the respiratory tract at the ends of the bronchioles). The respiratory system is thus an organ in unavoidable contact with air pollutants, inasmuch as an average adult breathes well over 12,000 liters of air per day. This organ is also furnished with several mechanical and immunological mechanisms (e.g., filtration in nasal cavity, sneezing) devoted to keeping itself free from invading particles or microorganisms. In particular, there are small hair-like appendages termed *cilia* located in the respiratory tract that can sweep foreign particles out of the airways, and up to the throat through which these foreign particles may enter the GI.

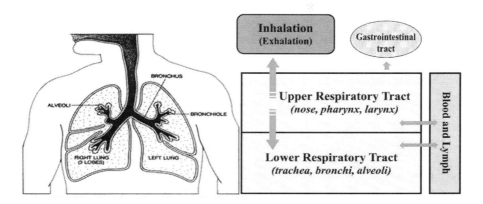

Figure 7.5. Uptake of Xenobiotics through the Human Respiratory Tract
(*lung image from public domain at www.freeclipartnow.com*)

C. Gastrointestinal (GI) Absorption

Figure 7.6 presents a simplified schematic overview of the human GI tract, along with the *enterohepatic circulation* (that of bile from the liver to the small intestine) and the *portal venous system* (Figure 7.7). The GI tract may be treated as a long tube running from the mouth to the anus, with its contents external to the rest of the organism's body system. Aside from dietary exposure, the oral route of toxicological concern is generally limited to accidental or deliberate ingestion of toxicants.

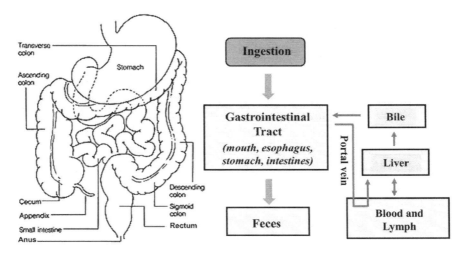

Figure 7.6. Absorption of Xenobiotics through the Human Gastrointestinal Tract (GI)
(*GI image from public domain at www.freeclipartnow.com*)

7.4. Distribution and Excretion of Toxicants

Figures 7.4 through 7.6 above offer not only a simplified overview of the uptake and absorption of toxicants by humans, but also a rather brief account of their distribution via the bloodstream and the lymphatic system. Note that in the skin, it is the inner layer *dermis* that provides maximum opportunity for further transport of toxicants once they have penetrated through the epidermis or the skin appendages (e.g., sweat glands, hair follicles). This opportunity owes to the fact that dermis is the place that harbors most of the blood vessels (and nerve endings). It is also important to note that the *portal venous system* (Figure 7.7) is the component responsible for directing blood from parts (predominately the small intestine) of the GI tract to the liver, where the absorbed toxicant will be *processed* (Chapter 8) prior to their distribution to the cardiovascular system.

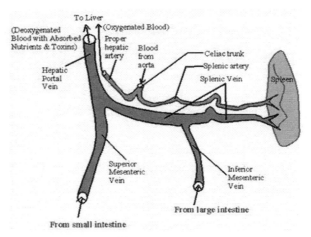

Figure 7.7. Portal Venous System *(courtesy of and permission from www.GenericLook.com)*

7.4.1. Distribution via the Bloodstream

Body fluids in humans (and in many other mammalians) are composed of three main components: *intracellular fluid*, ~40% of (human) body weight; *interstitial fluid* (a.k.a. *tissue fluid)*, ~20% of body weight; and *intravascular fluid* (a.k.a. *blood plasma*), ~4% of body weight. Of the three, intravascular fluid plays the most significant role in the distribution of absorbed toxicants, as human blood plasma accounts for over 50% of total blood volume. Lymph is the roughly 10% of the plasma and tissue fluids left behind for taking out the cellular wastes. The transport of toxicants by lymph is comparatively insignificant, in that lymph flow is many times slower than blood flow.

Following absorption, toxicants are usually distributed along with plasma proteins. If a toxicant is bound to a plasma protein, it usually becomes immobilized away from the site of (e.g., toxic) action. Toxicants are frequently distributed to the sites of storage (e.g., bones, fats), to the liver or kidneys for metabolic processing, or to the site of action (e.g., binding to the hemoglobin). In particular, lipophilic compounds such as PCBs, dioxins, and DDTs are stored mainly in the fats whereas fluoride (F) and lead (Pb), in the bones. It is important to note that whenever there is a large amount of a toxicant stored in one of the depots, it is a potential health hazard. This is because if and when certain biochemical or physiological disturbance occurs, a large amount of the stored toxicant can be suddenly released to become available for body distribution to *overload* the site of action.

7.4.2. Excretion of Toxicants

Despite the fact that elimination of toxicants is the process more for their degradation by metabolism within the body, in general it is used interchangeably with the term *excretion* to describe the chemical disposition phase whereby a substance is *removed* from the body. In any event, this phase is pivotal in determining the potential toxic effects of xenobiotics (or of their metabolites, as defined and discussed in Chapter 8). In a mammalian body, the primary routes of chemical elimination (i.e., excretion) are via urine, feces, and exhaled air. Minor routes include breast, saliva, milk, tears, semen, sweat, and hair.

A. Renal Excretion

The main function of a kidney is to remove urea, mineral salts, and waste materials from the blood. Its secondary but still crucial functions include the retentions of water, salts, and electrolytes (i.e., those substances containing free ions such as the potassium ion K^+), the excretions of these substances, as well as the regulation of blood pressure. The kidney therefore plays a vital role in eliminating toxicants from the body, in keeping the blood clean, and in regulating the amount of fluid in the body. The *nephron*, which is approximately one million in number in each of the two human kidneys, is the functional unit responsible for renal (i.e., that pertaining to the kidney) excretion. This functional unit has three main regions central to this primary route of excretion: *the glomerulus*; *the proximal (convoluted) tubule*; and *the distal (convoluted) tubule* (Figure 7.8). The tubular portion closer to the glomerulus is referred to as the *proximal* section.

Urine is composed of water, certain electrolytes, and various waste molecules that are filtered out of the renal blood system. The first phase in urine formation is filtration in the very vascular beginning of the nephron called glomerulus. Approximately 25% of the cardiac output passes through the human kidneys, of which about 20% is passively filtered via the numerous relatively large (~70 nm) glomerular pores. Small molecules, whether polar or lipid-soluble, thereby readily pass through this sieve-like filter into the nephron tubule. The amount of this filtrate is substantial, about 45 gallons per day in an adult human. The urine, as eliminated, represents only about 1% of the amount of fluid filtrated through the glomerulae into the renal tubules. Molecules too large to pass through, or those bound to proteins, must either be further altered or be eliminated by other processes or mechanisms. Tubular reabsorption is the second, and comparatively less crucial, phase that takes place in the proximal (convoluted) tubule. Nearly all of the water, glucose, K^+, and amino acids lost during the first phase (i.e., glomerular filtration) will re-enter the blood from this nephron section by passive diffusion (i.e., to their lower concentrations in the capillaries surrounding the tubule). The urine's pH is one key factor that can greatly affect this passive diffusion process as well as urinary excretion.

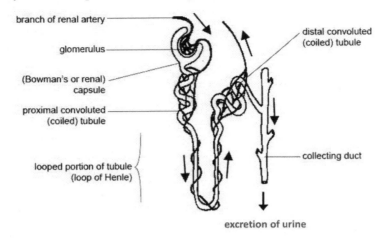

branch of renal artery

glomerulus

(Bowman's or renal) capsule

proximal convoluted (coiled) tubule

looped portion of tubule (loop of Henle)

distal convoluted (coiled) tubule

collecting duct

excretion of urine

Figure 7.8. Nephron – the Functional Unit *(modified from Wikibooks.org at http://en.wikibooks.org/wiki/File:Anatomy_and_physiology_of_animals_Kidney_tubule_or_nephron.jpg; permission under Creative Commons Attribution 3.0)*

Another secondary phase, in which solutes may be secreted into the kidney, occurs in the distal tubule. This mechanism permits passive but relies more on active transport of solutes from the peritubular capillaries into the tubular lumen. Solutes actively secreted into this lumen include H^+, K^+, as well as some polar and nonpolar substances.

In essence, a toxicant's renal excretion can be approximated as the *sum* of glomerular filtration *and* distal tubular secretion of the toxicant *minus* proximal tubular reabsorption of the toxicant. Small toxicants (both polar and lipid-soluble) are filtered with ease by the glomerulus. In some cases, large molecules (including some bound to plasma proteins) may be excreted by passive transfer from the blood and then cross both the capillary cell walls and the nephron tubular membranes to enter the urine.

B. Fecal Excretion

Elimination of toxicants in the feces relies on two physiological processes: *hepatic excretion* involving bile secretion; and *intestinal excretion*. Of the two, the biliary route is the more important. Bile is a complex fluid flowing through the biliary tract into the small intestine. It contains water, electrolytes, and a host of organic molecules including bile acids, cholesterols, and phospholipids. Many waste products, including bilirubin, are removed from the body by hepatic secretion into the bile and then into the duodenum (i.e., the beginning portion of the small intestine) for excretion in the feces. For certain types of substances (e.g., organic bases, organic acids, neutral compounds), the predominate means of excretion is via special active transport mechanisms. Some metals (e.g., Pb, Hg) are also secreted into the bile. However, substances that tend to be secreted into and through the bile are typically large size ionized molecules, such as large-molecular-weight conjugates (e.g., those discussed in Chapter 8).

Note that most of the substances secreted into and from the bile are water-soluble. Therefore, those substances are not likely to be reabsorbed as such from the small intestine back to the liver. Enzymes in the intestinal flora are capable of hydrolyzing some glucuronide and sulfate conjugates (Chapter 8) to produce smaller and less water-soluble compounds that can then be reabsorbed along the proximal and distal ileum (i.e., the terminal portion of the small intestine). This process of secretion into the small intestine via the bile, together with reabsorption along the ileum and then back to the liver by the portal circulation, is referred to as *enterohepatic circulation*. It is this process that prevents a relatively large amount of the bile acids from leaving the (human) body. In fact, roughly 95% of the bile acid molecules delivered to the duodenum are reabsorbed into the blood within the ileum, where the venous blood goes straight into the portal vein to allow thereby their repeated passage via the sinusoids (i.e., venous cavities) of the liver. As expected, continuous enterohepatic recycling can occur and therefore can lead to very long half-lives of some lipid-soluble toxicants in the body.

The other key mechanism of fecal elimination is by direct intestinal excretion. Despite the fact that this is not a major pathway of fecal elimination, a considerable number of toxicants can be excreted directly into and out of the intestinal tract and thus be eliminated directly through this route. Some substances, particularly those poorly ionized in the plasma (e.g., weak bases), may passively diffuse through the walls of the capillaries surrounding the intestinal tract and into the intestinal lumen to be eliminated in the feces. Intestinal excretion is not considered as a major pathway in that it is a slow process compared to hepatic excretion. It is an important elimination route only for those toxicants that cannot be easily metabolized or be easily eliminated by other excretion processes.

C. Pulmonary Excretion

The lower respiratory tract, particularly the alveolar region, represents a significant pathway for excretion of many volatile substances including their gaseous metabolites. As noted earlier, the main function of alveoli in the lungs is for exchange of oxygen (O_2) from the air with carbon dioxide (CO_2) from the blood. This gas(eous) exchange, also known as pulmonary respiration, is maintained predominantly by passive diffusion following a concentration gradient. Gaseous compounds with a low solubility in the blood are thereby more rapidly eliminated than those with a high solubility. Volatile liquid dissolved in the blood are also readily excreted as part of the exhaled air. The amount of a liquid excreted by the alveoli is proportional to its vapor pressure. Actually, exhalation can be an efficient route of excretion for some lipid-soluble toxicants. This is possible in that each alveolus is surrounded by a network of capillaries in such a way that the alveolar contents are separated from those in the capillaries only by an extremely thin alveolar membrane. Also, some substances can be removed directly by exhalation if they are taken into the respiratory system but have not yet diffused into the alveolar blood.

7.5. Toxicokinetics of Toxicants

For adverse effect as well as the associated toxic response to occur, both the amount and the way a toxicant is delivered to the site of action is foremost relevant. This type of pursuit is within the realm of toxicokinetics (TK), starting with the notion of reaction kinetics. Reaction kinetics is concerned with the rates and the tendency of chemical processing or, more specifically, with the changes in the reactant concentrations in chemical reactions. In essence, TK is the explanation as well as the study of the kinetics and the quantitative movement of toxicants in a living system. It deals with the time course of a toxicant *being handled* by the host organism's body. Its focus is on the *quantitative* aspects of toxicant disposition in an organism's body.

7.5.1. Principles and Models of Toxicokinetics

Much like pharmacokinetics (PK) dealing with the disposition kinetics of drugs and for lack of real time physiological data, TK relies heavily on mathematical models for explanation and prediction of a toxicant's disposition kinetics in the body of a biological system. The delivery of a toxicant to the site of action depends on two key disposition processes: *absorption* from the exposure site into the general circulation; and *distribution* via the circulation to the site of action as well as to all other body tissues. Within the *distribution* process, the toxicant's concentration at the site of action is affected greatly by the rate of elimination (including metabolism and excretion). For simplicity, the toxicant's concentrations in the general circulation, or the *central compartment* in TK modeling terms, are all that matters under the notion that such time-dependent concentrations can be used to reflect those levels at the action site or other tissues of concern. This is why a one-compartment open model (Figure 7.9) is frequently used to approximate the disposition kinetics of a chemical. If specific interests arise and additional parameter data become available for the disposition kinetics to be represented by additional compartments, then two (Figure 7.9) or more anatomic compartments are used.

One of the more complex compartment models is physiologically-based pharmacokinetics (PB-PK) model (e.g., Dong, 1994; Medinsky and Valentine, 2001), or more appropriately referred to as PB-*T*K model for *t*oxicokinetics. Fundamental to each PB-TK model is a set of tedious, if not complex, mathematical equations that presumably offer a comprehensive time course of the chemical disposition in several pre-selected anatomic compartments (e.g., kidneys, liver, lungs, muscle, brain). Each of these anatomic regions is supposed to have its own characteristic blood flow, metabolic and excretion rate constants, volume, and tissue-blood partition coefficient that collectively are deemed responsible for the chemical disposition in that body region. All models used in TK, whether PB-TK or one-compartment, are considered open in the sense that they each allow the chemical's elimination from the model. Given that the absorption rate of environmental toxicants is often uncertain, as the exact amount of environmental exposure does not seem to be known, the rate constant for elimination is more practical and more critical than that for absorption when investigating the time-course disposition of a toxicant.

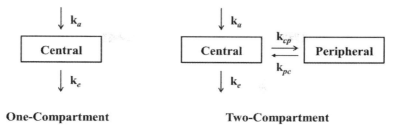

One-Compartment   **Two-Compartment**

Figure 7.9. Schematic Presentation of a One- and a Two-Compartment Open Model *(showing the kinetics parameters to be measured for the time-course disposition of a xenobiotic, where k_a is the absorption rate, k_e is the excretion rate, k_{cp} is the rate for distribution from the central [circulation] to peripheral [e.g., site of action] compartment, and k_{pc} is the rate for distribution from the peripheral to the central compartment)*

7.5.2. Basic Mathematical Concepts

The mathematical principles involved in TK analysis are complex and beyond the scope of this introductory text. Accordingly, no attempt is made to describe them in any detail in this chapter. Yet a few very basic concepts are thought worth introducing here in an effort to demonstrate the nature and complexity of the analysis involved. The numerical example in Box 7.1 that follows is for those more mathematically inclined. Regardless, it is important to note that, as hinted in the numerical example, knowing the chemical-specific values for some of the kinetics parameters may enable a toxicologist to estimate the amount of a toxicant that a victim has absorbed (i.e., has been exposed to).

A. Volume of Distribution

This parameter is also known as *apparent* volume of distribution (Vd), a term used to quantify the distribution of a toxicant throughout the body after intake or absorption. It is defined as the plasma volume that is apparently or presumably required to distribute the absorbed substance to the concentration so measured in the plasma (e.g., in the central compartment). Note that Vd is a hypothetical value only, as it does not represent the actual physiological volume of the plasma inside a body. For instance, when a lipophilic toxicant of a known amount enters a body and binds preferentially to the fatty tissues at the expense of the plasma, its measured concentration in the plasma can be very low. This can result in a huge value projected for Vd, which can be larger than the actual plasma volume in the body. This is possible because by definition Vd = [(total amount x of toxicant in plasma) ÷ (concentration Cp of toxicant in plasma)]; that is, Vd = x/Cp.

B. Toxicant Clearance

After intake or absorption, a toxicant is distributed among the tissues and fluids in the body and then all or a portion of it is eventually cleared or eliminated (predominantly by the liver and kidneys). This physiological process, referred to as toxicant or systemic clearance (CL), results in the toxicant's concentration in the plasma decreasing steadily, although at different rates for different substances in different species. More specifically, CL is defined as the plasma *volume* theoretically required for losing (clearing) its toxicant within a unit time, in order to account for an observed rate of the toxicant's elimination from the body. CL thereby expresses the rate or efficiency at which a toxicant is removed from the plasma and not the actual amount of the toxicant eliminated. Mathematically it can be expressed as the ratio of elimination rate Ke (e.g., in mg/min) to plasma concentration Cp (e.g., in mg/ml) of the toxicant; that is, $CL = Ke/Cp$.

C. Elimination Rate Constant

This constant (Kel) is a chemical-specific parameter used to characterize the *fraction* of a toxicant in the body eliminated per unit time. The value for this *constant* can be represented (approximated) by the slope of the line of the log plasma concentration versus time (i.e., plotted against time). It has the following relationship with the two terms discussed above: $Kel = CL/Vd$, in units of time^{-1} (e.g., min^{-1}, hr^{-1}). The elimination *rate* Ke of a toxicant (i.e., not the rate *constant*) is also proportional to its concentration, as elimination is typically a first-order process until it becomes saturated.

D. Area under the Curve

This term represents the total amount of a toxicant taken in by the host organism's body, irrespective of the rate of absorption. It is simply that *total* area under the curve (AUC) in a semi-log plot of toxicant concentration in the plasma against time. AUC can be used as a measure of toxicant exposure or the bioavailability of a drug or toxicant absorbed (usually via the oral route). It is mathematically related to the above three parameters Kel, CL, and Vd as follows: $AUC = Cp_0/Kel = (Cp_0)(Vd)/CL$, where Cp_0 is the toxicant's plasma concentration at (near) time zero serving as the initial point on the curve.

Box 7.1. Numerical Example for Clarification of Basic Disposition Kinetics

> Suppose there are x grams of grapefruit pulp (e.g., a toxicant) in a jar containing 10 ml water (e.g., plasma); and the entire content of the jar is poured into a tank (e.g., an animal body) prefilled with 990 ml water. The volume of distribution (Vd) of the pulp in the tank is then 1,000 ml [$= \{(x\ g) \div ((x\ g)/(10\ ml + 990\ ml))\}$].
>
> If, at each minute, 10 ml of the grapefruit pulp is emptied from the tank, discarded, and replaced with 10 ml of water added into the tank, then the clearance (CL) is 10 ml per min.
>
> The elimination rate constant Kel is $CL/Vd = (10\ ml/min) \div (1,000\ ml) = 0.01/min$ (or at the constant rate of 1% per minute).
>
> Note that the elimination half-life ($t_{1/2}$), which is the time for the pulp concentration in the tank water to fall to 50%, is 69 min, given that $t_{1/2} = [(\ln 2) \times (Vd)] \div (CL) = [(0.693) \times (1,000\ ml)] \div (10\ ml/min)$ and that $\ln 2 = $ natural log of $2 = 0.693$.

References

Christodoulakis NS, Menti J, Galatis B, 2002, Structure and Development of Stomata on the Primary Root of *Ceratonia siliqua* L. *Ann. Botany* 89:23-29.

Dong MH, 1994. Microcomputer Programs for Physiologically-Based Pharmacokinetic (PB-PK) Modeling. *Comput. Methods Programs Biomed.* 45:213-221.

Humble GD, Raschke K, 1971. Stomatal Opening Quantitatively Related to Potassium Transport: Evidence from Electron Probe Analysis. *Plant Physiol.* 48:447-453.

Jinno N, Kuraishi S, 1982. Acid-Induced Stomatal Opening in *Commelina communis* and *Vicia-faba. Plant & Cell Physiol.* 23:1169-1174.

Kim DJ, Lee JS, 2007. Current Theories for Mechanism of Stomatal Opening: Influence of Blue Light; Mesophyll Cells, and Sucrose. *J. Plant Biol.* 50:523-526.

Kvesitadze G, Khatisashvili G, Sadunishvili T, Ramsden JJ, 2006. *Biochemical Mechanisms of Detoxification in Higher Plants: Basis of Phytoremediation.* Berlin, Heidelberg, Germany: Springer-Verlag.

Kvesitadze K, Sadunishvili T, Kvesitadze G, 2009. Mechanisms of Organic Contaminants Uptake and Degradation in Plants. *World Academy of Sci., Engineering & Technol.* 55:458-468.

Larcher W, 2003. *Physiological Plant Ecology: Ecophysiology and Stress Physiology of Functional Groups*, Fourth Edition. Berlin, Heidelberg, Germany: Springer-Verlag.

McCutcheon SC, Schnoor JL (Eds.), 2003. *Phytoremediation: Transformation and Control of Contaminants.* Hoboken, New Jersey, USA: Wiley/Interscience.

Medinsky MA, Valentine JL, 2001. Toxicokinetics. In *Casarett and Doull's Toxicology: The Basic Science of Poisons* (Klaassen CD, Ed.). New York, New York, USA: McGraw-Hill, Chapter 7.

Purves WK, Orians GH, Heller HC, 1995. *Life: The Science of Biology*, Fourth Edition. Sunderland, Massachusetts, USA: Sinauer Associates.

Schraudner M, Moeder W, Wiese C, van Camp W, Inzé D, Langebartels C, Sandermann H Jr, 1998. Ozone-Induced Oxidative Burst in the Ozone Biomonitor Plant, Tobacco Bel W3. *The Plant J.* 16: 235-245.

Taiz L, Zeiger E, 2006. *Plant Physiology*, Fourth Edition. Massachusetts, USA: Sinauer Associates.

Tarkowska JA, Wacowska M, 1987. The Significance of the Presence of Stomata on Seedling Roots. *Ann. Botany* 61:305-310.

Tsao D (Ed.), 2003. Phytoremediation (Advances in Biochemical Engineering/Biotechnology, No.78). Berlin, Heidelberg, Germany: Springer-Verlag.

Review Questions

1. Briefly explain why this chapter has its focus on systemic effects induced by environmental toxicants, rather than on localized effects.

2. Name the major biochemical events (phases) involved in the disposition of toxicants inside a biological system.

3. Briefly describe the five common mechanisms of entry enabling or aiding toxicants to get inside an organism's body or to cross the body's cellular membranes.

4. What are the two common ways in which terrestrial plants can take up environmental contaminants?

5. Why are biomembranes permeable to only certain toxicants?

6. Which *structural* component of a plant leaf (or root) is most responsible for uptake of environmental pollutants?

7. How is phytoremediation related to the uptake of toxicants by plant roots?

8. What type of toxicants tends to be absorbed easily by the human skin, and why?

9. Which of the three main human skin layers is most responsible for distributing the absorbed toxicants to the blood, and why?

10. In what way would inhaled foreign particles be removed from the respiratory tract to enter the gastrointestinal tract?

11. Briefly explain why a toxicant stored in a depot can become a serious health hazard or threat.

12. What are the primary functions of the portal venous system, and of the enterohepatic circulation?

13. What are the two main *disposition* processes that are primarily responsible for the delivery of a toxicant to the site of (toxic) action?

14. What is likely to be the elimination half-life $t_{1/2}$ if the toxicant clearance is 20 ml/min and the apparent volume of distribution is 2,000 ml?

15. What are the primary routes of chemical elimination in a mammalian body? And why one of them is the most important?

16. Of the three phases involved in renal excretion (as covered in this chapter), which is the most significant and why?

17. Under what circumstances is intestinal excretion more important than hepatic excretion for fecal elimination of toxicants?

18. What type(s) of toxicants in the blood is (are) eliminated more rapidly and easily via gaseous exchange in the alveolar region?

CHAPTER 8

Metabolism/Biotransformation of Xenobiotics

8.1. Introduction

Contrary to general perception, humans and other mammalians are not physiologically defenseless to the apparently countless environmental toxicants that they may be exposed to. Many environmental toxicants that the human body is exposed to are lipophilic, a biochemical property that enables many toxicants to penetrate various kinds of cellular membranes to some level. In humans, following uptake and absorption, these foreign substances are distributed via the bloodstream and the lymphatic system to various body parts, including the excretory organs where the xenobiotics can be eliminated. While the xenobiotics are in various body tissues and organs, many are known to undergo biotransformation, a process whereby a substance is transformed from one chemical form or species to another by one or more biochemical reactions.

Biotransformation of toxicants is commonly thought as synonymous with the biochemical process known as *metabolism* (a.k.a. *metabolic conversions*). Yet metabolism includes other biochemical events basic to cellular *homeostasis,* which is the tendency of a cell to maintain a stable internal environment. Further discussion on this distinction is given in Section 8.1.1 for a due appreciation of the basic attribute defining life. Closely related to this attribute is the set of nutritional factors that affects the biotransformation and hence the toxicity of toxicants. Biotransformation and metabolic reactions are mostly enzymatic in nature, as virtually all of them are catalyzed by one or more enzymes in the body. Accordingly, one important prerequisite to learning chemical biotransformation is a knowledge of the basic functions of enzymes. And it is for this very purpose that a brief introduction on (biotransforming) enzymes and their actions is given in Section 8.1.2.

8.1.1. Metabolism *vs.* Biotransformation

Biotransformation is for the most part limited to studying the chemical fate of xenobiotics that have entered the body. It is a topic directly and extremely relevant to toxicology. Metabolism, on the other hand, is a broader term used to define the sum total of all chemical processes and events occurring in living organisms that results in basic life functions such as growth, energy production, and elimination of waste materials. Therefore, along with growth and reproduction, metabolism is regarded as one of the most critical attributes that define life.

More specifically, metabolism refers to those biochemical reactions that take place in living cells so that the cells as well as the body can sustain their life by maintaining a homeostatic environment which requires, among other things, a constant energy supply to the body cells, a constant body temperature, and a constant blood sugar level. Insofar as cells in the body must perform a vast variety of chemical, mechanical, electrical, and osmotic activities, a continuous supply of energy for these basic body functions is indispensable. The two principal sets of metabolic conversions are known as *catabolism* and *anabolism*. Catabolism is the set of metabolic reactions that breaks down large molecules (e.g., the macronutrients carbohydrates, lipids, and proteins) into smaller units to release energy as a by-product. Many times, the term *catabolism* is loosely used interchangeably with *metabolism*. In contrast, anabolism is the set of metabolic reactions that synthesizes molecules from smaller units, usually powered by the energy released from catabolic reactions.

Metabolism is frequently studied under two closely related subspecialties: cellular (or cell) metabolism; and nutrient (or nutritional) metabolism. Cellular metabolism studies the sum of chemical reactions that transpire within cells. In contrast, nutrient metabolism is concerned with the molecular fate of nutrients and other dietary compounds in the body, including all facets of nutritional biochemistry that have crucial effects on chemical biotransformation (Section 10.3).

8.1.2. Biotransforming Enzymes and Their Actions

Enzymes are proteins mostly of globular shape and all capable of catalyzing biochemical reactions, and are common targets of drugs and environmental toxicants. Enzymes work by lower the energy required to activate certain biochemical events. This explains why some reaction rates can be millions of times faster when catalyzed by enzymes than when not, as in the case by the antioxidant enzyme *catalase* (Section 8.5.2). Enzymes are generally very specific to the reactions that they catalyze since part of their structure is used as the site (in some cases also known as receptor) where a specific substrate needs to fit in. For this reason, enzymes are each commonly name after the specific reaction or the specific substrate that they catalyze or interact with. Some enzymes can exert their catalytic function to their fullness without any additional component. Others require the binding with non-protein molecules termed *cofactors*. If the cofactor is an *organic* compound, it is more specifically referred to as *coenzyme*. Examples of (inorganic) cofactors and (organic) coenzymes in chemical biotransformation are given in Section 8.6.4.

Several groups of enzymes are regarded as particularly important to toxicologists studying chemical biotransformation. Accordingly, enzymes in these special groups are further characterized in some detail below, following Sections 8.2 and 8.3 given on the basic sequence and enzymatic processes involved in chemical biotransformation.

8.2. General Sequence/Processes of Biotransformation

Upon uptake or absorption, a xenobiotic (e.g., a toxicant) will most likely undergo a sequence of biochemical events referred to as *Phase I* (enzymatic) reactions, then likely followed by one or more *Phase II* (enzymatic) reactions. The typical outcome of a Phase I reaction is a *primary metabolite* that is slightly more polar (i.e., water-soluble) than the parent compound. This change in polarity is accomplished by enzymatically introducing a functional group (e.g., -OH, -SH, -COOH, -NH₂) to the parent compound (now termed *primary metabolite*). It is with or onto these functional groups that the Phase II enzymes (e.g., mostly transferases) and coenzymes (e.g., glucuronic acid) will conjugate, resulting in a complex called conjugate or *intermediate metabolite*. These conjugates are relatively more polar and hence can be more readily excreted from the body.

When the Phase II conjugation is through use of *u*ridine *di*phosphate glucuronic acid (UDP-glucuronic acid, or glucuronic acid for short) as the coenzyme, and (hence) *U*DP-glucuronyl *t*ransferase (UGT) as the enzyme, it is specifically termed *glucuronidation*. Other Phase II specific conjugations, which are not as predominant, are sulfation, methylation, acetylation, and conjugation with glutathione (GSH) or with amino acids (e.g., glycine, glutamine, serine). Note that some xenobiotics that already contain one or more of the required functional groups will bypass Phase I to directly undergo Phase II reactions. An example is phenol (C₆H₅-OH), which has one of the carbons in its benzene ring bonded to a hydroxyl group OH in place of a H atom.

The major aspects of xenobiotic biotransformation are outlined graphically below in Figure 8.1, followed by a discussion on their specifics and importance.

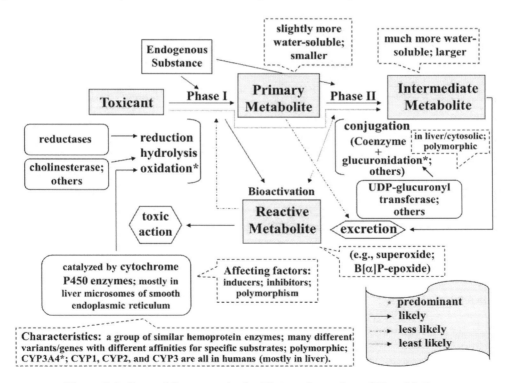

Figure 8.1. General Processes in the Biotransformation of Xenobiotics

8.2.1. Phase I Enzymatic Reactions

As shown in Figure 8.1, Phase I enzymatic reactions include predominantly *oxidation* and less so *reduction, hydrolysis, hydration, dehydrochlorination*, as well as several others. These reactions are catalyzed or mediated by enzymes available much more in the smooth-surfaced endoplasmic reticulum than in the cytosol or other organelles. For enzymes located in the endoplasmic reticulum, they are referred to as the microsomal kind.

A. Oxidation

This group typically involves the *addition* of one oxygen, the *removal* of one hydrogen, and a *loss* of electrons (thus resulting in an increase in valence as well as in binding capacity). The reactions in this group are mediated predominantly by cytochrome P450 enzymes and less so by other mixed-function oxidases (MFO), by alcohol dehydrogenase, or by aldehyde dehydrogenase. The predominant oxidative reaction is of the *mono-oxygenation* type (i.e., with the addition of *one* oxygen), as generalized in Reaction 8.1:

$$X\text{-}H + O_2 + 2H^+ + 2e^- \rightarrow X\text{-}OH + H_2O \tag{8.1}$$

where X-H is the xenobiotic (i.e., substrate), and X-OH is the resultant primary metabolite product. A closely related enzyme important to this type of oxidation, but not always necessary, is NADPH-cytochrome P450 reductase. This reductase can serve as an important electron donor for the oxygenase cytochrome P450. When a substrate binds to the active site (which is around the heme group) of cytochrome P450, such a binding favors the transfer of an electron from NADP-H (nicotinamide adenine dinucleotide phosphate) through the cytochrome reductase or another related reductase (Sligar *et al.*, 1979) to the heme group. The cytochrome P450 reductase contains both the flavin FAD (Section 8.6.4), which can accept electrons from $NADP^+$, and the flavin FMN (Section 8.6.4), which can donate electrons to the oxygenase cytochrome P450.

Oxidative reactions include numerous specific kinds, such as hydroxylation, dealkylation, deamination, and epoxidation. Hydroxylation adds the functional group -OH to the parent compound. Oxidative dealkylation involves the removal of an alkyl group, such as the methyl (CH_3) or ethyl (C_2H_5) group, from the parent compound. Oxidative deamination removes an amine (NH_3). Epoxidation requires the interaction with oxygen molecules. The substrate in this case is usually an alkene (i.e., an unsaturated chemical compound containing at least one carbon-carbon double bond). The resultant epoxide functional group consists of a three-member ring with an oxygen atom bonded to two carbon atoms that (usually) are already bonded to each other. Of the four oxidative reactions noted above, hydroxylation is the most predominate in Phase I reactions and produces a functional group that is most ready for Phase II reactions.

B. Reduction

This group chemically has the opposite outcome of oxidation. The reactions in this group each typically involve the *removal* of one oxygen, the *addition* of one hydrogen, and a *gain* of electrons. Some representative enzymes are NADPH-cytochrome P450 reductase, nitroreductase, and GSH (glutathione) reductase. An example of this type of reactions is a nitro (NO_2) reduction in which the inexpensive perfume additive *nitrobenzene* (C_6H_5-NO_2) is reduced to the polyurethane precursor *aniline* (C_6H_5-NH_2).

C. Hydrolysis

This group involves the addition of a water molecule to split the substrate (e.g., a toxicant) into two smaller molecular fragments. Some enzymes responsible for Phase I hydrolysis are phosphatases (that removing a phosphate group PO_4^{3-}) and esterases (that splitting esters). Acetylcholinesterase is an esterase, of which highly excessive inhibition in humans (e.g., by organophosphate pesticides) can result in death (Chapters 9 and 15).

8.2.2. Phase II Enzymatic Reactions

Biotransformation reactions in this phase are conjugate or synthetic in action. They aim at attaching polar (hydrophilic) or ionizable (that tending to become an ion) groups to the primary metabolites (e.g., primarily from Phase I) to form products that are relatively larger but otherwise more water-soluble and thereby easier to be excreted in the urine. The coenzymes or endogenous substances that aid in providing the polar or ionizable groups include: UDP-glucuronic acid; S-adenosylmethionine (SAM); 3'-phosphoadenosine-5'-phosphosulfate (PAPS); acetyl coenzyme A (acetyl CoA); GSH (glutathione); and certain amino acids (e.g., glutamine, glycine, serine).

A. Glucuronidation

As discussed earlier, this type of reactions is so termed because the enzyme and coenzyme involved are UGT (UDP-glucuronosyltransferase) and UDP-glucuronic acid, respectively. Glucuronidation is the most predominant type of Phase II reactions in part because the functional group for conjugation is -OH, which is readily produced by hydroxylation (the predominant type of oxidation occurring in Phase I biotransformation). The coenzyme glucuronic acid is highly soluble in water.

B. Sulfation, Methylation, Acetylation, and Others

Phase II includes other specific types of reactions termed *sulfation, methylation, acetylation, amino acid conjugation,* and *GSH (glutathione) conjugation*. The enzymes involved in sulfation, methylation, and acetylation are *sulfo*transferase (SULT), *methyltransferase* (MeT), and *N-acetyltransferase* (NAT), respectively. The coenzymes required are PAPS (3'-phosphoadenosine-5'-phosphosulfate), SAM (S-adenosylmethionine), and acetyl CoA, respectively. The enzyme responsible for GSH conjugation is called glutathione-*S-t*ransferase (GST). GSH, an antioxidant, is a tripeptide consisting of the amino acids *glutamic acid, glycine,* and *cysteine*. For amino acid conjugation, the enzymes involved are not necessarily a transferase. For example, with the amino acid *serine*, it is an enzyme named seryl-t(ransfer)RNA synthetase that is responsible for mediating the ser-ine conjugation of an aromatic hydroxylamine (Parkinson, 2001).

8.3. Other Sequences/Processes of Biotransformation

As depicted in Figure 8.1, not all Phase I reactions lead to the detoxification of toxicants. Phase I may result in the *(bio)activation* of certain toxicants. It is also probable, though not nearly as frequent, to find that certain Phase II reactions can lead to a *reactive* metabolite. Another type of biotransformation involving neither detoxification nor bioactivation is the routine breakdown (more correctly catabolism) of *endogenous* substances.

8.3.1. Bioactivation of Toxicants

A familiar example of toxicant bioactivation is the biotransformation of the naturally occurring mycotoxin aflatoxin B_1 to an epoxide metabolite (aflatoxin B_1-2,3-epoxide), which is more reactive than its parent compound with the mutagenicity of causing (liver) cancer. It was thought that the aflatoxin B_1-DNA adducts found in liver cells was due to the tendency of this epoxide to bind to nuclear DNA (e.g., Croy *et al.*, 1978; Swenson *et al.*, 1977). A DNA adduct, which involves a piece covalently bonded to a foreign molecule, is believed to be a critical intermediate on the pathway of chemical carcinogenesis. After all, it is then a DNA in a damaged form and thus with a much greater potential for miscarriage of genetic information for cell division or cell growth (Chapter 18).

Benzo[α]pyrene (BαP), often found in incomplete burning of cigarette smoke and coal, is another chemical that may undergo Phase I reactions to yield a reactive epoxide (BαP-7,8-dihydrodiol-9,10-epoxide), which is believed to act as an ultimate carcinogen (e.g., Smart, 2004). The main difference between the two bioactivation mechanisms is that for BαP, it is a two-step epoxidation whereas for aflatoxin B_1, a direct one.

Still another familiar case is the bioactivation of carbon tetrachloride (CCl_4) to the tri-chloromethyl free radical $CCl_3 \cdot$ leading to the initiation of lipid peroxidation (Chapter 9) and later to the formation of lipid-protein adducts (Parinandi *et al.*, 1990; Trostchansky and Rubbo, 2007). Lipid peroxidation refers to a biochemical phenomenon in which un-saturated lipids undergo oxidative degradation, as initiated by a free radical stealing electrons from the lipids on nearby cell membranes to cause structural damage there.

A third pathway leading to bioactivation of toxicants is *N*-hydroxylation, which is a special kind of hydroxylation involving specifically the oxidation of the N atom in the NH_2-group of an organic compound. *N*-hydroxylation is the initial step in activating the aromatic amine benzidine ($(C_6H_4NH_2)_2$) (Morton *et al.*, 1979), which was linked to bladder cancer and used in high quantities in the past to produce dyes in cloth, paper, and leather.

8.3.2. Biotransformation of Endogenous Substances

Both the Phase I and Phase II reactions can biotransform not only xenobiotics but also endogenous substances. The cytochrome P450 enzymes in Phase I are involved in the oxidative metabolism of many endogenous substances. Bile acids are synthesized in the liver by oxidation of cholesterol mediated by cytochrome P450. Many other endogenous substances like thyroid hormones and bilirubin can undergo glucuronidation. Both glucuronidation and sulfation of the sex hormone testosterone were demonstrated in human livers (e.g., Pacifici *et al.*, 1997). Strictly speaking, these types of Phase I and Phase II reactions are *metabolic conversions*, not part of the typical *biotransformation* processes.

8.4. Characteristics of Cytochrome P450 Enzymes

As reflected in Section 8.2.1, the most important and common enzyme group responsible for biotransformation in Phase I is cytochrome P450 enzymes (a.k.a. P450 enzymes, CYP 450s, or P450s for short). P450 enzymes are a large and diverse superfamily of hemoproteins found in most tissues of most living organisms. These enzymes, of which the most common is the monooxygenase kind, use either exogenous or endogenous substances as substrates in the catalytic reactions. P450 enzymes represent most of the monooxygenases known (which are also referred to as *mixed*-function oxidases in that each of the two oxygen atoms in Reaction 8.1 is used for a *different* function). In most situations, P450 enzymes play a key role in the detoxification of xenobiotics. These enzymes derived their popular name P450 from the complex between their ferrous (Fe^{2+}) heme center and the carbon monoxide (CO) molecule that absorbs light maximally at wavelength 450 nm. Their official name now is CYP (standing for *cy*tochrome *P*450).

8.4.1. Families of Cytochrome P450

There are numerous genetic variants (i.e., isoforms) of P450s (i.e., numerous forms with each derived from a specific gene) which are classified according to the similarities of their amino acid sequences *genetically* encoded by the DNA in the body. The *family* names for all CYP isoforms (also called CYP iso[en]zymes) are *numbered*, such as CYP*2* or CYP*3*. There are over 70 families used to describe the P450s, of which about 20% have been identified in humans. The CYP families have their own *sub*families each identified by a *letter*, such as CYP2*C* and CYP3*A*. The subfamilies in turn have their specific genes each identified by a *number* again, such as CYP3A*4* and CYP2B*29*. Among the diverse *human* CYP enzyme genes, CYP3A4 is the most abundant and most important in oxidative reactions (e.g., Keshava *et al.*, 2004; Eichelbaum and Burk, 2001).

8.4.2. Catalytic Activities and Cellular Locations

The catalytic activities of P450s vary greatly in different people as well as in different races. Genetic variation in a population group is termed *polymorphism* when both alleles (variant forms of the same gene pair) exist with a frequency of at least 1 percent. Such a (genetic) polymorphism may have profound clinical consequences, given that people with different CYP genotypes may need to follow different dosage schemes for certain drug treatments. Many P450s can be *induced* (i.e., with their catalytic activities speeded up) by drugs (e.g., phenobarbital), insecticides (e.g., mirex), and polycyclic aromatic hydrocarbons (e.g., BαP). Yet more importantly, many of the same or other P450s can be *inhibited* (slowed down) by drugs (e.g., certain antifungals), substances in tobacco smoke (e.g., BαP), and natural products (e.g., a constituent of grapefruit juice).

Although P450s (and most Phase II and other Phase I enzymes as well) are found in virtually all body tissues in most mammalians, their highest concentrations involved in the biotransformation of toxicants are present in the hepatic (i.e., liver) microsomes (i.e., those small vesicles) of the smooth-surfaced endoplasmic reticulum (*see* Figure 9.1), with small quantities contained in the cytosol (i.e., the soluble fraction of the cytoplasm). The mitochondria, lysosomes, and nuclei in the hepatic cell each contain even smaller quantities of this versatile group of biotransforming enzymes.

8.5. Characteristics of Other Relevant Enzyme Groups

Many specific enzyme groups other than cytochrome P450 are also involved in the biotransformation of xenobiotics. Many Phase I enzymes other than cytochrome P450 are not as commonly known in the general discussion of chemical biotransformation, but in some cases are equally important. For example, like NADPH-dependent cytochrome P450 reductase (Section 8.2.1.A), carbonyl reductase also belongs to the family of oxidoreductases. This reductase, located primarily in the cytosol, can catalyze the reduction of ketones (e.g., pentoxifylline) to secondary alcohols (Parkinson, 2001). Another example is epoxide hydrolase, which is located largely in the microsomes and cytosol. It belongs to a subcategory of the hydrolytic enzyme group that includes esterases, dehalogenases, and phosphatases. This hydrolase can play the dual role in activating BαP to a tumorigenic epoxide and in detoxifying BαP's other epoxide to a more stable, less toxic product (Parkinson, 2001). Carboxylesterase and (acetyl)cholinesterase are esterases involved in the Phase I hydrolysis. The basic mechanism for the latter's enzymatic inhibition that can lead to severe health effects is discussed in Chapters 9 and 15.

Those enzymes that are naturally involved in Phase II reactions, along with antioxidant enzymes and a monooxygenase encoded by the CYP1A1 gene, are considered as either highly relevant to the biotransformation of xenobiotics or particularly intriguing to environmental toxicologists. Their characteristics are thus specifically highlighted below.

8.5.1. Enzymes in Phase II Reactions

As with cytochrome P450s, and almost an exception among all Phase II enzymes, UGTs (UDP-glucuronyl transferases) are located predominately in hepatic microsomes. Other Phase II enzymes are primarily cytosolic, as they are not bound to membranes but occur free within the cytoplasm. At least 15 variants of human UGTs have been identified (Tukey and Strassburg, 2000). Depending on the level involved, a (hereditary) deficiency in this enzyme can cause hyperbilirubinemia known either as Gilbert's syndrome involving *mild* jaundice or as Crigler-Nijar syndrome involving *severe* jaundice.

Sulfotransferases (SULTs) are widely distributed in tissues, of which at least three isoforms have been identified in humans. Although these enzymes act as a major detoxification system in the human adult and developing fetus, they are capable of bioactivating precarcinogens to reactive electrophile species which can potentially affect gene expression (Gamage *et al.*, 2006).

Methyltransferases (*N*-MeT, *O*-MeT, *S*-MeT) as a group are commonly found in the cytosol and microsomes but have a minor role in Phase II detoxification. This is because many functional groups (e.g., -*N*H, -*O*H, -*S*H) to which a MeT will transfer the methyl group (CH$_3$) from its coenzyme SAM are subject to Phase I oxidation first. Two distinct isoforms of *N*-acetyltransferases (NATs), known as NAT1 and NAT2, are found with overlapping substrate specificities in humans (e.g., Payton *et al.*, 2001). The two isozymes are able to mediate the detoxification of a number of arylamine and hydrazine drugs. A somewhat related form named acyl-CoA amino acid:*N*-acyltransferase is known to catalyze glycine and some other amino acid conjugations.

8.5.2. Antioxidant Enzymes

Antioxidants are molecules or substances capable of preventing or slowing down the oxidative stress to body cells. Oxidation reactions tend to produce free radicals to start a chain reaction by stealing electrons from neighboring molecules which then become free radicals. Antioxidants can either inhibit oxidation reactions by being oxidized themselves or terminate these chain reactions by removing free radical intermediates. This explains why they are frequently referred to as *free radical scavengers*. Vitamin E, vitamin C, β-carotene (precursor of vitamin A), and the chemical element selenium (Se) are the most common antioxidants found in human foods. Phytochemicals known to have antioxidant function include: allyl sulfides (e.g., *as from* onions, garlic); carotenoids (e.g., fruits, carrots); flavonoids (e.g., fruits, vegetables); and polyphenols (e.g., tea, grapes).

Another group of antioxidants are certain enzymes, which are endogenous substances as they are synthesized within the body. Superoxide dismutase (SOD), GSH peroxidase (GPx), and catalase (CAT) are the three mostly investigated antioxidant enzymes. Other less common enzymes with antioxidant activity include GSH reductase, thioredoxin reductase, and heme oxygenase.

As its name implies, SOD (superoxide dismutase) has the ability to convert *two* superoxide anion radicals (O$_2^-$·) into one hydrogen peroxide (H$_2$O$_2$) and one oxygen (O·). However, without the further removal of hydrogen peroxide by GPx or CAT, the dismutation by SOD generally would be of little value since hydrogen peroxide is a strong oxidant. There are three major families of SOD, depending on the metal(s) it has in its reactive center as the cofactor(s): the Cu (copper) and Zn (zinc) type; the Fe (iron) or Mn (manganese) type; and the Ni (nickel) type. In humans (and in all other mammals and most chordates), three forms of SOD are present: SOD1 containing Cu and Zn, located in the cytoplasm; SOD2 containing Mn, located in the mitochondria; and SOD3 containing also Cu and Zn, but located outside the cell. The physiological importance of the various forms of SOD was evident from the severe pathologies found in mice genetically engineered to lack these enzymes. For instance, mice lacking SOD2 were found death several days after birth, amid massive oxidative stress (Li *et al.*, 1995). *Drosophila* lacking SOD1 had a dramatically shortened lifespan (Reveillaud et al, 1994; Woodruff *et al.*, 2004); and these flies lacking SOD2 died hours after birth (Duttaroy *et al.*, 2003).

Catalase (CAT) is found in nearly all living aerobic organisms where it functions to catalyze the decomposition of hydrogen peroxide (H_2O_2) to water and oxygen (Chelikani *et al.*, 2004). This antioxidant is a heme-containing redox (oxidation-reduction) enzyme present in high concentrations in a cellular compartment called peroxisome. It has one of the highest turnover rates of all enzymes. One molecule of CAT is reportedly capable of converting millions of H_2O_2 molecules to water and oxygen per second (Allaby, 2009). Hydrogen peroxide is a harmful by-product of many normal cellular reactions.

As noted earlier, a glutathione peroxidase (GPx) can also break down hydrogen peroxide. Glutathione peroxidase is the general name for members in the enzyme family with peroxidase activity. Its main function is to protect living organisms against oxidative stress (and hence damage) by breaking down hydrogen peroxide and by reducing lipid hydroperoxides to their corresponding alcohols. Hydroperoxides are monosubstitution products of hydrogen peroxide having the basic structure of RO-OH, where R is any organyl group. There are several GPx isozymes encoded by different genes, with most containing selenium as the cofactor. In mammalians, at least 5 GPx isoforms (as GPx1 through GPx5) have been reported (Singh *et al.*, 2006). The GPx1 isoform is reportedly the most abundant in mice (de Haan *et al.*, 1998; Potter *et al.*, 2005), and has been linked to an increased risk of cardiovascular events in humans (Blankenberg *et al.*, 2003).

8.5.3. EROD (7-Ethoxyresorufin *O*-Deethylase)

EROD is a P450-dependent monooxygenase encoded for by the CYP1A1 gene (e.g., Kerzee and Ramos, 2001). These days, EROD is known more commonly as an assay, rather than as an enzyme, used to monitor the induced activity of CYP1A1. The activity of EROD *per se* is widely used as a biomarker for exposure of wildlife and fish to polycyclic aromatic hydrocarbons (PAHs) as well as to structurally similar compounds such as PCBs (polychlorinated biphenyls) and dioxins. The receptive site in certain cellular proteins is specifically prone to bind with this type of organic compounds and is thereby called *a*ryl *h*ydrocarbon (Ah) receptor. Activation of Ah binding with PAH type compounds, particularly with dioxin, was reported to be one of the (first) steps leading to the induction of CYP1A1 in the body (Ma, 2001).

More specifically, when the body is exposed to a PAH type compound, the Ah receptors in the body cells will aggressively bind to that compound's molecules. Such bindings will mediate an increased concentration of CYP1A1 in the body. And such a mediation in turn will increase the catalytic activity of CYP1A1 on EROD. Therefore, a measured increase in EROD should reflect an increased exposure to the PAH type compound under study. The application of EROD activity as an exposure assessment technique in this way has increased in recent years. The increased acceptance of EROD's application to monitor the enzymatic activity of CYP1A1 is largely due to the relatively inexpensive and rapid techniques available for measuring this P450-dependent monooxygenase (e.g., Kennedy and Jones, 1994; Pohl and Fouts, 1980).

8.6. Factors Affecting Biotransformation

Many factors that affect the adverse action of toxicants, which is the topic covered extensively in Chapter 10, are also ones that affect the relative effectiveness and efficiency of chemical biotransformation. These factors, applying across most species, include: dose levels; exposure duration; species; age; gender; genetic variability; health status; nutrition; and exposure to inducers or inhibitors of Phase I and Phase II enzymes.

When compared to cytochrome P450s, most other Phase I and most Phase II enzymes are also polymorphic although in most cases to a less extent. The activities of these non-P450 enzymes too can be induced or inhibited by certain cofactors, coenzymes, or other substances. In addition to vitamin E, vitamin C, GSH, and selenium, several antioxidant enzymes discussed in Section 8.5.2 play a key role in the defense against free radical-mediated cellular damage. Certain xenobiotics, such as sodium fluoride (NaF), are found to have the ability to induce or inhibit SOD or GPx, depending on the species involved (e.g., Guo *et al.*, 2003; Lawson and Yu, 2003; Sun *et al.*, 1997).

8.6.1. Genetic Polymorphism

As noted in Section 8.4.2, genetic polymorphism in cytochrome P450s comes with profound clinical consequences. To this date, the main concern with polymorphic P450 expression reportedly has been very much on the development of preclinical drugs (e.g., Pirmohamed and Park, 2003). This is largely owing to the common observation that extensive interindividual variability exists in the biotransformation of drug candidates that are substrates for many of the polymorphic enzymes predominant in Phase I (and at times in Phase II) reactions.

In humans, CYP2D6, CYP2C9, and CYP2C19 polymorphisms reportedly account for the most frequent variations in Phase I metabolism of drugs, as up to 80% of the drugs in use today are metabolized by these three enzymes. Some Africans/African-Americans (~8%), some Caucasians (~7%), and some Asians (~1%) are poor metabolizers as they lack (effective) CYP2D6 in their body (e.g., Abernethy and Flockhart, 2000; Zhou *et al.*, 2009). CYP2C9 is another clinically significant enzyme in that its multiple genetic variants can have variable functional impacts on the efficacy and adverse effects of drugs that the enzyme is responsible for in their elimination from the body (Zhou *et al.*, 2009). CYP2C19 is responsible for the metabolism of a variety of drugs, particularly those that help reduce gastric acid production (Goldstein and de Morais, 1994).

Genetic polymorphism in Phase II enzymes are also found to give rise to abnormal drug biotransformation and greater susceptibility to carcinogens or toxicants in various subpopulations. In particular, an epidemiological study showed that compared to the 197 controls, 97 lung cancer patients in central south China had higher frequencies of GST_{M1}-null or GST_{T1}-null genotype, or both (Chen *et al.*, 2006). Another study showed that the frequency of individuals carrying the GST_{T1}-null genotype was approximately fourfold higher among Egyptian patients with chronic myeloid leukemia than among the controls (Mahmoud *et al.*, 2010).

Among the antioxidant enzymes, SOD appears to be the most investigated to date for its genetic polymorphism effects, particularly those of Mn-SOD in humans. One study showed that this SOD2 polymorphism, along with those of NADPH oxidase and endothelial nitric oxide synthase, significantly increased the risk of hypertension in a group of Taiwanese living in an area known as hyperendemic of arsenic (Hsueh *et al.*, 2005).

8.6.2. Enzyme Inhibitors

Studies showed that many xenobiotics have the ability to inhibit the catalytic activities of Phase I and Phase II enzymes. Many of these xenobiotics are drugs whereas some are phytochemicals or pesticides. These findings have significant clinical implications, in that nearly all drugs used today are metabolized by Phase I or Phase II enzymes and that phytochemicals are treated by many people as nutrients or drug substitutes.

Although medicinal drugs are usually not regarded as environmental toxicants, they may be considered as factors that can affect significantly the biotransformation of toxicants. For instance, patients taking a Phase I enzyme inhibitor drug are expected to have a lower catalytic activity of that enzyme in detoxifying or activating an environmental toxicant in their body. Several chemical inhibitors of GSTs were investigated under this principle for their potential of surpassing or attenuating the resistance of anticancer drugs (e.g., Johansson *et al.*, 2007; Mahajan and Atkins, 2005; Mathew *et al.*, 2006; Pratt *et al.*, 1994; Townsend and Tew, 2003).

Drugs and phytochemicals are not the only groups of xenobiotics capable of inhibiting the activities of Phase I and Phase II enzymes. Certain pesticides and their metabolites are notorious inhibitors of some of these enzymes. In particular, the organochlorine pesticide methoxychlor is known to interfere with the catalytic activity of CYP2B6 (Hodgson and Rose, 2007). Examples of Phase I and Phase II enzyme inhibitors, including methoxychlor, are listed in Table 8.1.

8.6.3. Enzyme Inducers

Also included in Table 8.1 are examples of drugs and non-medicinal substances having the ability to *induce* the catalytic activities of Phase I and Phase II enzymes. Among these enzyme inducers, the predominant group appears to be drugs again such as ritonavir (anti-HIV) and fluconazole (antifungal) that are actively used today. On the non-drug list, mirex and kepone represent some of the strong Phase I enzyme inducers. These two organochlorine pesticides are reportedly capable of inducing CYP2B1 in mouse hepatic microsomes (Lewandowski *et al.*, 2006).

Table 8.1. Select Inhibitors and Inducers of Phase I and Phase II Enzymes in
the Biotransformation of Xenobiotics

Substance	Type/Source	Affected Enzyme(s)[a,b]
	A. Enzyme Inhibitors	
fluconazole	antifungal	CYP2C19 (a)
disulfiram	antabuse	CYP2E1 (a)
fluoxetine	antidepressant	CYP2D6 (a), CYP3A4 (b)
ritonavir	anti-HIV	CYP3A4 (a, b)
dicofenac	anti-inflammatory	UGT (c, d)
probenecid	uricosuric	UGT (c)
flunitrazepam	sedative	UGT (d)
ethacrynic acid	diuretic	GST (e)
TLK99	Anti-hematologic	GST (e)
safrole	black pepper	CYP1A2 (f), CYP2A6 (f), CYP2E1 (f)
resveratrol	grape skin, wine	CYP1A1 (g), UGT1A1 (g)
silybin	milk thistle	CYP2C9 (h), CYP3A4 (h)
silymarin	milk thistle	UGT (i)
flavonoids	grapefruit juice	CYP3A4 (j)
methoxychlor	organochlorine pesticide	CYP2B6 (k)
	B. Enzyme Inducers	
phenobarbital	anticonvulsant	CYP2B6 (a), CYP3A4 (a)
rifampin	antibiotic	CYP2B6 (a), CYP2C19 (a), CYP3A4 (a)
carbamazepine	anticonvulsant	CYP3A4 (a)
phenytoin	anticonvulsant	CYP2B6 (a), CYP3A4 (a, b)
ethanol	alcohol	CYP2E1 (a)
glucosinolate	cruciferous vegetables	CYP1A2 (a, j)
PAHs[b]	charcoal-broiled meat[b]	CYP1A2 (a, j)
isoflavones	phytochemical	Phase II enzymes (l, m, n)
sulforaphane	cruciferous vegetables	Phase II enzymes (o)
mirex	organochlorine pesticide	CYP2B1 (p)
kepone	organochlorine pesticide	CYP2B1 (p)

[a]as reported in: (a) Parkinson (2001); (b) Zhou (2008); (c) Uchaipichat *et al.* (2004); (d) Ghosal *et al.* (2004); (e) Mathew *et al.* (2006); (f) Ueng *et al.* (2005); (g) Leung *et al.* (2009); (h) Jančová *et al.* (2007); (i) D'Andrea *et al.* (2005); (j) Ensom and Blouin (2006); (k) Hodgson and Rose (2007); (l) Appelt and Reicks (1999); (m) Froyen *et al.* (2009); (n) Mikulcik and Fischer (2001); (o) Fahey and Talay (1999); (p) Lewandowski *et al.* (2006).

[b]CYP = cytochrome P450 (Phase I); UGT = UDP-glucuronosyltransferase (Phase II); GST = glutathione S-transferase (Phase II); PAHs = polycyclic aromatic hydrocarbons, also from tobacco smoke.

Inducers of Phase II enzymes apparently have not been investigated to the same extent. Nonetheless, isoflavones in soy, primarily genistein and quercetin, have been under extensive investigation for their potential as inducers in protecting Phase II enzyme activities (e.g., Appelt and Reicks, 1999; Froyen *et al.*, 2009; Mikulcik and Fischer, 2001). Sulforaphane, an anticancer as well as an antimicrobial chemical, is also considered as a strong inducer of Phase II enzymes (e.g., Fahey and Talalay, 1999). This chemical is an organosulfur compound extractable from cruciferous vegetables, particularly broccoli.

8.6.4. Enzyme Cofactors and Coenzymes

In general, most enzymes including those in Phase I and Phase II occur in two biochemical forms termed *apoenzymes* and *holoenzymes*. Apoenzymes are those not bound to a cofactor and not biochemically active, whereas holoenzymes are those bound to one or more required cofactors (e.g., Sauke *et al.*, 2001). In chemical biotransformation, a cofactor is more specifically defined as any *inorganic* substance required to ensure the enzyme's full biochemical capacity. Such a cofactor is referred to as the prosthetic group to the apoenzyme, and is generally *tightly* bound to the enzyme (now called holoenzyme). Many cofactors are metal ions, such as Cu^{2+}, Fe^{2+}, Fe^{3+}, Mg^{2+}, and Zn^{2+}.

If the substance so required is a non-protein *organic* compound, it is commonly called *coenzyme* and is typically bound *loosely* to the enzyme. Some common coenzymes such as glucuronic acid, SAM, and PAPS are introduced in Section 8.2.2. Many other common ones are either vitamins or their derivatives: biotin; vitamin C; CoA (coenzyme A) from vitamin B_5; NAD^+ (nicotine adenine dinucleotide) and $NADP^+$ (nicotine adenine dinucleotide phosphate) from niacin (vitamin B_3); and FMN (flavin mononucleotide) and FAD (flavin adenine dinucleotide) from riboflavin (vitamin B_2). Examples of other coenzymes not vitamin-based and not specific to Phase II enzymes include: heme; ATP (adenosine-5'-triphosphate); GSH (glutathione); and CoB (coenzyme B).

References

Abernethy DR, Flockhart DA, 2000. Molecular Basis of Cardiovascular Drug Metabolism: Implications for Predicting Clinically Important Drug Interactions. *Circulation* 101:1749-1753.

Allaby M, 2009. Catalase. *Oxford Dictionary of Zoology*, Third Edition. New York, New York, USA: Oxford University Press.

Appelt LC, Reicks MM, 1999. Soy Induces Phase II Enzymes But Does Not Inhibit Dimethylbenz[a]anthracene-Induced Carcinogenesis in Female Rats. *J. Nutri.* 129:1820-1826.

Blankenberg S, Rupprecht HJ, Bickel C, Torzewski M, Hafner G, Tiret L, Smieja M, Cambien F, Meyer J, Lackner KJ, 2003. Glutathione Peroxidase 1 Activity and Cardiovascular Events in Patients with Coronary Artery Disease. *NEJM* 349:1605-1613.

Chelikani P, Fita I, Loewen PC, 2004. Diversity of Structures and Properties among Catalases. *Cell. Mol. Life Sci.* 61:192–208.

Chen HC, Cao YF, Hu WX, Liu XF, Liu QX, Zhang J, Liu J, 2006. Genetic Polymorphisms of Phase II Metabolic Enzymes and Lung Cancer Susceptibility in a Population of Central South China. *Dis. Markers* 22:141-52.

Croy RG, Essigmann JM, Reinhold VN, Wogan GN, 1978. Identification of the Principal Aflatoxin B1-DNA Adduct Formed *in vivo* in Rat Liver. *Proc. Natl. Acad. Sci.* USA 75:1745-1749.

D'Andrea V, Perez LM, Pozzi EJS, 2005. Inhibition of Rat Liver UDP-Glucuronosyltransferase by Silymarin and the Metabolite Silibinin-Glucuronide. *Life Sci.* 77:683-692.

de Haan JB, Bladier C, Griffiths P, Kelner M, O'Shea RD, Cheung NS, Bronson RT, Silvestro MJ, Wild S, Zheng SS, Beart PM, Hertzog PJ, Kola I, 1998. Mice with a Homozygous Null Mutation for the Most Abundant Glutathione Peroxidase, Gpx1, Show Increased Susceptibility to the Oxidative Stress-Inducing Agents Paraquat and Hydrogen Peroxide. *J. Biol. Chem.* 273: 22528-22536.

Duttaroy A, Paul A, Kundu M, Belton A, 2003. A Sod2 Null Mutation Confers Severely Reduced Adult Life Span in *Drosophila. Genetics* 165:2295-2299.

Eichelbaum M, Burk O, 2001. CYP3A Genetics in Drug Metabolism. *Natl. Med.* 7:285-287.

Ensom MH, Blouin RA, 2006. Dietary Influences on Drug Disposition. In *Applied Pharmacokinetics and Pharmacodynamics: Principles of Therapeutic Drug Monitoring* (Burton ME, Shaw LM, Schentag JJ, Evans WE, Eds.), Fourth Edition. Baltimore, Maryland, USA: Lippincott Williams & Wilkins, Chapter 12.

Fahey JW, Talalay P, 1999. Antioxidant Functions of Sulforaphane: A Potent Inducer of Phase II Detoxication Enzymes. *Food Chem. Toxicol.* 37:973-979.

Froyen EB, Reeves JL, Mitchell AE, Steinberg FM, 2009. Regulation of Phase II Enzymes by Genistein and Daidzein in Male and Female Swiss Webster Mice. *J. Med. Food* 12:1227-1237.

Gamage N, Barnett A, Hempel N, Duggleby RG, Windmill KF, Martin JL, McManus ME, 2006. Human Sulfotransferases and Their Role in Chemical Metabolism. *Toxicol. Sci.* 90:5-22.

Ghosal A, Hapangama N, Yuan Y, Achanfuo-Yeboah J, Iannucci R, Chowdhury S, Alton K, Patrick JE, Zbaida S, 2004. Identification of Human UDP-Glucuronosyltransferase Enzyme(s) Responsible for the Glucuronidation of Ezetimibe (Zetia). *Drug Metab. Disp.* 32:314-320.

Goldstein JA, de Morais SM, 1994. Biochemistry and Molecular Biology of the Human CYP2C Subfamily. *Pharmacogenetics* 4:285-299.

Guo X-Y, Sun G-F, Sun Y-C, 2003. Oxidative Stress from Fluoride-Induced Hepatotoxicity in Rats. *Fluoride* 36:25-29.

Hodgson E, Rose RL, 2007. The Importance of Cytochrome P450 2B6 in the Human Metabolism of Environmental Chemicals. *Pharmacol. Ther.* 113:420-428.

Hsueh Y-M, Lin P, Chen H-W, Shiue H-S, Chung C-J, Tsai C-T, Huang Y-K, Chiou H-Y, Chen C-J, 2005. Genetic Polymorphisms of Oxidative and Antioxidant Enzymes and Arsenic-Related Hypertension. *J. Toxicol. Environ. Health* 68:1471-1484.

Jančová P, Anzenbacherová E, Papoušková B, Lemr K, Lužná P, Veinlichová A, Anzenbacher P, Šimánek V, 2007. Silybin Is Metabolized by Cytochrome P450 2C8 *in vitro. Drug Metab. Disp.* 35:2035-2039.

Johansson K, Ahlen K, Rinaldi R, Sahlander K, Siritantikorn A, Morgenstern R, 2007. Microsomal Glutathione Transferase 1 in Anticancer Drug Resistance. *Carcinogenesis* 28:465-470.

Kennedy SW, Jones SP, 1994. Simultaneous Measurement of Cytochrome P4501A Catalytic Activity and Total Protein Concentration with a Fluorescence Plate Reader. *Biochemistry* 222:217-223.

Kerzee JK, Ramos KS, 2001. Constitutive and Inducible Expression of Cyp1a1 and Cyp1b1 in Vascular Smooth Muscle Cells: Role of the Ahr bHLH/PAS Transcription Factor. *Circulation Res.* 89:573-582.

Keshava C, McCanlies EC, Weston A, 2004. CYP3A4 Polymorphisms – Potential Risk Factors for Breast and Prostate Cancer: A HuGE Review. *Am. J. Epid.* 160:825-841.

Lawson P, Yu MH, 2003. Fluoride Inhibition of Superoxide Dimutase (SOD) from the Earthworm *Eisenia fetida*. *Fluoride* 36:143-151.

Leung HY, Yung LH, Shia G, Lua A-L, Leung LK, 2009. The Red Wine Polyphenol Resveratrol Reduces Polycyclic Aromatic Hydrocarbon-Induced DNA Damage in MCF-10A Cells. *Nutri. Toxicol.* 102:1462-1468.

Lewandowski M, Levi P, Hodgson E, 2006. Induction of Cytochrome P-450 Isozymes by Mirex and Chlordecone. *J. Biochem. Toxicol.* 4:195-199.

Li Y, Huang TT, Carlson EJ, Melov S, Ursell PC, Olson JL, Noble LJ, Yoshimura MP, Berger C, Chan PH, Wallace DC, Epstein CJ, 1995. Dilated Cardiomyopathy and Neonatal Lethality in Mutant Mice Lacking Manganese Superoxide Dismutase. *Natl. Genet.* 11:376-381.

Ma Q, 2001. Induction of CYP1A1. The AhR/DRE Paradigm: Transcription, Receptor Regulation, and Expanding Biological Roles. *Curr. Drug Metab.* 2:149-164.

Mahajan S, Atkins WM, 2005. The Chemistry and Biology of Inhibitors and Pro-Drugs Targeted to Glutathione S-Transferases. *Cell. Mol. Life Sci.* 62:1221-1233.

Mahmoud S, Labib DA, Khalifa RH, Abu Khalil RE, Marie MA, 2010. CYP1A1, GSTM1 and GSTT1 Genetic Polymorphism in Egyptian Chronic Myeloid Leukemia Patients. *Res. J. Immunol.* 3:12-21.

Mathew N, Kalyanasundaram M, Balaraman K, 2006. Glutathione S-Transferase (GST) Inhibitors. *Expert Opinion on Therap. Patents* 16:431-444.

Mikulcik EM, Fischer JG, 2001. Possible Mechanism for Protective Effect of the Flavonoid Quercetin. *J. Am. Diet. Assoc.* 101(Suppl):A35.

Morton KC, King CM, Baetcke, KP, 1979. Metabolism of Benzidine to N-Hydroxy-N, N'-Diacetylbenzidine and Subsequent Nucleic Acid Binding and Mutagenicity. *Cancer Res.* 39:3107-3113.

Pacifici GM, Gucci A, Giuliani L, 1997. Testosterone Sulphation and Glucuronidation in the Human Liver: Interindividual Variability. *Eur. J. Drug Metab. Pharmacokinet.* 22:253-258.

Parinandi NL, Weis BK, Natarajan V, Schmid HH, 1990. Peroxidative Modification of Phospholipids in Myocardial Membranes. *Arch. Biochem. Biophy.* 280:45-52.

Parkinson A, 2001. Biotransformation of Xenobiotics. In *Casarett and Doull's Toxicology: The Basic Science of Poisons* (Klaassen CD, Ed.) New York, New York, USA: McGraw-Hill, Chapter 6.

Payton M, Mushtaq A, Yu T-W, Wu L-J, Sinclair J, Sim E, 2001. Eubacterial Arylamine N-Acetyltransferases – Identification and Comparison of 18 Members of the Protein Family with Conserved Active Site Cysteine, Histidine and Aspartate Residues. *Microbiology* 147:1137-1147.

Pirmohamed M, Park BK, 2003. Cytochrome P450 Enzyme Polymorphisms and Adverse Drug Reactions. *Toxicology* 192:23-32.

Pohl RJ, Fouts JR, 1980. A Rapid Method for Assaying the Metabolism of 7-Ethoxyresorufin by Microsomal Subcellular Fractions. *Anal. Biochem.* 107:150-155.

Potter SM, Mitchell AJ, Cowden WB, Sanni LA, Dinauer M, de Haan JB, Hunt NH, 2005. Phagocyte-Derived Reactive Oxygen Species Do Not Influence the Progression of Murine Blood-Stage Malaria Infections. *Infect. & Immun.* 73:4941-4947.

Pratt WB, Ruddon RW, Ensminger WD, Maybaum J, 1994. *The Anticancer Drugs*. New York, New York, USA: Oxford University Press (p.329).

Reveillaud I, Phillips J, Duyf B, Hilliker A, Kongpachith A, Fleming JE, 1994. Phenotypic Rescue by a Bovine Transgene in a Cu/Zn Superoxide Dismutase-Null Mutant of *Drosophila* Melanogaster. *Mol. Cell. Biol.* 14:1302-1307.

Sauke DJ, Metzler DE, Metzler CM, 2001. *Biochemistry: The Chemical Reactions of Living Cells*, Second Edition. San Diego, California, USA: Harcourt/Academic.

Singh A, Rangasamy T, Thimmulappa RK, Lee H, Osburn WO, Brigelius-Flohé R, Kensler TW, Yamamoto M, Biswal S, 2006. Glutathione Peroxidase 2, the Major Cigarette Smoke-Inducible Isoform of GPX in Lungs, Is Regulated by Nrf2. *Am. J. Respir. Cell Mol. Biol.* 35:639-650.

Sligar S, Cinti DL, Gibson GG, Schenkman JB, 1979. Spin State Control of the Hepatic Cytochrome P-450 Redox Potential. *Biochem. Biophy. Res. Commun.* 90:925-932.

Smart RC, 2004. Chemical Carcinogenesis. In *A Textbook of Modern Toxicology* (Hodgson E, Ed.), Third Edition. Hoboken, New York, USA: John Wiley & Sons, Chapter 13 (p.243).

Sun GF, Yu M-H, Ding GY, Shen HY, 1997. Lipid Peroxidation and Changes in Antioxidant Levels in Aluminum Plant Workers. *Environ. Sci.* 5:139-144.

Swenson DH, Lin J-K, Miller EC, Miller JA, 1977. Aflatoxin B1-2,3-Oxide as a Probable Intermediate in the Covalent Binding of Aflatoxins B1 and B2 to Rat Liver DNA and Ribosomal RNA *in vivo. Cancer Res.* 37:172-181.

Townsend DM, Kenneth D, Tew KD, 2003. The Role of Glutathione-S-Transferase in Anticancer Drug Resistance. *Oncogene* 22:7369-7375.

Trostchansky A, Rubbo H, 2007. Lipid Nitration and Formation of Lipid-Protein Adducts: Biological Insights. *Amino Acids* 32:517-522.

Tukey RH, Strassburg CP, 2000. Human UDP-Glucuronosyltransferases: Metabolism, Expression, and Disease. *Ann. Rev. Pharmacol. Toxicol.* 40:581-616.

Uchaipichat V, Mackenzie PI, Guo X-H, Gardner-Stephen D, Galetin A, Houston JB, Miners JO, 2004. Human UDP-Glucuronosyltransferases: Isoform Selectivity and Kinetics of 4-Methylumbelliferone and 1-Naphthol Glucuronidation, Effects of Organic Solvents, and Inhibition by Diclofenac and Probenecid. *Drug Metab. & Disp.* 32:412-423.

Ueng YF, Hsieh CH, Don MJ, 2005. Inhibition of Human Cytochrome P450 Enzymes by the Natural Hepatotoxin Safrole. *Food Chem. Toxicol.* 43:707-712.

Woodruff RC, Phillips JP, Hilliker AJ, 2004. Increased Spontaneous DNA Damage in Cu/Zn Superoxide Dismutase (SOD1) Deficient *Drosophila. Genome* 47:1029-1035.

Zhou S-F, 2008. Drugs Behave as Substrates, Inhibitors and Inducers of Human Cytochrome P450 3A4. *Curr. Drug Metab.* 9:310-322.

Zhou S-F, Liu J-P, Chowbay B, 2009. Polymorphism of Human Cytochrome P450 Enzymes and Its Clinical Impact. *Drug Metab. Rev.* 41:89-295.

Review Questions

1. Briefly describe the main differences between chemical metabolism and xenobiotic biotransformation.

2. What are the main differences between a primary and an intermediate metabolite produced in xenobiotic biotransformation?

3. What are enzymes? Briefly characterize their general actions and functions.

4. Which of the following is generally regarded as the predominant form of oxidation in Phase I reactions? a) epoxidation; b) hydroxylation; c) deamination; d) dealkylation.

5. What is a monooxygenation type of oxidative reactions?

6. How does NADPH-dependent cytochrome P450 reductase biochemically induce the catalytic activity of a cytochrome P450 oxygenase?

7. Which of the following is the most predominant Phase II reactions? a) sulfation; b) methylation; c) glucuronidation; d) conjugation with glutathione; e) conjugation with amino acids.

8. Name three metabolites produced as a result of bioactivation in Phase I or Phase II reactions.

9. Which of the following cytochrome P450 enzymes is the most abundant as well as most important in humans? a) CYP2B6; b) CYP3A4; c) CYP2C19; d) CYP1A2.

10. Why and how is EROD (7-ethoxyresorufin *o*-deethylase) typically used as a biomarker for exposure of fish to certain polycyclic aromatic hydrocarbons?

11. Give three examples of the types of endogenous substances that can undergo biotransformation (i.e., Phase I or Phase II reactions).

12. Which of the following cell organelles in a human liver contains most of the cytochrome P450s? a) mitochondrion; b) lysosome; c) smooth endoplasmic reticulum; d) nucleus.

13. Name the Phase II enzyme in which a deficiency can cause Gilbert's syndrome.

14. Why is genetic polymorphism so important to the development of preclinical drugs, despite the fact that they are generally not regarded as environmental toxicants?

15. What are antioxidants? Name four that are (antioxidant) enzymes.

16. Match the Phase II enzymes (left column) to their required coenzymes (right column).

(1) UGT	(a) SAM
(2) SULT	(b) acetyl CoA
(3) MeT	(c) PAPS
(4) NAT	(d) GSH
(5) GST	(e) glucuronic acid

17. Identify the substances below, if any, that are: (1) Phase I enzyme inhibitors; (2) Phase II enzyme inhibitors; (3) Phase I enzyme inducers; (4) Phase II enzyme inducers.

(a) methoxychlor	(b) sulforaphane	(c) grapefruit juice
(d) genistein	(e) safrole	(f) charcoal-broiled meat
(g) ethanol	(h) TLK99	(i) silymarin
(j) mirex	(k) kepone	(l) ritonavir
(m) resveratrol	(n) glucosinolate	(o) phenobarbital

18. What are the main differences between enzyme cofactors and coenzymes, and between apoenzymes and holoenzymes?

19. Name one coenzyme that is derived from vitamin B_2, and two that are neither vitamin-based nor specific to Phase II enzymes.

CHAPTER 9

Adverse Action/Toxic Response

9.1. Introduction

Depending on the toxicological properties and the environmental level involved, an organism's exposure to a contaminant may or may not result in an adverse effect. Certain defense mechanisms in the organism's body also may or may not launch. For example, in humans, most airborne particles larger than 15 μm in diameter are filtered by the nasal hairs. If the particles are of the size and shape capable of passing through the nasal septum and deposit in sufficient amounts at a site where tonsils and adenoids are located nearby, immunological defense may kick in to protect against the substances filtered at that point. Immunological response is also a common mode through which the body protects its tissues and organs against microbial agents of certain toxicological properties. Still another mode of defense against certain toxicants that have entered the body is via the detoxification processes involved in chemical biotransformation (Chapter 8).

9.1.1. Site and Mechanism of Action

In humans and most other mammalians, many individuals respond to toxicants differently. The way in which an individual responds to a toxicant is affected by many factors, but mainly by those from within the four categories discussed in Chapter 10. Although some toxicants can damage any cell or tissue that they come in contact with, many affect specific tissues or organs only. Toxic damage can result from adverse biochemical, cellular, or macromolecular changes. The site where such changes occur is termed *site of (toxic) action*; and the specific biochemical interaction whereby a toxicant induces its effect is termed (its) *mechanism of (adverse) action*, or the affected site's *toxic response*.

This chapter follows the more conventional terminology that mechanism of action is a specific biochemical event underlying a mode of toxic action. For example, Carls and Meador (2009) treated baseline toxicity (e.g., narcosis) as a *mode* of toxic action (e.g., cytotoxicity, teratogenesis, endocrine disruption), rather than a mechanism of toxic action, because they contended that such an action lacks a *specific* receptor or platform. Yet some other scholars (e.g., Barron *et al.*, 2004) used the two terms interchangeably.

9.1.2. Basic Mechanisms of Action and Toxicodynamics

There are more mechanisms of (toxic) action than can be covered in even one book. However, many that are particularly relevant or challenging to a general environmental toxicologist may fall under the six common categories as follows: (1) direct damage to cellular structure; (2) toxic reactions mediated by free radicals; (3) modulation of receptor functions; (4) binding with a cell constituent; (5) adverse secondary or indirect actions; and (6) disruption of enzymatic activities. In this chapter, these six common mechanism categories are further divided into three groups to facilitate as well as to simplify the discussion, with the last two categories being on their own due to both their complexities and the unique cellular or molecular platform that they operate on.

Collectively these three broader groups of common mechanisms of action can induce, directly or indirectly, many types of adverse effects that are briefly introduced in Chapter 2. The wider spectrum of these toxic effects is further revisited in Section 9.5 below under the heading of toxicodynamics (TD), with the intent to offer a fuller appreciation of the mechanisms of action discussed. As further defined in Section 9.5, TD is about what toxicants can do to the body and thus is closely interrelated with toxicokinetics (TK), inasmuch as the latter is most concerned with the quantitative aspects of a toxicant's disposition kinetics (Chapter 7). In essence, how a toxic response takes its course is also contingent largely on the amount and the way a toxicant is delivered to the site of action.

9.2. Primary or Mediated Toxic Actions

Based on the conventional definition noted earlier, this chapter may not be correct to include *direct damage* as a mechanism of action category without qualification. The justification here is that whenever direct damage is considered, a rather specific biochemical site, receptor, or mechanism of action is implied, such as in direct DNA damage, direct oxidative damage, direct bacterial damage, direct UV (ultraviolet radiation) damage, and so forth. It is in this sense that the term *direct damage* is treated here as a mechanism (*vs.* mode) category that (environmental) toxicologists should be familiar with.

Also included in this first group are free radical-mediated actions. An appreciation is needed for this type of toxic actions in that reactive oxygen species (ROS) are inevitably and constantly produced during normal cellular metabolic processes. These and other free radicals are associated with many diseases, including cancer.

There is also a need for learning the modulation of receptor functions because in toxicology and biochemistry, receptors are protein molecules ubiquitously embedded in a cell's plasma membrane and within its cytoplasm. These receptors are usually attached to one or more specific kinds of signaling molecules. If the functions of these receptors are compromised, so are those of the signaling molecules such as certain hormones, neurotransmitters, drugs, or toxicants. The fourth and last mechanism category included in this first group is binding with a cell constituent. As evident from the discussion in Section 9.2.4 below, the binding of a toxicant such as carbon monoxide (CO) to a major cell constituent such as hemoglobin (Hb) can be extremely and acutely fatal.

9.2.1. Direct Damage to Cellular Structure

The consequence of direct damage can be readily seen on a plant's leaf surface. Many air pollutants are phytotoxic, such as sulfur dioxide (SO_2), nitrogen dioxide (NO_2), ozone (O_3), and particularly hydrogen fluoride (HF). At sufficiently high concentrations, these pollutants can directly cause leaf injuries leading to chlorosis or necrosis. Chlorosis is a condition in which leaves do not produce sufficient chlorophyll for their green appearance and thereby turn pale, yellow, or yellow-white. The affected leaf then has little or no ability to produce carbohydrates via photosynthesis to sustain its cell life. Necrosis is the condition in which death of plant tissues occurs, with the affected area generally turning black or brown. Many herbicides are phytotoxic by intent and design, since their only purpose is to get rid of unwanted plants (e.g., weeds).

As evident from several historical acute air pollution episodes, such as Donora smog of 1948 and London fog of 1952 (Chapter 12), certain air pollutants can also exert direct damage on the surface linings of the respiratory tract in humans (and other mammalians). In addition, the highly reactive free radicals (e.g., superoxide radical $O_2^-\cdot$) can react with protein or lipid molecules on the cell's membrane to damage the structure there.

9.2.2. Reactions Mediated by Free Radicals

Actions via this type of biochemical mechanism can result in oxidative stress and eventually damage of cellular components. One major serious consequence is lipid peroxidation, which refers to a more specific reaction process whereby highly reactive free radicals "steal" electrons from the cell membrane *lipid* molecules nearby. These lipid molecules generally are each of a polyunsaturated fatty acid (PURA) moiety. A general scheme involving PURA peroxidation is given below in Reactions 9.1a through 9.1c:

$$\text{PURA-H} + \text{X}\cdot \rightarrow \text{PURA}\cdot + \text{X-H} \tag{9.1a}$$

$$\text{PURA}\cdot + O_2 \rightarrow \text{PURA-OO}\cdot \tag{9.1b}$$

$$\text{PURA-OO}\cdot + \text{PURA-H} \rightarrow \text{PURA}\cdot + \text{PURA-OOH} \tag{9.1c}$$

where $\text{X}\cdot$ is an energetic one-electron oxidant (e.g., hydroxyl radical $\text{HO}\cdot$) and the lipid peroxyl radical $\text{PURA-OO}\cdot$ is the chain-carrying culprit (Wagner *et al.*, 1994).

Another chain reaction of this kind, which can occur inside or outside of a living organism, involves a highly reactive hydroxyl radical $\text{HO}\cdot$ generated by the iron-dependent Fenton reaction (Reaction 9.2) in which only inorganic reagents are required.

$$Fe^{2+} + H_2O_2 \rightarrow Fe^{3+} + \text{HO}\cdot + OH^- \tag{9.2a}$$

$$Fe^{3+} + H_2O_2 \rightarrow Fe^{2+} + HO_2\cdot + H^+ \tag{9.2b}$$

Note that the highly reactive hydroxyl radical generated from Reaction 9.2b can be used to oxidize organic contaminants in water or soil as a bioremediation stimulating or pretreatment agent (e.g., Crawford *et al.*, 2004). Studies suggested that antioxidants such as uric acid ($C_5H_4N_4O_3$) could readily suppress the oxidative activity of hydroxyl radical generation by the Fenton reaction (Howell and Wyngaarden, 1960; Simic and Jovanovic, 1989). Uric acid is produced when purines found in certain foods (e.g., liver, dried beans) and certain drinks (e.g., beer, wine) are broken down completely.

Another notorious toxic reaction mediated by a free radical, but not involving a chain propagation, is that by trichloromethyl free radical ($CCl_3^-\cdot$). This free radical can be generated from the dehydrogenation of carbon tetrachloride (CCl_4), and has been shown to cause hepatic injuries in several animal studies (Williams and Burk, 1990).

9.2.3. Modulation of Receptor Functions

Receptors of toxicological and biochemical concerns are protein molecules located on the plasma membrane separating its interior from its outside environment, located inside the cytoplasm of a cell, or located on the nuclear envelope (membrane) separating its nucleoplasm (that containing the nucleolus, chromatin, etc.) from its cytoplasm (*see* Figure 9.1). In most instances, the functions of a receptor are either blocked or activated by one or more specific kinds of endogenous or exogenous molecules referred to as ligands that bind to the receptor's proteinaceous structure. Upon binding, a series of signaling activities occurs in accordance with the receptor's structural characteristics. Unlike enzymes, regular protein receptors typically do not *catalyze* chemical changes in their ligands.

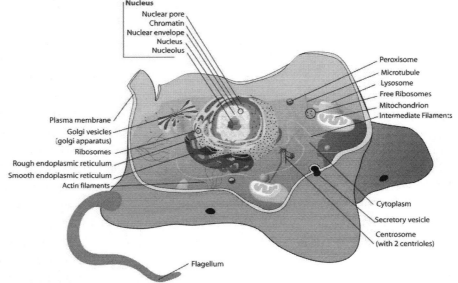

Figure 9.1. General Structure of an Animal Cell *(Commons.Wikimedia.org at http://en.wikipedia.org/wiki/File:Animal_cell_structure_en.svg; public domain image upon release by author Mariana Ruiz Villarreal)*

Intracellular receptors represent the most important class. They include those that respond to steroid hormones (primarily found in the liquid component of cytoplasm known as cytosol) and thyroid hormones (primarily found in the nucleoplasm). Once activated by ligands (e.g., toxicants), these receptors may be capable of entering the cell nucleus where they can alter gene expression (*see* example with AhR below in Figure 9.2, as further discussed later on).

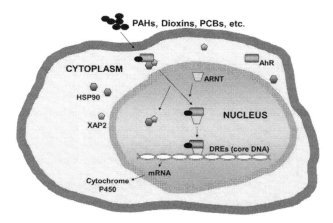

AhR = Aryl hydrocarbon receptor; ARNT = AhR nuclear translocator protein;
DREs = Dehydration-responsive elements (of the dioxin type); HSP90 and
XAP2 = cytoplasmic chaperonins; PAHs = polycyclic aromatic hydrocarbons

Figure 9.2. Current Concept of Mechanism Whereby Dioxins, PCBs, and PAH-like Compounds along with an Ah Receptor Can Cause Alteration of Gene Expression

Receptors located within a cell's plasma membrane (a.k.a. cell membrane) may be peripheral, but mostly integral, proteins (as illustrated in Figure 7.2). Integral protein receptors include those for hormonal functions and neurotransmission; and most fall into one of the two structural categories termed *ionotropic* and *metabotropic*. Ionotropic type transmembrane protein receptors are ligand-gated ion channels capable of permitting entry of ions when the central pore is open. Metabotropic type transmembrane receptors are coupled to *guanine* nucleotide-binding proteins (or G proteins for short), acting via various secondary pathways that involve specific ion channels and enzymes.

Ion channels are pore-forming proteins located on the plasma membrane to help facilitate or limit the diffusion of ions across a membrane in all living cells by allowing or restricting the flow of ions down their electrochemical gradient. The ions of most relevance are sodium (Na^+), potassium (K^+), chloride (Cl^-), and calcium (Ca^{2+}). Also located across the plasma membranes of certain cells (e.g., neurons, axons) are voltage-gated conductance ion channels (that to be activated by changes in electrical potential difference near the channel), as well as mechanosensitive ion channels which are open under the influence of stress, pressure, and the kind.

For the G protein-coupled receptors, their main function is to transduce extracellular stimuli into intracellular signals. These metabotropic receptors are involved in the modulation or regulation of a wide variety of physiological processes, including the mood and behavior center, the visual and smell senses, the immunological system, and the transmission in the autonomic nervous system. They are each activated by an external stimulus in the form of binding with a ligand or another signal mediator. Upon binding, the conformational change induced in the receptor will cause activation of the G protein to either activate or inhibit a specific enzyme which then produces a second messenger. It is this second messenger that initiates the destined cellular response.

In toxicology, the importance of protein receptors may be illustrated with the activation of the *aryl hydrocarbon receptor* (AhR). This cytosolic receptor is a member of the transcription factors that dictate the time at which genes are to be switched on or off (i.e., to be transcribed or not). The current concept is that the receptor is normally inactive until it is bound to a chemical ligand such as TCDD (2,3,7,8-tetrachlorodibenzo-*p*-dioxin). When its activated form is complexed with the cytoplasmic chaperonins HSP90 and XAP2, AhR can be translocated into the nucleus to dimerize (combine) with an AhR nuclear translocator (ARNT) protein. The activated AhR/ARNT heterodimer complex is then capable of interacting with DNA to cause (adverse) changes in gene transcription (*see* Figure 9.2). The ultimate biologic effect from this process can be carcinogenic.

9.2.4. Binding with a Cell Constituent

Hydrogen cyanide (HCN), CO, and certain epoxides are molecules having a strong binding affinity to a particular cell constituent and hence capable of interfering with the normal function of that constituent. Two physiologically important cell constituents are *n*uclear deoxyribonucleic acid (*n*DNA or frequently DNA for short) and Hb (hemoglobin). Hb is the metalloprotein found in all red blood cells and contains a ferrous iron (Fe^{2+}) in its heme unit to allow the transportation of oxygen vital to many cellular functions. DNA is contained within the nucleus of each eukaryotic cell. Working together with their *m*essenger ribonucleic acid (*m*RNA), nDNA molecules will encode many more specific enzymes and other proteins than those DNA in the mitochondria will.

Hydrogen cyanide is an extremely poisonous gas, which can be produced when synthetic polymers (e.g., nylon, polyacrylonitrile, polyurethane) in clothes and furnishings are burned. Once it is taken into the bloodstream, over 90% of the cyanide (CN^-) will occupy the oxygen-binding site in Hb, thus making the Hb unable to transport oxygen to the body's various tissues and organs. Moreover, while arriving in the form of Hb-CN, CN^- will preferentially bind to cytochrome *c* oxidase's heme unit in the host tissue to inhibit electron transport and thereby will deprive the cells there of oxygen use.

The gaseous molecule CO is likewise very poisonous, given that its binding affinity to Hb (in the oxygenated Fe^{2+} form) is around 220 times stronger compared to oxygen's affinity to Hb (in the Fe^{2+} form). When existing in the Hb-CO bound form, the metalloprotein is incapable of carrying oxygen to cells in all other tissues.

As noted in Chapter 8, aflatoxin B_1-8,9-epoxide and benzo[α]pyrene-7,8-dihydrodiol-9,10-epoxide are capable of binding covalently to DNA. These DNA adducts can lead to the initiation of cancerous cells.

9.3. Major Adverse Secondary or Indirect Actions

The presence of a xenobiotic in a body may mechanistically cause the release or production of certain substances that in turn can harm the cells in that body. Highlighted below are four example categories included in this group: (1) allergic response; (2) side effects of medications; (3) complexation; and (4) microbic invasion.

9.3.1. Allergic Response

This type of responses by (or in) the body comes around when the body's immunological system responds to the presence of a normally innocuous agent (e.g., pollen, dust) that comes in contact with lymphocytes specific for that agent (more technically termed *antigen*). Lymphocytes are a special group of white blood cells capable of producing antibodies (called immunoglobulins or Ig's for short) and other substances to fight infectious and other types of diseases. The allergic response frequently includes the release of a large amount of a biogenic amine (i.e., an organic compound with an amine group) termed *histamine* which may then result in two major allergic symptoms: inflammation and contraction of smooth muscle (e.g., walls of blood vessels or the gastrointestinal tract). In certain allergic response, the release of histamine can be so much that it will cause anaphylactic (hypertensive) shock which can lead to death in a matter of minutes.

9.3.2. Side Effects of Medications

All medications come with side effects, of which some are due to specific secondary reactions. For example, some medicines contain dextromethorphan (DXM) as the active ingredient for cough suppression. However, in recent years, DXM is notoriously known as a drug of abuse. This is because DXM can potentiate the level of the endogenous neurotransmitter called serotonin in the brain (e.g., Schwartz *et al.*, 2008), at times to the point that it is sufficient to induce the so-called serotonin syndrome. The syndrome starts with euphoria, hallucinations, and excitability, but at sufficiently high dosage can end in life-threatening seizures. Many drugs of abuse, such as ecstasy, LSD (lysergic acid diethylamide), and cocaine, also have been linked to serotonin syndrome.

9.3.3. Complexation

This mechanism can refer to the tight-binding or, more commonly, chelation of a ligand with a substrate. The substrate in chelation usually is a mineral or metal, whereas the ligand is typically an organic compound. The resultant complex is referred to as a chelate complex. The ligand has many names, such as chelator, chelant, or chelating agent. In medicine, chelation is a therapy in that it can be used to remove excess toxic metals before they can cause harm to the body. The removal can be done effectively because the undesired substrate (e.g., a toxic metal) can be removed along with the ligand as a single entity, with the former being held tightly by the latter. The resultant complex that contains the ligand and the substrate, though somewhat larger than the ligand itself, is still comparatively easier to be excreted from the body.

Chelation can be a toxic reaction, however. In addition to causing some common side effects (e.g., headaches, skin irritation, fever, fatigue, tissue damage), it can remove excess amounts of essential elements or metals (e.g., selenium, iron, zinc) from the body along the way. In particular, the use of EDTA has been associated with kidney damage (Cranton, 2001). EDTA is a synthetic amino acid named *ethylenediaminetetraacetate* (a.k.a. edetate disodium). There has been a controversy over EDTA's use as chelation therapy for reducing the risk of cardiovascular diseases (Seely *et al.*, 2005). The Asian herb cilantro is a chelator even more readily available in the environment. The herb has been actively use in recent years to remove mercury (Hg) absorbed from amalgam dental fillings and other sources. As with EDTA and other chelators, cilantro comes with side effects when overused, including excess removal of essential minerals and metals.

9.3.4. Microbic Invasion

While many bacterial and viral infections are contagious, the two types exert their pathogenic effects via different invasive mechanisms (Chapter 17). For bacterial invasions, some are actually beneficial to the host organism particularly if the colonization is not aggressive. Whether a bacterial invasion can cause an infectious disease or not depends on the interplay between the bacterium's ability to proliferate in the host's body and the degree to which the host's body is able to defend the invasion. Most bacterial infections begin with the adherence of the pathogens (the bacteria) to specific cells on the mucous membranes of the respiratory, gastrointestinal, or genitourinary tract, followed by penetration of the epithelium to generate pathogenicity as the next stage. The third critical pathogenesis stage is for the bacteria to colonize by binding to specific tissue surface receptors and to overcome any nonspecific or immunological host defenses. Some bacteria produce highly potent and lethal endotoxins or exotoxins upon invasion. Exotoxins are proteins (e.g., botulinum toxin) that may act at tissue sites away from the colonization site as they are extracellular diffusible. Endotoxins are lipopolysaccharides localized on the outer membrane of bacteria. They are less potent compared to exotoxins and are not released until the pathogens are killed by the host's defense system.

Viruses are much smaller than bacteria and can multiply only inside a host cell. Each virus particle called virion consists of its own genetic materials (typically the RNA kind) surrounded by a protective coat of protein called capsid. As viruses are acellular and do not grow via cell division or cell proliferation on their own, they produce multiple copies of themselves and their destructive enzymes by inserting their genetic materials into the host cell to basically hijack the latter's cell division materials and functions. When sufficient copies of a virus are so bioengineered, the new virions will burst out of the host cell, killing it and moving onward to infect other cells in the host organism.

9.4. Disruption of Enzymatic Activities

The general characteristics of enzymes and their basic actions crucial to biochemical processes in a living system are highlighted in Chapter 8. Also given in that chapter is a list of substances known or suspected as capable of preventing or slowing down the catalytic abilities of certain enzymes. Although there are several ways in which enzyme inhibition can take place, for simplicity they may be broadly subsumed under two general modes as follows: (1) those inhibition mechanisms in which the required coenzyme or cofactor is inactivated or becomes less bioactive; and (2) those inhibitions in which the target enzyme's active site is blocked, disrupted, or otherwise less bioavailable.

9.4.1. Inhibition of Cofactors or Coenzymes

The function of a coenzyme can be inactivated by one or more specific toxicants. One toxicant with this ability is warfarin, an anticoagulant widely used at one time as a pesticide to kill rodents (Chapter 15). To avert life-threatening hemorrhaging, thrombin (one of the clotting enzymes) must be sufficiently available in the body. Thrombin is made available from its precursor prothrombin binding with a calcium ion (Ca^{2+}) in the liver. However, prothrombin is not available in the form ready for Ca^{2+} binding unless it is activated by the *coenzyme* vitamin K, which also occurs in an inactive form as vitamin K-2,3-epoxide in the liver. Warfarin, along with many other anticoagulants, is capable of antagonizing the functions of vitamin K. This inhibition is made possible likely owing to warfarin's ability to bind to vitamin K-2,3-epoxide reductase (Gregus and Klaassen, 2001; Odenburg *et al.*, 2006). This reductase enzyme is responsible for catalyzing the transformation of the vitamin K epoxide to the active form of vitamin K.

For inactivation of cofactors critical to an enzyme's activation, the application of liquid citrate ($C_3H_5O[COO]_3^{3-}$) contained in a test tube for measuring prothrombin time (PT) serves as a good example. PT is a measure reflecting the clotting tendency of blood. It can be measured using blood plasma drawn into a test tube in which the citrate acts as an anticoagulant by binding to the Ca^{2+} in the sample. The time that the sample takes to clot is measured after an excess amount of the Ca^{2+} *cofactor* (of prothrombin leading to thrombin formation, as noted above) is added to reverse the effects of citrate.

As another example, the enzyme Mg^{2+}-ATPase needs to be activated with the cofactor Ca^{2+} or magnesium (Mg^{2+}) ion before it can catalyze the hydrolysis of ATP (adenosine-5'-triphosphate) to ADP (adenosine diphosphate). This hydrolytic conversion plays a key role in supplying energy for many biochemical processes in most life forms. Mg^{2+}-ATPase is also referred to as Ca^{2+}/Mg^{2+}-ATPase or Ca^{2+}-ATPase, depending on its location in the organism's body (Ritsuko *et al.*, 1994; Zhao *et al.*, 1991). The toxic metal cadmium (Cd^{2+}) can compete with Ca^{2+} and Mg^{2+} for the binding site on Mg^{2+}-ATPase when under conducive conditions (e.g., with proper temperature, proper concentration) in certain species, including algae, sugar beet, mussel, and rat (e.g., Jeanne *et al.*, 1993; Lindberg and Wingstrand, 1985; Pivovarova and Lagerspetz, 1996; Zhao *et al.*, 1991).

9.4.2. Inhibition/Inactivation of the Active Site

Like the active site of a protein receptor, that of an enzyme reserved for a specific substrate can be blocked or deformed. As depicted in Figure 9.3, the Krebs cycle (a.k.a. the citric acid cycle or the tricarboxylic acid cycle) is a complex series of enzymatic reactions in all cells that use oxygen as part of their respiration process. It is in this respiration process that the energy-rich compound ATP is produced.

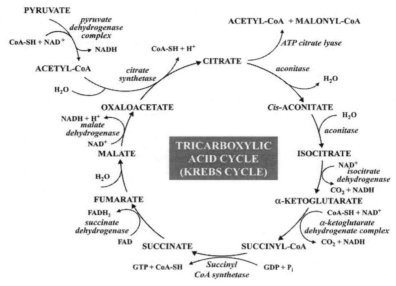

Figure 9.3. The Krebs Cycle *(a.k.a. the Citric Acid or Tricarboxylic Acid Cycle)*

The organic compound fluorocitrate ($FC_3H_4O[COO]_3^{3-}$) is a potent Krebs cycle inhibitor by converting to 4-hydroxy-*trans*-aconitate which can bind tightly to the enzyme aconitase in the cycle (Lauble *et al.*, 1996). The inhibition of this enzyme shuts down the Krebs cycle crucial to many biological processes in aerobic organisms. Fluorocitrate can be produced as an intermediate from the rodenticide fluoroacetate ($FCH_2CO_2^-$) under the process commonly termed *lethal synthesis*, in that a highly toxic compound is synthesized from a relatively nontoxic precursor. The precursor fluoroacetate can also be found in certain South African plants known to cause livestock poisoning.

Organophosphates (OPs) and carbamates (CBs) are among other groups of pesticides (Chapter 15) also known for their ability to inhibit important enzymes. The notorious effects of OP and CB pesticides come about through their ability of binding to the active site of the enzyme acetylcholinesterase (AChE) at the brain synapses and neuromuscular junctions, where the substrate acetylcholine (ACh) acts as the neurotransmitter (i.e., substance required for stimulating the muscle to move) there. AChE is the enzyme that hydrolyzes (breaks down) the neurotransmitter ACh following stimulation of a nerve; it is thus the enzyme that subsequently terminates the stimulation upon considerable degradation of ACh. Accordingly, inhibition or depression of AChE allows the neurotransmitter to accumulate and result in initially excessive stimulation, but with death being a possible outcome when the inhibition is continuous at a sufficiently high level or duration.

Some drugs (e.g., donepezil, tacrine) developed mainly for treatment of Alzheimer's disease are known AChE inhibitors.

Metals such as lead (Pb), Hg (mercury), Cd (cadmium), and silver (Ag) are also potent enzyme inhibitors due to their high affinity for the thiol (-SH) groups present on enzymes. Many enzymes are made of peptide chains rich in cysteine ($HO_2CCH[NH_2]CH_2$-SH, or Cys-SH for short), an amino acid with a thiol (a.k.a. sulfhydryl) group on its side. When enough of the hydrogen (H) atoms in these -SH groups are replaced by the metal (M) ions (as shown in Reactions 9.3 and 9.4), the tertiary structure of the enzyme's protein chain can easily be altered enough that the shape of its active site is also seriously affected, often to the point that the target substrate can no longer bind to this site.

$$Cys\text{-}SH + M^+ \rightarrow Cys\text{-}S\text{-}M + H^+ \tag{9.3}$$

$$2(Cys\text{-}SH) + M^{2+} \rightarrow Cys\text{-}M\text{-}Cys + 2H^+ \tag{9.4}$$

Lead is notorious for its ability to inhibit the essential enzyme *delta*-aminolevulinic acid dehydratase (δ-ALAD or ALAD) via a mechanism implicit in Reaction 9.4 (Patrick, 2006; Schafer *et al.*, 2005). The enzyme is crucial to the biosynthesis of heme, the prosthetic group of hemoglobin that carries oxygen molecules around in the blood. For most life forms, heme is also a key building block used for various biological functions in virtually every tissue in the body. Inhibition of δ-ALAD has been proposed for use as a biomarker to monitor environmental lead pollution (e.g., Kutlu and Sümer, 1998) or lead-induced effects in the heme biosynthesis pathway (e.g., Ahamed *et al.*, 2006; Alimonti and Mattei, 2008; Sakai, 2000).

9.5. Toxicodynamics of Toxicants

Toxicodynamics (TD) is defined (IUPAC, 1997) as "*The study of toxic actions on living systems, including the reactions with and binding to cell constituents, and the biochemical and physiological consequences of these actions.*" Its focus is therefore on the adverse effects and the associated toxic responses, and on the underlying mechanisms of action (Hodgson *et al.*, 1998). Again, inasmuch as dosage is considered as the most crucial factor affecting toxicity, TD is interrelated closely with TK (toxicokinetics; Sections 7.5 and 9.1.2). In their simplest terms, TD attempts to explain how the body *reacts* to a toxicant, whereas TK is concerned with how the body *handles* the toxicant.

9.5.1. Basic, Nonspecific Types of Adverse Effects

Table 9.1 below summarizes the various types of adverse effects (or responses) that are relevant to TD in terms of environmental *exposure* concerns. In addition to these effects (or responses) and the common underlying mechanisms of toxic action highlighted in Sections 9.2 through 9.4, other aspects relevant to TD are dose-response relationship and chemical interaction. The toxicity of a xenobiotic in an organism can be increased or decreased by a consecutive or simultaneous exposure to one or more other toxic or harmless agents. The joint effects of additivity, synergism, potentiation, and antagonism due to chemical interaction are among the many affecting factors discussed in Chapter 10.

Table 9.1. Basic Types of Adverse Effects or Responses as Relevant to Toxicodynamics, in Terms of Environmental *Exposure* Concerns

Type of Effects/ Responses	General Characteristics
Local	Toxic effect/response occurring at the site of contact with the toxicant
Systemic	Toxic effect to/response by the entire body or a particular body region other than the portal of entry
Reversible	Effect that is temporary, reparable from (tissue) injury, or otherwise reversible
Irreversible	Effect that is permanent, not reparable from (tissue) injury, or otherwise irreversible
Immediate	Response or effect that develops rapidly after acute or a single exposure
Delayed	Response that develops following a short latent period from typically an acute exposure
Acute	Similar to immediate effect, but typically reserved for the kind that is usually of the severe type
Chronic	Response or effect that is developed after repeated exposures, or that lasts for a long time
Allergic	Effect requiring prior sensitization by an agent or by one similar in structure or chemical properties
Idiosyncratic	Effect or response related to abnormally high susceptibility to a specific toxicant

While its analysis serves as a key health risk assessment component (Chapter 23), in general terms dose-response relationship refers to a quantitative relationship between exposure to a toxicant and the severity or incidence of a toxic response. An important assertion or precaution in the analysis of dose-response relationship is that there is almost always an exposure level or dose below which no adverse effect (and thus no response) occurs or can be observed. A second assertion is that once a maximum response is reached, any further increase in the exposure will not result in any increase in the effect.

In addition to carcinogenicity which generally assumes a non-threshold tumorigenic effect, allergic reaction (Table 9.1) is one adverse effect or response that does not seem to fit well into the above generalization. This type of effects is treated as an overreaction or inappropriate response of the immunological system; it is not truly a *toxic* response. The main difference between allergy and toxic reaction is that a toxic effect is directly the result of the toxicant acting at the site of action. In contrast, allergic response is typically the result of a harmless xenobiotic (termed *allergen*) stimulating the body to release a protective antibody called IgE (immunoglobulin E) which will then induce an observable effect of concern. As it is often said, in an allergic reaction the xenobiotic at best acts as the trigger only, not the bullet. Once a person has had an allergic reaction (i.e., once sensitized to the allergen), even a very limited exposure to a very small dose of the allergen can trigger a life-threatening allergic reaction (e.g., anaphylaxis).

Also of special concern here is the *systemic* type effect listed in Table 9.1, which represents a very broad category on its own (e.g., Section 9.5.2.F). It includes all that can be on all of the body's internal organs and tissues. Toxicants with systemic effects typically have their own target organs or tissues in which they accumulate and exert their effect(s). Many of these effects cannot be observed until a critical body burden is reached.

9.5.2. Specific/Mechanism-Based Adverse Effects

In Chapter 2, adverse health effects from environmental exposure are introduced as environmental diseases by category and in the form of concerns with their environmental impacts. Below are those and additional adverse effects characterized in relation to the more specific mechanisms of action, more unique sites of action, or more prominent toxicants that they are involved in or with. The adverse effects included in this (sub)section are necessarily selective and brief due to space limitation, but otherwise with the dual purpose of delineating the boundary of TD while at the same time adding a place for some background material relevant to physiological toxicology.

A. Irritation and Corrosive Effects

Irritation is a state of inflammation and painful reactions involving cell-lining damage. In most situations, it represents a localized inflammatory effect resulting from a topical exposure of an external organ (primarily the eye, skin, respiratory, and genital) of the body to an agent commonly termed *irritant*. Inflammation is the complex biological response of vascular tissues to the irritant, a type of nonspecific immunological response involving the use of the body's leukocytes (i.e., white blood cells) to fight off the induced effect. This type of responses is a protective attempt by the body to remove the harmful irritant as well as to initiate the healing process for the damaged tissue.

Irritants can be of almost any kind or form, including biological (e.g., stings), chemical (e.g., phenol), mechanical (e.g., physical trauma), thermal (e.g., heat), and radioactive (e.g., ultraviolet light) stimuli. Corrosive effect refers to the production of irreversible tissue damage in the lining of the external tissues following topical exposure.

Chronic irritation is a medical term signifying the condition in which the inflammatory effect has been lingering on and off the same area of the body for some time. This chronic disorder was once regarded as a very serious condition in that the irritated tissue was thought to be highly susceptible to cancerous skin lesions (e.g., Mayo, 1914; Dyas, 1928). There are many toxic responses that can lead to chronic irritation, with the majority involving the skin and the respiratory tract.

B. Asphyxiation

Asphyxiation is a condition in which the body is deprived of oxygen, whereas asphyxia is the earlier but still fairly serious stage characterized by an extreme decrease in oxygen supply in the body. More common terms for asphyxia include suffocation and inability to breathe. Several gases, including CO and HCN noted in Section 9.2.4 above, can cause asphyxia by interfering with the transport or provision of oxygen to other tissues. Symptoms of asphyxia include breathing difficulty, hypertension (a.k.a. high blood pressure), cyanosis, rapid pulse, convulsion, and even death.

C. Narcotic and Anesthetic Effects

Narcosis, as caused by the effects of narcotics, is a condition of deep stupor or unconsciousness produced by chemical substances (including drugs) derived from opium and those causing opiate-like addiction, such as heroin, morphine, cocaine, and barbiturates. Anesthesia, as caused by the effects of anesthetics, is a condition in which the body's sensation (including pain) in a specific anatomic region or in the entire system is blocked or temporarily taken away. Although the mechanisms of action for the two conditions are not precisely known, both mechanisms are believed to involve primarily the effects (inhibition or activation) of narcotic or anesthetic agents on their target receptors in the brain (e.g., Dabbagh *et al.*, 2007; Dean *et al.*, 2009; Perkins, 2005).

D. Carcinogenic Effects

These adverse biologic effects can lead to carcinogenesis, the process by which normal cells are transformed into cancer cells. The process is caused by mutations or adverse changes of the genetic materials in normal cells, resulting in the upset of the normal balance between cell proliferation (as a result of cell growth or cell division) and programmed cell death (termed *apoptosis*). Agents that cause carcinogenesis are called carcinogens; and those causing mutagenesis are called mutagens. Irreparable DNA molecules, as from damage by being "adducted" by an epoxide (Section 9.2.4), can disrupt the genetic programming that regulates the cell proliferation or apoptosis process. A fuller discussion on carcinogenesis and mutagenesis is given in Chapter 18.

E. Teratogenic Effects

These biologic effects can lead to teratogenesis, the process involving the production of abnormalities prior to birth. Agents that can cause birth defects or abnormalities in the embryo or fetus are specifically called teratogens. These agents can be viruses, radiation, and chemicals (e.g., pesticides, drugs). The mechanisms of action for most teratogens are not well understood. A teratogen usually causes a specific structural or functional effect when exposure occurs within a definite, short time window after conception. Adverse effects may result when teratogens alter the normal function of DNA. Toxicants that inhibit certain enzymatic activity, that deprive the embryo or fetus of energy or oxygen supply, or that alter the placental permeability can cause birth defects. Teratogenesis can also occur in plants leading to, for example, flower abnormalities (e.g., Meyer, 1966).

F. Effects on Target Body Organs or Systems

For humans and many other mammalians, the body organs and systems of toxicological concern generally include the reproductive system, cardiovascular system, nervous system, respiratory system, immunological system, liver, kidneys, eyes, skin, blood, and the endocrine network, not necessarily in that order. This list represents much of the basic and vital body organs and systems in a human. The mechanisms of action vary greatly for toxicants exerting their effects on these body parts. Collectively they include, but are not limited to, those discussed in Section 9.2.

Toxicants that affect the male or female reproductive system may ultimately cause effects on the reproductive function of that sex, or indirectly even of the opposite sex (i.e., of the sex partner). For example, both the human papilloma virus (Walboomers *et al.*, 1999) and cigarette smoke (Pate Capps *et al.*, 2009) are risk factors, if not etiological agents, strongly associated with cervical cancer. Any practical treatment of invasive cervical cancer necessarily comes with certain risk of infertility due to some loss of the structural and functional integrity of the cervical proper. Even a small biopsy operation to remove a cone-shaped area where the cancer develops has some risk of cervical stenosis. With the stenotic cervix becoming very narrow and stiffened, the mucus-producing glands there become compromised and thus the survival of sperms is adversely affected (Frishman 2002). On the males side, it has been demonstrated (Kluwe *et al.*, 1983) that the pesticide DBCP (1,2-dibromo-3-chloropropane) can reduce fertility in male rats by acting at a site in the genital tract beyond the testis.

The cardiovascular system consists of the heart and the blood vessels (e.g., arteries, arterioles, capillaries, venules, veins). Although the heart is not a common target organ of toxic insult, its myocytes can be damaged by some pharmaceutical agents such as the cancer therapeutic drug imatinib mesylate (Kerkelä *et al.*, 2006). There are other agents that can cause cardiotoxicity: certain natural products (e.g., animal toxins); certain solvents (e.g., toluene found in paint and certain household products); certain metals, such as cobalt (Co), Cd, Pb, and Hg; and certain halogenated hydrocarbons (e.g., freon). Some compounds in the pharmaceutical and metal groups, along with some gaseous pollutants such as automobile exhausts, CO, nitric oxide (NO), and O_3, are found especially harmful to the vascular portion. For example, a study in Korea (Kim *et al.*, 2005) has implicated that Hg could induce an increase of cholesterol in blood as a risk factor of both myocardial infraction and cardiovascular disease.

In humans and other mammalians, the nervous system consists of the central and peripheral parts, together representing a network of specialized cells called neurons (i.e., nerve cells) that coordinate the body's biological actions and its transmission of signals across various tissues and organs. The central nervous system (CNS), which consists of the brain and the spinal cord, has a blood-brain barrier to restrict the influx of substances in the blood to the brain. However, this and the peripheral nervous system are still susceptible to damage from a variety of chemical toxicants and microbial toxins, especially in young children whose blood-brain barrier is not yet fully developed. Neurotoxicants such as certain metals (e.g., Pb, Hg) and pesticides (e.g., organophosphates, pyrethroids, organochlorine insecticides) are of high concern to environmental toxicologists. Death, hallucination, seizure, paralysis, and coma are some of the apparent as well as severe or fatal health outcomes associated with poisoning of the nervous system.

Some toxic airborne residues that exist in the form of gases, vapors, liquid droplets, or solid particulate matter can induce not only localized effects on the respiratory tract, but also systemic effects after inhalation intake and distribution to other tissues. Cigarette smoke is one ill-known example of environmental toxicants that can cause cancer in general and lung cancer in particular. Respiratory diseases can be broadly classified into two types: *obstructive*, that impeding the air flow (e.g., asthma, bronchiolitis); or *restrictive*, that characterized by reduction in lung volume (e.g., lung cancer, pulmonary fibrosis). Causes of this disease group range from infectious agents and other environmental exposure to allergens and genetic origin.

The immunological system is a network of special proteins, cells, tissues, and organs working together to protect the host against foreign objects (e.g., microbes, cells, substances) by using its antibodies. From this system (including bone marrow, spleen, and lymph nodes in humans), various lymphocytes and other cells with different functions are derived. Many agents are known to suppress immunological function, leading to reduced control of abnormal tissue growth or lowered host resistance to infections. Some toxicants may provoke exaggerated responses causing systemic or localized effects, or eventually autoimmune reactions. Responses of the immunological system to toxicants generally fall into four hypersensitivity types: (1) *anaphylactic reactions* (Type I: acute, allergy); (2) *cytolytic reactions* (Type II: antibody-dependent); (3) *immunological complex reactions* (Type III: involving mostly IgG antibodies with soluble antigens); and (4) *delayed reactions* (Type IV: T cell-mediated, antibody-independent). Environmental allergens of concern include: ozone (O_3); certain metals (e.g., Pb, Hg); certain aromatic hydrocarbons (e.g., benzene); and certain pesticides (e.g., certain OPs).

The liver is both the largest and a highly complex organ in the body. As a metabolism center for most nutrients, drugs, and other xenobiotics, it is the common target organ of many toxicants. Many of these toxicants at high doses can induce a variety of harmful effects on different organelles in the hepatic (i.e., liver) cells: steatosis (fatty liver); hepatic cell death; cholestasis (reduction or impaired secretion of bile or its components); liver cirrhosis (liver scarring); liver cancer; and hepatitis (liver inflammation). Hepatotoxicants of environmental health concern include: ethanol; arsenic (As); organic arsenicals; CCl_4 (carbon tetrachloride); vinyl chloride; and aflatoxins.

The kidney is also a major target organ of toxic effects, insomuch as urine is the principal route by which many toxicants are (eventually) excreted from the body. Environmental toxicants of nephrotoxic concern include certain: metals (e.g., Hg, Cd); halogenated hydrocarbons (e.g., CCl_4, chloroform); herbicides (e.g., paraquat); persistent organic pollutants (e.g., PCBs, TCDD); and mycotoxins (e.g., aflatoxins). Their mechanisms of toxic action include: interaction with receptors; inhibition of oxidative phosphorylation (e.g., the process forming the energy-rich compound ATP in the Krebs cycle); injuries to cell membranes; and disturbance of calcium (Ca^{2+}) homeostasis (e.g., Commandeur and Vermeulen, 1990; Tarloff and Wallace, 2008; Wang *et al.*, 2009).

In addition to skin irritation noted above, dermal contact with certain environmental toxicants can result in various types of dermal toxicity: sensitization; allergic dermatitis (including the photoallergic type); contact dermatitis (including the phototoxic type); skin lesions; skin cancer; and a variety of *systemic* effects after dermal absorption and distribution to other body tissues. Environmental toxicants that can induce dermal toxicity include: ultraviolet radiation (with effects including phototoxicity and photoallergy); persistent organochlorines such as PCBs and dioxins (with effects including notably chloracne); pesticides such as propargite and permethrin (both with effects including dermatitis); and metals such as nickel (Ni) and Hg (both with effects including allergic dermatitis), and arsenic (with effects including skin cancer).

Substances that can injure the cornea and its nearby iris include acids, alkalis, detergents, solvents, and smog. A number of toxic agents are known to compromise the transparency integrity of the lens, frequently ending in cataract formation. In addition to certain drugs (Meier-Ruge, 1972) and a host of medical conditions (e.g., diabetes, arterial hypertension, HIV-1 disease), environmental exposure to chemicals such as carbon disulfide (Sugimoto *et al.*, 1978) and 4,4′-methylenedianiline aerosols (Leong *et al.*, 1987) can damage the retina in humans and animals. This in turn will adversely affect visual acuity as retina is the light sensitive tissue lining the inner surface of the eye.

In addition to HCN and CO noted in Section 9.2.4, nitrate (NO_3^-) and hydrosulfide (HS^-) can adversely affect the hemoglobin's ability to serve as an oxygen-carrier. When the HS^- or NO_3^- ion binds to the metalloprotein to form sulfhemoglobin (sulfHb) or methemoglobin (metHb), respectively, the F^{2+} ion in the heme is converted to F^{3+} thus losing its ability to bind to an oxygen molecule. A number of environmental toxicants (e.g., arsine, benzene, copper, Pb, methyl chloride) can cause (acquired) hemolytic anemia, a condition with destruction of red blood cells at an abnormally high rate causing the victim to experience fatigue, dizziness, confusion, and other symptoms. In particular, exposure to benzene is linked to leukemia, a cancer of the blood or bone marrow.

The endocrine network controls development, growth, and regulation within the body. The network consists of endocrine glands and the natural chemical messengers termed *hormones*. Some basic mechanisms of action for endocrine disruptors involving receptor binding are reflected in Section 9.2.3 above. A fuller discussion on chemical disruption of the endocrine system is given in Chapter 19.

References

Ahamed M, Verma S, Kumar A, 2006. Delta-Aminolevulinic Acid Dehydratase Inhibition and Oxidative Stress in Relation to Blood Lead among Urban Adolescents. *Human & Exper. Toxicol.* 25:547-553.

Alimonti A, Mattei D, 2008. Biomarkers for Human Biomonitoring. In *Biological Monitoring: Theory & Applications – Bioindicators and Biomarkers for Environmental Quality and Human Exposure Assessment* (Conti ME, Ed.). Billerica, Massachusetts, USA: WIT Press, Chapter 6.

Commandeur JNM, Vermeulen NPE, 1990. Molecular and Biochemical Mechanisms of Chemically Induced Nephrotoxicity: A Review. *Chem. Res. Toxicol.* 3:171-194.

Cranton EM, 2001. Kidney Effects of Ethylene Diamine Tetraacetic Acid (EDTA): A Literature Review. In *A Textbook on EDTA Chelation Therapy* (Cranton EM, Ed.), Second Edition. Charlottesville, Virginia, USA: Hampton Roads, Chapter 26.

Crawford RL, Hess TF, Paszczynski A, 2004. Combined Biological and Abiological Degradation of Xenobiotic Compounds. In *Biodegradation and Bioremediation* (Singh A, Ward OP, Eds.). Berlin, Heidelberg, Germany: Springer-Verlag, Chapter 11.

Dabbagh A, Dahi-Taleghani M, Elyasi H, Vosoughian M, Malek B, Rajaei S, Maftuh H, 2007. Duration of Spinal Anesthesia with Bupivacaine in Chronic Opium Abusers Undergoing Lower Extremity Orthopedic Surgery. *Arch. Iranian Med.* 10:316-320.

Dean R, Bilsky EJ, Negus SS (Eds.), 2009. *Opiate Receptors and Antagonists: From Bench to Clinic.* New York, New York, USA: Humana Press.

Dyas FG, 1928. Chronic Irritation as a Cause of Cancer. *JAMA* 90:457.

Frishman GN, 2002. Treatment of Cervical Stenosis. In *Office-Based Infertility Practice* (Seifer DB, Collins RL, Eds.). New York, New York, USA: Springer-Verlag, Chapter 14.

Gregus Z, Klaassen CD, 2001. Mechanisms of Toxicity. In *Casarett and Doull's Toxicology: The Basic Science of Poisons* (Klaassen CD, Ed.). New York, New York, USA: McGraw-Hill, Chapter 3.

Hodgson E, Mailman RB, Chambers JE (Eds.), 1998. *Dictionary of Toxicology.* New York, New York, USA: Grove's Dictionaries Inc.

Howell R, Wyngaarden J, 1960. On the Mechanism of Peroxidation of Uric Acids by Hemeoproteins. *J. Biol. Chem.* 235:3544-3550.

IUPAC (International Union of Pure and Applied Chemistry), 1997. Compendium of Chemical Terminology (compiled by McNaught AD and Wilkinson A), Second Edition. London, Great Britain: Royal Society of Chemistry.

Jeanne N, Dazyl AC, Moreau A, 1993. Cadmium Interactions with ATPase Activity in the Euryhaline Alga *Dunaliella bioculata. Hydrobiologia* 252:245-256.

Kerkeläl R, Grazette L, Yacobi R, Iliescu C, Patten R, Beahm C, Walters B, Shevtsov S, Pesant S, Clubb FJ, Rosenzweig A, Salomon RN, Van Etten RA, Alroy J, Durand J-B, Force T, 2006. Cardiotoxicity of the Cancer Therapeutic Agent Imatinib Mesylate. *Nature Med.* 12:908-916.

Kim DS, Lee EH, Yu SD, Cha JH, Ahn SC, 2005. Heavy Metal as Risk factor of Cardiovascular Disease – An Analysis of Blood Lead and Urinary Mercury. *J. Prev. Med. Public Health* 38:401-407.

Kluwe WM, Lamb JC IV, Greenwell AE, Harrington FW, 1983. 1,2-Dibromo-3-Chloropropane (DBCP)-Induced Infertility in Male Rats Mediated by a Post-Testicular Effect. *Toxicol. App. Pharmacol.* 71:294-298.

Kutlu M, Sümer S, 1998. Effects of Lead on the Activity of δ-Aminolevulinic Acid Dehydratase in *Gammarus pulex*. *Bull. Environ. Contam. Toxicol.* 60:816-821.

Lauble H, Kennedy MC, Emptage MH, Beinert H, Stout CD, 1996. The Reaction of Fluorocitrate with Aconitase and the Crystal Structure of the Enzyme-Inhibitor Complex. *Proc. Natl. Acad. Sci. USA* 93:13699-13703.

Leong BKJ, Lund JE, Groehn JA, Coombs JK, Sabaitis CP, Weaver RJ, Griffin RL, 1987. Retinopathy from Inhaling 4,4′-Methylenedianiline Aerosols. *Fund. Appl. Toxicol.* 9:645-658.

Lindberg S, Wingstrand G, 1985. Mechanism for Cd^{2+} Inhibition of $(K^+ + Mg^{2+})$ ATPase Activity and K^+ $(^{86}Rb^+)$ Uptake Join Roots of Sugar Beet (*Beta vulgaris*). *Physiologia Plantarum* 63:181-186.

Mayo WJ, 1914. Chronic Irritation A Cause of Cancer. *The New York Times*, 10 April.

Meier-Ruge W, 1972. Drug-Induced Retinopathy. *CRC Crit. Rev. Toxicol.* 1:325-360.

Meyer VG, 1996. Flower Abnormalities. *The Botanical Rev.* 32:165-218.

Oldenburg J, Bevans CG, Müller CR, Watzka M, 2006. Vitamin K Epoxide Reductase Complex Subunit 1 (VKORC1): The Key Protein of the Vitamin K Cycle. *Antioxidants & Redox Signaling* 8:347-353.

Pate Capps NJ, Stewart A, Shaw CB, 2009. The Interplay between Secondhand Cigarette Smoke, Genetics, and Cervical Cancer: A Review of the Literature. *Biol. Res. Nursing* 10:392-399.

Patrick L, 2006. Lead Toxicity Part II: The Role of Free Radical Damage and the Use of Antioxidants in the Pathology and Treatment of Lead Toxicity – Lead. *Altern. Med. Rev.* 11:114-127.

Perkins B, 2005. How Does Anesthesia Work? *Scientific America*, 7 February.

Pivovarova NB, Lagerspetz KYH, 1996. Effect of Cadmium on the ATPase Activity in Gills of *Anodonta cygnea* at Different Assay Temperatures. *J. Therm. Biol.* 21:77-84.

Ritsuko M, Mitsuoa H, Masatakaa A, Taizoua I, Hisashi T, 1994. Evidence that Both $Ca2^+$-ATPase and $(Ca^{2+} + Mg^{2+})$-ATPase Activities in the Plasma Membrane-Rich Fraction from Bovine Parotid Gland Reside on the Same Enzyme Molecule. *Inter. J. Biochem.* 26:287-229.

Sakai T, 2000. Biomarkers of Lead Exposure. *Ind. Health* 38:127-142.

Schafer JH, Glass TA, Bressler J, Todd AC, Schwartz BS, 2005. Blood Lead Is a Predictor of Homocysteine Levels in a Population-Based Study of Older Adults. *Environ. Health Perspect.* 113:31-35.

Schwartz AR, Pizon AF, Brooks DE, 2008. Dextromethorphan-Induced Serotonin Syndrome. *Clin. Toxicol.* 46:771-773.

Seely DR, Wu P, Mills EJ, 2005. EDTA Chelation Therapy for Cardiovascular Disease: A Systematic Review. *BMC Cardiovasc. Disord.* 5:32 (online journal).

Simic M, Jovanovic S, 1989. Antioxidation Mechanisms of Uric Acid. *J Am. Chem. Soc.* 11:5778-5782.

Sugimoto K, Goto S, Kanda S, Taniguchi H, Nakamura K, Baba T, 1978. Studies on Angiopathy due to Carbon Disulfide. Retinopathy and Index of Exposure Dosages. *Scand. J. Work Environ. Health* 4:151-158.

Tarloff JB, Wallace AD, 2008. Biochemical Mechanisms of Renal Toxicity: In *Molecular and Biochemical Toxicology* (Smart RC, Hodgson E, Eds.), Fourth Edition. Hoboken, New Jersey, USA: John Wiley & Sons, Chapter 29.

Wagner BA, Buettner GR, Burns CP, 1994. Free Radical-Mediated Lipid Peroxidation in Cells: Oxidizability Is a Function of Cell Lipid bis-Allylic Hydrogen Content. *Biochemistry* 33:4449-4453.

Walboomers JM, Jacobs MV, Manos MM, Bosch FX, Kummer JA, Shah KV, Snijders PJ, Peto J, Meijer CJ, Muñoz N, 1999. Human Papillomavirus Is a Necessary Cause of Invasive Cervical Cancer Worldwide. *J. Pathol.* 189:12-19.

Wang L, Cao J, Chen D, Liu X, Lu H, Liu Z, 2009. Role of Oxidative Stress, Apoptosis, and Intracellular Homeostasis in Primary Cultures of Rat Proximal Tubular Cells Exposed to Cadmium. *Biol. Trace Element Res.* 127:53-68.

Williams AT, Burk RF, 1990. Carbon Tetrachloride Hepatotoxicity: An Example of Free Radical-Mediated Injury. *Semin Liver Dis.* 10:279-284.

Zhao D, Elimban V, Dhalla NS, 1991. Characterization of the Purified Rat Heart Plasma Membrane Ca^{2+}/Mg^{2+}ATPase. *Mol. Cell. Biochem.* 107:151-160.

Review Questions

1. Briefly define the toxicological terms *site of (toxic) action* and *mechanism of (toxic) action*.

2. What are the six categories of common mechanisms of toxic action that are important to a general environmental toxicologist (and thereby discussed in this chapter)?

3. What is the key role of the lipid peroxyl radical in lipid peroxidation?

4. Briefly characterize the two types of transmembrane receptors.

5. What are ion channels? And in these channels, what are the most relevant ions in terms of receptor modulation?

6. Briefly describe the general mechanisms in which hydrogen cyanide and carbon monoxide can adversely affect the normal functions of hemoglobin.

7. How is allergic response different from a typical toxic effect?

8. In terms of *adverse action*, what is something that can be regarded as *common* to the use of medications and the use of chelation therapy?

9. How does bacterial invasion mechanistically differ from viral invasion?

10. What are the two basic modes in which enzymatic activities can be inhibited?

11. Name a cation that is a competitive inhibitor of Mg^{2+} for the binding site on Mg^{2+}-ATPase.

12. Briefly explain why fluorocitrate is a potent Krebs cycle killer (blocker).

13. How does lead (Pb) biochemically inhibit the enzymatic activity of δ-ALAD?

14. What is the basic difference between toxicodynamics and toxicokinetics?

15. Briefly characterize the following: a) acute effect; b) delayed effect; c) idiosyncratic effect.

16 How are cell proliferation and apoptosis mechanistically relevant to carcinogenesis?

17. Why was (is) chronic irritation considered an important medical condition?

18. What is one most prominent target organ of the pesticide DBCP in male rats?

19. Name the body organs and systems on which mercury (Hg) can exert its adverse effects (as mentioned in this chapter).

20. Name an agent that can cause: a) chloracne; b) photoallergic dermatitis; c) retinopathy.

21. Name the agent(s) that can cause both hepatotoxicity and nephrotoxicity.

CHAPTER 10

Factors and Conditions Affecting Toxicity

10.1. Introduction

Today the term *toxicity* is coined as the state or quality of being poisonous or as the degree of an agent's toxic strength, a subject matter of foremost relevance to toxicologists in all branches. Aside from its toxicological properties, a toxicant's *actual* adverse effect on or to the body of an organism depends predominantly on three interrelated conditions: (1) the way in which the toxicant is disposed in the organism's body; (2) the toxicant's bioavailability at the site of action; and (3) the extent to which the organism's body can defend against the toxic action. These three contingencies are not mutually exclusive but somewhat convoluted. For example, the extent to which the organism responds to a toxic action depends largely on how and how much the toxicant is delivered to the site of action. At the same time, the toxicant's bioavailability at the site of action is largely contingent on the organism's ability to eliminate, detoxify, or weaken the toxicant during the course of the toxicant's disposition in the body.

10.1.1. Extrinsic Factors

There are a vast number of extrinsic factors available that can affect one or more of the three contingencies noted above, with many involving the mechanism of (toxic) action. To facilitate the discussion in this chapter, these external factors are broadly subsumed under three source categories as follows, listed somewhat in the order of their most relevance to environmental toxicology: (1) environmental factors; (2) nutritional factors; and (3) physicochemical factors.

The above three categories are neither mutually exclusive, considering that as an example the nutritional constituents of a diet that can affect toxicity are also those coming from the environment or available as food products to consumers. Another reality is that despite the notion that a toxicant's physicochemical properties tend to be intrinsic in nature, these intrinsic properties are greatly affected by the environmental conditions in which the toxicant is present. As discussed specifically in Section 10.4 below, a toxicant's chemical properties include its reactivity with other substances co-existing in the environment. It is in this sense that many physicochemical properties may be treated as involving certain extrinsic elements, if not truly as extrinsic environmental factors.

10.1.2. Intrinsic Cofactors

In contrast, biological factors such as age, gender, and species differences are intrinsic in nature and are not everyday variables that fall within the realm of environmental toxicology. This is not to suggest that these intrinsic factors are not of concern or relevance to any branch of toxicology. It only means that in practice, environmental toxicology is much more preoccupied or masterminded with finding ways to control and prevent *external* factors that affect human health and the environment. This notion is consistent with the concept of environmental health advocated by the World Health Organization (WHO), a point made explicitly in Chapter 2.

Biological factors are included in this chapter, nonetheless, not only for a sense of completeness but also for their important role acting in many ways at least as *co*factors of the extrinsic variables discussed in this chapter. After all, it is not a perception, but rather a reality, that children being younger are generally more vulnerable to environmental exposure than adults are. One apparent reason for such a difference is that children's brain and other body parts are not yet fully developed to withstand as much of the comparatively larger load of environmental exposure. Another reality is that there are now more clinical data available to support the emergence of gender dimorphic profiles, at least in terms of drug efficacy and adverse drug reactions (e.g., Nicolson *et al.*, 2010).

10.2. Environmental Factors

In many cases within a practical range, a positive correlation exists between the level of exposure to a toxicant and the amount or the severity of the adverse effect that the toxicant exerted on an organism, leading to the notion of dose-response relationship consistently asserted by people in the health risk assessment sector. Whether being measured directly or indirectly, environmental exposure is a function of the toxicant's concentration and the way in which the exposure is encountered. There is the consensus that for most toxic effects their manifestation requires the dose to reach a threshold, and that beyond the maximum level no further increase in toxicity will result (Section 9.3.1). It is also intuitive that before a toxic response can be induced, there has to be exposure. Many etiological hypotheses from epidemiological studies are built on this concept. In the case of *environmental* exposure, the toxicant's concentration in a medium becomes the most influential factors affecting its toxicity. In fact, all regulatory mitigation measures proposed or developed for environmental exposure are based on this notion.

Inasmuch as environmental exposure is almost always an involuntary act, other exposure-related environmental variables such as control measures in effect, exposure duration, and exposure frequency are all crucial and relevant. Nonexposure-related environmental factors that can affect toxicity include the environmental medium's pH, temperature, and many other meteorological variables.

10.2.1. Level of Environmental Exposure

There are ample cases and experimental data supporting Paracelsus' notion of dose-response relationship (Chapter 1), which asserts that a contaminant's toxicity is strongly related to its environmental exposure level (though usually within a practical range only). Four such cases are discussed in this (sub)section for illustration purposes, with each selected to intentionally represent a unique toxicity situation or platform.

A. London Fog of 1952

In December 1952, London and its greater metropolitan area in Great Britain were severely polluted with heavy smog containing high levels of sulfur dioxide (SO_2). As discussed in Chapter 11, SO_2 is not only highly toxic to plants but also a potent pulmonary irritant to humans. This air pollution episode resulted in as many as 4,000 excess (premature) deaths and 100,000 extra cases of cardiovascular- or respiratory-related illnesses in the metropolitan area. As later reassessed by Bell and Davis (2001), the weekly mortality estimated for Greater London was highly and positively correlated with the weekly air concentrations of SO_2 occurring in that area, even beyond the episode period during the first week of December 1952 (Figure 10.1). The strong positive correlation should be interpreted with some caution, however, in that certain confounding effects might be inevitable as SO_2 might not be the only smog pollutant present at the time.

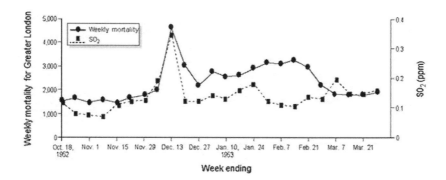

Figure 10.1. Approximate Weekly Mortality and Air Concentrations of Sulfur Dioxide (SO_2) in Greater London, 1952-1953 *(reproduced from Bell and Davis [2001] with implicit permission for public domain materials published in a U.S. Government journal)*

B. Uptake of Soil Cadmium and Arsenic

Cadmium (Cd) and arsenic (As) are phytotoxic metals known to retard plant growth (e.g., Anastasia and Kender, 1973; John *et al.*, 2008; Sheppard, 1992; Woolson, 1973). In one pot-culture experiment (Sun *et al.*, 2008) on deadly nightshade (*Solanum nigrum* L.), which is a hyper-accumulator of Cd, the data showed that the accumulation of the metal increased with increasing soil concentration except when As was also present at a sufficiently high level in the same soil pot. As shown in Table 10.1, mean levels were increased up to *three*fold for Cd accumulation in the *S. nigrum* stems when the spike with Cd in the soil was increased *five*fold (i.e., from Cd-10 to Cd-50), except when the soil was also spiked with As at the highest spike level of 250 mg/kg (i.e., except at As-250).

Table 10.1. Mean Concentrations of Cadmium (Cd) Measured in the Stems of *Solanum nigrum* Growing in Pot Soils Spiked with Various Levels of Cd and Arsenic (As)[a]

Treatment	Concentration of Cd (mg/kg)		
	Cd-10	Cd-25	Cd-50
As-0	122	208	387
As-50	170	184	385
As-250	106	124	102

[a]modified from Table 1 in Sun *et al.* (2008); spike As-50 = 50 mg/kg of As added, spike Cd-25 = 25 mg/kg of Cd added, and so forth.

C. LC_{50} of Polychlorinated Biphenyls for Fish

Polychlorinated biphenyls (PCBs) were sold in the United States under the eight trade names Aroclor 1221, 1232, 1242, 1248, 1254, 1260, 1262, and 1268. Their individual LC_{50} values (i.e., the lethal concentrations that killed 50% of a study population) were determined by Stalling and Mayer (1972) for three fish species using the intermittent-flow bioassay method (Adams, 1995; Chandler *et al.*, 1974; *see* also Section 22.2.2). These acute toxicity data, reproduced in Table 10.2, showed that while varying greatly among the eight PCB products and the three fish species tested, the LC_{50} values decreased with increasing days of exposure (and thereby with increasing exposure).

Table 10.2. Acute Toxicity of Aroclors (PCBs) to Three Fish Species[a]

Aroclor	Species	Median Lethal Concentration (LC_{50}, in μg/L)					
		5 days	10 days	15 days	20 days	25 days	30 days
1254	Trout	156	8	–	–	–	–
1260	Trout	–	240	94	21	–	–
1242	Bluegills	154	72	54	–	–	–
1248	Bluegills	307	160	76	10	–	–
1254	Bluegills	–	443	204	135	54	–
1260	Bluegills	–	–	–	245	212	151
1242	Catfish	–	174	107	–	–	–
1248	Catfish	–	225	127	–	–	–
1254	Catfish	–	–	741	300	113	–
1260	Catfish	–	–	–	296	166	137
1248[b]	Bluegills	137	76	–	–	–	–
1248[b]	Catfish	–	94	57	–	–	–

[a]modified from Stalling and Mayer (1972); temperature, 20° C (except noted otherwise); alkalinity, 260; pH, 7.4; days are duration of exposure; Aroclor is the trade name for polychlorinated biphenyl (PCB) products sold in the United States.

[b]temperature at 27° C.

D. Cigarette Consumption in Japan

An epidemiological study was conducted in which the death rate (i.e., mortality) of lung cancer in Japan was correlated with cumulative amount of cigarettes consumed and measured at the national level (Yamaguchi *et al.*, 2000). Cumulative consumption was defined as the total number of cigarettes consumed in a person's life up to a certain age. Figure 10.2 shows that in each of the eight 5-year birth cohorts (from ages 35-39 to 70-74), lung cancer death rate increased linearly and significantly with increasing cumulative cigarette consumption, as evident from the mostly high coefficient of determination R^2 values obtained. The data also suggested that other factors might have played a role in more recent years, as the R^2 values were comparatively lower for the two youngest age (35-39 and 40-44) groups. Coincidentally or not, according to the investigators, the dietary habits in Japan had changed rapidly and more recently (i.e., in the 1960s and 1970s).

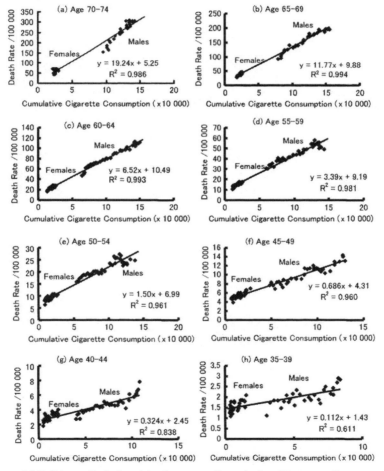

Figure 10.2. Linear Relationships between Cumulative Cigarette Consumption and Lung Cancer Mortality for Eight Japanese Birth Cohorts
(reproduced from Yamaguchi et al. [2000] with permission from the publisher Oxford Journals)

10.2.2. Other Exposure-Related Factors

In addition to exposure level, other common relevant exposure-related factors include mode of contact with the toxicant and control measures that are in effect. There are many other factors that in some cases have a strong influence on exposure, such as employment type and work experience. These other variables are not treated as straightly environmental in nature within the context of this book. In many cases, frequency of exposure and duration of exposure are key determinants of exposure level, as in the above two cases with PCBs (Table 10.2) and cigarette consumption (Figure 10.2). They are nevertheless treated as separate, distinct factors momentarily for the consideration given below.

A. Frequency and Duration of Exposure

Both exposure frequency and exposure duration are collaborative with environmental exposure level, especially for chronic effects resulting from exposure at lower levels. Here by collaborative, it means that the effect of dose, including that of environmental exposure, *presumably* obeys Haber's law (e.g., Gaylor, 2000). This law asserts the effect e equivalency of any two sets of dose concentrations c_i and exposure times t_i, as long as the mathematical products of the two sets are equivalent. That is, if $c_1 \times t_1 = c_2 \times t_2$, then $e_1 = e_2$. It is apparent that such an assertion cannot hold true for all cases. For example, suppose for simplicity $t_2 = t_1 + t_1$ (i.e., twice as long as t_1). Then $c_1 = c_2 + c_2$ (i.e., twice as high as c_2) in order for $e_1 = e_2$. However, if the toxicant from exposure at the lower level c_2 can be sufficiently eliminated from the host's body by t_1 and the effect can be induced only from exposure at levels exceeding c_2, then no effect would likely result from the second exposure scenario. Note that in exposure assessment, duration of exposure is commonly defined as the *period* of each exposure event (e.g., 1 day) whereas frequency of exposure, as the *number* of exposure events (e.g., daily, biweekly, annually).

In reality, the adverse effect of any given exposure is much more dynamic than what can be explained mathematically and tends to obey Haber's law within some constraints. Both the data in Figure 10.2 and Table 10.2 demonstrated that exposure frequency is a crucial factor. In the case with cumulative cigarette consumption (Figure 10.2), it is clear that the lung cancer death rate increased with increasing years of consumption. In the case with the acute toxicity of PCBs to fish (Table 10.2), the data showed that at least for the fish species and the bioassay conditions studied, longer exposure days were required for lower exposure concentrations in order for the various PCB products each to have a concrete median lethal concentration (i.e., LC_{50}).

B. Mode of Contact and Control Measure

These two factors are more *subtle* compared to environmental concentration or exposure time and can be highly interrelated. An example for supporting this notion is the case of young children playing on a residential lawn treated with an herbicide. At what time post-application and in what manner these children are allowed to play on a treated lawn may depend on the health conscience of their parents concerning the herbicide's harmful effects. In general, a parent's knowledge on a pesticide's toxicity comes from product labeling which serves as some form of control measure.

Control measure can have a substantial impact on the environmental exposure of certain (groups of) toxicants. A case in point is the state law in California, effective New Year's Day of 2010 and as discussed in Chapter 4 (Section 4.2.2.C), for banning the use of trans fats in restaurants. Other case examples for mitigating exposure via control measure can also be found in Chapter 4, such as those related to lead on toys (Section 4.2.1.B), plastic bags (Section 4.2.3.A), pharmaceutical wastes (Section 4.2.3.B), and cleanup at the United Heckathorn Superfund toxic site (Section 4.2.3.C).

Nonetheless, in reality it is very difficult to assess the magnitude of children's exposure when it comes to something like lead on toys, as it all depends on *their* individual personality and habits. Touching the supposedly low levels of lead coated on toys is generally not a significant exposure route. However, infants up to about 3 years of age often chew on their toys and put their hands in their mouths. Exposure from object-to-mouth or hand-to-mouth will increase considerably the intake of a substance compared to routine dermal contact. In most cases, the dermal absorption and acquisition of a topical dose in an incremental manner is supposedly less potent than the oral absorption and acquisition of a bolus (oral) dose (e.g., Ross *et al.*, 2000). There are ample data supporting this assertion. For example, where available the *oral* LD_{50} (the lethal dose that killed 50% of a test population) is almost always much lower (i.e., much more potent) than the respective *dermal* LD_{50} listed in the Material Safety Data Sheet (commonly known by its acronym MSDS) specifically for each ingredient (e.g., a pesticide) in a product.

For environmental exposures of relatively long duration and high frequency, people can be exposed to more than one contaminant with the same adverse effect of concern. It is for this potential that the Food Quality Protection Act (FQPA) of 1996 directs U.S. EPA to consider the *cumulative* adverse effect from exposures to pesticides sharing a common mechanism of toxicity. This type of public health concern has strengthened and expanded U.S. EPA's practice in its pesticide risk assessment to perform *aggregate* exposure as well for each target population, by considering exposures to the same pesticide from work, foods, drinking water, as well as other sources and routes. Further discussion on this topic is given in Chapter 23. What is important to know here is that the route of exposure to (i.e., the mode of contact with) an environmental toxicant is not always well defined. This problem is not unique to the human species. Large fish can take in a persistent toxic substance not only from the contaminated water, but also from eating smaller fish that each might already have had a considerable amount of the substance accumulated in their tissues. The two familiar terms relating to this kind of environmental exposure are *bioaccumulation* and *biomagnification*, which are discussed extensively in Chapter 6.

10.2.3. Nonexposure-Related Factors

Environmental factors that are influential but not as directly related to exposure include the medium's pH, temperature, humidity, light, and other meteorological variables.

Temperature variations may cause a physiological stress to the host or lead to a substantial difference in a toxicant's physicochemical properties and hence its toxicological profile as well. As shown in Table 10.2, the LC_{50} of Aroclor 1248 for both catfish and bluegills were reduced twofold when the temperature in the bioassay was increased from $20°$ C to $27°$ C. Other studies have also implicated that temperature has a significant effect on a chemical's toxicity, though mostly in insects and other invertebrates (e.g., Barson, 1983; Bat *et al.*, 2000; Boina *et al.*, 2009; Khan *et al.*, 2007; Li *et al.*, 2006; Viswanathan and Murti, 1989). High temperature can affect the release and transport of airborne substances that may trigger an allergic reaction (Jacobson and Morris, 1976; Viswanathan and Murti, 1989). Moreover, it is a familiar practice to many farmers that plants are not to be sprayed with lime sulfur at a field temperature above $29°$ C ($85°$ F), as then the fungicide would become a burning agent to the foliage instead.

The effects of humidity and moisture on toxicity, like those of temperature, are not as well understood in humans and other mammalians as in insects. One reason is that chemicals like pesticides are not intended to get rid of humans and other mammalians. There tend to be greater motivations for investigating the effects of temperature and humidity on insects because a pesticide's efficacy is at stake for marketing purposes. In any case, there was one very relevant study in which beetles (*Oryzaephilus surinamensis*) were exposed to each of three organophosphorus insecticides at various (30, 50, 70, 90% relative) humidity levels (Barson, 1983). The study found that the mortality of the test beetles increased with increasing humidity at each test temperature ($5°$ to $30°$ C at $5°$ C intervals). It was thought that the increase in lethal effect was due to high ambient humidity's capability to cause swelling of the stratum corneum of invertebrates and thereby to allow greater penetration of chemicals through their skin (Suskind, 1977).

The toxicities of many metals and other chemicals were reportedly affected by the pH in the aqueous test solution (e.g., Franklin *et al.*, 2000; Ho *et al.*, 1999; Kobayashi and Kishino, 1980; Michnowicz and Weaks, 1984; Sawyer *et al.*, 2007). However, this factor or condition may not be of immediate concern for terrestrial organisms.

High altitude areas are those on the Earth's surface high above sea level (e.g., above 5,000 ft), where the temperature is cold and the atmospheric pressure is low compared to those at sea level. Altitude effects on the toxicological properties of environmental substances are not well understood. Nonetheless, studies have been published showing that the toxicities of some chemicals can be affected considerably in humans treated and animals dosed at high altitude (e.g., Fischer, 1941; Singh *et al.*, 2001; Vats *et al.*, 2008). It is likely that these altitude-related changes in toxicity were due to the effect on the test subject's physiological response, rather than to any modulation directly on the toxicity of the test material. Regardless, it is a known fact that in humans, the risk of carbon monoxide (CO) poisoning is proportionate to high altitude (among other variables). This however is likely (also) due to the fact that less oxygen per breath is available at high altitude.

Light is a variable that can affect a host's diurnal rhythm or the physicochemical (and thereby likely the toxicological) properties of a toxicant. For instance, atmospheric SO_2

in the presence of sunlight and water vapor can readily form sulfuric acid (H_2SO_4), which is a major acidic component found in acid rain (Chapter 5). Many chemicals are subject to photolysis (i.e., chemical decomposition induced by light or other radiant energy; *see* Chapter 5). Both light quality and light quantity have been shown to affect herbicide toxicity to plants (e.g., Erickson *et al.*, 1972; Pollak and Crabtree, 1976). It is apparent that temperature is closely related to (sun)light.

Many studies have been conducted to analyze the interactions between light and the hormone melatonin (Chapter 19) in humans, animals, and plants. In humans and certain mammalians, melatonin regulates the circadian rhythms of several biological functions by varying its circulating levels in a daily cycle. Secretion of certain hormones including melatonin is reportedly influenced by light exposure (e.g., Bellastella *et al.*, 1998; Boyce and Kennaway, 1987; Hymer *et al.*, 2009; Kasuya *et al.*, 2008; Reiter *et al.*, 2007).

10.3. Nutritional Factors

Nutrition as a science refers to the study dealing with the physiological process by which an organism nourishes itself, or is nourished, with food for growth and health maintenance. Food toxicology is the branch of toxicology or nutrition concerned with toxicants (including especially toxins) found in foods, whereas nutritional toxicology is the branch with its focus on nutritional status affected by the interactions between toxicants and nutrients in the diet (Omaye, 2004). Nourishing ingredients found in foods are known as nutrients, which in general biochemical terms include proteins, lipids, carbohydrates, vitamins, and minerals. The focus of this section is on nutrition-related factors or conditions tending to modulate the adverse effects of environmental toxicants. Such nutritional variables can be broadly divided into two groups: (1) those nutrients capable of modulating a toxicant's effect; and (2) nutritional status of the host body.

10.3.1. Nutritional Status

Malnutrition, starvation, fasting, obesity, and nutritional disorders all reflect the nutritional status of the host in which a toxicant is present; that is, all representing a common nutritional state that the host is in. Any of these nutritional conditions can modulate considerably the adverse effect that the toxicant has on its host. For instance, malnutrition can increase substantially the toxicity of some metals (e.g., cadmium; Prasad and Nath, 1995), some pesticides (e.g., naled; Kaloyanova and Tasheva, 1983), and some other substances (e.g., hexachlorocyclohexane; Agrawal *et al.*, 1992).

Starvation can be caused by famine, poverty, severe gastrointestinal disorders, coma, stroke, the eating disorder anorexia nervosa, and fasting, with the last two being largely a voluntary act. In all cases, this nutritional condition can modulate the toxicity of xenobiotics what malnutrition can do and more, as it represents the worse and more dangerous form of the latter. In particular, an animal study (Dave, 1981) showed that adult fathead minnows starved for 80 days were twice more susceptible to the acute toxicity of endrin which, like hexachlorocyclohexane (HCH), is an organochlorine pesticide with high lipophilicity. During starvation, lipids stored in the fatty tissues are utilized before other sources such as proteins and fats in the muscle (Czesny et al., 2003). This event suggests that starvation can cause lipophilic toxicants such as endrin and HCH to become less available in the adipose tissue and hence more available at the site of toxic action instead.

10.3.2. Macro- and Micro-Nutrients

Nutrients are generally divided into macronutrients and micronutrients according to the quantity in which they are needed by the organism's body to sustain essential biological functions. Accordingly, *micro*nutrients such as potassium (K) and phosphorus (P) for mammalians (especially humans) are actually *macro*nutrients for plants. Macronutrients for humans generally include proteins, carbohydrates, and lipids. Water is a macronutrient by definition, but frequently excluded from consideration as a nutritional factor not only due to its unique importance to life but also due to its abundance. Micronutrients for humans include a number of vitamins, minerals, and metals, of which some are more essential than others. Many nutrients have the ability to modulate the activities of certain Phase I and Phase II enzymes (Chapter 8) and hence the potential to affect considerably the toxicity of xenobiotics as well. Below is a brief overview of some studies that support this notion which is largely species-specific.

A. Macronutrients in Mammalians

Protein deficiency in quantities is a major kind of malnutrition and thus has much of the effects on toxicity as malnutrition in general has. Biochemically, these malnutrition effects are likely due to, as induced by protein deficiency, an alteration in the liver's ability to biotransform the xenobiotic (Czygan et al., 1974; Hayes et al., 1973; Kawano and Hiraga, 1980). In addition, low quality of dietary protein can be treated as a special form of protein deficiency. Protein quality refers to how well the essential amino acids in a protein can compensate for those required by the body. Studies showed that the quality of dietary protein correlated positively with cytochrome P450 activities in the rat liver (Campbell and Hayes, 1976; Kato et al., 1981; Miranda and Webb, 1973), thereby enhancing either the detoxification or the bioactivation of certain toxicants. In particular, a study by Schulsinger et al. (1989) showed that either low quantity or poor quality of protein intake was equally effective in inhibiting the development of aflatoxin B_1-induced hepatic preneoplastic lesions.

Low levels of carbohydrate intake, whether along with alcohol (Korourian et al., 1999; Tsukada et al., 1998) or with high fat (Yoo et al., 1991) in the diet, can elevate the hepatic level of CYP2E1 in the rat. And modulation of this P450 enzyme level will have a crucial effect on the toxicity of some environmental toxicants, in that the enzyme plays a key role in xenobiotic biotransformation . In contrast, high dietary carbohydrates in the male rat with low fat but normal protein content reportedly resulted in a noticeable decrease in microsomal P450 enzymes in the liver (Sonawane et al., 1983).

Other studies showed that high levels of polyunsaturated fats in diets to rats generally also brought about an increase in the activity of microsomal cytochrome P450 in the liver (Century, 1973; Clinton *et al.* 1984; Marshall and McLean, 1971; Wade and Norred, 1976). In particular, dietary lipids containing a high concentration of certain unsaturated fatty acids, such as the *Omega*-6 linoleic acid, were shown to induce a higher elevation of the P450 enzyme activity (Saito *et al.*, 1990). These findings all supported the notion that lipid quality too can affect considerably the toxicity of xenobiotics.

B. Micronutrients in Mammalians

The effects of vitamins, minerals, and metals on the toxicity of xenobiotics can be appreciated from their role as a coenzyme or cofactor of certain Phase I and Phase II enzymes. Among the vitamins found in humans, vitamins A (e.g., retinol), B_1 (thiamine), B_2 (riboflavin), C (ascorbic acid), and E (e.g., tocopherol) are the more prominent ones known to affect the activities of Phase I enzymes. Some other vitamins are themselves affected by the activities of certain cytochrome P450s. For example, in humans vitamin D is bioactivated to its hormonal form by some P450s. And the cause of vitamin K deficiency can be attributed to an induction of P450s by some anticonvulsants.

Experiments with vitamin C-deficient guinea pigs consistently showed a decreased hepatic microsomal P450 content in animals fed on diets not supplemented with the vitamin (e.g., Rikans, 1982; Sato and Zannoni, 1976). A study with rats also found that vitamins C and E were protective against alcohol-induced liver injury and capable of modulating hepatic and plasma lipid peroxidation (Ramírez-Farías *et al.*, 2008).

In general, deficiencies in vitamins A and E can cause a *decrease* in cytochrome P450 activity in animal livers (Iwasaki *et al.*, 1994; Miranda *et al.*, 1979). In contrast, vitamin B_1 deficiency has been associated with an *increased* content of CYP2E1 in the rat liver (Yoo *et al.*, 1990); and vitamin B_2 deficiency has been linked to an *increase* in the hepatic contents of cytochrome P450s and cytochrome b_5, but a *decrease* in the hepatic content of NADPH-dependent cytochrome P450 reductase (Taniguchi, 1980). Other members in the vitamin B group (e.g., biotin, niacin, pantothenic acid, pyridoxine, folic acid, choline, cyanocobalamin) either do not affect the activities of Phase I or Phase II enzymes, or have not been actively investigated for such or similar effects.

Overall, a decrease in the contents or activities of P450 enzymes has been linked to a deficiency in dietary magnesium (Mg), calcium (Ca), copper (Cu), and zinc (Zn), or to an excess intake of iron (Fe) and iodine (I). In particular, Zn deficiency can alter the activities of certain Phase II enzymes (Jagadeesan and Oesch, 1988). Even though zinc is essential for all living forms, an excess intake of this metallic element can be harmful to the human body (Fosmire, 1990). For example, excessive intake of zinc can suppress copper absorption (Fosmire, 1990; Oestreicher and Cousins, 1985), thus indirectly affecting the activities of certain cytochrome P450 enzymes through the effects of copper deficiency. Studies have shown that copper has the ability to inhibit or retard the catalytic functions of CYP1A1, CYP1A2, CYP3A4, and NADPH-dependent cytochrome P450 reductase in hepatic microsomes (Kim *et al.*, 2002; Korashy and El-Kadi, 2005; Letelier *et al.* 2009). This however does not seem to be the case with zinc *per se* (Kim *et al.*, 2002).

Like zinc and copper, molybdenum (Mo) is an essential trace element for virtually all life forms. In humans, this element functions as a cofactor for sulfite oxidase, xanthine oxidase, and aldehyde oxidase. The last two enzymes reportedly play a key role in the biotransformation of certain xenobiotics (Eckhert, 2006). Significant increases were observed in brain mitochondrial and microsomal P450 contents in rats treated with magnesium (Liccione and Maines, 1989). One study (Yasukochi *et al.*, 1977) showed that the P450 contents were depressed considerably in rats injected with cobalt (Co), a key component of vitamin B_{12}. Another study (Shivarajashankara *et al.*, 2001) found that an excess of dietary fluoride (F) caused an increase in brain and hepatic levels of glutathione S-transferase (GST), an important Phase II enzyme, in the rat. Some effects of selenium (Se) deficiency were observed on the hepatic microsomal cytochrome P450 system in the rat (Burk and Masters, 1975). At the present time, it is unclear what effects, if any, that other micronutrients (e.g., boron, chloride, chromium, potassium, sodium) can have on the biotransformation of xenobiotics.

10.4. Physicochemical Factors

Most of a toxicant's physicochemical properties are actually its nature and are what have made up its basic toxicological profile. For instance, as noted earlier, in humans most airborne particles larger than 15 μm in diameter are filtered by the nasal hairs and thereby unable to exert their toxic effects at the lower region of the lung. And sulfur spray fungicide will burn the foliage if it is applied to plants at a field temperature above 29° C (85° F), although this second point may be viewed as due to an environmental condition with high temperature rather than to a chemical or physical factor. Strictly speaking, chemical property is any of a material's properties that has the potential to alter the chemical nature of matter during a chemical reaction by virtue of the material's chemical composition. A material's chemical properties thus include its toxicity, chemical stability, flammability, and reactivity with or against other substances. Of these, the material's *reactivity* is the variable that can affect greatly its own toxicity or that of another, and thereby is the focus of this section. This reactivity, of which chemical interaction is the main part, may result in a joint toxic effect that falls into one of the four patterns: (1) additivity or additive effects; (2) synergism; (3) potentiation; and (4) antagonism.

10.4.1. Additivity of Toxic Effects

In toxicology, especially in health risk assessment, this term refers to the combined effect that is expected from two toxicants; that is, additive in nature. For additive effects, the joint exposure to one toxicant with a toxicity level of 1 unit and concurrently or subsequently to another toxicant with a toxicity level of 2 units would result in a combined toxicity level of 3 units. This result implies that neither toxicant has any apparent effect on the other's toxicity. One desired consequence from this additivity effect is that in its absence, the effect of the toxicant at issue may be below the threshold of exerting harm to the host's body. It has been reported that when two organophosphate insecticides are applied together, the resultant joint AChE (acetylcholinesterase) inhibition is likely additive (e.g., Eaton and Klaassen, 2001).

Dose-addition is currently the default approach used to determine cumulative risks from exposures to multiple toxicants that are suspected or expected to share a common mechanism of toxicity (e.g., Chen *et al.*, 2001). These days, the concerns with cumulative risks by regulatory entities come about from largely two developments: (1) mandate of the FQPA of 1996 (Sielken, 2000); and (2) use of toxic equivalency factors advocated by WHO for estimation of health risks from dioxin-like substances (Chapter 16). The validity of this cumulative risk approach has remained controversial until recently, when there is now more evidence emerging to support the dose-additive effects of the pyrethroid pesticides (Chapter 15) on motor activity in rats (Wolansky *et al.*, 2009).

10.4.2. Synergism of Toxic Effects

The term *synergism* (of toxic effects) refers to the joint effect of two toxicants that is greater than additive. Numerically, the combined toxicity level would be greater than 3 units for the example with the two hypothetical toxicants given in Section 10.4.1 above on additivity. This also implies that one toxicant has an effect on the toxicity of the other, with a consequence potentially being much worse than expected. An example is the concurrent exposures to the two hepatotoxic compounds ethanol (C_2H_5-OH) and carbon tetrachloride (CCl_4) that together produce much more liver injury than what would be expected from adding their individual hepatic effects (Eaton and Klaassen, 2001).

Another example of synergism is the lung cancer risk from joint exposure to asbestos and cigarette smoking. Estimates of the joint effect of the two agents were found to exceed the sum of their individual carcinogenic effects observed in each of the 12 epidemiological studies revisited by Erren *et al.* (1999). A pot experiment (Agrawal *et al.*, 1981) also revealed that synergistic effect of plant injury occurred when rice plants were fumigated jointly with O_3 (ozone) and SO_2 (sulfur dioxide). In that experiment, the plant injury was measured in terms of the reductions in chlorophylls *a* and *b* as well as in total contents of chlorophyll and carotenoid in leaves.

10.4.3. Potentiation of Toxic Effects

In keeping with the definition of the verb *potentiate* being to make (more) potent or to enhance an effect, here the term *potentiation* refers to an interaction in which one substance's presence makes the other substance toxic or more toxic to a body organ or tissue. It means that the potentiator (i.e., potentiating agent) has little or no toxic effect on that body part, but has an enhancing effect on the toxicity of the other substance. This assertion is based on the notion that if the potentiator has similar toxic effects on the same body part, then by definition the joint effect should be treated as additive or synergistic.

Regardless, isopropanol and acetone have been shown able to potentiate the hepato-toxicity of CCl_4 in rats (Plaa *et al.*, 1982), as neither potentiator is a hepatotoxicant. And the relatively nontoxic ascorbic acid (vitamin C) has been implicated for potentiating the cytotoxicity of the anticancer therapeutic drug arsenic trioxide (As_2O_3) in human leuke-mia cells (Yedjou *et al.*, 2009). In addition, two cases of acute occupational poisoning have been reported (Manno *et al.*, 1996), in which severe hepatonephrotoxicity was de-veloped from inhalation of CCl_4 present at high concentrations in the fire extinguishing liquid. The toxicity of CCl_4 was reportedly potentiated by alcohol abuse by the two pa-tients. The study's conclusion was based on the observation that the rest of the co-workers showed no signs of the toxicity even for those that were exposed to CCl_4 under the same working conditions but were verified as non-alcohol abusers. Since *nephro*toxi-city was involved, alcohol and not CCl_4 was concluded as more likely the potentiator.

10.4.4. Antagonism of Toxic Effects

Of the four types of chemical interaction discussed here, antagonism is the most de-sirable from a medical standpoint, given that this type is the basis of many therapeutic developments. The term refers to a chemical interaction between two substances where-by the joint effect is less than what one would expect from the sum of their individual ef-fects. Antagonism itself can be subdivided into four major forms or subtypes. Chelation therapy, as discussed in Section 9.3.3, is an example of the *chemical* form of antagonism. Treatment of CO (carbon monoxide) poisoning with hyperbaric oxygen is a therapy rely-ing on the increased removal of CO from hemoglobin. This competition for receptor sites is an example of the *receptor* or *competitive* form of antagonism.

Functional or *physiological* antagonism is the third major form which occurs when two agents produce opposite effects on the same physiological system or function there-by effectively counteracting each other agent's effect. A historical account of this form of antagonism between calcium (Ca) and magnesium and between a few other ions can be found in the paper by Haag and Palmer (1928), which credited its importance in main-taining a physiological balance among the elements entering the animal diet. The fourth form is *dispositional* in nature, involving the alteration of chemical disposition whereby the agent at issue becomes less bioactive or bioavailable at the site of action. Dietary cal-cium is a dispositional antagonist known to lower the intestinal absorption of lead (Pb) in humans (Peraza *et al.*, 1998). In a way, the hyperbaric oxygen used in the treatment of CO poisoning can be classified additionally as a dispositional antagonist.

10.5. Biological Factors

As with the three main groups of extrinsic factors discussed above, there is a vast number of biological factors capable of affecting the toxicity of xenobiotics in an organ-ism. The more crucial ones include gender, age, health status, disease condition, species, strain, race, genetic makeup, and physiological state, with some being highly interrelated.

These biological factors individually or in combination play a key role in setting the effects that the extrinsic factors have on the toxicity of xenobiotics. Considering that these biological factors are all intrinsic in nature, perhaps the most effective way to attenuate their effects on the toxicity of concern is to avoid coming in contact with the toxicant.

10.5.1. Age, Gender, and Health Status

In terms of effects on toxicity, age does matter a lot. In 2003, WHO launched a campaign on environmental health specifically for children (Chapter 2), with the concern that these future citizens possess unique biological, developmental, and behavioral vulnerabilities; and they indeed do. One argument in point is that the blood-brain barrier cellular structure in infants is not fully developed to be able to restrict the passage of many harmful substances from their blood to their brain. An example for age effect in a different direction is that in the plant kingdom, young leaves of certain plants (e.g., Cucurbitaceae) were reportedly more resistant to injury from acute exposure to SO_2, whereas mature leaves were more sensitive to such exposure (e.g., Sekiya *et al.*, 1982).

Gender can also affect greatly the toxicity of certain environmental toxicants. A study showed that the oldest females were the most difficult wild house mice to be killed by the anticoagulant warfarin compared to the males and the younger females (Rowe and Redfern, 1964, 1967). Another study showed that in a population of small insectivorous passerine birds living around a copper smelter, the males had a 33% higher local survival probability, whereas the local survival rate of the females did not differ between those living in the polluted and the unpolluted environment (Eeva *et al.*, 2006). Still another example is the discovery, which is widely known to many toxicologists, that unleaded gasoline was capable of inducing kidney tumors only in male rats but not in females or in either sex of mice. This species- and sex-specific disorder was later confirmed to be attributed to the much higher levels of the protein $\alpha_{2\mu}$-globulin present in male rats only, and hence is now referred to as $\alpha_{2\mu}$-globulin nephropathy. A paper by Swenberg (1993) compiled a long list of chemical substances (including certainly unleaded gasoline) that were reported as capable of causing $\alpha_{2\mu}$-globulin nephropathy.

Health status and disease condition, both of which can lead to a certain physiological state of the body, are simply two terms referring to the same thing but viewing it from the opposite end of the same spectrum. Either case can affect considerably the activities of certain Phase I and Phase II enzymes and thereby the toxicity of certain xenobiotics. For example, a study showed that the blood level of CYP3A4 mRNA (i.e., CYP3A4 gene expression) in a group of patients correlated positively with the progression of their viral liver diseases (Horiike *et al.*, 2005). CYP3A4 is one of the most important human cytochrome P450 enzymes involved in the biotransformation of xenobiotics. There is a body of evidence supporting the correlation between the expression of CYP3A4 mRNA and the metabolic activity of the enzyme in the human liver (Watanabe *et al.*, 2004). Kidney is quantitatively the second major organ that can increase the toxic potential of environmental pollutants, mainly by causing slower elimination of the pollutants from the body. Renal failure can adversely affect not only the elimination, but also the transport and metabolism of xenobiotics (e.g., Sun *et al.*, 2006).

As is true of people who are sick, unhealthy plants too are more susceptible to attack by pests, pathogens, and chemical agents. Compared to the leaves of healthy plants, those of chlorotic plants (e.g., caused by iron-deficiency) generally show more signs of oxidative stress despite the idea that oxidative injury may not be as definitive or transparent (e.g., Salama *et al.*, 2009; Tewari *et al.*, 2005). In plants, oxidative stress refers to the adverse condition leading to excessive production of ROS (reactive oxygen species) in their cells, likely caused by the loss of some of their physiological antioxidant mechanisms.

10.5.2. Species, Strain, Race, and Genetics

An example of species variation as a definite toxicity-affecting variable was given earlier concerning $\alpha_{2\mu}$-globulin nephropathy on rats but not on mice. Even within the same species, the potency of an environmental toxicant can vary greatly among strains. For example, the LD_{50} of thiourea ($[NH_2]_2CS$) was found to differ nearly 300-fold from one strain of rats to another (e.g., tame Norway *vs.* wild Alexandrine *vs.* wild Norway) when the animals were dosed under identical conditions (Dieke and Richter, 1945). Thiourea, an antioxidant, has been used in the modification of textile and dyeing auxiliaries, in the leaching of ores, as well as in the synthesis of pesticides and drugs.

As noted in Section 8.6.1, around 7% of Caucasians are considered as "poor" metabolizers because they lack CYP2D6 or its function in their body. This cytochrome P450 is one of the most important Phase I enzymes in xenobiotic biotransformation, as it is responsible for catalyzing the oxidative metabolism of many drugs and many other chemicals in the human body. Yet there is a considerable variability of its genetic expressions in the liver, with some losing entirely its ability to oxidize many xenobiotics. In essence, genetic variations in CYP2D6 activity alone can influence the toxicity of many xenobiotics, especially drugs. The P450 enzymes in other families are also highly polymorphic as they too are subject to considerable genetic variation.

In the plant kingdom, many species vary in their tolerance to and uptake of metals. In particular, in the 99 pea genotypes tested (Belimov *et al.*, 2003; Metwally *et al.*, 2005), large variability was found in their uptake of heavy metals and tolerance to cadmium.

References

Adams WJ, 1995. Aquatic Toxicology Testing Methods. In *Handbook of Ecotoxicology* (Hoffman DJ, Rattner BA, Burton GA, Cairns J, Eds.). Boca Raton, Florida, USA: Lewis/CRC Publishers, pp.25-46.

Agrawal D, Sultana P, Gupta GSD, Gopal K, Khanna RN, Anand M, 1992. Effect of Hexachlorocyclohexane on Biochemical Parameters of Rats on a Protein Deficient Diet. *Toxicol. Environ. Chem.* 35:109-114.

Agrawal M, Nandi PK, Rao DN, 1981. Effect of Ozone and Sulphur Dioxide Pollutants Separately and in Mixture on Chlorophyll and Carotenoid Pigments of *Oryza sativa*. *Water, Air, Soil Pull.* 18:449-454.

Anastasia FB, Kender WJ, 1973. The Influence of Soil Arsenic on the Growth of Low-Bush Blueberry. *J. Environ. Qual.* 2:335-337.

Arthur FH, 1999. Effect of Temperature on Residual Toxicity of Cyfluthrin Wettable Powder. *J. Econ. Entomol.* 92:695-699.

Barson G, 1983. The Effects of Temperature and Humidity on the Toxicity of Three Organophosphorus Insecticides to Adult *Oryzaephilus surinamensis* (L.). *Pest. Magnt. Sci.* 14:145-152.

Bat L, Akbulut M, Mehmet Çulha M, Gündoğdu A, Satilmiş HH, 2000. Effect of Temperature on the Toxicity of Zinc, Copper and Lead to the Freshwater Amphipod *Gammarus pulex* (L., 1758). *Turk. J. Zool.* 24:409-415.

Belimov AA, Safronova VI, Tsyganov VE, Borisov AY, Kozhemyakov AP, Stepanok VV, Martenson AM, Gianinazzi-Pearson V, Tikhonovich IA, 2003. Genetic Variability in Tolerance to Cadmium and Accumulation of Heavy Metals in Pea (*Pisum sativum* L.). *Euphytica* 131:25-35 (revised version published online in August 2006).

Bell ML, Davis DL, 2001. Reassessment of the Lethal London Fog of 1952: Novel Indicators of Acute and Chronic Consequences of Acute Exposure to Air Pollution. *Environ. Health Perspect.* 109(Suppl 3):389-394.

Bellastella A, Pisano G, Iorio S, Pasquali D, Orio F, Venditto T, Sinisi AA, 1998. Endocrine Secretions under Abnormal Light-Dark Cycles and in the Blind. *Hormone Res.* 49:153-157.

Boina DR, Onagbola EO, Salyani M, Stelinski LL, 2009. Influence of Posttreatment Temperature on the Toxicity of Insecticides against *Diaphorina citri* (Hemiptera: Psyllidae). *Hort. Entomol.* 102:685-691.

Boyce P, Kennaway DJ, 1987. Effects of Light on Melatonin Production. *Biol. Psych.* 22:473-478.

Burk RF, Masters BSS, 1975. Some Effects of Selenium Deficiency on the Hepatic Microsomal Cytochrome P-450 System in the Rat. *Arch. Biochem. Biophys.* 170:124-131.

Campbell TC, Hayes JR, 1976. The Effect of Quantity and Quality of Dietary Protein on Drug Metabolism. *Fed. Proc.* 35:2470-2474.

Castillo LS, Timiras PS, 1964. Electroconvulsive Responses of Rats to Convulsant and Anticonvulsant Drugs during High Altitude Acclimatization. *J. Pharmacol. Exp. Ther.* 146:160-166.

Century B, 1973. A Role of the Dietary Lipid in the Ability of Phenobarbital to Stimulate Drug Detoxification. *J. Pharmacol. Exp. Ther.* 185:185-194.

Chandler JH, Sanders HO, Walsh DF, 1974. An Improved Chemical Delivery Apparatus for Use in Intermittent-Flow Bioassays. *Bull. Environ. Contam. Toxicol.* 12:123-128.

Chen JJ, Chen Y-J, Rice G, Teuschler LK, Hamernik K, Protzel A, Kodell RL, 2001. Using Dose Addition to Estimate Cumulative Risks from Exposures to Multiple Chemicals. *Regul. Toxicol. Pharmacol.* 34:35-41.

Clinton SK, Mulloy AL, Visek WJ, 1984. Effects of Dietary Lipid Saturation on Prolactin Secretion, Carcinogen Metabolism and Mammary Carcinogenesis in Rats. *J. Nutri.* 114:1630-1639.

Czesny S, Rinchard J, Abiado MAG, Dabrowski K, 2003. The Effect of Fasting, Prolonged Swimming, and Predator Presence on Energy Utilization and Stress in Juvenile Walleye (*Stizostedion vitreum*). *Physiol. Behav.* 79:597-603.

Czygan P, Greim H, Garro A, Schaffner F, Popper H, 1974. The Effect of Dietary Protein Deficiency on the Ability of Isolated Hepatic Microsomes to Alter the Mutagenicity of a Primary and a Secondary Carcinogen. *Cancer Res.* 34:119-123.

Dave G, 1981. Influence of Diet and Starvation on Toxicity of Endrin to Fathead Minnows (*Pimephales promelas*). EPA-600/S3-81-048. U. S. Environmental Protection Agency, Environmental Research Laboratory, CERI, Duluth, Minnesota, USA.

Dieke SH, Richter CP, 1945. Acute Toxicity of Thiourea to Rats in Relation to Age, Diet, Strain and Species Variation. *J. Pharmacol. Exp. Ther.* 83:195-202.

Eaton DL, Klaassen CD, 2001. Principles of Toxicology. In *Casarett and Doull's Toxicology: The Basic Science of Poisons* (Klaassen CD, Ed.). New York, New York, USA: McGraw-Hill, Chapter 2.

Eckhert C, 2006. Other Trace Elements. In *Modern Nutrition in Health and Disease* (Shils ME, Shike M, Ross AC, Caballero B, Cousins RJ, Eds.), Tenth Edition. Philadelphia, Pennsylvania, USA: Lippincott, Williams & Wilkins, pp.338-350.

Eeva T, Hakkarainen H, Laaksonen T, Lehikoinen E, 2006. Environmental Pollution Has Sex-Dependent Effects on Local Survival. *Biol. Lett.* 2:298-300.

Erickson DH, Erickson LC, Seely CI, 1972. Effects of Light Quantities and Glucose on 2,4-D Toxicity to Canada Thistle. *Weed Sci.* 20:384-386.

Erren TC, Jacobsen M, Piekarski C, 1999. Synergism between Asbestos and Smoking on Lung Cancer Risks. *Epidemiology* 10:405-411.

Farooqi ZR, Iqbal MZ, Kabir M, Shafiq M, 2009. Toxic Effects of Lead and Cadmium on Germination and Seedling Growth of *Albizia Lebbeck* (L.) Benth. *Pak. J. Bot.* 41:27-33.

Fischer E, 1941. Prophylaxis against Lethal Effect of High Altitude by Means of a Digitalis Glycoside (Gitalin). *Am. Heart J.* 21:545-550.

Fosmire GJ, 1990. Zinc Toxicity. *Am. J. Clin. Nutri.* 51:225-227.

Franklin NM, Stauber JL, Markich SJ, Lim RP, 2000. pH-Dependent Toxicity of Copper and Uranium to a Tropical Freshwater Alga (*Chlorella* sp.). *Aquatic Toxicol.* 48:275-289.

Gaylor DW, 2000. The Use of Haber's Law in Standard Setting and Risk Assessment. *Toxicology* 149:17-19.

Haag JR, Palmer LS, 1928. The Effect of Variations in the Proportions of Calcium, Magnesium, and Phosphorus Contained in the Diet. *J. Biol. Chem.* 76:361-365.

Hayes JR, Mgbodile MUK, Campbell TC, 1973. Effect of Protein Deficiency on the Inducibility of the Hepatic Microsomal Drug-Metabolizing Enzyme System – I: Effect on Substrate Interaction with Cytochrome P-450. *Biochem. Pharmacol.* 22:1005-1014.

Ho K, Kuhn A, Pelletier M, Hendricks T, Helmstetter A, 1999. pH Dependent Toxicity of Five Metals to Three Marine Organisms. *Environ. Toxicol.* 14:235-240.

Horiike N, Abe M, Kumagi T, Hiasa Y, Akbar SMF, Michitaka K, Onji M, 2005. The Quantification of Cytochrome P-450 (CYP 3A4) mRNA in the Blood of Patients with Viral Liver Diseases. *Clin. Biochem.* 38:531-534.

Hymer WC, Welsch J, Buchmann E, Risius M, Whelan HT, 2009. Modulation of Rat Pituitary Growth Hormone by 670 nm Light. *Growth Horm. IGF Res.* 19:274-279.

Iwasaki M, Iwama M, Miyata N, Iitoi Y, Kanke Y, 1994. Effects of Vitamin E Deficiency on Hepatic Microsomal Cytochrome P450 and Phase II Enzymes in Male and Female Rats. *Intern. J. Vitam. Nutr. Res.* 64:109-112.

Jacobson AR, Morris SC, 1976. The Primary Air Pollutants: Viable Particulates, Their Occurrences, Sources and Effects. In *Air Pollution* (Stern AC, Ed.), Third Edition. New York, New York, USA: Academic Press, Vol.1, pp.169-196.

Jagadeesan V, Oesch F, 1988. Effects of Dietary Zinc Deficiency on the Activity of Enzymes Associated with Phase I and II of Drug Metabolism in Fischer-344 Rats: Activities of Drug Metabolising Enzymes in Zinc Deficiency. *Drug Nutr. Interact.* 5:403-413.

John R, Ahmad P, Gadgill K, Sharma S, 2008. Effect of Cadmium and Lead on Growth, Biochemical Parameters and Uptake in *Lemna polyrrhiza* L. *Plant Soil Environ.* 54:262-270.

Kaloyanova F, Tasheva M, 1983. Effect of Protein Malnutrition on Toxicity of Pesticides. In *Pesticide Chemistry, Human Welfare, and the Environment* (Miyamoto J, Kearney PC, Eds.) – Volume 3: Mode of Action, Metabolism, and Toxicology. Oxford, London, UK: Pergamon Press, pp.527-529.

Kasuya E, Kushibiki S, Yayou K, Hodate K, Sutoh M, 2008. Light Exposure during Night Suppresses Nocturnal Increase in Growth Hormone Secretion in Holstein Steers. *J. Anim. Sci.* 86: 1799-1807.

Kato N, Tani T, Yoshida A, 1981. Effect of Dietary Quality of Protein on Liver Microsomal Mixed Function Oxidase System, Plasma Cholesterol and Urinary Ascorbic Acid in Rats Fed PCB. *J. Nutri.* 111:123-133.

Kawano S, Hiraga K, 1980. Effect of Dietary Protein Deficiency on Rat Hepatic Drug-Metabolizing Enzyme System. *Japan J. Pharmacol.* 30:75-83.

Khan MA, Ahmed SA, Salazar A, Gurumendi J, Khan A, Vargas M, von Catalin B, 2007. Effect of Temperature on Heavy Metal Toxicity to Earthworm *Lumbricus terrestris* (Annelida: Oligochaeta). *Environ. Toxicol.* 22:487-494.

Kim J-S, Ahn T, Yim S-K, Yun C-H, 2002. Differential Effect of Copper (II) on the Cytochrome P450 Enzymes and NADPH-Cytochrome P450 Reductase: Inhibition of Cytochrome P450-Catalyzed Reactions by Copper (II) Ion. *Biochemistry* 41:9438-9447.

Kobayashi K, Kishino T, 1980. Effect of pH on the Toxicity and Accumulation of Pentachlorophenol in Goldfish. *Bull. Japan. Soc. Sci. Fish* 46:167-170.

Korashy HM, El-Kadi AOS, 2005. Regulatory Mechanisms Modulating the Expression of Cytochrome P450 1A1 Gene by Heavy Metals. *Toxicol. Sci.* 88:39-51.

Korourian S, Hakkak R, Ronis MJ, Shelnutt SR, Waldron J, Ingelman-Sundberg M, Badger TM, 1999. Diet and Risk of Ethanol-Induced Hepatotoxicity: Carbohydrate-Fat Relationships in Rats. *Toxicol. Sci.* 47:110-117.

Letelier ME, Faúndez M, Jara-Sandoval J, Molina-Berríos A, Cortés-Troncoso J, Aracena-Parks P, Marín-Catalán R, 2009. Mechanisms Underlying the Inhibition of the Cytochrome P450 System by Copper Ions. *J. Appl. Toxicol.* 29:695-702.

Li H, Feng T, Liang P, Shia X, Gao X, Jiang H, 2006. Effect of Temperature on Toxicity of Pyrethroids and Endosulfan, Activity of Mitochondrial Na^+- K^+-ATPase and Ca^{2+}- Mg^{2+}-ATPase in *Chilo suppressalis* (Walker) (Lepidoptera: Pyralidae). *Pest. Biochem. Physiol.* 86:151-156.

Liccione JJ, Maines MD, 1989. Manganese-Mediated Increase in the Rat Brain Mitochondrial Cytochrome P-450 and Drug Metabolism Activity: Susceptibility of the Striatum. *J. Pharmacol. Exp. Ther.* 248:222-228.

Manno M, Rezzadore M, Grossi M, Sbrana C, 1996. Potentiation of Occupational Carbon Tetrachloride Toxicity by Ethanol Abuse. *Human Exp. Toxicol.* 15:294-300.

Marshall WJ, McLean AEM, 1971. A Requirement for Dietary Lipids for Induction of Cytochrome P-450 by Phenobarbitone in Rat Liver Microsomal Fraction. *Biochem. J.* 122:569-573.

Metwally A, Safronova VI, Belimov AA, Dietz K-J, 2005. Genotypic Variation of the Response to Cadmium Toxicity in *Pisum sativum* L. *J. Exp. Botany* 56:167-178.

Michnowicz CJ, Weaks TE, 1984 Effects of pH on Toxicity of As, Cr, Cu, Ni and Zn to *Selenastrum capricornutum* Printz. *Hydrobiologia* 118:299-305.

Miranda CL, Webb RE, 1973. Effects of Dietary Protein Quality on Drug Metabolism in the Rat. *J. Nutri.* 103:1425-1430.

Miranda CL, Mukhtara H, Benda JR, Chhabra RS, 1979. Effects of Vitamin A Deficiency on Hepatic and Extrahepatic Mixed-Function Oxidase and Epoxide Metabolizing Enzymes in Guinea Pig and Rabbit. *Biochem. Pharmacol.* 28:2713-2716.

Nicolson TJ, Mellor HR, Roberts RR, 2010. Gender Differences in Drug Toxicity. *Trends Pharmacol. Sci.* 31:108-114.

Oestreicher P, Cousins RJ, 1985. Copper and Zinc Absorption in the Rat: Mechanism of Mutual Antagonism. *J. Nutri.* 115:159-166.

Omaye ST, 2004. *Food and Nutritional Toxicology*, Boca Raton, Florida, USA: CRC Press, Chapter 1 (p.3).

Peraza MA, Ayala-Fierro F, Barber DS, Casarez E, Rael LT, 1998. Effects of Micronutrients on Metal Toxicity. *Environ. Health Perspect.* 106(Suppl 1):203-216.

Plaa GL, Hewitt WR, du Souich P, Caill G, Lock S, 1982. Isopropanol and Acetone Potentiation of Carbon Tetrachloride-Induced Hepatotoxicity: Single *versus* Repetitive Pretreatments in Rats. *J. Toxicol. Environ. Health* 9(Part A):235-250.

Pollack T, Crabtree G, 1976. Effect of Light Intensity and Quality on Toxicity of Fluorodifen to Green Bean and Soybean Seedlings. *Weed Sci.* 24:571-574.

Prasad R, Nath R, 1995. Cadmium-Induced Nephrotoxicity in Rhesus Monkeys (*Macaca mulatta*) in Relation to Protein Calorie Malnutrition. *Toxicology* 100:89-100.

Ramírez-Farías C, Madrigal-Santillán E, Gutiérrez-Salinas J, Rodríguez-Sánchez N, Martínez-Cruz M, Valle-Jones I, Gramlich-Martínez I, Hernández-Ceruelos A, Morales-Gonzaléz JA, 2008. Protective Effect of Some Vitamins against the Toxic Action of Ethanol on Liver Regeneration Induced by Partial Hepatectomy in Rats. *World J. Gastroenterol.* 14:899-907.

Reiter RJ, Tan DX, Korkmaz A, Erren TC, Piekarski C, Tamura H, Manchester LC, 2007. Light at Night, Chronodisruption, Melatonin Suppression, and Cancer Risk: A Review. *Crit. Rev. Oncog.* 13:303-328.

Rikans LE, 1982. NADPH-Dependent Reduction of Cytochrome P-450 in Liver Microsomes from Vitamin C-Deficient Guinea Pigs: Effect of Benzphetamine. *J. Nutri.* 112:1796-1800.

Ross JH, Dong MH, Krieger RI, 2000. Conservatism in Pesticide Exposure Assessment. *Regul. Toxicol. Pharmaco.* 31:53-58.

Rowe FP, Redfern R, 1964. The Toxicity of 0.025% Warfarin to Wild House Mice (*Mus muscultu* L.). *J. Hyg., Camb.* 62:389-393.

Rowe FP, Redfern R, 1967. The Effect of Sex and Age on the Response to Warfarin in a Non-Inbred Strain of Mice. *J. Hyg., Camb.* 65:55-60.

Saito M, Oh-Hashi A, Kubota M, Nishide E, Yamaguchi M, 1990. Mixed Function Oxidases in Response to Different Types of Dietary Lipids in Rats. *Br. J. Nutr.* 63:249-257.

Salama Z, El-Beltagi H, El-Hariri D, 2009. Effect of Fe Deficiency on Antioxidant System in Leaves of Three Flax Cultivars. *Not. Bot. Hort. Agrobot. Cluj.* 37:122-128.

Sato PH, Zannoni VG, 1976. Ascorbic Acid and Hepatic Drug Metabolism. *J. Pharmaco. Exp. Ther.* 198:295-307.

Sawyer TW, Vair C, Nelson P, Shei Y, Bjarnason S, Tenn C, McWilliams M, Villanueva M, Burczyk A, 2007. pH-Dependent Toxicity of Sulphur Mustard *in vitro*. *Toxicol. Appl. Pharmacol.* 221:363-371.

Schulsinger DA, Root MM, Campbell TC, 1989. Effect of Dietary Protein Quality on Development of Aflatoxin B1-Induced Hepatic Preneoplastic Lesions. *JNCI* 81:1241-1245.

Sekiya J, Wilson LG, Filner P, 1982. Resistance to Injury by Sulfur Dioxide: Correlation with Its Reduction to, and Emission of, Hydrogen Sulfide in Cucurbitaceae. *Plant Physiol.* 70:437-441.

Sheppard SC, 1992. Summary of Phytotoxic Levels of Soil Arsenic. *Water, Air, Soil Poll.* 64:539-550.

Shivarajashankara YM, Shivashankara AR, Bhat PG, Rao SH, 2001. Effect of Fluoride Intoxication on Lipid Peroxidation and Antioxidant Systems in Rats. *Fluoride* 34:108-113.

Sielken RL, 2000. Risk Metrics and Cumulative Risk Assessment Methodology for the FQPA. *Regul. Toxicol. Pharmacol.* 31:300-307.

Singh SN, Vats P, Kumria MML, Ranganathan S, Shyam R, Arora MP, Jain CL, Sridharan K, 2001. Effect of High Altitude (7,620 m) Exposure on Glutathione and Related Metabolism in Rats. *Europ. J. Appl. Physiol.* 84:233-237.

Sonawane BR, Coates PM, Yaffe SJ, Koldovsky O, 1983. Influence of Dietary Carbohydrates (Alpha-Saccharides) on Hepatic Drug Metabolism in Male Rats. *Drug Nutr. Interact.* 2:7-16.

Stalling DL, Mayer FL Jr, 1972. Toxicities of PCBs to Fish and Environmental Residues. *Environ. Health Perspect.* 1:159-164.

Sun H, Frassetto L, Benet LZ, 2006. Effects of Renal Failure on Drug Transport and Metabolism. *Pharmacol. Ther.* 109:1-11.

Sun Y, Zhou Q, Diao C, 2008. Effects of Cadmium and Arsenic on Growth and Metal Accumulation of Cd-Hyperaccumulator *Solanum nigrum* L. *Bioresource Technol.* 99:103-1110

Suskind RR, 1977. Environment and the Skin. *Environ. Health Perspect.* 20:27-37.

Swenberg JA, 1993. Alpha 2μ-Globulin Nephropathy: Review of the Cellular and Molecular Mechanisms Involved and Their Implications for Human Risk Assessment. *Environ. Health Perspect.* 101(Suppl 6):39-44.

Taniguchi M, 1980. Effects of Riboflavin Deficiency on Lipid Peroxidation of Rat Liver Microsomes. *J. Nutr. Sci. Vitaminol.* 26:401-413.

Tewari RK, Kumar P, Neetu, Sharma PN, 2005. Signs of Oxidative Stress in the Chlorotic Leaves of Iron Starved Plants. *Plant Sci.* 169:1037-1045.

Tsukada H, Wang P-Y, Kaneko T, Wang Y, Nakano M, Sato A, 1998. Dietary Carbohydrate Intake Plays an Important Role in Preventing Alcoholic Fatty Liver in the Rat. *J. Hepatol.* 29:715-724.

Vats P, Singh VK, Singh SN, Singh SB, 2008. Glutathione Metabolism Under High-Altitude Stress and Effect of Antioxidant Supplementation. *Aviation, Space Environ. Med.* 79:1106-1111.

Viswanathan PN, Murti CRK, 1989. Effects of Temperature and Humidity on Ecotoxicology of Chemicals. In *Ecotoxicology and Climate* (Bourdeau P, Haines JA, Klein W, Murti CRK, Eds.). New York, New York, USA: John Wiley & Sons.

Wade AE, Norred WP, 1976. Effect of Dietary Lipid on Drug-Metabolizing Enzymes. *Fed. Proc.* 35:2475-2479.

Watanabe M, Kumai T, Matsumoto N, Tanaka M, Suzuki S, Satoh T, Kobayashi S, 2004. Expression of CYP3A4 mRNA Is Correlated with CYP3A4 Protein Level and Metabolic Activity in Human Liver. *J. Pharmacol. Sci.* 94:459-462.

Wolansky MJ, Gennings C, DeVito MJ, Crofton KM, 2009. Evidence for Dose-Additive Effects of Pyrethroids on Motor Activity in Rats. *Environ. Health Perspect.* 117:1563-1570.

Woolson EA, 1973. Arsenic Phytotoxicity and Uptake in Six Vegetable Crops. *Weed Sci.* 21:524-527.

Yamaguchi N, Mochizuki-Kobayashib Y, Utsunomiyac O, 2000. Quantitative Relationship between Cumulative Cigarette Consumption and Lung Cancer Mortality in Japan. *Intern. J. Epidemiol.* 29:963-968.

Yasukochi Y, Nakamura M, Minakami S, 1977. Effect of Cobalt on the Synthesis of Liver Microsomal Cytochromes. *J. Biochem.* 81:1005-1009.

Yedjou C, Thuisseu L, Tchounwou C, Gomes M, Howard C, Tchounwou P, 2009. Ascorbic Acid Potentiation of Arsenic Trioxide Anticancer Activity against Acute Promyelocytic Leukemia. *Arch. Drug Inf.* 2:59-65.

Yoo JH, Ning SM, Pantuck CB, Pantuck EJ, Yang CS, 1991. Regulation of Hepatic Microsomal Cytochrome P450IIE1 Level by Dietary Lipids and Carbohydrates in Rats. *J. Nutri.* 121:959-965.

Yoo JS, Park HS, Ning SM, Lee MJ, Yang CS, 1990. Effects of Thiamine Deficiency on Hepatic Cytochromes P450 and Drug-Metabolizing Enzyme Activities. *Biochem. Pharmacol.* 39:519-525.

Review Questions

1. What can be considered as the most important environmental factor in terms of potential for affecting the toxicity of environmental contaminants?

2. How were the weekly air concentrations of SO_2 related to the weekly mortality in the Greater London area during October 1952 through March 1953?

3. What some other factors might have been responsible for the lower R^2 values observed for the two youngest birth cohorts in Japan in correlating their lung cancer death rates with their cumulative cigarette consumptions at the national level?

4. Explain why the LC_{50} of Aroclor 1248, as shown in Table 10.2, could have such a wide range as from 10 µg/L to 307 µg/L.

5. Give a numerical example (along with certain assumptions) for the potential fallacy of using Haber's law to estimate environmental exposure.

6. Why is it important to understand the mode of contact and the control measure in effect when estimating environmental exposure?

7. How can temperature, humidity, or altitude affect the toxicity of certain environmental contaminants?

8. How is light related to the diurnal rhythm in humans that can affect their exposures to certain environmental toxicants?

9. What is likely the common biochemical mode whereby many nutrients can affect the toxicity of environmental toxicants?

10. How can dietary lipids that contain linoleic acid biochemically affect the toxicity of certain environmental toxicants?

11. Briefly describe how high and low levels of dietary carbohydrates can affect the toxicity of certain environmental toxicants.

12. Give an example for the possibility that Zn intake can indirectly affect the toxicity of certain environmental toxicants.

13. Give a chemical example for each of the following joint toxic effect patterns: a) additivity; b) potentiation; c) synergism; d) dispositional form of antagonism; e) chemical form of antagonism.

14. Explain why kidney tumors can be induced by unleaded gasoline in only male but not female rats.

15. Briefly explain how kidney disease can affect the toxicity of an environmental toxicant?

16. Briefly explain why genetic polymorphism of CYP2D6 is a clinically important issue to human health.

CHAPTER 11

Air Pollutants – I: Inorganic Gases

11.1. Introduction

All air pollutants of concern are confined to the troposphere, which is the lowest layer of the Earth's atmosphere extending to about 10 miles above sea level. This air zone, in which almost all of the Earth's weather occurs, contains about 75 to 80% of the atmosphere's mass and 99% of its water (H_2O) vapor and dust particles. The cooler, second major layer of Earth's atmosphere is the stratosphere, just above the troposphere and below the mesosphere. The air that people breathe is present in the troposphere and is a mixture of gaseous substances containing about 78.1% nitrogen (N_2) and 20.9% oxygen (O_2) molecules. The other gaseous substances in the remaining 1% or so include: ~0.9% argon (Ar); ~0.03% carbon dioxide (CO_2); and ~0.04% of collectively H_2O vapor, trace gases such as helium (He) and neon (Ne), as well as all air pollutants. It is with such an atmospheric composition that in most situations, any pollutant found in the air that people breathe is considered as having low enough concentrations not to pose any *immediate* or *acute* health threat. Otherwise, inhalation is a major route of environmental exposure insomuch as an average adult inhales well over 12,000 liters of air per day.

11.1.1. Hazardous Air Pollutants

Over 200 hazardous air pollutants have been detected in the ambient air. These toxic air pollutants, also referred to as air toxics, are substances that can cause cancer or other serious health effects. Where appropriate, some of these air toxics are discussed in the chapters that follow. For instance, airborne residues such as those of the fumigant methyl bromide and the industrial chemical asbestos are discussed in Chapters 15 and 20, respectively. The list of air toxics considered by U.S. EPA, as mandated by the U.S. Clean Air Act Amendments of 1990, does not include such commonly found air pollutants as the particulate matter (PM) and volatile organic compounds (VOCs) covered in the next two chapters (respectively) or the inorganic gases discussed in this chapter.

11.1.2. Criteria Inorganic Gaseous Pollutants

The air pollutants that U.S. EPA has found to occur commonly over the United States include sulfur dioxide (SO_2), nitrogen oxides (NO_x), ozone (O_3), carbon monoxide (CO), lead (Pb), and PM. These six air pollutants are also referred to as the "criteria air pollutants" due to the U.S. Clean Air Act mandate that U.S. EPA needs to adopt a National Ambient Air Quality Standard (NAAQS) for each of these six air pollutants. According to the U.S. Clean Air Act, airborne particles of lead compounds are also considered as air toxics. Lead is discussed in Chapter 14, along with other toxic metals.

In this chapter, the four criteria inorganic gaseous pollutants (i.e., SO_2, NO_x, O_3, CO) are considered separately in their respective sections. The discussion on each of these four inorganic gases focuses primarily on the same three fundamental aspects: (1) its sources of pollution; (2) its characteristics and physicochemical properties; and (3) its toxic effects on humans, animals, and plants, where appropriate or applicable.

Several other inorganic gases, such as ammonia (NH_3), hydrogen sulfide (H_2S), chlorine (Cl_2), hydrogen chloride (HCl), and hydrogen fluoride (HF), are also harmful or with some even more so. However, due to their relatively infrequency in occurrence and space limitation, these other inorganic gases are not specifically discussed in this or other chapters.

11.2. Sulfur Dioxide

Sulfur dioxide (SO_2) is the most predominant member of a group of highly reactive gases known as sulfur oxides (SO_x). Another SO_x member that is also a significant but less common air pollutant is sulfur trioxide (SO_3). Historically, SO_2 was responsible for several acute air pollution episodes, including those occurring in Meuse Valley in October of 1930, in Donora in December of 1948, and in London in December of 1952. Again (Section 10.2.1.A), the London fog of 1952 resulted in 4,000 excess deaths and over 100,000 extra illness cases due to the smog's effects on their respiratory or cardiovascular system. The smog was reportedly the result of the cold, stagnant fog contaminated with chimney smoke, particulates from vehicle exhausts, and other pollutants including particularly SO_2. The death tolls from the two earlier smog disasters noted above were on a much smaller scale, with 60 to 70 deaths occurring in the densely populated valley near Liege, Belgium and about 20 deaths in the American mill town Donora, Pennsylvania.

11.2.1. Sources of Pollution

In the United States, about 95% of all SO_2 emissions from anthropogenic sources are from fossil fuel combustion at electric power plants (66%) and other industrial facilities (29%). The remaining 5% includes from industrial processes (e.g., extracting metals from ore), paper and pulp manufacturing, and the burning of high sulfur-containing fuels by trains, large ships, and some diesel trucks (U.S. EPA, 2009).

Environmental exposure to SO_2 is usually at its highest outdoors in the summer months, when smoke pollutants can react more readily and more actively with the sun and hot temperature to form smog. Levels of SO_2 in the air are usually higher than normal within or near facilities that release the air pollutant through heavy industrial activities (e.g., copper smelting, processing or combustion of coal and petroleum oil at electric power plants). People may also be exposed to SO_2 if they work in or are around places producing sulfuric acid (H_2SO_4), paper, pulp, fertilizers, or food preservatives.

Sulfur dioxide is commonly used as a food preservative for many dried fruits, vegetables, and alcoholic drinks owing to its strong antimicrobial and antioxidant properties. It also has the following uses: as a disinfectant; as an intermediate for making other chemicals; for bleaching flour, textile fibers, and glue; for winemaking; and for water treatment. Sulfur dioxide is a high-volume product used in the United States, with an annual production exceeding 1 million pounds.

Natural pollution sources of SO_2 include biological or plant decays and volcanoes. Although emissions of SO_2 caused by human activity far exceed its natural emissions in the developed countries, natural processes are responsible for half of the world's atmospheric sulfur (S). Along with CO_2 and HF, SO_2 is the volcanic gas posing the greatest potential hazard to humankind and ecosystems. Large explosive eruptions can result in a tremendous volume of sulfur aerosols injected into the stratosphere, where the aerosols can promote depletion of the ozone layer and eventually cause lower, undesired temperatures on the Earth's surface.

11.2.2. Characteristics and Properties

Sulfur dioxide is a nonflammable, colorless, irritating, liquefied compressed gas when packaged in cylinders under its own vapor pressure (35 psig at 21.1° C). It has a pungent, acidic, and suffocating odor, detectable at around 3 to 5 ppm (parts per million); and at around 0.5 to 1 ppm, it leaves an acidic taste in the mouth. This gas can cause severe chemical burns if inhaled or upon skin contact at sufficiently high doses. Its general physicochemical properties are listed in Table 11.1.

Table 11.1. General Physicochemical Properties of Sulfur Dioxide (SO_2)

Molecular weight	64.1
Vapor pressure	35 psig (at 21.1° C)
Boiling point	−10° C (at 1 atm)
Vapor density (specific gravity)	2.25 (with air = 1)
Freezing point	−75.5° C (at 1 atm)
Gas density	0.293 kg/m^3, at 0° C and 1 atm

In the laboratory, SO_2 gas can be formed by addition of hydrochloric acid (HCl·H_2O) to solid sodium sulfite ($NaSO_3$). Commercially or more commonly, the gas can be produced by burning the element S (sulfur), by combusting hydrogen sulfide (H_2S), or by roasting of sulfide ores such as iron pyrite (FeS_2) and copper chalcocite (Cu_2S), as illustrated below in Reactions 11.1 through 11.4 (where s = solid, g = gas):

$$S\ (s) + O_2\ (g) \rightarrow SO_2\ (g) \tag{11.1}$$

$$2\ H_2S\ (g) + 3O_2\ (g) \rightarrow 2H_2O\ (g) + 2SO_2\ (g) \tag{11.2}$$

$$4FeS_2 \ (s) + 9O_2 \ (g) \rightarrow 2Fe_2SO_3 \ (s) + 6SO_2 \ (g) \tag{11.3}$$

$$2Cu_2S \ (s) + 3O_2 \ (g) \rightarrow 2Cu_2O \ (s) + 2SO_2 \ (g) \tag{11.4}$$

In essence, SO_2 gas is formed whenever sulfur-containing fuels, such as coal and oil, are burned. Iron disulfide (a.k.a. iron pyrite) is the most common of the sulfide minerals. This mineral is commonly found coexisting with other sulfides or oxides, such as chalcopyrite ($CuFeS_2$). Chalcopyrite and chalcocite are the most abundant minerals found in copper (Cu) ores and hence in copper smelting plants as well.

Oxidation of SO_2 with oxygen, in the presence of a catalyst, forms H_2SO_4. For example, when the catalyst used is vanadium pentoxide (V_2O_5), SO_3 is formed first which is then hydrated into the acid, as shown below in Reaction 11.5 (where l = liquid).

$$2SO_2 \ (g) + O_2 \ (g) \rightarrow 2SO_3 \ (g) \tag{11.5a}$$

$$SO_3 \ (g) + H_2O \ (l) \rightarrow H_2SO_4 \ (g) \tag{11.5b}$$

In the troposphere, atmospheric SO_2 can be readily oxidized to SO_3 by hydroxyl radical ($HO^{\cdot}$) followed by O_2, as discussed in Section 5.2.3.C (e.g., Reactions 5.8 through 5.10). The resultant H_2SO_4 then becomes the principal acidic component of acid rain. The hydroxyl radical can readily become available as a by-product component of the photochemical smog reaction discussed in Section 5.2.3.B.

11.2.3. Toxic Effects and Advisories

Sulfur dioxide is both a potent phytotoxicant and a strong respiratory irritant. It is largely due to such concerns that U.S. EPA (2010) has set an arithmetic mean of 0.03 ppm and a maximum 24-hour average of 0.14 ppm as the *primary* NAAQS (National Ambient Air Quality Standard) for protection of public health from SO_2 exposure. The guideline values set forth by the World Health Organization (WHO, 2006) are 20 and 500 $\mu g/m^3$ (i.e., 0.008 and 0.19 ppm) for a maximum 24-hour and a 10-minute average, respectively. For *secondary* NAAQS, which is for public welfare that includes protection against reduced visibility and damage to animals, vegetation, crops, and buildings, U.S. EPA has set a maximum 3-hour average of 0.5 ppm as the limit. The guideline values set forth by WHO (2000a) for vegetation protection are an average of 30 $\mu g/m^3$ for annual exposure and an average of 100 $\mu g/m^3$ for a 24-hour exposure.

In the United States, a 71% decrease in the national average level of SO_2 from 1980 (0.01 ppm) to 2008 (0.003 ppm) was observed (U.S. EPA, 2009). Yet despite such a significant decline in the national levels of SO_2 in the country (and in many of the other western countries), the air pollutant still represents a threat to public health and vegetation in certain local areas. For instance, it was estimated (Schneider, 2004) that in the early 2000s, the 17 coal plants in the state of Texas collectively emitted close to 500,000 tons of SO_2 annually. These emissions were reportedly responsible for over 1,000 annual cases in total of heart attacks, deaths, and related excess hospital admissions in Texas.

A. Effects on Humans and Animals

In humans and many other mammalians, inhalation is the major route of exposure to SO_2 which is readily converted to sulfite (SO_3^-) and bisulfite (HSO_3^-) in the moist mucous membrane of the upper respiratory tract. Exposure to high levels (≥ 100 ppm) can be life threatening, especially for asthmatic children. Otherwise, common symptoms from acute exposure include wheezing, chest tightness, and shortness of breath. From chronic exposure at 0.5 to 3.0 ppm, the effects include respiratory illness, modulation of the defense mechanisms in the lungs, and aggravation of existing cardiovascular diseases.

At least two health organizations (ATSDR, 1998; WHO, 2006) had extensively evaluated the large volumes of epidemiological and animal toxicity data available concerning environmental exposure to SO_2. Their reviews came down to three common points. First, it was not certain if the chronic effects observed in workers were attributed to SO_2 exposure alone since these people might have been exposed to other pollutants as well. Second, the thresholds for the health effects of SO_2 were highly variable, depending on the nature of local sources, the prevailing meteorological conditions, and the victim's asthmatic status. And third, which is more certain, studies in a range of animal species supported strongly the human data on airway damage (e.g., epithelial hyperplasia) and pulmonary effects (e.g., bronchoconstriction) from chronic exposure to SO_2.

According to ATSDR (1998), there does not seem to be any conclusive evidence supporting the reproductive or developmental effects of SO_2 exposure in humans, in part because again those human study subjects exposed to SO_2 were exposed to other air pollutants as well. Another reason is that the animal data on developmental or maternal effects of SO_2 showed either negative or inconclusive support for extrapolation to humans.

B. Effects on Plants

Uptake of SO_2 by plants is primarily via the stomata (i.e., the microscopic pores) located between the guard cells on leaf surfaces shielded by the epidermis (Figure 7.3). The symptoms associated with acute injury appear as necrotic lesions on both leaf surfaces that usually occur between veins, with the color of the injured areas ranging from light tan or bleached white to reddish brown, depending on the prevailing environmental conditions present and the plant species affected. With chronic injury, the affected plants usually have chlorotic leaves from paling to yellow with green veins.

Both the enlarging and older leaves tend to be more resistant to acute SO_2 injury, whereas the younger and fully expanded ones are typically the most sensitive (Daines, 1968). Studies showed inter- and intra-species variations in plant sensitivity to SO_2 injury. Such variations can occur in part because SO_2 usually needs to first enter the stomata before leaf injury can take place. And the stomatal aperture is affected considerably by the specific environmental conditions that the plant is in. It has been reported (Griffiths,

2003; Schubert, 1984) that certain crops (e.g., alfalfa, sweet clover), certain flowers (e.g., cosmos, violet, zinnia), certain trees (e.g., apple, American elm, pear), and certain vegetables (e.g., radish, carrot) tend to be more susceptible to SO_2 injury.

C. Effects of Acid Rain

Rain that falls on the ground as wet deposition may contain acidic components such as H_2SO_4 (sulfuric acid), a mineral liquid readily formed by oxidation of SO_2 in the troposphere. This type of rain, more formally termed *acid rain* or *acid deposition*, has significant toxic effects on the environment by acidifying soils, aquatic systems, and infrastructures. Acid rain can also reduce visibility. It was largely due to these environmental concerns that U.S. Congress passed the Acid Deposition Act in 1980.

When falling on the plants, acid rain can damage their leaves ending in necrotic lesions or chlorotic tissues. In most situations, acid rain can reduce or inhibit plant germination and growth. When the soil is acidified, the plant roots can be severely damaged, along with a high potential for leaching of their nutrients (e.g., calcium, potassium) present in the soil nearby. Moreover, many soil microbes and their enzymes can be denatured by the high acidity generated. Otherwise, through their enzymes, these microbes can help release nutrients from decaying leaves and other debris on the soil.

Acid rain can adversely affect many aquatic organisms and land animals. Fish and other aquatic biota are particularly more vulnerable, inasmuch as they all need water to breathe. When the water is acidified, an aquatic organism's life and its reproductive function can be endangered. In particular, water acidity may cause a reduction of the calcium (Ca) levels in the female fish to the point that either these creatures can no longer produce eggs, or their eggs will fail to pass through from their ovaries. Even when the eggs are fertilized, the freshly hatched larvae will not develop normally when the aquatic environment that they are in has an unfavorably low pH (U.S. EPA, 1980).

Acids, including particularly H_2SO_4, have a corrosive effect on limestone and marble buildings. Marble and limestone are made of calcium carbonate ($CaCO_3$) which, when reacting with H_2SO_4 long enough, will get dissolved. H_2SO_4 is also corrosive to copper and the metal's alloys (e.g., bronze). It is due to such concerns that Harvard University now hides its bronze Large Four Piece Reclining Figure (by Henry Moore) for the winter in waterproof swaddling, which otherwise has reclined on the grass in front of the university's Lamont Library for well over 20 years (*Harvard Magazine*, 2000).

11.3. Nitrogen Oxides: Nitrogen Dioxide

Nitrogen dioxide (NO_2) and nitric oxide (NO) are the most predominant members of a group of highly reactive gases known as nitrogen oxides (NO_x). This section has its focus on NO_2 because NO can be readily converted to NO_2 in the presence of O_2 (Reaction 11.6). Both NO_2 and NO, along with their related compounds ozone (O_3) and PAN (peroxyacetylnitrate), are involved in the photochemical smog reaction described in Section

5.2.3.B. These oxidants were responsible for several acute air pollution episodes occurring in the greater Los Angeles area in the mid-1950s. More recent photochemical smog episodes, though on smaller scales, can still be found in other parts of the world where traffic congestion is an issue, such as in Hong Kong (Wang *et al.*, 2006), Jakarta (Suhadi *et al.*, 2005), and Santiago (Rubio *et al.*, 2005).

11.3.1. Sources of Pollution

Whether from natural or anthropogenic sources, it does not seem fair to discuss NO_2 without considering NO, as both are the predominant components of NO_x present almost always together and in large quantities. The two oxides are produced from a variety of natural processes in the air, soil, and water. Atmospheric nitrogen fixation is one such process whereby diatomic nitrogen (N_2) in the air is separated by lightning into monatomic N which can then react with O_2 in the air to form NO_x (Section 5.2.3.D). Biological nitrogen fixation is another in which N_2 is converted to mostly NH_3 and (then to) NO_x via the actions of certain algae in water or certain bacteria in soil and plants.

The primary anthropogenic sources of NO_x are automobile exhaust fumes and emissions from electric utilities or other industrial processes. Although exhaust fumes have more NO than NO_2, the NO released into the air readily reacts with atmospheric O_2 to form NO_2 (Reaction 11.6). In 2005, 92% of the 18.3 million tons of national NO_x emissions in the United States were from on-road automobiles (35.5%), non-road engines (22.8%), electricity generation (20.7%), and fossil fuel combustion (13.0%). The remaining 8% were from numerous minor sources such as residential wood combustion, waste disposal, solvent use, fires, fertilizers, and livestock (U.S. EPA, 2009).

On-road traffic is likewise the major source of NO_x emissions in Europe, accounting for over half of the annual total emissions there (EEA, 2002). In certain European cities such as London, it accounts for 75% of the total toll in that area (Holman, 1999).

Unlike SO_2, considerable levels of NO_2 gas are commonly found indoors in places burning fuel. The primary indoor sources of NO_2 include kerosene heaters, gas heaters, gas stoves, wood-burning fireplaces, and tobacco smoke. Due to these sources, the indoor levels can exceed those in the outdoor ambient air. An Ethiopian study found that season of the year, fire use characteristics, housing conditions, frequency of cooking, and agroecological (biomass) factors were the most important determinants of indoor NO_2 concentration (Kumie *et al.*, 2009). That study's findings were based on over 17,000 air samples collected in 3,300 rural local residences during a two-year investigation period.

11.3.2. Characteristics and Properties

At above room temperature (21.1° C), NO_2 is present as a reddish brown gas with a pungent odor. It is nonflammable, but accelerates burning of combustible materials. This gas typically arises via the oxidation of NO by O_2 in the air (Reaction 11.6).

$$2NO + O_2 \rightarrow 2NO_2 \tag{11.6}$$

Nitrogen dioxide and other NO_x are precursors of a number of highly toxic secondary (i.e., second-generation) air pollutants such as O_3 and the organic nitrate PAN. The general physicochemical properties of NO_2 are listed in Table 11.2.

Table 11.2. General Physicochemical Properties of Nitrogen Dioxide (NO_2)

Molecular weight	46.0
Boiling point	21.1° C (at 1 atm)
Vapor density (specific gravity)	1.58 (with air = 1)
Freezing point	−11.2° C (at 1 atm)
Gas density	3.4 kg/m^3 at 22° C, 1 atm

Nitrogen dioxide is a strong oxidizing agent and readily reacts with H_2O vapor in the air to form corrosive nitric acid (HNO_3), which is one of the major acidic constituents of acid rain (Reaction 11.7) and a precursor of certain components found in PM (particulate matter). Another pathway through which NO_2 can form HNO_3 is by reacting with the hydroxyl radical (HO·) from photochemistry in the atmosphere (Reaction 11.8).

$$3NO_2 + H_2O \rightarrow 2HNO_3 + NO \tag{11.7}$$

$$NO_2 + HO· \rightarrow HNO_3 \tag{11.8}$$

11.3.3. Toxic Effects and Advisories

Like SO_2, NO_2 is not only a potent phytotoxicant but also a strong respiratory irritant. The HNO_3 in acid rain formed from NO_2 is corrosive to building materials at high concentrations. The organic nitrate PAN generated from NO_2 as a secondary air pollutant can cause haze to reduce visibility. The presence of NO_2 makes smog in summer look brownish. In the United States, the health-based NAAQS for NO_2 is an annual average of 0.053 ppm. U.S. EPA (2010) recently has set a new 1-hour national standard of 0.1 ppm for short-term exposure to NO_2, despite a 46% decrease observed (U.S. EPA, 2009) in national average emission of NO_2 from 1980 (0.028 ppm) to 2008 (0.015 ppm). The WHO (2006) guideline values for NO_2 are 200 µg/m^3 (0.11 ppm) for 1 hour and 40 µg/m^3 (0.021 ppm) for an annual average.

A. Effects on Humans and Animals

Nitrogen dioxide can irritate and burn the skin, the eyes, the nose, the throat, or the lungs, depending on the air concentrations in place. Inhalation of NO_2, especially by children, can decrease the lung's ability to defend against bacteria and viruses and thereby increase the risk of respiratory infection. Exposure to NO_2 may also aggravate asthma or cause poorer pulmonary function in later life. Symptoms from low levels of exposure to NO_2 may include coughing, shortness of breath, tiredness, nausea, and fluid buildup in the lungs. Exposure at very high levels can result in the following effects: rapid burning and spasms of tissues in the upper respiratory tract; interference with transport of oxygen across body tissues; buildup of fluid in the lungs; collapse; and even death.

Continued exposure to high enough levels of NO_2 may lead to permanent lung damage. There is evidence linking atmospheric levels of NO_2 to increases in daily mortality (Burnett et al., 2004) and daily hospital admissions for pulmonary disease (Linn et al., 2000). There are also studies showing that exposure to NO_2 can cause damage in the developing fetus (Brauer et al., 2008) and decrease fertility in men (Wiwanitkit, 2007). A case-control study showed that average outdoor levels of NO_2 were significantly linked to sudden infant death syndrome (Klonoff-Cohen et al., 2005). Another epidemiological study found an association between daily indoor exposures to NO_2 and asthmatic symptoms in children (Smith et al., 2000).

Nitrogen dioxide is not only a precursor of HNO_3, but can also increase atmospheric deposition of nitrogen (N_2). Nitrogen is the element most responsible for eutrophication, a term used for over-enrichment of nutrients in aquatic systems to the point that it will cause a substantial reduction in the amount of O_2 available in the water. This environmental effect, along with the effect of acid rain, provides an aquatic ecosystem that can be highly destructive to fish and other aquatic creatures.

B. Effects on Plants

Nitrogen dioxide can induce a highly detrimental effect on photosynthesis in plants. Symptoms from this type (and certain other types) of plant injury include random necrotic spots between leaf veins. Brownish-yellow spots can be seen on the marginal areas of broad leaves, whereas in coniferous leaves the browning typically occurs on their tips or mid-sections. NO_2 can suppress plant growth.

One study in bean plants showed that when 8-day old seedlings were exposed to NO_2 at 0.02 to 0.5 ppm for 6 hours daily for 15 days, shoot growth was inhibited (Srivastava and Ormrod, 1986). Another study showed that when Pinto bean and Pearson-improved tomato seedlings were exposed to NO_2 at levels less than 1.0 mg/m^3 continuously for 10 to 22 days, significant growth suppression was observed, along with an increase in green color (total chlorophyll content) and distortion of leaves (Taylor and Eaton, 1966). When SO_2 or O_3 was also present, the adverse effects caused jointly with NO_2 on plant growth were found to be synergistic, or at least additive, for certain species (Reinert and Gray, 1981; Tingey et al., 1971; White et al., 1974).

The effects of NO_2 on plants appear to be species- and dose-specific. For example, it was shown that exposure of *Mulukhiya* plants to NO_2 at 0.05 ppm in a controlled chamber promoted both vegetative growth and flowering (Adam et al., 2008a). At least two other studies also showed that at ambient levels, NO_2 stimulated the vegetative growth of lettuce, sunflower, cucumber, and pumpkin (Adam et al., 2008b; Takahashi et al., 2005). As hypothesized by the investigators, inasmuch as flowering is controlled by developmental and environmental signals, at the appropriate levels NO_2 might act as a signaling molecule rather than as a destructive pollutant.

11.4. Tropospheric Ozone

Ozone (O_3) is a gas found at substantial levels in both the troposphere and the stratosphere. In the troposphere, O_3 is a potent air pollutant to human health and ecosystems. In the stratosphere, the O_3 layer extends upward from about 10 to 30 miles to form a shield protecting life on the Earth from the sun's harmful ultraviolet (UV) rays. Like PAN, O_3 is (largely) a secondary air pollutant, generated predominantly from the photolysis of NO_2. As such, both of these secondary pollutants along with NO_2 are involved in most air pollution episodes identified as caused by photochemical oxidants.

11.4.1. Sources of Pollution

Given that NO_2 is a precursor of most O_3 found in the troposphere, the sources of O_3 are similar to those of NO_x discussed in Section 11.3.1. Accordingly, many urban areas tend to have high levels of O_3 in their environment, especially in the summer months. However, O_3 is subject to long-range transport carried by winds and thereby can also be found at considerable levels in some rural areas. Both CO and VOCs are also precursors of O_3 produced in the tropospheric environment (Reactions 11.9 and 11.10).

Natural sources of O_3 include the small amounts from hydrocarbons (HCs) released by plants and soil as well as from those very small amounts in the stratosphere that occasionally migrate down to the Earth's surface. In addition, O_3 can be produced by generating high-power electrical discharges in air or oxygen. Due to its strong oxidation properties, O_3 has been produced for use in medicine, as a food disinfectant or sanitizer, and for cleaning or detoxification purposes. This gas is gaining popularity as a "green" alternative to chlorine for treatment of pool water. Generators that yield a high concentration of O_3 are preferentially used by restaurants and hotels for removing foul odors in the shortest time in order to satisfy their (arriving) customers.

11.4.2. Characteristics and Properties

Under normal conditions, O_3 is an unstable gas with a strong, irritating, chlorine-like odor. It is a powerful oxidant as well as a strong corrosive agent and hence overall a highly toxic air pollutant. O_3 has a bluish color in either the gas or the liquid state. The gas changes to a liquid at $-111.9°$ C and to a bluish-black solid at $-193°$ C.

The formation of tropospheric O_3 from a VOC precursor may involve the two steps in Reaction 11.9, where VOC being a HC compound is often denoted by RC with the symbol C representing a carbon atom to which an oxygen (O) atom may attach.

$$RC + O^\bullet + O_2 \rightarrow RCO + O_2 \rightarrow RCO_3{}^\bullet \qquad\qquad (11.9a)$$

$$O_2 + RCO_3{}^\bullet \rightarrow RCO_2 + O_3 \qquad\qquad (11.9b)$$

Note that the highly reactive $O^\bullet$ atom in Reaction 11.9a can come from the photodissociation of NO_2 into this reactive species plus NO (Section 5.2.3.B). And the peroxide radical $RCO_3 \cdot$ has the (counter) effect of enhancing the formation of NO_2 by reacting with NO. Meantime, $O \cdot$ can easily react with O_2 to form O_3 (Reaction 5.4).

For tropospheric CO as the precursor, the formation of O_3 begins by reacting with the radical $HO \cdot$ in the air. The reaction of hyperoxy radical $HO_2 \cdot$ with NO forms NO_2 and $HO \cdot$. That is, CO can form tropospheric O_3 by enhancing the formation of $O \cdot$ via its formation of NO_2 (Reaction 11.10) and then via the photolysis of NO_2 (Section 5.2.3.B).

$$CO + HO \cdot \rightarrow CO_2 + H^+ \tag{11.10a}$$

$$H^+ + O_2 \rightarrow HO_2 \cdot \tag{11.10b}$$

$$HO_2 \cdot + NO \rightarrow HO \cdot + NO_2 \tag{11.10c}$$

For O_3 in the stratosphere, it is generated at the expense of breaking the stratospheric diatomic oxygen (O_2) apart into two monatomic oxygen ($O \cdot$) ions upon absorption of an UV photon (whose wavelength is shorter than 240 nm). Each of the two $O \cdot$ ions then combines with a separate, nearby O_2 molecule to form an O_3 molecule.

The physical and chemical properties of O_3 are very different from those of diatomic oxygen. Its general physicochemical properties are listed in Table 11.3.

Table 11.3. General Physicochemical Properties of Tropospheric Ozone (O_3)

Molecular weight	48.0
Boiling point	$-111.3°$ C (at 1 atm)
Vapor density (specific gravity)	1.612 (with air = 1)
Freezing point	$-192.5°$ C
Gas density	2.141 kg/m^3 ($0°$ C, 1 atm)

11.4.3. Toxic Effects and Advisories

In the United States, both the primary and secondary NAAQS for ground-level (i.e., tropospheric) O_3 are 0.08 ppm as the daily maximum 8-hour average and 0.12 ppm as the maximum 1-hour average (U.S. EPA, 2010). The WHO (2006) guideline value is 100 μg/m^3 (0.05 ppm) for 8 hours. A 25% decrease in the national average of ground-level O_3 was observed in the United States from 0.1 ppm in 1980 to 0.075 ppm in 2008 (U.S. EPA, 2009). In the recent years, southern Europe observed the worst summer ozone levels in 2003, followed by those in 2006 (EEA, 2007). In summer 2006, a large number of southern European nations experienced a 1-hour O_3 level that exceeded Europe's long-term alert threshold of 240 μg/m^3, with the highest of 370 μg/m^3 occurring in Italy.

A. Effects on Humans and Animals

Exposure to (ground-level) O_3 can trigger a wide variety of health problems including airway irritation, chest pain, coughing, wheezing, shortness of breath, and sunburn-like inflammation of the skin. It can aggravate asthma, bronchitis, emphysema, and other respiratory disorders. In addition, O_3 exposure can impair lung function and inflame the linings of the respiratory tract.

Prolonged exposure of O_3 may permanently scar lung tissue. There are many animal toxicity studies supporting the association between permanent damage to the human lung and chronic exposure to O_3 at various levels below 0.25 ppm (for around 8 to 10 hours a day), particularly those conducted in rats (Grose *et al.*, 1989; Huang *et al.*, 1988) and monkeys (Hyde *et al.*, 1989; Tyler *et al.*, 1988). There are also human data linking long-term exposure of O_3 at ambient air levels to the incidence (Beeson *et al.*, 1998) and mortality (Abbey *et al.*, 1999) of lung cancer in nonsmoker male adults.

B. Effects on Plants

Ozone at high concentrations can cause more harm to plants and ecosystems than all other air pollutants combined. It can injury the leaves of trees and other types of plants, suppress their growth, depress flowering, or reduce crop yields. O_3 can interfere with the ability of sensitive plants to produce or store food and can make them more susceptible to certain diseases, insects, other pollutants, and harsh weather.

The symptoms from plant injuries caused by O_3 include various types of chlorotic markings and necrotic lesions, including flecking (e.g., silver, yellow), stippling (e.g., light tan, red), bronzing, and reddening. There is evidence that certain plant species such as alfalfa, cotton, and soybean are more susceptible to yield loss caused by O_3 (Heagle, 1989; Rich and Tomlinson, 1974). Studies showed that SO_2 and O_3 had synergistic damage in tobacco plants (Macdowall and Cole, 1971; Menser and Heggestad, 1966). However, the interaction observed between SO_2 and O_3 in hybrid poplar plants (*Populus deltoids* Bartr. x *P. trichocarpa* Torr. and Gray) was rather antagonistic, as SO_2 actually reduced the toxic O_3 effect on leaf growth in the hybrids tested (Noble and Jensen, 1980).

11.5. Carbon Monoxide

Carbon monoxide (CO) is an odorless, colorless, tasteless, and potentially lethal gas. As such, it can kill a person before he or she is aware of its presence. It is for this reason that CO is nicknamed the silent killer. This gas is highly toxic to humans at high concentrations because its binding affinity to the metalloprotein hemoglobin (Hb) is about 220 times greater than that of oxygen to Hb (Section 9.2.4). When existing in the Hb-CO bound form, the metalloprotein is incapable of carrying oxygen to cells in other body tissues. As its sources of pollution being so numerous indoors as well as outdoors, CO is both an indoor poisonous gas and a notorious outdoor air pollutant. Historically, one acute outdoor episode was documented linking CO air pollution to daily mortalities observed in Los Angeles County during the years 1962 to 1965 (Hexter and Goldsmith, 1971). In two other acute outdoor episodes occurring around that period (December 1962 and October 1963), CO (along with SO_2 and total hydrocarbons) was also implicated for causing family illness in New York City (Ingram *et al.*, 1965). Note that in more recent reports concerning O_3 air pollution, such as that occurring in southern Europe in 2006 (Section 11.4.3), CO can actually be treated as a culprit inasmuch as it is one of the precursors for formation of tropospheric O_3 (Section 11.4.2).

11.5.1. Sources of Pollution

Carbon monoxide is formed wherever incomplete combustion of a carbonaceous fuel occurs. This means that in a place where oxygen supply is not proportionally in its fullness, burning a fossil fuel or the kind can result in a substantial amount of CO in the area. Fossil fuels include coal, petroleum, and natural gas, which are all rich in carbon. Even wood, tobacco, and kerosene are HC (hydrocarbon) materials thus highly rich in carbon. In any case, in unvented areas where oxygen supply is limited, worn or poorly maintained combustion devices can be a significant source of CO. Burning devices that are commonly found to use carbonaceous fuel indoors include wood stoves, fireplaces, kerosene heaters, gas furnaces, gas heaters, and any gasoline-powered equipment.

Automobile exhausts around the garages, nearby roadways, and parking areas are major outdoor sources of CO. This is especially true of exhausts from diesel engines which are powered directly by controlling the fuel rather than air supply. Even for vehicles using non-diesel fuels, the air-to-fuel ratios can be too low in the engine during starting or when the automobile is not maintained properly. These concerns are the main reasons why in many countries including the United States, on-road vehicles are each required to be equipped with a catalytic converter to help reduce the emission of CO and other by-product toxic substances coming off their engine.

In the United States, even with the catalytic converter requirement in effect for well over 20 years, on-road motor vehicle exhausts continue to contribute about 60% of all CO emissions nationwide. A much higher percentage (85 to 95%) from this source can be seen in cities with heavy traffic congestion. One explanation for such high percentages still being seen from vehicle exhausts is that the number of vehicles on the road and the miles that they have driven have doubled in the past 20 years. Other sources of CO emissions include non-road engines (e.g., boats), industrial processes (e.g., metal smelting), wildfires, and residential wood burning.

11.5.2. Characteristics and Properties

In addition to its special characteristics being odorless, colorless, and tasteless, CO is a flammable, non-irritating gas soluble in ethanol (C_2H_6O) and benzene (C_6H_6) but only sparingly in water. This inorganic gas has considerable industrial importance due to its widespread use as a fuel and as a reducing agent. Among other things, CO can be used to make aldehydes (R-CHO, where R = any organyl group) which can be used to make detergents or to be mixed with methanol (CH_3OH) to form acetic acid (CH_3COOH). Acetic acid in turn can be used to make certain polymers to be applied in paints and adhesives.

The general physicochemical properties of CO are listed in Table 11.4. Its flammable range is 12.5 to 74%, with the characteristic that when mixed with air, it will quickly ignite in the presence of a spark or flame.

Table 11.4. General Physicochemical Properties of Carbon Monoxide (CO)

Molecular weight	28.0
Boiling point	$-191.5°$ C (at 1 atm)
Vapor density (specific gravity)	0.97 (with air = 1)
Freezing point	$-205°$ C
Gas density	1.25 kg/m^3 ($0°$ C, 1 atm)

Several methods can be used to produce CO in the laboratory, including dehydration of formic acid (HCO_2H) with H_2SO_4 (Reaction 11.11) and heating calcium carbonate ($CaCO_3$) with zinc (Zn) metal (Reaction 11.12).

$$HCO_2H + H_2SO_4 \rightarrow CO + H_2O + H_2SO_4 \qquad (11.11)$$

$$CaCO_3 + Zn \rightarrow ZnO + CaO + CO \qquad (11.12)$$

The most common method for industrial production of CO is by combustion of carbon (C) in air at high temperatures with an excess of C over O_2 supply (Reaction 11.13).

$$O_2 + 2C \rightarrow 2CO \ (>800° \text{ C}) \qquad (11.13a)$$

$$2CO \leftrightarrows CO_2 + C \ (\leftarrow \text{ when at temperatures } >800° \text{ C}) \qquad (11.13b)$$

11.5.3. Toxic Effects and Advisories

In the United States, no federal standards have been reached yet for CO in indoor air. The NAAQS for outdoor air nationwide is set at 9 ppm (40 mg/m^3) for 8 hours, and 35 ppm for 1 hour (U.S. EPA, 2010). Average CO levels in residential areas without gas stoves reportedly range from around 0.5 to 5 ppm. Yet levels near properly- and poorly-adjusted gas stoves reportedly are as high as 15 ppm and above 30 ppm, respectively. The outdoor levels of CO generally peak during the colder months when inversion conditions are more frequent. During those moments, the air pollutant would likely get trapped near the ground beneath a layer of warm air. The WHO (2000b) guideline values for CO are 10 ppm for 8 hours and 90 ppm for 15 minute.

A. Effects on Humans and Animals

Carbon monoxide is known as the most potent and common asphyxiant, as it can deprive Hb (hemoglobin) of the ability to carry oxygen to cells in various body tissues. The adverse effects of CO exposure can vary considerably from person to person, especially at lower levels. At low levels of exposure, CO generally causes mild effects that are often mistaken for the common flu without fever. Symptoms from mild effects include headaches, disorientation, dizziness, nausea, and tiredness, with no motivation to work. The health threat from CO at low levels is most serious for those persons suffering from cardiovascular diseases, such as angina pectoris or congestive heart failure.

At moderate levels, angina, vision impairment, and reduced brain function may result, whereas at high levels even healthy people will be affected. The symptoms from high levels of exposure include vision impairment, disorientation, headaches, dizziness, nausea, confusion, and death. Acute fatal effects are mainly due to asphyxiation.

Carbon monoxide at ambient air concentrations may trigger serious respiratory problems largely due to its contribution to the formation of ground-level ozone smog. In a person with a cardiovascular disease, even a short-term exposure to CO at ambient air levels may cause chest pain and suppress that person's ability to work. Prolonged exposure even at low levels may induce other cardiovascular effects in that person.

B. Effects on Plants

Under most conditions, CO is not harmful to plants in that it can be rapidly oxidized to form CO_2 which is quickly used for photosynthesis. The increase in atmospheric CO_2 actually should have a substantial positive environmental effect, as atmospheric CO_2 can fertilize plants thus enabling them to grow faster as well as larger and to withstand drier climates. Studies showed that CO induced not only the initiation or stimulation of root formation in certain plant species (Cao *et al.*, 2007; Zimmerman *et al.*, 1993), but also a change in the sex expression pattern in certain (other) plant species (Heslop-Harrison and Heslop-Harrison, 1957; Minina and Tylkina, 1947). There is nonetheless evidence that CO also has the potential to inhibit the enzymatic activity of cytochrome oxidase in plant tissues and thereby can damage the cellular respiratory function there (Webster, 1954).

References

Abbey DE, Nishino N, McDonnell WF, Burchette RJ, Knutsen SF, Beeson WL, Yang JX, 1999. Long-Term Inhalable Particles and Other Air Pollutants Related to Mortality in Nonsmokers. *Am. J. Respir. Crit. Care Med.* 159:73-382.

Adam SEH, Abdel-Banat BMA, Sakamoto A, Takahashi M, Morikawa H, 2008a. Effect of Atmospheric Nitrogen Dioxide on Mulukhiya (*Corchorus olitorius*) Growth and Flowering. *Am. J. Plant Physiol.* 3:180-184.

Adam SEH, Shigeto J, Sakamoto A, Takahashi M, Morikawa H, 2008b. Atmospheric Nitrogen Dioxide at Ambient Levels Stimulates Growth and Development of Horticultural Plants. *Botany* 86:213-217.

ATSDR (U.S. Agency for Toxic Substances and Disease Registry), 1998. Toxicological Profile for Sulfur Dioxide. U.S. Department of Health and Human Services, Atlanta, Georgia, USA.

Beeson WL, Abbey DE, Knutsen SF, 1998. Long-term Concentrations of Ambient Air Pollutants and Incident Lung Cancer in California Adults: Results from the ASHMOG Study. *Environ. Health Perspect.* 106:813-823.

Brauer M, Lencar C, Tamburic L, Koehoorn M, Demers P, Karr C, 2008. A Cohort Study of Traffic-Related Air Pollution Impacts on Birth Outcomes. *Environ. Health Perspect.* 116:680-686.

Burnett RT, Stieb D, Brook JR, Cakmak S, Dales R, Raizenne M, Vincent R, Dann T, 2004. Associations between Short-Term Changes in Nitrogen Dioxide and Mortality in Canadian Cities. *Arch. Environ. Health* 59:228-236.

Cao Z-Y, Xuan W, Liu Z-Y, Li X-N, Zhao N, Xu P, Wang Z, Guan RZ, Shen W-B, 2007. Carbon Monoxide Promotes Lateral Root Formation in Rapeseed. *J. Int. Plant Biol.* 49:1070-1079.

Daines RH, 1968. Sulfur Dioxide and Plant Response. *J. Occup. Environ. Med.* 10:516-524.

EEA (European Environment Agency), 2002. Annual European Community CLR-TAP Emission Inventory 1990-2000 (Technical Report No. 91). Copenhagen, Denmark.

EEA (European Environment Agency), 2007. Air Pollution by Ozone in Europe in Summer 2006 (Technical Report No. 5). Copenhagen, Denmark.

Griffiths H, 2003. Air Pollution on Agricultural Crops. Ministry of Agriculture, Food & Rural Affairs, Ontario, Canada.

Grose EC, Stevens MA, Hatch GE, Jaskot RH, Selgrade MJK, Stead AG, Costa DL, Graham JA, 1989. The Impact of a 12-Month Exposure to a Diurnal Pattern of Ozone on Pulmonary Function, Antioxidant Biochemistry and Immunology. In *Atmospheric Ozone Research and Its Policy Implications* (Schneider T, Lee TS, Wolters GJR, Grant LD, Eds.). Nijmegen, The Netherlands: Elsevier, pp.535-544.

Harvard Magazine, 2000. Art under Wrap. Vol.102, March-April.

Heagle AS, 1989. Ozone and Crop Yield. *Ann. Rev. Phytopathol.* 27:397-423.

Heslop-Harrison J, Heslop-Harrison Y, 1957. The Effect of Carbon Monoxide on Sexuality in *Mercurialis ambigua* L. fils. *New Phytol.* 56:352-355.

Hexter AC, Goldsmith JR, 1971. Carbon Monoxide: Association of Community Air Pollution with Mortality. *Science* 172:265-267.

Holman C, 1999. Sources of Air Pollution. In *Air Pollution and Health* (Holgate ST, Samet JM, Koren HS, Maynard RL, Eds.). London, UK: Academic Press.

Huang Y, Chang LY, Miller FJ, Graham JA, Ospital JJ, Crapo JD, 1988. Lung Injury Caused by Ambient Levels of Oxidant Air Pollutants: Extrapolation from Animal to Man. *Am. J. Aerosol. Med.* 1:180-183.

Hyde DM, Plopper CG, Harkema JR, St. George JA, Tyler WS, Dungworth DL, 1989. Ozone-Induced Structural Changes in Monkey Respiratory System. In *Atmospheric Ozone Research and Its Policy Implications*, (Schneider T, Lee TS, Wolters GJR, Grant LD, Eds.). Nijmegen, The Netherlands: Elsevier, pp.523-534.

Ingram W, McCarroll JR, Cassell EJ, Wolter D, 1965. Health and the Urban Environment: Air Pollution and Family Illness. II. Two Acute Air Pollution Episodes in New York City. *Arch. Environ. Health* 10:364-366.

Klonoff-Cohen H, Lam P, Lewis A, 2005. Outdoor Carbon Monoxide, Nitrogen Dioxide, and Sudden Infant Death Syndrome. *Arch. Dis. Child.* 90:750-753.

Kumie A, Emmelin A, Wahlberg S, Berhane Y, Ali A, Mekonen E, Worku A, Brandstrom D, 2009. Sources of Variation for Indoor Nitrogen Dioxide in Rural Residences of Ethiopia. *Environ. Health* 8:51 (online journal).

Linn WS, Szlachcic Y, Gong H Jr, Kinney PL, Berhane KT, 2000. Air Pollution and Daily Hospital Admissions in Metropolitan Los Angeles. *Environ. Health Perspect.* 108:427-434.

Macdowall FDH, Cole AFW, 1971. Threshold and Synergistic Damage to Tobacco by Ozone and Sulfur Dioxide. *Atmosph. Environ.* 5:553-554.

Menser HA, Heggestad HE, 1966. Ozone and Sulfur Dioxide Synergism: Injury to Tobacco Plants. *Science* 153:424-425.

Minina EG, Tylkina LG, 1947. Physiological Study of the Effect of Gases upon Sex Differentiation in Plants. *Compt. Rend. Acad. Sci. URSS* 55:169-172.

Noble RD, Jensen KF, 1980. Effects of Sulfur Dioxide and Ozone on the Growth of Hybrid Poplar Leaves. *Am. J. Bot.* 67:1005-1009.

Reinert RA, Gray TN, 1981. The Response of Radish to Nitrogen Dioxide, Sulfur Dioxide, and Ozone, Alone and in Combination. *J. Environ. Qual.* 10:240-243.

Rich S, Tomlinson H, 1974. Mechanisms of Ozone Injury to Plants. In *Air Pollution Effects on Plant Growth* (Dugger M, Ed.). Washington DC, USA: American Chemical Society, Chapter 6.

Rubio MA, Lissi E, Villena G, Caroca V, Gramsch E, Ruiz A, 2005. Estimation of Hydroxyl and Hydroperoxyl Radicals Concentrations in the Urban Atmosphere of Santiago. *J. Chil. Chem. Soc.* 50:471-476.

Schneider CG, 2004. Dirty Air, Dirty Power: Mortality and Health Damage due to Air Pollution from Power Plants. Clear Air Task Force, 77 Summer Street, Boston, Massachusetts, USA.

Schubert TS, 1984. Sulfur Dioxide Injury to Plants. Plant Pathology Circular No. 257. Division of Plant Industry, Florida Department of Agriculture and Consumer Services, The Capitol, Tallahassee, Florida, USA.

Smith BJ, Nitschke M, Pilotto LS, Ruffin RE, Pisaniello DL, Willson KJ, 2000. Health Effects of Daily Indoor Nitrogen Dioxide Exposure in People with Asthma. *Eur. Respir. J.* 16:879-885.

Srivastava HS, Ormrod DP, 1986. Effects of Nitrogen Dioxide and Nitrate Nutrition on Nodulation, Nitrogenase Activity, Growth, and Nitrogen Content of Bean. *Plant Physiol.* 81:737-741.

Suhadi DR, Awang M, Hassan MN, Abdullah R, Muda AH, 2005. Review of Photochemical Smog Pollution in Jakarta Metropolitan, Indonesia. *Am. J. Environ. Sci.* 1:110-118.

Takahashi M, Nakagawa M, Sakamoto A, Ohsumi C, Matsubara T, Morikawa H, 2005. Atmospheric Nitrogen Dioxide Gas Is a Plant Vitalization Signal to Increase Plant Size and the Contents of Cell Constituents. *New Phytol.* 168:149-154.

Taylor OC, Eaton FM, 1966. Suppression of Plant Growth by Nitrogen Dioxide. *Plant Physiol.* 41:132-135.

Tingey DT, Reinert RA, Dunning JA, Heck WW, 1971. Vegetation Injury from the Interaction of Nitrogen Dioxide and Sulfur Dioxide. *Phytopathol.* 61:1506-1511.

Tyler WS, Tyler NK, Last JA, Gillespie MJ, Barstow TJ, 1988. Comparison of Daily and Seasonal Exposures of Young Monkeys to Ozone. *Toxicology* 50:131-144.

U.S. EPA (U. S. Environmental Protection Agency), 1980. Acid Rain. EPA-600/9-79-036. Office of Research and Development, Washington DC, USA.

U.S. EPA (U. S. Environmental Protection Agency), 2009. 1970-2008 Average Annual Emissions, All Criteria Pollutants in MS Excel – June 2009. Office of Air Quality Planning and Standards, Research Triangle Park, North Carolina, USA.

U.S. EPA (U.S. Environmental Protection Agency), 2010. National Primary and Secondary National Ambient Air Quality Standards. *Code of Federal Regulations.* Title 40 (Protection of Environment), Part 50. Washington DC, USA.

Wang TJ, Lam KS, Xie M, Wang XM, Carmichael G, Li YS, 2006. Integrated Studies of a Photochemical Smog Episode in Hong Kong and Regional Transport in the Pearl River Delta of China. *Tellus* 50:31-40.

Webster GC, 1954. The Effect of Carbon Monoxide on Respiration in Higher Plants. *Plant Physiol.* 29:399-400.

White KL, Hill AC, Bennett JH, 1974. Synergistic Inhibition of Apparent Photosynthesis Rate of Alfalfa by Combination of Sulfur Dioxide and Nitrogen Dioxide. *Environ. Sci. Technol.* 8:574-576.

WHO (World Health Organization), 2000a. WHO Air Quality Guidelines for Europe, Second Edition: Effects of Sulfur Dioxide on Vegetation – Critical Levels (Chapter 10). WHO European Centre for Environment and Health, Bonn, Germany.

WHO (World Health Organization), 2000b. WHO Air Quality Guidelines for Europe, Second Edition: Carbon Monoxide (Chapter 5.5). WHO European Centre for Environment and Health, Bonn, Germany.

WHO (World Health Organization), 2006. WHO Air Quality Guidelines for Particular Matter, Ozone, Nitrogen Dioxide and Sulfur Dioxide: Global Update 2005, Summary of Risk Assessment. Geneva, Switzerland.

Wiwanitkit V, 2007. Sexual Fertility and Its Relationship to Occupational Hazards. *Sexual. & Disab.* 25:45-47.

Zimmerman PW, Crocker W, Hitchcock AE, 1933. Initiation and Stimulation of Roots from Exposure of Plants to Carbon Monoxide Gas. *Contrib. Boyce Thompson Inst.* 5:1-17.

Review Questions

1. Name the six criteria air pollutants designated by U.S. EPA.

2. When and where did the acute air pollution take place that resulted in 4,000 excess deaths and over 100,000 extra people getting sick largely due to the effects of SO_2-based smog on their respiratory or cardiovascular system?

3. In addition to SO_2, which two volcanic gases pose the greatest potential hazard to humans and ecosystems?

4. What are the major anthropogenic sources of SO_2 emissions in the United States?

5. Briefly explain how H_2SO_4 can be formed from SO_2 in the troposphere.

6. What may H_2SO_4 in acid deposition do chemically to limestone and marble buildings?

7. What is the primary anthropogenic source of NO_2, given that automobile exhaust fumes typically contain a lot more NO than NO_2 by volume?

8. Which of the inorganic gases discussed in this chapter is (are) also considered as a common indoor air pollutant? And what are its (their) primary indoor sources?

9. Briefly describe the adverse health effects of NO_2 to humans.

10. Briefly describe the symptoms from plant injury induced by exposure to NO_2, particularly when either SO_2 or O_3 is also present.

11. How are tropospheric and stratospheric O_3 generally formed?

12. Briefly describe the major characteristics of O_3.

13. What are the three common precursors of O_3? And in each case, with which chemical component in the air does the diatomic oxygen (O_2) molecule eventually react to form O_3?

14. With respect to joint effect on leaf growth, what is likely to happen to *hybrid poplar* plants that have been exposed to SO_2 and O_3 simultaneously?

15. Why is carbon monoxide nicknamed the silent killer? And how is it generally produced?

16. Briefly explain why on-road motor vehicle exhausts continue to contribute over 50% of all CO emissions nationwide in the United States, even when the nationwide catalytic converter requirement has been in effect for well over 20 years.

17. Briefly describe the symptoms with acute CO poisoning in humans.

18. Briefly describe the effects of CO on plants.

19. Briefly describe separately the beneficial effects of O_3 and of CO.

CHAPTER 12

Air Pollutants – II: Particulate Matter

12.1. Introduction

To many people, the word *aerosol* refers to an aerosol spray or the canister that contains the spray material. In atmospheric chemistry, aerosol actually refers to a suspension of fine solid particles, tiny liquid droplets, or a mixture of both in a gas medium; and by default, air is the gas medium of common interest. Particulate matter (PM), the subject matter of this chapter, is atmospheric aerosol without specifically referring to or considering the gas (typically air) medium portion. Otherwise, for all practical purposes, the terms *PM* and *(atmospheric) aerosol* are synonymous with each other.

With respect to air pollution, the various forms of aerosol under consideration generally include dust, smoke, smog, fume, haze, fog, and mist. Dust aerosol typically refers to tiny solid particles produced by disintegration or decomposition, whereas the relatively tinier smoke particles are generated from fire or spark of light. Fume particles are similar to smoke particles in size, but can be generated by any material coming in contact with air. Haze is an atmospheric phenomenon where dust, smoke, or other airborne matters are in amounts sufficient to obscure visibility. Mist and fog are composed of liquid droplets and differ from each other only in density and visibility. Smog is fog that has been polluted with smoke. In all cases, the solid particles and liquid droplets, namely the PM, that are of health concern include primarily those that as a group are directly or indirectly harmful to human health or the environment. And by convention, they are collectively treated as a single air pollutant entity. Due to its common occurrence across the United States, PM has been designated by U.S. EPA as one of the six criteria air pollutants.

12.1.1. Composition of Airborne Particulates

The composition of primary airborne particulates can vary greatly depending on their sources. In areas such as the tropical and desert regions, wind-blown solid dust aerosol is the main source of particulate loading. This type is generally composed of mineral oxides and other materials blown from the Earth's crust. Another common source is sea spray, with the particulates consisting of largely the sodium chloride (NaCl) salt along with small quantities of organic compounds and other mineral constituents of sea salt.

By definition, PM includes biological particles, such as viruses, bacteria, molds, and any tiny metallic, radioactive, or carcinogenic substance carried by these microbes (or vice versa, depending on their size and other variables such as physicochemical properties). Secondary particulates typically stem from the oxidation of primary gases, such as from oxidation of sulfur oxides (SO_x) into sulfuric acid (H_2SO_4) and of nitrogen oxides (NO_x) into nitric acid (HNO_3). In the presence of ammonia (NH_3), secondary particulates take the form of ammonium salts (e.g., ammonium sulfate NH_2SO_4, ammonium nitrate NH_4NO_3). Organic matter (OM) is a collection of primary and secondary particulates, with the former being biogenic or anthropogenic in origin. Secondary OM particulates usually derive from the oxidation of VOCs (volatile organic compounds). Another significant particulate group consists mainly of black (i.e., elemental) carbon and is commonly called soot. Soot and OM together constitute the carbonaceous portion of particulates.

12.1.2. Basic Characteristics of Airborne Particulates

These days, most PM under consideration ranges from 0.01 μm (micron or micrometer) to less than 100 μm in diameter. As a point of reference, tobacco smoke particles are in the middle of this size range. It is of note that, as with biological particulates, particles in tobacco smoke are capable of picking up many tiny substances such as indoor radon and its progenies (Chapter 14). Most airborne particulates will eventually fall onto the ground or get washed down by precipitation. However, certain airborne particles are able to rise to (almost) the highest levels of the atmosphere, stay for a long time, or travel for long distances. In general, the lighter and smaller (<1 μm) a particle is, the longer (in weeks) it will stay in the atmosphere. In contrast, heavier and larger particles tend to settle onto the ground by gravity in a matter of hours. Some particulates such as diesel aerosol are usually found at their peak concentrations near the emission source.

Not all airborne particulates are harmful. Because most aerosols reflect sunlight back into space, they have a positive global cooling effect by lowering the amount of solar radiation that is to reach the Earth's surface. Particulates containing sulfates and nitrates are strong light-scatters due to the larger sizes of these components that make the particulate proper more effectively as a deflector. OM can affect the atmospheric radiation field by light absorption or scattering. And soot includes strong light-absorbing materials capable of yielding a large positive radiative forcing (i.e., a large positive balance between radiations traveling into and out of the atmosphere). Atmospheric deposition of particulates is also a significant source of nutrients (e.g., minerals, trace metals) to open oceans where carbon sequestration and aquatic productivity can then be enhanced.

12.2. Sizes of Particulate Matter

As alluded to earlier, PM includes many types of substances that together can cause a wide spectrum of toxic effects to human health and the ecosystem. Yet in spite of such a concern, these substances are almost always treated as a single complex mixture. This is because to many health regulatory entities, it is not the types of particulates involved that matters the most. Rather, it is their size that is deemed relevant to health threats. This notion is based on the large body of evidence (e.g., Section 12.4) supporting the strong link between the size of airborne particles and their potential for causing health problems.

Even though airborne particles have irregular shapes with geometric diameters difficult to measure, for simplicity and by convention their behavior in the immediate space is typically expressed in terms of the aerodynamic diameter of an idealized spherical particle. Airborne particles are thereby generally collected and characterized in terms of their aerodynamic equivalent diameter which is used to represent their size. The aerodynamic diameter of a spherical particle is roughly equal to the square root of the mathematical product of its diameter and density. In any case, this does not mean that airborne particles with the same aerodynamic diameter will necessarily have the same dimension or shape.

12.2.1. Sizes of Regulatory Importance

There are broadly four particulate size categories used by the health regulatory sector to characterize PM in relation to its impacts on environmental health. These four categories are: (1) non-inhalable coarse particles; (2) inhalable coarse particles; (3) fine particles; and (4) ultrafine or nano particles. However, in practice, not all agencies care to use these four sizes to the fullness. For example, U.S. EPA initially was concerned with airborne particles that were only 10 μm in (henceforth aerodynamic) diameter or smaller because the agency then concluded that these were the ones capable of passing through at least a human's upper respiratory tract. That is, U.S. EPA's position then was that those airborne particles larger than 10 μm were non-inhalable (as well as coarse) and therefore would have no apparent health threats as an air pollutant entity. The agency now has a focus on particulates in both the inhalable coarse and the fine particle groups, which by sampling limitations include automatically those in the ultrafine group.

By convention, inhalable coarse particles in the atmosphere are those each have a diameter between 2.5 and 10 μm and are put in the category denoted by $PM_{2.5-10}$. Fine particles are those that are also inhalable (as due to their size) but each have a diameter of 2.5 μm or smaller and accordingly are denoted by $PM_{2.5}$. For fine particles each with a diameter of 0.1 μm or less and now known to have greater health implications, they are specifically termed *ultrafine particles* (UFPs) and denoted by $PM_{0.1}$. Nanoparticles, denoted by PM_{nano}, are considered to have a similar particle size range as the UFPs have, except to a small group of scholars (e.g., Chang *et al.*, 2008) who specifically refer to particles having a diameter of 0.056 μm (i.e., 56 nm) or smaller as nanoparticles. As explained in Section 12.2.5, the sources of UFPs and of PM_{nano} may be treated as somewhat different, at least to some scholars. In any event, it is more certain that PM_{10} used to be the size group having the most regulatory attention. This group refers to all inhalable particles with a diameter of 10 μm *or smaller* and may include the fine, ultrafine, or nano particles depending on the context. Lastly, non-inhalable coarse particles as a group are denoted by PM_{10+}, which is not a notation used enough by the health and aerosol science sectors since the health concern with particles in this group is minimal.

Particle size is of regulatory importance because it is the principal parameter governing the motions and depositions of aerosols by affecting the inertial, gravitational, or Brownian diffusional force that applies. For airborne particles on the micron (μm) scale, inertial and gravitational forces dominate. Inertia is the tendency of a moving object to resist acceleration without settling down until it runs into another object (e.g., the walls of an airway conduit) resulting in an impaction or interception. Gravitational force occurs when the object's motion is governed or affected by gravity leading to sedimentation. As particle size decreases into the nano scale, diffusional force dominates, with the particles acting much like a gas or vapor. Diffusion occurs when smaller particles are in Brownian (i.e., jiggling-like) motion to hit another object's surface. The general composition and basic properties of particulates in $PM_{2.5-10}$, $PM_{0.1-2.5}$, and $PM_{0.1}$ are summarized in Table 12.1. More specific characteristics of airborne particulates in the various size groups, starting with those of PM_{10+}, are discussed separately in the (sub)sections that follow.

12.2.2. Non-Inhalable Coarse Particles (PM_{10+})

The terms *non-inhalable* and *inhalable* are somewhat subjective (e.g., Kumar, 2008; Raabe, 1982). About 50% of the particles with a diameter of around 10 μm (irrespective of their shape) were historically found to be capable of penetrating down below the pharynx region and hence are now treated as inhalable for size cutoff and monitoring purposes. However, some literature has also considered particles of 15 to 30 μm (e.g., cotton fiber) to be inhalable in the sense that they can penetrate through the nose or the mouth. Another inconsistency in usage is that, according to U.S. Occupational Safety and Health Administration and U.S. Mine Safety and Health Administration, respirable dust particles are those small enough to penetrate deep into the lung; and, as defined by the two agencies, they all have a diameter less than 10 μm. In contrast, U.S. EPA includes the 10 μm particles in its inhalable group. Adding to the confusion, in some places such as Europe, *fine* particles are denoted by PM_{10-}, not $PM_{2.5-}$ (e.g., van Zelma *et al.*, 2008).

Traditionally, for air monitoring purposes and therefore by sampling preference, only those airborne particles with a diameter of around 100 μm or less are collected as total suspended particles or particulates (TSP) which as a group are a collective and an inclusive term for a mixture of solid particles and liquid droplets measured in the air. Yet in reality, particles in PM_{10+} often have an upper-bound diameter of around 40 or 50 μm instead. This is because particles larger than 50 μm have a tendency to settle quickly (in hours) and thus likely near their sources of emission not readily collectible.

The group called TSP is actually an archaic regulatory measure of the *mass* concentration of all particles collected in an area's ambient air. As the monitoring interest then was mostly in the total *weight* of all airborne particles collected in a sample, the air samplers were typically designed without preference in particle size other than the filter's capacity to capture and retain particles in a certain size range. Many high volume air samplers have the ability to retain particles up to 100 μm (e.g., U.S. EPA, 1999). Unfortunately, the actual size cut varies with wind speed and wind direction in the field, thereby frequently ending with an actual capture of lighter particles of 50 μm or less.

With a size-select *inlet* to the filter collecting the airborne particles, even a high volume air sampler (U.S. EPA, 1999) can be used to collect particles of 10 μm or smaller in

Table 12.1. Comparison of Coarse and Fine Inhalable Airborne Particulates[a]

	PM$_{2.5}$ (Fine)		PM$_{2.5-10}$ (Coarse)
	PM$_{0.1}$ (Ultrafine)	PM$_{0.1-2.5}$ (Accumulation)	
Formation processes	Combustion, high-temperature processes/ atmospheric reactions		Break-up of large solids and droplets
Formation	Nucleation Condensation Coagulation	Condensation Coagulation Reaction of gases in or on particles Evaporation of cloud/fog droplets in which gases have dissolved and reacted	Mechanical disruption (crushing, grinding, abrasion of surfaces) Evaporation of sprays Suspension of dust reactions of gases in or on particles
Composition	Sulfate Elemental (black) carbon Metal compounds Organics with very low saturation vapor pressure at ambient temperature	Sulfate, nitrate, ammonium, and hydrogen ions Elemental (black) carbon Large variety of organic compounds Metals: compounds of lead, of cadmium, of nickel copper, of vanadium, of zinc, of manganese, of iron, etc. Particle-bound water	Suspended soil or street dust Fly ash from uncontrolled combustion of coal, oil, or wood Nitrates/chlorides from hydrochloric acid/nitric acid Oxides of crustal elements (silicon, aluminum, iron titanium) Calcium carbonate, sea salt, sodium chloride Pollen, molds, fungal spores Plant/animal fragments Tire, brake pad, or road wear debris
Solubility	Probably less than those of PM$_{0.1-1}$	Often soluble, hygroscopic and deliquescent	Largely insoluble and non-hygroscopic
Sources	Combustion Atmospheric transformation of sulfur dioxide or some organic compounds High-temperature processes	Combustion of coal, of oil, of gasoline, of diesel fuel, of wood Atmospheric transformation products of nitrogen oxides, of sulfur dioxide, or of organic carbon (e.g., terpenes) High-temperature processes, smelters, steel mills, etc.	Resuspension of industrial dust or of soil tracked onto roads and streets Suspension from disturbed soil (e.g. farming, mining, unpaved roads) Construction or demolition Uncontrolled coal or oil combustion Ocean spray Biological sources
Half-life (in air)	Minutes to hours	Days to weeks	Minutes to days
Removal processes	By growing in accumulation mode Diffusion to raindrops	Formation of cloud droplets and then deposition in rain Dry deposition	Dry deposition by fallout Scavenging by falling rain drops
Travel distance	<1 to 10s of km	100s to 1,000s of km	<1 to 100s of km

[a] adapted from WHO (2006b).

(again, aerodynamic equivalent) diameter. The level and the mass of PM_{10+} thus can be analyzed by subtraction of the PM_{10} level from the TSP level measured. Consequently, PM_{10+} generally contains particles collectible as TSP with a diameter >10 but practically <50 μm. The depositions of most PM_{10+} particles are by gravitational sedimentation, with a residence time in minutes to hours and a travel distance close to their emission source.

12.2.3. Inhalable Coarse Particles ($PM_{2.5-10}$)

Airborne particles in this group are almost the largest among all the inhalables; they are mostly produced by decomposition or disintegration of larger solid particles or liquid droplets, such as by crushing, grinding, spray evaporation, or suspensions of dusts from construction and agricultural operations. The particulates are inhalable but are also the coarse fraction of the PM_{10} (which by definition includes the fine and smaller particle fractions unless the notation is specifically intended for particles of exactly 10 μm). PM_{10} *per se* is known as the inhalable group as well as the thoracic fraction. This is because the particles in this group are considered to have the ability to penetrate into at least the larynx region. The cutoff for the low end for coarse particles is 2.5 μm because energy considerations normally limit coarse particle sizes to greater than 2 μm.

Examples of $PM_{2.5-10}$ particles include dust particles, bacteria, molds, pollen, spores, fly ash, and insect parts. The residence time of these inhalable coarse particles in the atmosphere, at least in certain regions such as Europe, is about 1 to 6 days (van Zelma *et al.*, 2008), with a travel distance less than 10 km (6.2 miles). In the United States, the NAAQS (National Ambient Air Quality Standards) for PM_{10} is set at 150 μg/m^3 averaged over a 24-hour period (U.S. EPA, 2010). The World Health Organization (WHO, 2006a) guideline values for this size group are 50 and 20 μg/m^3 averaged over a 24-hour and a one-year period, respectively.

12.2.4. Fine Particles ($PM_{0.1-2.5}$)

Airborne particles in this size group are different from those in $PM_{2.5-10}$ both in origin and in physicochemical properties. Once inhaled, these $PM_{0.1-2.5}$ fine particles can reach into the gas-exchange (alveolar) region of the lung and hence are also referred to as the *respirable* fraction. In addition to evaporation of fog or cloud droplets being a major source, these particles can be originated from a gas nucleated into a particle of ultrafine size. The gas may come from either an anthropogenic or a natural source. The UFPs (ultrafine particles) so generated can then become fine particles by growing up to a size of about 1 μm or greater via condensation or coagulation. In condensation, additional gas is required to condensate on the ultrafine particles generated from nucleation. Coagulation is the process whereby multiple ultrafine particles gather to form larger ones.

$PM_{0.1-2.5}$ particles are composed of various combinations of carbon (C) compounds, sulfate compounds (SO_4^{2-}), nitrate compounds (NO_3^-), ammonium (NH_4^+), hydrogen ion (H^+), polycyclic aromatic hydrocarbons (PAHs) and other organic compounds, metals (e.g., Pb, Cd, Ni, Cr, Mn), and particle-bound water. The major sources of $PM_{0.1-2.5}$ are fossil fuel combustion, burning of vegetation, and the smelting as well as processing of metals. Unlike the inhalable coarse $PM_{2.5-10}$, they tend to be soluble in water.

The residence time of $PM_{0.1-2.5}$ is from days to weeks, with a travel distance ranging from hundreds to over thousands of kilometers (1 kilometer = 0.6 mile). In the United States, the NAAQS for $PM_{2.5}$ are 35 $\mu g/m^3$ averaged over a 24-hour period and 15 $\mu g/m^3$ over a one-year period (U.S. EPA, 2010). The WHO (2006a) guideline values for $PM_{2.5}$ are 25 and 10 $\mu g/m^3$ averaged over a 24-hour and a one-year period, respectively.

12.2.5. Ultrafine or Nano Particles ($PM_{0.1}$)

Airborne particles in this group have the size of a molecule or virus which is less than 100 nm (0.1 μm) or approximately one-thousandth the width of a human hair. For consistency with other PM groups, oftentimes their diameters are still expressed in units of micrometers (microns). These UFPs (ultrafine particles) can be either carbon-based or metallic. Within each class, they can be further subdivided according to their magnetic properties. Both their presence and concentrations can be measured using a condensation nucleus counter (e.g., McMurry, 2000) which can detect particles as small as about 2 nm in diameter. The morphology of these nanoparticles can be observed using transmission electron microscopy under certain physical laboratory conditions.

Ultrafine particles are found in the atmospheric environment where they originate from combustion sources (e.g., vehicle exhaust fumes, forest fires) and volcanic activity. These tiny particles are frequently the end products of a wide variety of physical, chemical, and biological processes, of which some are commonplace and traditional whereas some others are novel and radically different (Aitken *et al.*, 2004). UFPs can originate from nucleation, an initial physical reaction stage whereby a gas becomes a particle with a size on the nano scale. As noted earlier, the gas may come from an anthropogenic or a natural source. These ultra-tiny particles are the principal constituents of airborne particulates. Due to their vast quantities found in the atmosphere and their strong ability to penetrate deep into the human lungs, they are a major health concern.

In some literature, there appears to be a technical difference between nano and ultrafine particles, although the two groups are practically in the same size range. To some scholars, the term *nanoparticles* refers to solely those particles manufactured intentionally for their specific material properties. These are usually some forms of polymers or metals that can act as a thermal spray or coating for another material. In contrast, UFPs are referred to by these scholars as particles found in the natural environment (volcanic dusts) or produced unintentionally, such as during thermal processes (e.g., candlelight burning, welding, domestic heating) and machining of materials.

12.3. Issues with Urban Airborne Particulate Pollution

In the United States, the national annual average level of PM_{10} decreased 31% from 80.8 $\mu g/m^3$ in 1990 (the first year this index was used to replace TSP) to 55.9 $\mu g/m^3$ in

2008; and for the $PM_{2.5}$, the annual average decreased 19% from 13.5 $\mu g/m^3$ in 2000 to 10.9 $\mu g/m^3$ in 2008 (U.S. EPA, 2009). Yet despite these downward trends, the environmental health problems with urban (airborne) particulate pollution remain an important issue in major cities. After all, the national annual averages that the Americans experienced in 2008 still exceeded the guideline values set forth by WHO (2006a).

Worldwide, the health problems with particulate pollution are due to the very fact that well over half of the global population lives in urban areas, a trend that is accelerating rapidly particularly in the developing countries. Urban cities tend to use large quantities of energy and synthetic materials, thereby leading to the generation of large quantities of waste materials and pollutants. Noteworthy is that for large urban cities around the world (e.g., Beijing, London, Los Angeles, Mumbai, New York, Tokyo), they are merging into huge megalopolitan areas, especially along highways with heavy traffic.

Air pollution in urban areas comes from a vast variety of sources. In general, fossil fuel combustion is the single most important source for PM, as well as for many other classic pollutants such as sulfur dioxide (SO_2), nitrogen oxides (NO_x), and carbon monoxide (CO) discussed in Chapter 11. Of particular importance is the burning of fuels for road transport and electricity generation. PM is both emitted directly and generated from SO_2, VOCs, and vehicle exhausts released into the atmosphere. PM particles that are emitted directly are called primary particulates, whereas those formed from gases and other compounds are referred to as secondary particulates. Anthropogenic sources of primary PM include transportation, industrial processes, coking, heating, burning of vegetation, and dust particles from disturbed land or soil surfaces. Natural sources include wind-blown dusts from deserts, natural vegetation, volcanoes, wildfires, and sea spray salt. Directly or indirectly, industrial developments and human-related events can have a significant influence on all these natural and anthropogenic emissions.

In more technical and simplified terms, there are three main source categories of air pollution in urban areas. These are mobile sources, stationary sources, and open-burning sources, which collectively can be further categorized into several more specific source groups such as motor traffic, industrial processes, power plants, and domestic fuel. The investigation published by Mage *et al.* (1996) determined that motor traffic was one of the major sources, if not the major source, of air pollution in megacities.

12.3.1. Episodes of Particulate Pollution

Urban pollution attributed to PM is inevitably an ongoing major environmental health problem, inasmuch as motor traffic remains a principal anthropogenic source of airborne particulates (and of ozone). As a case example, despite the extensive emission control efforts made to improve the air quality in Los Angeles for the past 30 years, thick hazes can still be seen today obscuring the metropolitan's skylines. In fact, the South Coast Air Basin, which includes all of Los Angeles and its nearby counties Riverside, Orange, and San Bernardino, is currently designated as one of the worst regions, if not the worst region, in the United States for nonattainment of PM_{10} (CARB, 2010).

In Europe, the year 2003 experienced several wintertime pollution episodes due to PM on the Paris Basin (Bessagnet *et al.*, 2005). In addition, according to a World Bank study in 1999 (Pandey *et al.*, 2006), about 85% of the 3,226 residential areas under investigation worldwide had an estimated annual average PM_{10} level exceeding the WHO (2006a) guideline limit of 20 $\mu g/m^3$, with 46% of these areas having levels exceeding by twofold or more. The residential areas included in this study were those in cities reported to the United Nations to each have a population larger than 100,000.

The findings from the World Bank study, which reflected the more recent state of air quality worldwide, further implicated PM_{10} as a major problem in all Asian countries except Japan. The study also found that many cities worldwide, such as Tegucigalpa and Montevideo in Latin America, experienced an annual average PM_{10} level well over 300 $\mu g/m^3$. Overall, the findings from this World Bank study were consistent with those observed by Baldasano *et al.* (2003), who similarly assessed the air quality for a number of principal cities in both the developed and the developing countries.

Motor traffic is not the only major source of PM pollution in urban areas. For instance, one large Asian city with the most serious urban particulate pollution problem is Beijing, the national capital of China. In addition to both the high volume of daily motor traffic in the city and the persistent industrial pollution from many large facilities (e.g., Capitol Steel Company) located there (Dillner *et al.*, 2006), each spring Beijing experiences dust storms that cause high levels of PM. One of the recent episodes reported in the news worldwide occurred on 28 February 2013, when Beijing residents reportedly woke up that morning to only find the capital blanketed in yellow dusts, amidst a sandstorm sweeping relentlessly into the city. The sweep was reportedly in a manner similar to the ones experienced by residents living in Sydney, Australia on 23 September 2009 and 11 January 2013. The two huge outback dust storms swept across much of Australia and blanketed Sydney aggressively on those days, disrupting flights and ground transportation as well as forcing residents to stay indoors from the gale-force winds.

Still another major source of PM polluting urban areas is industrial processing. This is the case with Greece in its northwestern region where lignite mining operations and lignite-fired power stations are located. According to Triantafyllou *et al.* (2006) investigating the air quality of that region, the particulate pollution problems there with flying ashes and dusts were not only serious but also (not unexpectedly) more complicated as the region is located near the mining activities. Their analysis revealed that a complex system of sources (e.g., as due to additional contribution from urban pollution) coupled with poor meteorological conditions had worsened the particulate pollution in that region.

12.3.2. Monitoring of Particulate Matter

The term *urban air pollution episode* generally implies a short-term increase in ambient pollution that is greater than what would be expected as part of a day-to-day variation. In their most extreme form, urban air pollution episodes are accompanied by physical discomfort, disruption of daily living, public fear, illness, and in some instances even death. In any event, it is important to have the airborne particulate levels monitored periodically for all urban areas.

As summarized in Table 12.1, different size particulates (e.g., $PM_{2.5-10}$, $PM_{0.1-2.5}$) have different properties especially with respect to their deposition patterns and penetration in the human respiratory tract. In addition to size and physical properties, the biological or chemical composition of PM can influence considerably its adverse health effects. For example, metals such as vanadium (V), cobalt (Co), iron (Fe), and copper (Cu) are reportedly the major contributors of cellular response induced by ambient PM (Chen *et al.*, 1999). Therefore, monitoring of PM even at ambient levels is important.

Mass measurements of PM were first made in the late 1800s by drawing ambient air through filter paper that was weighed before and after sampling. In the United States, measurements of TSP (total suspended particulates) for radioactivity analyses were first performed during the 1950s to evaluate the effects of tests for above-ground nuclear weapons. The technology was soon adopted for measuring mass concentrations of particulates in major urban areas. The availability of these data was the basis for designating TSP (i.e., all those particles with a practical aerodynamic diameter of <40 μm) as the first indicator of PM for the NAAQS adopted in the United States in 1970.

Measurement of PM concentrations, identification of their sources, and evaluation of the effects of emission-reduction measures are difficult tasks under any circumstance, particularly in developing countries where many small industries lack the appropriate pollution-control devices to provide an emission inventory. Many urban areas in those countries still use some unquantifiable combination of fuel sources (e.g., bottled gas, natural gas) for cooking and heating. Burning of vegetation and waste incineration are also common events even in places where such activities are prohibited. For these and other reasons, TSP remains to be the only practical, yet less accurate, particulate measurement available in many developing countries (Krzyzanowski and Schwela 1999).

12.3.3. Airborne Microbes

As noted earlier repeatedly, airborne particulates are not confined to chemical matters. They may include biological materials (e.g., bacteria, molds, viruses, along with indoor radon and the kind that these microbes carry). Although under normal conditions air does not contain the nutrients and moisture required for the growth of airborne microbes, it can still abound in their numbers in that microbes can be evaporated or blown off from soils or other dry decomposed materials on the ground (e.g., excrete).

Microbes in decomposed materials or in soils can become an important source of particulates contaminating food products and places such as schools and hospitals. Such contaminations can cause food spoilage and diseases when the spoiled food products are ingested. People can also be exposed to airborne microbes via inhalation.

Still a more active exposure pathway is the transmission of airborne microbes from person to person through coughs and sneezes. During a sneeze, millions of tiny droplets of water and mucus containing the microbes can be sprayed into the air. Even though the droplets initially are each about 10 to 100 μm, they can rapidly dry to the more floatable, inhalable droplet nuclei of less than 5 μm. These tiny nuclei can still contain the microbial particles. Environmental diseases transmitted in this manner include Legionnaire's disease, SARS (severe acute respiratory syndrome), and H1N1 flu of 2009.

The ultimate fate of airborne microbes is governed by a complex set of conditions involving many variables such as sunlight, temperature, size and nature of the particulate carriers, adaptability of a particular microbe species to the new physical environment, and the ability of microbes to form resistant spores. Even the slightest air current can extend the residence time of airborne microbes to a sufficiently long one.

Both the quantity and quality of airborne microbes vary considerably with location as well as with time of the day, month, and year. For example, the microbial flux and hence the microbial quantity in the air are likely conditioned on a solar environment that affects the release of microbes into the air (Karra and Katsivela, 2007; Lighthart, 2000). Phylogenetic analyses showed that the atmospheric microbial community structure was linked to particle size (Polymenakou *et al.*, 2008).

Limited information is available concerning the natural microbial community in the urban areas and their relationship to the particulates in ambient air. In general and as expected, the ambient air in a congested urban area tends to harbor a greater number of microbes. An ambient air monitoring for about four months in 2003 revealed that the airborne particulates from two American cities (Austin and San Antonio) in the state of Texas contained over 1,800 diverse bacterial species, a richness reportedly approaching that of the bacterial communities in the soil (Brodie *et al.*, 2007). The study also showed that meteorological and temporal factors tended to be more important determinants than location in shaping the composition of airborne biological materials.

In terms of absolute quantity, it has been estimated that as many as a quarter of the total particulates present above ground are made up of biological materials ranging from 0.02 to 100 μm in (diameter) size (Jones and Harrison, 2004). In general, viruses are smaller than 0.3 μm and bacteria are mostly between 0.3 and 8 μm. Pollen and fungal spores tend to be larger, up to 60 μm (Stanley and Linskins, 1974).

At the moment, studies focusing on bioaerosols in urban ambient air are limited. Of the few published, one was a cross-sectional study conducted to assess the microbial counts (expressed as cfu = colony forming units) and the PM_{10} levels in air samples collected from roadsides of the Bangkok Fashion City Area in Thailand ((Mopuang *et al.*, 2005). The study showed that ~5% of the bacterial counts and ~26% of the PM_{10} levels exceeded the recommended targets of 1,000 cfu/m^3 and 120 μg/m^3, respectively.

Another study was conducted to determine the size distribution of airborne microbes over a coastal city along the eastern Mediterranean Sea during an intensive north African dust storm (Polymenakou *et al.*, 2008). This Mediterranean study showed that airborne microbes of particle size >3.3 μm were predominately spore-forming bacteria, whereas those respirable and smaller than 3.3 μm were bacteria commonly found in the soil or widely distributed in the environment.

Still another more recent study (Zheng *et al.*, 2009) was conducted to examine the average content of airborne microbes in 8 of the 16 cities located in China in the region known as Pearl River Delta Urban Agglomeration. The region covering 47,525 km^2 has become one of the most flourishing places in economic development in China. In that study, the average content of airborne microbes (mainly bacteria and fungi) measured was statistically correlated with each of the environmental factors investigated. The factors under investigation included wind speed, humidity, temperature, TSP, rate of pedestrians or car trafficking, and population density. These factors were found to have either a significantly negative or a significantly positive effect on the microbial content.

12.4. Toxic Effects of Airborne Particulates

The link between airborne particulate pollution and mortality goes back to at least 1930, when the then heavily industrialized areas in Meuse Valley in Belgium were blanketed by thick fog during the first week of December in that year. That air pollution episode reportedly caused more than 60 deaths in the valley, an area located east of the city of Liege. Although SO_2 and H_2SO_4 were the respiratory irritants blamed for causing those deaths, fine soot particles such as those found in diesel exhaust were also considered as a possible contribution (Nemery *et al.*, 2001). Those fine diesel-like particles were thought to have been coated with much of the ultrafine particulate sulfates formed from oxidation of SO_2 in the atmosphere.

Other historical links included pollution episodes occurring in the mill town Donora, Pennsylvania in 1948, in London in 1952, in New York in 1953, and in London again in 1962. Among these episodes, the London fog of 1952 has since become a notorious landmark in air pollution epidemiology as it led to the most excess deaths (4,000) and most excess morbidity (over 100,000) of this kind in history. Several studies also demonstrated a specific link between increase in daily mortality and exposure to low levels of PM_{10} and $PM_{2.5}$. Those studies included notably a time series analysis by Daniel *et al.* (2000), which supported the findings by others showing a positive link between daily mortality and particulate pollution, even at levels below regulatory limits.

Recent epidemiological studies on urban particulate pollution have all pointed to the direction that inhalation of particulates, particularly those of the $PM_{2.5}$ portion, has serious chronic health effects in humans and is a major cause of premature death worldwide. According to the WHO (2006b) estimation, each year about 350,000 attributable deaths reported in 25 European countries are due to PM exposure. In the United States, particulate pollution is estimated to cause 24,000 deaths each year (Mokdad *et al.*, 2004).

Available data all suggest that the mortality and the morbidity that were linked to particulate pollution may fall under three adverse effects categories as follows: those related or due to (1) effects on the respiratory tract; (2) effects on the cardiovascular system; and (3) other serious health effects such as cancer and sudden infant death syndrome (SIDS). Particulate air pollution can also have serious adverse effects on the environment, such as prevention of photosynthesis in plants, impairment of visibility, and soiling of surface materials such as those on building structures.

12.4.1. Mechanisms and General Trends

According to the report by Lippmann *et al.* (2003), many issues related to the underlying mechanisms of toxic action were investigated in epidemiological and toxicological studies in an effort to further the understanding of the health effects associated with PM exposure. And such collaborations had led to the development of certain common mechanism hypotheses (e.g., Section 12.4.3), and certain common toxic endpoints for testing such as lung function, heart rate, arterial oxygen saturation, tissue biomarkers of effects, cardiac dysrhythmias, and respiratory symptoms. Results from these collaborations repeatedly revealed strong links between $PM_{2.5}$ exposures and a variety of acute responses, implicating that $PM_{2.5}$ is biologically active at current peak exposure levels.

Several of the studies also demonstrated higher PM-associated health risks for certain susceptible subpopulations such as the elderly or those with preexisting cardiopulmonary diseases. Results from those studies showed specifically that while socioeconomic factors and race did not affect susceptibility to PM-associated mortality, females were found to be at a greater risk (e.g., Zanobetti and Schwartz 2000). Children were also found to be more susceptible to PM exposures, particularly for those with asthma. There were data showing that an increment of 10 $\mu g/m^3$ in PM_{10} or in $PM_{1.0}$ would increase the children's risk of having asthma symptoms by 11% or 18%, respectively (Yu *et al.*, 2000).

Diabetics too were identified as a major susceptible subpopulation. In several single-city studies, the risk of PM-associated hospitalization for cardiovascular diseases for diabetics was found two times higher than that for the general population (Zanobetti and Schwartz 2001, 2002). Persons having other types of diseases were also at a higher risk of the disease at issue. For example, heart failure and respiratory disorders reportedly elevated the risks of hospital admission for chronic obstructive pulmonary disease (COPD) and for cardiovascular diseases, respectively, from PM exposure (Zanobetti *et al.* 2000).

12.4.2. Effects on the Respiratory Tract

Airborne particulates of special concern to the protection and maintenance of pulmonary health are those known as fine particles ($PM_{2.5}$), which each by strict notation have an aerodynamic diameter of 2.5 μm *or smaller*. Fine particles are easily inhaled deep into the gas-exchange (alveolar) region of the lung, where they can enter the bloodstream or remain embedded in the recessed areas for a long time. The particle's size is a main determinant governing the location at which the particle would come to rest in the respiratory tract once inhaled. Larger particles are generally filtered in the nose or in the throat and therefore do not cause much health concern other than potential nuisance. In contrast, particulates smaller than about 10 μm (i.e., PM_{10}) can settle in the bronchi as well as the lungs and can thereby cause health problems. As noted earlier, the 10 μm size does not represent a strict cutoff between those that are inhalable and non-inhalable, but has been followed by most regulatory agencies for monitoring purposes. Regardless, tiny particles on the nano scale are those most capable of passing through the human lung to affect other organs and tissues including the brain.

According to a time series analysis (Anderson *et al.*, 2004) performed for WHO, an increase of 10 µg/m^3 in PM$_{10}$ level would cause a 1.3% increase in mortality from respiratory disease. It is important to remember that even levels of particulates that otherwise might not affect healthy people could cause breathing difficulties for people with asthma or pulmonary disease (e.g., COPD), especially for children. Particulate pollution can in fact trigger asthma attacks and cause wheezing, coughing, as well as respiratory irritation. It can aggravate respiratory conditions in individuals with sensitive airways. In particular, individuals with chronic bronchitis can experience a worsening of their pulmonary conditions upon exposure to dust or smoke.

Recent studies have repeatedly linked increase of premature death with exposure to relatively low levels of PM. As noted earlier, individuals at a greater risk are the elderly and those with preexisting respiratory disorder or heart disease. The elderly are typically more susceptible in part because they are likely to have preexisting lung or heart disease. Cigarette smokers, especially those smoking for years, generally have reduced lung function and thus may be affected more seriously by particulate pollution.

Children tend to be more susceptible to particulate pollution because their lungs and immunological system are still being developed. These youngsters are the ones found frequently engaging in vigorous outdoor activities, thus making them more vulnerable to particulate pollution compared to healthy adults. In the recent past, a number of studies were published linking airborne particulate pollution with various adverse health effects specifically on children; these various adverse effects included reduced lung function, asthma exacerbation, impairment of lung function growth, increased episodes of coughing and breathing difficulty, and premature death (e.g., Avol *et al.*, 2001; Gauderman *et al.*, 2000, 2002, 2004; Kaiser *et al.*, 2004; Woodruff *et al.*, 1997, 2006; Yu *et al.*, 2000).

12.4.3. Effects on the Cardiovascular System

A nationwide study on 204 urban counties in the United States showed that people with short-term exposure to PM$_{2.5}$ had an increased risk of hospital admission not only for respiratory but also for cardiovascular diseases (Dominici *et al.*, 2006). The highest admission increase observed was for heart failure, with a 1.3% increase in risk of hospitalization per 10 µg/m^3 increase in same-day PM$_{2.5}$ concentration. The study also showed that the risk of cardiovascular diseases tended to be higher in counties located in the Northeast, the Southeast, the Midwest, and the South of the United States.

In addition, according to a literature review by Brook *et al.* (2004), several epidemiological studies revealed a consistent elevated risk of cardiovascular events in relation to short-term and long-term exposures to PM at ambient levels. The review ended with a discussion of several plausible pathophysiological mechanisms (e.g., enhanced thrombosis, propensity for arrhythmias, acute arterial vasoconstriction) for the increased risk.

In particular, an animal study indicated that mice inhaling air polluted with $PM_{2.5}$ had more plaque (i.e., fatty deposits) in their arteries than those breathing filtered air (Sun *et al.*, 2005). The health effects of $PM_{2.5}$ exposure in this mouse study were found to be more dramatic when the test animals were put on a high-fat diet.

12.4.4. Other Serious Health Effects

Some UFPs (ultrafine particles) can be found in diesel exhaust fumes and fireplace soot. These particles may even be more damaging to the pulmonary or cardiovascular system than previously speculated by some scientists. There is strong evidence that particles <100 nm can pass through cell membranes to migrate into other body tissues. Studies showed that airborne particulates in this size range were able to cause brain damage similar to those found in patients with Alzheimer's disease. In addition to their ability to disrupt cellular processes, these tiny particles can bypass the respiratory tract's natural defense mechanisms to become embedded in the deepest recesses of the lung. It is important to note that in terms of *number* of particles, many more UFPs than $PM_{2.5-10}$ are inhaled into the lungs. This is because it takes well over 1 million particles of 100 nm to have the same *mass* as one particle of 10 μm (Oberdorster *et al.*, 1995).

Particles found in diesel exhausts, known more commonly as diesel particulate matter (DPM), are typically in the size range of 100 nm. DPM is made up of inorganics, hydrocarbons, but predominately carbon particles; it thus has the nickname *soot* or *black carbon* particulate matter. Soot is a principal component of diesel exhausts emitted by on-road (e.g., trucks, buses) and off-road (e.g., ships, trains, construction equipment) diesel engines. U.S. EPA (2005) has estimated that each year soot pollution causes a total of about 4,700 early deaths in nine major American cities (Boston, Detroit, Los Angeles, Philadelphia, Phoenix, Pittsburgh, San Jose, Seattle, St. Louis). As with many biological agents, soot particles can serve as carriers for those tinier carcinogenic components (e.g., benzopyrenes from tobacco smoke) adsorbed onto their surfaces.

Several studies showed that long-term exposure to airborne particulates significantly (Avol *et al.*, 2001; Gauderman *et al.*, 2000, 2002) and permanently (Gauderman *et al.*, 2004) impaired lung function growth in children. Some other studies linked PM to SIDS (sudden infant death syndrome) and to postneonatal infant mortality (Kaiser *et al.*, 2004; Woodruff *et al.*, 1997, 2006). SIDS is defined as the sudden death of a one-year old infant or younger, for which the cause remains unexplainable even after a thorough case analysis and a complete autopsy investigation (Willinger *et al.*, 1991).

A study by Woodruff *et al.* (1997) estimated that American infants had a 12% greater risk of SIDS for each 10 μg/m³ increase in PM_{10}. Based on the risk factors derived in that study, the Environmental Working Group (EWG, 1997) later redetermined that around 500 SIDS cases occurring in the United States each year were linked to airborne particulate pollution. Their re-analysis further revealed that PM_{10} pollution was associated with nearly one out of every five SIDS cases in the top 12 metropolitan areas (leading by Los Angeles) where SIDS and particulate pollution were more severe. However, some other more recent studies (e.g., Dales *et al.*, 2004; Tong and Colditz, 2004; Woodruff, 2006) were unable to find any significant link between particulate pollution and SIDS.

12.4.5. Effects on the Environment

Plants exposed to wet and dry deposition of airborne particulates can be injured when certain other air pollutants are also present. The leaves of the plants can be coated with PM that falls onto their surfaces to block their gas-exchange function and thereby to reduce their exposure to sunlight for photosynthesis which is a life-sustaining process for plants. This type of coating may also cause abrasion and radiative heating and may reduce the active photon flux reaching the photosynthetic sites. In addition, strong acidic or alkaline materials included in the PM can cause direct damage to the leaf surface.

Some investigators consider the rhizosphere (i.e., the soil zone surrounding the plant roots) as a more probable route for uptake of nutrients by plants and thereby to have a greater impact on vegetation and ecosystems. For example, those toxic metals present in the particulates, when deposited onto the soil, can inhibit the process in the soil that makes nutrients available to plants. On the other hand, the availability of alkaline cation and aluminum is affected by soil pH which may be altered considerably by the various types of particles in PM deposited onto the soil. For terrestrial ecosystems, in most cases particulate pollution has its greatest impact in the vicinity of its emission source.

It is a well-known fact that particulates in acid precipitation can contribute to the soiling and erosion of property and other structural materials including notably surface paint. These environmental effects can lead to a considerable increase in cleaning and maintenance costs, as well as a substantial loss of properties. When acidic particulates eventually settle onto lakes, rivers, or oceans, they can acidify the water there to a pH level less suitable for aquatic life. These acid particulates can also have similar adverse effects on forests and crops that are sensitive to an acidic climate.

Moreover, fine particulates have the ability to scatter light, thereby having the greatest impact on visibility impairment which has negative effects on property values and traffic safety. When light is scattered away or absorbed, such as by certain fine particulates, both the clarity and the color of what can be visioned are reduced. In the United States, fine particulates are blamed for causing the Brown Cloud that has remained a complex urban pollution problem for the metropolitan area in Denver, Colorado for well over three decades. The thick, smoggy brownish cloud that hovers above that area typically occurs in the winter days as part of a seasonal air inversion. In the meantime, on the other side of the globe in the Delhi city in India, visibility impairment is reportedly caused more by carbonaceous particulates followed by sulfate (Singh *et al.*, 2008).

References

Aitken RJ, Creely KS, Tran CL, 2004. Nanoparticles: An Occupational Hygiene Review. Health and Safety Executive Research Report 274, prepared by the Institute of Occupational Medicine, Research Park North, Riccarton, Edinburgh, UK.

Anderson HR, Atkinson RW, Peacock JL, Marston L, Konstantinou K, 2004. Meta-Analysis of Time Series Studies and Panel Studies of Particulate Matter (PM) and Ozone (O$_3$). Report of a WHO Task Group. WHO Regional Office for Europe, Copenhagen, Denmark.

Avol EL, Gauderman WJ, Tan SM, London SJ, Peters JM, 2001. Respiratory Effects of Relocating to Areas of Differing Air Pollution Levels. *Am. J. Respir. Crit. Care Med.* 164:2067-2072.

Baldasano JM, Valera E, Jiménez P, 2003. Air Quality Data from Large Cities. *Sci. Total Environ.* 307:141-165.

Bessagnet B, Hodzic A, Blanchard O, Lattuati M, Le Bihan O, Marfaing H, Rouil L, 2005. Origin of Particulate Matter Pollution Episodes in Wintertime over the Paris Basin. *Atmos. Environ.* 39: 6159-6175.

Brodie EL, DeSantis TZ, Parker JPM, Zubietta IX, Piceno YM, Andersen GL, 2007. Urban Aerosols Harbor Diverse and Dynamic Bacterial Populations. *Proc. Natl. Acad. Sci. USA* 104:99-304.

Brook RD, Barry Franklin B, Cascio W, Hong Y, Howard G, Lipsett M, Luepker R, Mittleman M, Samet J, Smith SC Jr, Tager I, 2004. Air Pollution and Cardiovascular Disease. *Circulation* 109:2655-2671.

CARB (California Air Resources Board), 2010. Analysis of the South Coast Air Basin PM$_{10}$ Redesignation Request, Maintenance Plan, and Conformity Budgets (Staff Report). California Environmental Protection Agency, Sacramento, California, USA.

Chang L-P, Tsai J-H, Chang K-L, Lin JJ, 2008. Water-Soluble Inorganic Ions in Airborne Particulates from the Nano to Coarse Mode: A Case Study of Aerosol Episodes in Southern Region of Taiwan. *Environ. Geochem. Health* 30:291-303.

Chen LC, Su WC, Qu Q, Cheng TJ, Chan CC, Hwang JS, 1999. Composition of Particulate Matter as the Determinant of Cellular Response. In *Proceedings of the Third Colloquium on Particulate Air Pollution and Human Health,* prepared for and sponsored by the California Air Resources Board, California Environmental Protection Agency, Sacramento, California, USA.

Dales R, Burnett RT, Smith-Doiron M, Stieb DM, Brook JR, 2004. Air Pollution and Sudden Infant Death Syndrome. *Pediatrics* 113:628-631.

Daniels MJ, Dominici F, Samet JM, Zeger SL, 2000. Estimating Particulate Matter – Mortality Dose-Response Curves and Threshold Levels: An Analysis of Daily Time-Series for the 20 Largest US Cities. *Am. J. Epidemiol.* 152:397-406.

Dillner AM, Schauer JJ, Zhang Y, Zeng L, Cass GR, 2006: Size-Resolved Particulate Matter Composition in Beijing during Pollution and Dust Events. *J. Geophys. Res.* 111:D05203.

Dominici F, Peng RD, Bell ML, Pham L, McDermott A, Zeger SL, Samet JM, 2006. Fine Particulate Air Pollution and Hospital Admission for Cardiovascular and Respiratory Diseases. *JAMA* 295:1127-1134.

EWG (Environmental Working Group), 1997. Particulate Pollution and Sudden Infant Death Syndrome in the United States, published 10 July on Environmental Working Group (http://www.-ewg.org).

Gauderman WJ, McConnell R, Gilliland F, London S, Thomas D, Avol E, Vora H, Berhane K, Rappaport EB, Lurmann F, Margolis HG, Peters J, 2000. Association between Air Pollution and Lung Function Growth in Southern California Children. *Am. J. Respir. Crit. Care Med.* 162:1383-1390.

Gauderman WJ, Gilliland GF, Vora H, Avol E, Stram D, McConnell R, Thomas D, Lurmann F, Margolis HG, Rappaport EB, Berhane K, Peters JM, 2002. Association between Air Pollution and Lung Function Growth in Southern California Children: Results from a Second Cohort. *Am. J. Respir. Crit. Care Med.* 166:76-84.

Gauderman WJ, Avol E, Gilliland F, Vora H, Thomas D, Berhane K, McConnell R, Kuenzli N, Lurmann F, Rappaport E, Margolis H, Bates D, Peters J, 2004. The Effect of Air Pollution on Lung Development from 10 to 18 Years of Age. *NEJM* 351:1057-1067.

Jones AM, Harrison RM, 2004. The Effects of Meteorological Factors on Atmospheric Bioaerosol Concentrations – A Review. *Sci. Total Environ.* 326:151-180.

Kaiser R, Romieu I, Medina S, Schwartz J, Krzyzanowski M, Künzli N, 2004. Air Pollution Attributable Postneonatal Infant Mortality in U.S. Metropolitan Areas: A Risk Assessment Study. *Environ. Health* 3:4 (online journal).

Karra S, Katsivela E, 2007. Microorganisms in Bioaerosol Emissions from Wastewater Treatment Plants during Summer at a Mediterranean Site. *Water Res.* 41:1355-1365.

Krzyzanowski M, Schwela D, 1999. Patterns of Air Pollution in Developing Countries. In *Air Pollution and Health* (Holgate ST, Samet JM, Koren HS, Maynard RL, Eds.). San Diego, California, USA: Academic Press.

Kumar RS, 2008. Cotton Dust – Impact on Human Health and Environment in the Textile Industry. *Textile Magazine* 49:55-60.

Lighthart B, 2000. Mini-Review of the Concentration Variation Found in the Alfresco Atmospheric Bacterial Populations. *Aerobiologia* 16:7-16.

Lippmann M, Frampton M, Schwartz J, Dockery D, Schlesinger R, Koutrakis P, Froines J, Nel A, Finkelstein J, Godleski J, Kaufman J, Koenig J, Larson T, Luchtel D, Liu L-J, Oberdörster G, Peters A, Sarnat J, Sioutas C, Suh H, Sullivan J, Utell M, Wichmann E, Zelikoff J, 2003. The U.S. Environmental Protection Agency Particulate Matter Health Effects Research Centers Program: A Midcourse Report of Status, Progress, and Plans. *Environ. Health Perspect.* 111:1074-1092.

Mage D, Ozolins G, Peterson P, Webster A, Orthofer R, Vandeveerd V, Gwynne M, 1996. Urban Air Pollution in Megacities of the World. *Atmos. Environ.* 30:681-686.

McMurry PH, 2000. The History of Condensation Nucleus Counters. *Aerosol Sci. Technol.* 33:297-322.

Mokdad AH, Marks JS, Stroup DF, Gerberding JL, 2004. Actual Causes of Death in the United States, 2000. *JAMA* 291:1238-1245.

Mopuang M, Kongtip P, Sujirarat D, Luksamijarulkul P, 2005. Microbial Count and Particulate Matter Level in Roadside Air of Bangkok Fashion City. *Thai Environ. Engr. J.* 20:31-34.

Nemery B, Hoet PH, Nemmar A, 2001. The Meuse Valley Fog of 1930: An Air Pollution Disaster. *The Lancet* 357(3 Mar):704-708.

Oberdorster G, Gelein RM, Ferin J, Weiss B, 1995. Association of Particulate Air Pollution and Acute Mortality: Involvement of Ultrafine Particles? *Inhal. Toxicol.* 7:111-124

Pandey KD, Wheeler D, Ostro B, Deichmann U, Hamilton K, Bolt K, 2006. Ambient Particulate Matter Concentrations in Residential and Pollution Hotspot Areas of World Cities: New Estimates Based on the Global Model of Ambient Particulates (GMAPS). The World Bank, Washington DC, USA.

Polymenakou PN, Mandalakis M, Stephanou EG, Tselepides A, 2008. Particle Size Distribution of Airborne Microorganisms and Pathogens during an Intense African Dust Event in the Eastern Mediterranean. *Environ. Health Perspect.* 116:292-296.

Raabe OG, 1982. Comparison of the Criteria for Sampling 'Inhalable' and 'Respirable' Aerosols. *Ann. Occup. Hyg.* 26:33-44.

Singh T, Khillare PS, Shridhar V, Agarwal T, 2008. Visibility Impairing Aerosols in the Urban Atmosphere of Delhi. *Environ. Monit. Assess.* 141:67-77.

Stanley RG, Linskins HF, 1974. *Pollen: Biology, Chemistry and Management.* Berlin, Germany: Springer Verlag.

Sun Q, Wang A, Jin X, Natanzon A, Duquaine D, Brook RD, Aguinaldo J-G, Fayad ZA, Fuster V, Lippmann M, Chen LC, Rajagopalan S, 2005. Long-Term Air Pollution Exposure and Acceleration of Atherosclerosis and Vascular Inflammation in an Animal Model. *JAMA* 294:3003-3010.

Tong S, Colditz P, 2004. Air Pollution and Sudden Infant Death Syndrome: A Literature Review. *Paediatr. Perinat. Epidemiol.* 18:327-335.

Triantafyllou AG, Zoras S, Evagelopoulos V, 2006. Particulate Matter over a Seven Year Period in Urban and Rural Areas Within, Proximal and Far from Mining and Power Station Operations in Greece. *Environ. Monit. Assess.* 122:41-60.

U.S. EPA (U.S. Environmental Protection Agency), 1999. Sampling of Ambient Air for Total Suspended Particulate Matter (SPM) and PM_{10} Using High Volume (HV) Sampler. Compendium Method IO-2.1, EPA/625/R-96/010a. Office of Research and Development, Cincinnati, Ohio, USA.

U.S. EPA (U.S. Environmental Protection Agency), 2005. Particulate Matter Health Risk Assessment for Selected Urban Areas. EPA 452/R-05-007A. Office of Air Quality Planning and Standards, Research Triangle Park, North Carolina, USA.

U.S. EPA (U.S. Environmental Protection Agency), 2009. 1970-2008 Average Annual Emissions, All Criteria Pollutants in MS Excel – June 2009. Office of Air Quality Planning and Standards, Research Triangle Park, North Carolina, USA.

U.S. EPA (U.S. Environmental Protection Agency), 2010. National Primary and Secondary National Ambient Air Quality Standards. *Code of Federal Regulations.* Title 40, Part 50. Washington DC, USA.

van Zelma R, Huijbregtsa MAJ, den Hollanderc HA, van Jaarsveldd HA, Sautere FJ, Struijsb J, van Wijnenc HJ, van de Meent D, 2008. European Characterization Factors for Human Health Damage of PM_{10} and Ozone in Life Cycle Impact Assessment. *Atmospheric Environ.* 42:441-453.

WHO (World Health Organization), 2006a. WHO Air Quality Guidelines for Particular Matter, Ozone, Nitrogen Dioxide and Sulfur Dioxide: Global Update 2005, Summary of Risk Assessment. Geneva, Switzerland.

WHO (World Health Organization), 2006b. Health Risks of Particulate Matter from Long-Range Transboundary Air Pollution. WHO Regional Office for Europe, Copenhagen, Denmark.

Willinger M, James LS, Catz C, 1991. Defining the Sudden Infant Death Syndrome (SIDS): Deliberations of an Expert Panel Convened by the National Institute of Child Health and Human Development. *Pediatr. Pathol.* 11:677-684.

Woodruff TJ, Grillo J, Schoendorf KC, 1997. The Relationship between Selected Causes of Postneonatal Infant Mortality and Particulate Air Pollution in the United States. *Environ. Health Perspect.* 105:608-612.

Woodruff TJ, Parker JD, Schoendorf KC, 2006. Fine Particulate Matter (PM$_{2.5}$) Air Pollution and Selected Causes of Postneonatal Infant Mortality in California. *Environ. Health Perspect.* 114: 786-790.

Yu O, Sheppard L, Lumley T, Koenig JQ, Shapiro GG, 2000. Effects of Ambient Air Pollution on Symptoms of Asthma in Seattle-Area Children Enrolled in the CAMP Study. *Environ. Health Perspect.* 108:1209-1214.

Zanobetti A, Schwartz J, 2000. Race, Gender, and Social Status as Modifiers of the Effects of PM$_{10}$ on Mortality. *J. Occup. Environ. Med.* 42:469-474.

Zanobetti A, Schwartz J, 2001. Are Diabetics More Susceptible to the Health Effects of Airborne Particles? *Am. J. Respir. Crit. Care Med.* 164:831-833.

Zanobetti A, Schwartz J, 2002. Cardiovascular Damage by Airborne Particles: Are Diabetics More Susceptible? *Epidemiology* 13:588-592.

Zanobetti A, Schwartz J, Gold D, 2000. Are There Sensitive Subgroups for the Health Effects of Airborne Particles? *Environ. Health Perspect.* 108:841-845.

Zheng Z, Xie X, Ouyang Y, Wang C, Zeng H, Chen Y, Chen T, 2009. Study on the Relativity between Airborne Microbes and Environmental Factors in Pearl River Delta' Urban Agglomeration, Guangdong. *J. Sustain. Develop.* 2:106-113.

Review Questions

1. What do the terms *dust*, *smoke*, *smog*, *fume*, *haze*, *fog*, and *mist* refer to in relation to atmospheric aerosol pollution?

2. What are the main differences between particulates formed from wind-blown dust particles in tropical or desert regions and those from sea spray?

3. What are the main differences between primary and secondary particulate matter?

4. Briefly characterize the various sizes of airborne particulate matter that are of regulatory importance.

5. Which of the following is nonhygroscopic and likely has an atmospheric half-life of minutes to days? a) PM$_{0.1}$; b) PM$_{0.1-1}$; c) PM$_{2.5}$; d) PM$_{2.5-10}$.

6. Give at least three examples for the sources of PM$_{2.5-10}$.

7. Briefly describe the two processes *condensation* and *coagulation* for the formation of PM$_{0.1}$.

8. What might be the *technical* differences between ultrafine and nano particles?

9. What is generally the single most important source of PM in urban areas? And what is the more specific, major source of PM in megacities?

10. Name a region in the United States that currently is designated as (one of) the worst for nonattainment of PM$_{10}$.

11. Name three recent episodes of urban airborne particulate pollution that were caused by dust storms or industrial processing, as covered in this chapter.

12. Briefly discuss some of the major issues, concerns, or problems with monitoring PM concentrations, particularly in the developing countries, as discussed in this chapter.

13. Briefly explain why airborne microbes may or should be regarded as a major and significant constituent of urban airborne particulate pollution.

14. What particles were considered as responsible for causing the deaths in the acute air pollution episode that occurred in Meuse Valley, Belgium in 1930?

15. List the human subpopulations that tend to be more susceptible to PM-associated health problems.

16. According to the WHO estimation, each year approximately _____ attributable deaths in 25 European countries are due to PM exposure: a) 24,000; b) 50,000; c) 100,000; d) 350,000.

17. Briefly explain why children are especially susceptible to adverse health effects of PM on their respiratory system.

18. What may be a plausible mechanism that promotes atherosclerosis leading to cardiovascular diseases when humans or mice are subjected to chronic exposure to air polluted by $PM_{2.5}$, especially when the exposure is coupled with a high-fat diet?

19. What is the main determinant that would direct or cause an airborne particle to rest in the respiratory tract once inhaled?

20. Briefly explain what diesel particulate matter is, and briefly describe its impacts on human health.

21. List the major types of adverse effects on the environment that can be caused by airborne particulate pollution.

CHAPTER 13

Volatile Organic Compounds

13.1. Introduction

In general terms, volatile organic compounds (VOCs) refer to a huge group of diverse hydrocarbon (and hence organic) solid or liquid substances that readily evaporate and remain in the air as gases at ambient temperature. These compounds, including those fully halogenated, generally have sufficiently high vapor pressures with boiling points between 50° to 250° C (122° to 248° F). Substances in this group thus include a wide variety of biological compounds from plants, synthetic chemicals from industrial processes, ingredients of consumer products found in homes, and ingredients of protective coatings and paints from building or other structural materials. Or to put it more bluntly, VOCs of environmental health concern can be found virtually everywhere indoors and outdoors, such as in the air, water, soil, household goods, and industrial products. Yet in practice, as due to limited resources, many regulatory agencies (e.g., U.S. EPA) focus on only a very few that have been determined to pose considerable potential threats to human health while at the same time occurring with alarmingly high frequency.

13.1.1. As Precursors of Ozone and Particulate Matter

As noted in Chapters 11 and 12, some VOCs are precursors of ozone (O_3) and secondary particulate matter (PM). The formation of O_3 with VOCs as precursors can occur via the reaction between oxygen (O_2) and peroxyacyl radicals $R\text{-}CO_3{}^\bullet$, where R stands for any organic substituent group (Reaction 11.9). Many atmospheric VOCs can also react directly with nitrogen oxides (NO_x) and sunlight to form O_3.

In the urban environment, the most abundant secondary species of PM include sulfate, nitrate, ammonium, and secondary organic matter (SOM). The formation of SOM from oxidation of atmospheric VOCs can contribute significantly to the airborne particulate load. Even though the formation of SOM is not well understood due to the perturbation with the wide array of VOCs available, one accepted mechanism is the oxidation of hydrocarbons (HCs) with six or more carbon atoms to form products with sufficiently low(er) vapor pressure. When such an atmospheric VOC is oxidized (e.g., by hydroxyl radical $HO^\bullet$), the oxidation product has relatively higher polarity and lower volatility due to the addition of oxygen or nitrogen to the parent compound regardless of the species involved. Because of their lower volatility, these "semi-volatile" oxidation products will eventually condense on pre-existing PM. Some of these oxidation products can nucleate directly and homogeneously to form new tiny particles (Seinfeld and Pankow, 2003).

13.1.2. Sources of Pollution

As VOCs are available in a wide array of products, nearly every person is inevitably exposed to these compounds to some level. Smokers and those individuals working at dry cleaners, photograph laboratories, industrial facilities, or similar settings tend to face the greatest risk. In addition to consumer products such as automotive cleaners, spot removers, and degreasing fluids, many VOCs can be found in groundwater.

Contamination of groundwater with VOCs can be traced to sources such as industrial facilities, home septic tanks, municipal landfills, and hazardous waste dumps. VOCs can also be found in groundwater when fuel such as gasoline is spilled on the ground or leaks from an underground storage tank. These compounds can readily evaporate into indoor air when contaminated water is used for drinking or during cooking, showering, and washing dishes, especially when the water is heated. Accordingly, the levels of VOCs can be higher indoors than in the ambient air, sometimes by as much as tenfold or more under certain circumstances such as in a confined, closed-door area.

There are two prominent groups of VOCs when all common anthropogenic sources are considered: (1) chlorinated solvents; and (2) fuel components. Chlorinated solvents are widely used in industry and as common consumer products, such as carbon tetrachloride (CCl_4), methylene chloride (CH_2Cl_2), tetrachloroethylene ($Cl_2C=CCl_2$), trichloroethylene ($HC=CCl_3$), and vinyl chloride ($CH_2=CHCl$). Fuel components, those found largely in petroleum, include benzene (C_6H_6), toluene ($C_6H_5CH_3$), the isomers of xylene ($C_6H_4C_2H_6$), and methyl *tert(iary)*-butyl ether ($C_5H_{12}O$). VOCs can also be by-products from indoor combustion or certain natural processes, such as formaldehyde (CH_2O). Other by-products of less concern to environmental health include those formed by chlorination in water treatment, such as chloroform ($CHCl_3$).

13.2. Use Standards and Environmental Concerns

In the United States, no federal *use* standards have been established for VOCs in nonindustrial settings. However, U.S. EPA has set maximum contaminant levels (MCLs) for many VOCs in groundwater. Also, U.S. Occupational Safety and Health Administration (OSHA) has regulated formaldehyde as a carcinogen, by adopting a permissible exposure limit (PEL) of 0.75 ppm (parts per million) for exposure in the workplace.

13.2.1. Standards for Consumer/Commercial Products

For consumer or commercial products sold in the United States, California was the first state passing laws in the year 2000 to limit the VOC contents in paints and coatings. Arizona, New Jersey, New York, and Texas were the other states that followed suit to adopt their own limits on similar products. In April 2004, the European Union (EU) finalized the EU-wide VOC content limits on solvent paints, varnishes, and automobile refinishing products. The EU legislation limits the VOC contents in 12 categories of decorative paints and varnishes and in 5 categories of products used in vehicle refinishing.

Effective 1 January 2009, the states of California, Maine, Maryland, Michigan, New Jersey, and Pennsylvania all impose more stringent limits for product categories already covered in their existing VOC regulations, while in some cases also expanding their list of product categories per existing regulation (Balek, 2009). The VOC limits in California (actually effective 31 December 2008) are 1% of the product content by weight for non-aerosol sanitizers, disinfectants, and bathroom or tile cleaners. There does not appear to be any guidance or limit set for VOCs in consumer products outside of the United States, except for those proposed by the Canadian government (Environment Canada, 2013).

13.2.2. Select Compounds of Environmental Concern

Aside from being the precursors of O_3 and secondary PM, VOCs as a group have a wide range of health effects on humans ranging from being carcinogenic to relatively harmless. For a considerable number of these HC-based compounds, long-term exposure can damage the liver, the kidneys, and the nervous system. Due to their use mostly being an ingredient in consumer and commercial products, their toxic effects on plants, vegetation, and wildlife generally receive less public health attention. It is with this notion that the characteristics, sources, and health effects of the six select VOCs are discussed in this chapter. The select six are formaldehyde, benzene, methyl *tert*-butyl ether, methylene chloride, tetrachloroethylene, and trichloroethylene; all have been selected due to their certain unique applications, large production, and relatively high toxicity.

The chemical structures of the six select VOCs are given in Figure 13.1. Their physicochemical and toxicological properties are discussed separately in the sections that follow. For their physicochemical and toxicological properties, much of the information given here is from the individual documents prepared for their toxicological profiles by the U.S. Agency for Toxic Substances and Disease Registry (ATSDR). Main sources for supplementary information are U.S. EPA and the World Health Organization (WHO).

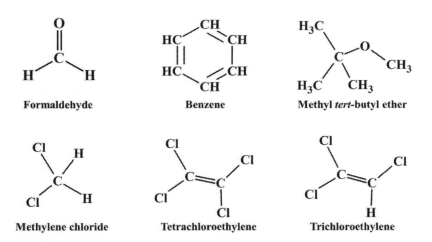

Figure 13.1. Chemical Structures of Six Select Volatile Organic Compounds

It is of note that this chapter has a special concern with formaldehyde mainly because it is a chemical commonly used to manufacture a variety of consumer and textile products found in homes. With benzene, the concern is that its use in the United States ranks in the top 20 in terms of production volume for synthesis of other chemicals, not only is it a natural component of crude oil, gasoline, and cigarette smoke. Methyl *tert*-butyl ether was (is) produced in huge quantities in (and outside) the United States for use once predominately as a fuel additive (i.e., as an oxygenate) in motor gasoline. The other three VOCs (methylene chloride, tetrachloroethylene, trichloroethylene) are among the handful toxic chlorinated solvents still being used widely in the industry today.

13.3. Formaldehyde

At ambient temperature, formaldehyde (CH_2O) is a flammable, nearly colorless gas with a pungent, suffocating smell. It is the simplest aldehyde (R-CHO, where R is an organyl group and here a hydrogen atom instead), and is known by several other names including formic aldehyde, methanal, and methyl aldehyde. This VOC is soluble in water but does not stay in a water solution for long. In sunlight, most of its molecules in the air will decompose into formic acid (CH_2O_2). While formaldehyde does not accumulate in animals or plants, it is produced in small quantities in the human body. In liquid ($\geq 37\%$ solution), it has a vapor pressure of ~25 mm Hg at 25° C and a boiling point of 96° C.

13.3.1. Sources and Use

Formaldehyde is used in many industrial processes. It is a component of many consumer products (e.g., automobile body polishes, synthetic resins, carpets, medicines, disinfectants, personal care products, cosmetics). It is a common building block for the synthesis of many other more complex materials, especially for the production of polymers. The annual global production of formaldehyde in 2005 was estimated at around 21 million tons (IARC, 2006).

Formaldehyde gas at room temperature readily converts to a variety of derivatives that are used extensively in the industry. One important derivative is the stable cyclic 1,3,5-trioxane ($C_3H_6O_3$). This cyclic trimer is commonly used as a stable source of anhydrous formaldehyde and for polymerization of certain thermoplastics (e.g., polyacetal). A longer polymer formed from formaldehyde is termed *paraformaldehyde* ($OH[CH_2O]_nH$; typically n = 9 to 100). When reacting with certain chemicals (e.g., melamine, phenol, urea), formaldehyde produces resins that have wide applications as adhesives and binders in wood product, pulp and paper, and fiberglass industries. The textile industry uses formaldehyde-based resins as finishers to make fabrics crease-resistant.

Formaldehyde can be formed naturally in the environment with atmospheric carbon (C), hydrogen (H), and oxygen (O_2). This natural source may account for as much as 90% of its total volume in certain environment. The gas is a major intermediate in the combustion of methane (CH_4) and many other HCs (e.g., those in wildfires, automobile exhausts, tobacco smoke). Formaldehyde (CH_2O) can be a major component of photo-chemical smog when accumulated in the air following the oxidation of atmospheric CH_4 (Reactions 13.1) and other HCs, provided that O_3 (ozone), nitric oxide (NO), sunlight (*hv*), and water (H_2O) vapor are all available.

$$O_3 + hv \rightarrow O_2 + O^{\bullet} \qquad\qquad\qquad (13.1a)$$

$$O^{\bullet} + H_2O \rightarrow 2HO^{\bullet} \qquad\qquad\qquad (13.1b)$$

$$CH_4 + HO^{\bullet} \rightarrow CH_3^{\bullet} + H_2O \qquad\qquad\qquad (13.1c)$$

$$CH_3^{\bullet} + O_2 \rightarrow CH_3O_2^{\bullet} \qquad\qquad\qquad (13.1d)$$

$$CH_3O_2^{\bullet} + NO \rightarrow CH_3O^{\bullet} + NO_2 \qquad\qquad\qquad (13.1e)$$

$$CH_3O^{\bullet} + O_2 \rightarrow CH_2O + HO_2^{\bullet} \qquad\qquad\qquad (13.1f)$$

Subreactions (or more correctly Steps) 13.1a and 13.1b above are part of those given in Section 5.2.3.B for photochemical reaction. The three methane-based radicals involved in the above subreactions are methyloxy radical ($CH_3O^{\bullet}$), methyl peroxy radical ($CH_3O_2^{\bullet}$), and methyl radical ($CH_3^{\bullet}$). As cyclic and complex as the process seems, following formaldehyde formation (Subreaction 13.1f), the resultant hyperoxy radical $HO_2^{\bullet}$ can combine with NO to form hydroxyl radical $HO^{\bullet}$ and nitrogen dioxide (NO_2).

Formaldehyde is used widely as a disinfectant due to its capability of getting rid of most fungi, most bacteria, and certain viruses. Topical solutions containing formaldehyde derivatives as active ingredients are applied as medicines for treatment of warts and some other skin conditions. Some topical creams, cosmetics, and personal hygiene products specifically contain formaldehyde derivatives for prevention of bacterial infection. For example, methenamine ($N_4[CH_2]_6$), a cyclic HC compound that in acid medium can be hydrolyzed into ammonia (NH_3) and formaldehyde, is commonly used to prevent and treat urinary tract infections. In addition, this VOC has been widely used as an embalming agent for the temporary preservation of human and animal remains from decay.

13.3.2. Exposures and Toxic Effects

As far back as in the 1980s, animal studies revealed that long-term exposure to formaldehyde caused nasal cancer in rats (ATSDR, 1999; NCI, 2009). Since some 25 years later, after all the carcinogenicity data have been reassessed thoroughly by its 26 scientists from 10 countries, WHO's International Agency for Research on Cancer (IARC, 2006) has classified formaldehyde as a human (Group 1) carcinogen. The IARC experts have reached the conclusion that there is now sufficient evidence linking formaldehyde exposure to the development of nasopharyngeal cancer in humans, which is a rare cancer occurring predominantly in the developed countries. The IARC working group has also found limited evidence linking formaldehyde exposure to leukemia.

The main concern with formaldehyde exposure is for workers in the facilities manufacturing or processing the chemical. It is estimated that over 1 million workers are exposed to some level of this VOC across the EU (IARC, 2006). Occupational exposure to formaldehyde is from three major sources: during (1) decomposition of formaldehyde-based resins; (2) emission of formaldehyde from embalming fluids or other aqueous solutions; and (3) production of formaldehyde via the combustion of a variety of organic compounds (e.g., in automobile exhaust fumes). In addition to carcinogenic harm, formaldehyde can cause allergy and other short-term adverse health effects. Inasmuch as its resins are used in so many textile and construction materials, formaldehyde is one of the common indoor air pollutants. When present in the air at levels exceeding 0.1 ppm, it can irritate the eyes and mucous membranes. As a result, some people may experience watery eyes, burning sensations (in the eyes, nose, or throat), coughing, wheezing, nausea, and skin irritation. Certain people are particularly sensitive to formaldehyde. For these sensitive individuals, exposure to even very small amounts of formaldehyde can trigger asthma symptoms or cause breathing difficulties. It is for these health concerns that EU has banned the commercial use of formaldehyde since September 2007.

In the United States, at least three incidents were reported to have been caused by exposure to formaldehyde-based resins used to build trailers and mobile homes. The occupants were victims of Hurricane Katrina in 2005, Hurricane Rita in 2005, and the Iowa floods in 2008. The trailers and mobile homes that the victims moved into were provided by the U.S. Federal Emergency Management Agency in response to the evacuation crises. Some of the trailer occupants complained of violent coughing, nosebleeds, breathing difficulties, and persistent headaches. Tests showed that the formaldehyde levels in some of these trailers exceeded U.S. EPA's recommended limits of 16 ppb (parts per billion).

13.4. Benzene

Benzene (C_6H_6) is a colorless, flammable liquid with a sweet (aromatic) smell. It is a *mono*aromatic (i.e., that with *one* benzene ring) HC (hydrocarbon) available as a natural constituent of crude oil and can be synthesized from other chemicals present in petroleum. This VOC is structurally famous for its highly polyunsaturated *benzene* ring which is constructed with just one hydrogen atom for each of the six carbon atoms forming the ring (Figure 13.1). Benzene is insoluble in water (0.19% at 25° C), but miscible with many organic solvents (e.g., alcohol, carbon disulfide, chloroform, oils). It has a boiling point of 80.1° C and a vapor pressure of 75 mm Hg at 20° C.

13.4.1. Sources and Use

Benzene is a VOC commonly found in automobile exhausts, tobacco smoke, industrial emissions, fumes from automobile service stations, and household products such as glues, detergents, and paint strippers. Because the VOC recently has been more actively considered as a human carcinogen, its use as an additive in gasoline is now limited in many countries. However, it is still widely used as an industrial solvent and a precursor in the production of drugs, dyes, plastics, rubbers, and pesticides.

Many important chemicals are derived from benzene by replacing one or more of its hydrogen atoms with functional groups (e.g., $-NH_2$, $-OH$, $-CH_3$). Examples of simple benzene derivatives include toluene ($C_6H_5CH_3$), the isomers of xylenes ($C_6H_4C[CH_3]_2$), and phenol (C_6H_5OH). Linking two benzene rings gives the biphenyl molecule ($C_6H_5-C_6H_5$), as present in PCBs (polychlorinated biphenyls). Further loss of the two H and C atoms at the linkage gives the "fused" two-ring aromatic HC called naphthalene ($C_{10}H_8$). Anthracene ($C_{14}H_{10}$) is a fused three-ring aromatic HC (with one of its three rings being fused to the other two at its opposite sides). All HCs with more than one benzene ring are termed *polycyclic* or *polynuclear aromatic hydrocarbons* (PAHs). Note that in *heterocycles* (i.e., *hetero*cyclic compounds), at least one carbon atom in the benzene ring is replaced with another chemical element (e.g., nitrogen).

Gasoline used to contain a small percent of benzene as antiknock additive until it was replaced by tetraethyl lead ($[CH_3CH_2]_4Pb$) in the 1950s. Yet these days with the worldwide phase-out of leaded gasoline, benzene has been used once again as a gasoline additive in some countries. In Europe (Ubrich and Jeuland, 2007) and the United States (U.S. EPA, 2006), recent concerns over benzene's adverse health effects and the potential for its entering groundwater have led to more stringent regulations of its content in all forms of gasoline, with national limits set at 1% and 0.62% by content, respectively.

Benzene is now used principally as an intermediate to synthesize other chemicals, with styrene ($C_6H_5CH=CH_2$) being one of the most widely produced derivatives. Styrene, also known as vinyl benzene, is commonly used to make polystyrene (a thermoplastic substance) and copolymers (those made from two or more monomeric species). Other benzene derivatives include phenol and the fully saturated cyclohexane (C_6H_{12}). Phenol is widely used for resins and adhesives, and is an important precursor for large groups of herbicides and pharmaceuticals. Cyclohexane is used mostly as raw material for producing nylon.

In laboratory research, toluene is now commonly used in place of benzene. Although the chemical properties of the two monoaromatics are similar, toluene has a wider liquid range and, due to its methyl group ($-CH_3$), is less toxic. The methyl group in toluene is subject to rapid oxidation, thereby causing the aromatic to undergo a relatively more rapid enzymatic degradation to result in a lower observed toxicity.

13.4.2. Exposures and Toxic Effects

Exposure to benzene may come from several sources. Outdoor air may contain some low levels of benzene from tobacco smoke, wildfires, automobile exhausts, fumes from automobile service stations, and industrial emissions. Air with higher levels of benzene can be found around toxic waste dumps or near older, not well-constructed gas stations.

The indoor sources naturally include indoor smoking and vapors from household products that contain the VOC as one of their ingredients.

Workers in various industries using or producing benzene are at a greater risk for exposure to this carcinogenic aromatic. Industries engaging in the use of benzene include rubber production, paint production, shoe making, leather manufacturing, oil refinery, and adhesive production. In the United States, OSHA has set a PEL of 1 ppm for an 8-hour workday, 40-hour workweek exposure (i.e., on a time-weighted average basis), and a short-term exposure limit of 5 ppm for 15 minutes. (Note that discussion on OSHA's PEL is given in Chapter 20 concerning occupational toxicology.)

At times, water and soil contaminations are also major sources of exposure to benzene. For example, the water supply to the greater city of Harbin in China (the tenth largest in the nation with a population of nearly 10 million people) was shut down for five days in November 2005 due to a chemical explosion occurring 10 days earlier in a petrochemical plant located nearby (UNEP, 2005). The explosion led to a chemical spill of roughly 100 tons of toxic mixture of benzene, nitrobenzene ($C_6H_5NO_2$), and aniline into the nearby Songhua River supplying the city's drinking water. Also, in the United States, federal regulations require that reports be submitted to U.S. EPA for spills or accidental releases of benzene into the environment if they each amount to 10 pounds (4.5 kg) or more. According to a U.S. EPA report (GWPC, 2007), over 100,000 underground storage tank sites across the United States have involved groundwater or soil contamination by some types of benzene as a result of industrial seepage. In the United States, the MCL of benzene in drinking water has been set at 5 µg/L (U.S. EPA, 2009).

Human exposure to benzene is a worldwide health concern. This monoaromatic targets several vital body organs including the liver, kidneys, lungs, heart, and brain. It can also cause breakage of DNA strand as well as damage to chromosomes. The main health concern with benzene exposure, however, is the chemical's effects on the blood. The chemical is known to cause leukemia, a cancer involving the blood-forming organs. Chronic exposure to benzene can cause bone marrow damage, lower white blood cell count, and a decrease in red blood cells that can lead to anemia. The VOC can cause excessive bleeding and increase the chance of infection by depressing the immunological system. Benzene is also linked to other hematological malignancies (i.e., those cancers that affect the blood, bone marrow, and lymph nodes). Overall, there does not appear to be any controversy or dispute over the body of evidence linking benzene to acute myeloid leukemia or to acute nonlymphocytic leukemia. According to the toxicological profile prepared by ATSDR (2007), several studies collectively showed that benzene caused cancer in both sexes of multiple species of animals exposed via various routes. IARC (1987) has long classified benzene as a human (Group 1) carcinogen.

In humans, benzene is biotransformed into several metabolites including *trans, trans*-muconic acid ($C_6H_6O_4$) which can be accurately measured in the urine if the test is performed shortly following exposure. Although this urine test may not be sufficiently specific for benzene exposure, as the metabolite may come from other sources as well, it is a practical and relatively inexpensive biomonitoring tool. Pure benzene in the human body may also be oxidized to produce a metabolite named benzene epoxide. This epoxide is not readily excreted out of the body, but can readily interact with a guanine base on the DNA to form a DNA adduct which has the potential to cause cancer.

Acute exposure to benzene at high levels can lead to unconsciousness (as it can cause narcosis) and hence even death, whereas at low levels it can cause drowsiness, dizziness, rapid heart rate, tremors, and confusion. If exposure is via drinking water or eating foods with high levels of benzene, the symptoms can include vomiting, nausea, and irritation of the stomach.

13.5. Methyl *tert*-Butyl Ether

Methyl *tert(iary)*-butyl ether ($C_5H_{12}O$), known to the general public more commonly by its acronym MTBE, is a volatile, flammable, and colorless liquid. MTBE has a minty odor somewhat reminiscent of diethyl ether ($[CH_3\text{-}CH_2]_2O$), leading to unpleasant taste and odor in water. This VOC is only moderately soluble in water (4.8% at 20° C), but miscible with gasoline and certain organic solvents (e.g., alcohol, other ethers). It has a boiling point of 55.2° C and a vapor pressure of 245 mm Hg at 25° C.

13.5.1. Sources and Use

MTBE is commonly used as an oxygenate in gasoline to raise the octane rating. However, due to newer environmental health concerns, its production in the United States has declined substantially in recent years. Recently, the gasoline additive has been found to pollute easily and quickly large quantities of groundwater when gasoline oxygenated with MTBE is spilled or leaked at gas service stations. This VOC is currently being investigated for potential use as an inexpensive solvent to dissolve gallstones by applying a special surgical tube to deliver it directly to the patient's gall bladder.

MTBE can be produced via the chemical reaction of methanol (CH_3OH) with isobutylene (C_4H_8). Methanol is derived from natural gas whereas isobutylene can be made available from butane (C_4H_{10}) in crude oil or natural gas, thereby qualifying MTBE as a (semi-)fossil fuel. In the United States, MTBE was produced in huge quantities during its high use as a fuel additive, with over 200,000 barrels per day in 1999. Its production has reduced considerably since the early 2000s, however, after numerous states banned its use as a gasoline oxygenate. These state bans were enacted in response to concerns over the widespread contamination by MTBE-containing gasoline detected in many drinking water aquifers within the affected states. The widespread releases of MTBE-containing gasoline reportedly came from underground storage tanks, with the most infamous cases being in Santa Monica and South Lake Tahoe (both located in California).

To some extent, the decline of MTBE production in the United States is also due to the alternative ethanol-derived ethyl *tert*-butyl ether ($C_6H_{14}O$) being given a more favorable tax break in many states. The use and production of MTBE are declining in western

Europe at a similar rate. However, MTBE's market is expected to continue to grow in other parts of the world (e.g., countries in Asia and Latin America) that together contributed to about 50% of the VOC's global production in 2004.

As an organic solvent, MTBE possesses a distinct advantage over most other ethers by having a higher boiling point coupled with a much lower tendency to form explosive organic peroxides. The ether is biodegradable to carbon dioxide (CO_2) and water molecules under aerobic conditions with bacteria yet normally of the slow-growing type. Fortunately, MTBE can be rapidly and affordably removed from water to undetectable levels by means of a fluidized bed reactor designed to carry out multiphase chemical reactions.

13.5.2. Exposures and Toxic Effects

Given that MTBE offers water an unpleasant taste even at very low levels (e.g., ~10 µg/L), it can render large quantities of groundwater non-potable. MTBE is frequently introduced into water-supply aquifers either by leakage from underground storage tanks at gasoline stations or by MTBE-treated gasoline spilling onto the ground. Despite the fact that nowadays the storage tanks are much better designed and constructed than in the 1980s, a substantial number of accidental releases still occur since many of the older tanks are still being used. Due to its high solubility and persistence, MTBE travels faster and farther than many other gasoline components released into the same aquifer. Another reality is that MTBE's high water solubility will cause it to seep through the soil with ease, thereby polluting ground and surface waters rather quickly.

The views amongst scientists concerning the health effects of MTBE are inconsistent at the moment, in part because of the limited toxicity data available. The animal data reviewed by ATSDR (1996) supported the link between inhalation exposure to MTBE and certain respiratory effects. Acute health effects such as coughing, nose or throat burning, headaches, and nausea were reported by people exposed to the fuel vapors while pumping MTBE-treated gasoline into automobile tanks or while driving on the road (ATSDR, 1996; NRC, 1996). Yet there was the contention that symptoms of this type as observed in the human studies could come from exposure to other gasoline components.

IARC (1999a) has classified MTBE as a Group 3 carcinogen (i.e., an agent not classifiable as to its carcinogenicity to humans; *see* Section 18.3.3 for the classification scheme used by IARC). U.S. EPA (1997) has reached a different decision on the VOC's carcinogenicity to humans, however. It has classified MTBE as a potential human carcinogen at high doses, after receiving the support of an interagency assessment (Melnick *et al.*, 1997). The data available to U.S. EPA showed that when test animals inhaled high doses of MTBE, some of them experienced various noncancerous health effects including depression of the central nervous system (CNS), decreased muscle tone, impaired treadmill performance, labored respiration, ataxia, abnormal gait, and decreased hind-limb grip. At any rate, U.S. EPA has not yet set a national health advisory limit for MTBE in drinking water, with the explanation that the limited animal data on hand were insufficient to quantify the VOC's health risks from low exposure levels expected in drinking water.

13.6. Methylene Chloride

The molecular formula of methylene chloride (MC) is CH_2Cl_2. Therefore, this chlorinated solvent is also chemically known as *dichloro*methane (DCM). MC is a colorless, nonflammable liquid widely used as an industrial solvent. This VOC is slightly soluble in water (20 g/L at 20° C), but fairly miscible with many organic solvents (e.g., acetone, alcohol, carbon tetrachloride, chloroform). MC has a sweet aroma, a boiling point of 40° C, and a vapor pressure of 349 mm Hg at 20° C.

13.6.1. Sources and Use

Methylene chloride is a useful solvent for many industrial processes owing to its low boiling point and high solvency power to dissolve a wide array of organic compounds. The chlorinated solvent is used principally as a paint remover, as an aerosol spray propellant, as a degreasing agent, and in the manufacture of pharmaceuticals (e.g., antibiotics, steroids, vitamins, tablet coating). In the food industry, it is used as an extraction solvent for coffee decaffeination as well as for hops and other flavorings. Some consumer products in aerosol form may contain the solvent as an ingredient, such as in room deodorants and household cleaners. MC is used in the garment screen printer industry for removal of heat-seal transfers on garments. The VOC is also used for cleaning metal surfaces. Due to its chemical ability to weld plastic parts, the chlorinated solvent is commonly used to seal the casing of electric meters.

It has been estimated that over 500,000 tons of MC are produced worldwide each year, of which about 50% is used in the western Europe (WHO, 2000a). In the United States, the annual MC production has been estimated at around 400 million pounds (ATSDR, 2000). However, recent concerns over MC's health effects have led various sectors in many countries to search for alternatives to many of its industrial applications. Measures have been approved recently by EU to ban MC in paint strippers used by consumers and professionals outside of the industrial premises (European Parliament, 2009). The MC limit in Europe is 0.1% by weight in a product, with an effective date as early as 2010 depending on the type of business involved.

13.6.2. Exposures and Toxic Effects

Methylene chloride can be an air pollutant of great health concern, considering the assessment by WHO (2000a) that up to 80% of the solvent's global production is released into the atmosphere. A similar annual percentage release of the MC production is experienced in the United States (ATSDR, 2000). Although MC may be formed from natural sources, these sources reportedly do not make a significant contribution compared to the global release. In the atmosphere, MC generally has a residence life of about six months prior to complete degradation with photochemically-produced hydroxyl radical (WHO, 2000a). Accordingly, the main environmental exposure concern for the general population is inhalation of ambient air. For workers and consumers, indoor exposure to this VOC is expected to be much higher, particularly during the formulation of paint strippers and other spray aerosols. In the United States, it was estimated that over 1 million workers in the 1980s were potentially exposed to MC vapors (U.S. EPA, 1985; Zahm *et al.*, 1987). All in all, the exposure and release estimates given above might not be too far off from the actual data experienced in recent years, as thus far no substantial decrease in the annual MC production has been observed in the United States or worldwide.

Methylene chloride is among the many chlorinated solvents known to impair the CNS if inhaled at high doses. The solvent used to be a general anesthetic until fatalities were reported (IPCS, 1997). Like those of other VOCs, MC vapors are more harmful to humans when present in poorly ventilated areas. Despite the fact that it is the least toxic of the chloromethane group (IPCS, 1997), the solvent still has a potential for acute inhalation hazard owing to its high volatility. For one thing, inhalation of MC vapors at high concentrations can potentially lead to CO (carbon monoxide) poisoning since the solvent will be biotransformed to CO and chloride (Cl⁻) ion in the body. Acute inhalation exposure to MC can lead to severe optic neuropathy (Kobayashi *et al.*, 2008) and hepatitis (Cordes *et al.*, 1988), whereas dermal contact with the solvent in sufficient amount and duration can cause chemical burns on the skin (Wells and Waldron, 1984).

Laboratory studies showed that the solvent induced liver and lung cancers in several animal species. Based on this body of evidence, IARC (1999b) and U.S. EPA (2010) have classified MC as a possible human (Group 2B) carcinogen and as an agent "likely to be carcinogenic in humans (Group B)", respectively.

It is noteworthy that even though the primary adverse health effect associated with short-term exposure to MC is impairment of CNS functions, such does not normally produce permanent disability. The acute toxicity of MC by inhalation or other routes is thus not expected to be substantial. Chronic exposure to MC was found to associate with induction of fatty liver in guinea pigs (Morris *et al.*, 1979), as well as with increased incidences of hepatic hemosiderosis, necrosis, granulomatous inflammation, and bile duct fibrosis in rats (NTP, 1986). Other animal studies (Narotsky *et al.*, 1992; Nishio *et al.*, 1984; WHO, 2000a) implicated MC's potential harm for its ability to cross the placental barrier, although the VOC was not found to be teratogenic in rats and mice at high doses.

13.7. Tetrachloroethylene

Tetrachloroethylene ($Cl_2C=CCl_2$) is also known by its IUPAC (International Union of Pure and Applied Chemistry) name tetrachloroethene, but is preferentially referred to as perchloroethylene (with *per*-chloro = *all* chlorinated) largely due to its acronym PCE or PERC being distinguishable from TCE which is customarily reserved for its structurally related cousin trichloroethylene (Section 13.8 below). PCE is a colorless, nonflammable liquid widely used for dry cleaning of fabrics, and hence is nicknamed *the* dry-cleaning fluid. This VOC is slightly soluble in water (0.15 g/L at 25° C), but miscible with many organic solvents (e.g., alcohol, benzene, ether). It has a boiling point of 121° C, a vapor pressure of 18.5 mm Hg at 25° C, and a sweet odor detectable by most people at ≥1 ppm.

13.7.1. Sources and Use

Tetrachloroethylene is used in the dry cleaning industry as a degreaser and as an ingredient in other industrial and consumer products. PCE is used largely in dry cleaning, especially in the small-business sector, owing to its excellent solvency for organic materials. When included in a mixture with other chlorohydrocarbons, its application is then mainly to degrease metal parts in the automotive and other metalworking shops. The chlorinated solvent has a long history of use in spot removers and paint strippers.

Although PCE has been the dry cleaning fluid of choice for many decades, in recent years it has suffered a dramatic reduction in global production, by 70 to 80% from 1990 to 2005 (Lacson and Toki, 2006). In the United States, the decrease in PCE use for dry cleaning from 1990 (103,000 tons) to 2005 (17,000 tons) was 83%. The reductions over the same time period in Japan and the western Europe were around 75% and 70%, respectively. The recent reduction in global production of PCE has been reportedly due to more efficacious work practices coupled with the utilization of more efficient equipment designed to minimize losses of the solvent.

It has been estimated that about 85% of PCE produced is released into the environment, primarily into the atmosphere (ATSDR, 1997a). In the atmosphere, PCE is degraded by hydroxyl radical (HO$^\cdot$), yielding phosgene (COCl$_2$), trichloroacetyl chloride (C$_2$Cl$_4$O), hydrogen chloride (HCl), and other by-products. The half-life of PCE in the air varies with latitude, season, and level of atmospheric HO$^\cdot$, but typically between 1 and 8 months (ATSDR, 1997a; WHO, 2000b). In water, PCE is degraded very slowly by hydrolysis, and is persistent under aerobic conditions. PCE can be degraded via reductive dechlorination under anaerobic conditions, yielding dichloroethylene (C$_2$H$_2$Cl$_2$), trichloroethylene (C$_2$HCl$_3$, *see* Section 13.8 below), vinyl chloride (CH$_2$=CHCl), and other by-products. Release of PCE into the environment is mainly through industrial emissions, but may also be from building materials and consumer products. When released onto surface water and land in sewage sludge, PCE readily evaporates to the atmosphere owing to its relatively low solubility in water and moderately high mobility in soil.

13.7.2. Exposures and Toxic Effects

Because of PCE's pervasiveness and ability to persist under certain conditions, the potential for human exposure to this VOC can be substantial. The major routes of exposure for the general population are inhalation of ambient air and consumption of contaminated drinking water. Available data suggest that dermal uptake is not a principal route for most people. Exposure to PCE from inhalation of ambient air can vary considerably depending on location. In general, levels of PCE in the air are higher in urban areas and places near point sources than in rural areas. As expected, PCE poses the greatest risk to workers in dry cleaning facilities. This chlorinated solvent is also a common soil contaminant, owing to the high volume of its discharges from industrial use.

According to the toxicity data reviewed by ATSDR (1997a), the adverse health effects from PCE exposure include mainly neurological problems, damage to the liver and kidneys, and cancer. At high concentrations, PCE vapor is both a potent anesthetic agent and a cardiac epinephrine sensitizer. Teratogenicity studies in rats, rabbits, and mice collectively suggested that PCE could cause fetotoxicity and embryotoxicity at high doses. Inconclusive adverse reproductive effects from occupational exposure were reported. As supported mechanistically by several animal studies, a handful of epidemiological studies on dry cleaning workers implicated increased risks from PCE exposure for several types of cancer including liver, kidney, and leukemia. Based on this body of evidence, IARC (1995) has classified PCE as a probable human (Group 2A) carcinogen.

Like many other chlorinated hydrocarbons, PCE can dissolve fats from the human skin with the potential for skin irritation. Intense irritation of the upper respiratory tract was observed in human volunteers exposed to high concentrations (>1,000 ppm) of PCE (Carpenter 1937; Rowe *et al.*, 1952). A population-based study of 198 twin pairs, along with available relevant animal data, provided substantial circumstantial evidence linking PCE as well as TCE to Parkinson's disease (Goldman, 2010).

13.8. Trichloroethylene

Trichloroethylene ($ClCH=CCl_2$) is also known as trichloroethene (TCE) under its systematic (i.e., IUPAC) name. This VOC is a clear liquid with a sweet smell. It is not soluble in water, but miscible with many organic solvents (e.g., alcohol, chloroform, ether). TCE is nonflammable under normal conditions. It has a boiling point of $86.7°$ C and a vapor pressure of 74 mm Hg at $25°$ C.

13.8.1. Sources and Use

Trichloroethylene is an effective solvent for a variety of organic materials, having many of the chemical functions and industrial applications offered by PERC (a.k.a. PCE) and DCM (a.k.a. MC). As such, TCE is an excellent extraction solvent for greases, oils, fats, tars, waxes, and the kind. Up to 90% of its use is for degreasing and cold cleaning of metal parts (WHO, 2000c). The remaining 10% or so of its use is largely for printing, printing ink production, paint production, textile printing, and large-scale industrial drycleaning (*vs.* small business type for PCE). The textile industry has used TCE to scour fabrics (e.g., cotton, wool) and as a solvent in waterless dyeing and finishing operations. As a solvent or a component of solvent blends, TCE is used in pesticides, adhesives, lubricants, paint strippers, and cold metal cleaners (ATSDR, 1997b).

Virtually all (99%) TCE from industrial and consumer uses is released into the environment, primarily into the atmosphere with only a negligible percentage entering the water (WHO, 2000c). Owing to its relatively high vapor pressure, this VOC can readily evaporate from surface waters when contaminated from direct industrial discharges. TCE in soil has the potential to seep into groundwater due to its moderate water solubility. Some low levels of TCE are therefore commonly found in drinking water supplied by groundwater aquifers. TCE can be released into indoor air during the use of consumer products containing the solvent as an ingredient, or due to vapor migration (i.e., vapor intrusion) from subsurfaces such as underground walls or the water supply. In the United States, much of the TCE is released into the atmosphere from vapor degreasing operations. Even more so than for PCE and MC in the air, the predominant degradation process for atmospheric TCE is through reaction with hydroxyl radical (HO·), though with a much shorter atmospheric residence half-life of about one week (ATSDR, 1997b).

13.8.2. Exposures and Toxic Effects

According to ATSDR (1997b), the atmospheric levels of TCE, as with those of PCE, are much higher in industrial and populated places than in rural or remote areas. The general population is exposed to TCE through consumption or use of water contaminated by the chlorinated solvent, largely due to evaporation and leaching from waste disposal sites. In addition to consuming contaminated water, showering or bathing can be a significant source of indoor exposure to TCE. This is because TCE can readily volatilize into the air from hot water. Another source of (indoor) exposure is through use of consumer products containing the chlorinated solvent as an ingredient.

Inhalation is the major route through which workers are exposed to the highest levels of TCE, particularly those working in the degreasing industry. Workers may be exposed to TCE in facilities where the VOC is manufactured or processed. Bystanders may also be exposed to TCE from inhaling air around these facilities.

In humans, short-term and long-term inhalation exposures to TCE can affect the CNS, with the common signs and symptoms being drowsiness, dizziness, headaches, fatigue, facial numbness, and euphoria. Other adverse health effects, especially from chronic exposure, may include damage to the liver and kidneys as well as impairment to the developmental, immunological, and endocrine systems (ATSDR, 1997b).

When inhaled, TCE can induce CNS depression resulting in general anesthesia, but at a slow rate due to its high lipid solubility and consequently with less desirable effect as an anesthetic agent. The symptoms of acute non-medical exposure are similar to those of alcohol intoxication, starting with headaches, dizziness, and confusion. With increasing exposure, the effect can progress to unconsciousness. The associated respiratory and circulatory depression can result in death. TCE at low levels is relatively non-irritating to the respiratory tract. However, at high levels of exposure it can cause rapid breathing and lower the threshold for epinephrine-induced cardiac arrhythmias (WHO, 2000c).

Several epidemiological studies implicated a link between congenital heart defects and maternal exposure to TCE (Watson *et al.*, 2006; Yauck *et al.*, 2004). Increase in incidence of congenital cardiac defects was claimed in these studies with communities exposed to TCE contamination in groundwater, although the exact exposure levels involved were unclear. These findings were for the large part consistent with the adverse health effects observed in laboratory animals.

Some other epidemiological studies associated TCE exposure with several types of tumors in humans (e.g., cervical, kidney, lymphatic). Animal studies also linked TCE exposure to liver, kidney, and lung cancers in mice and rats (e.g., Fukuda *et al.*, 1983; Maltoni *et al.*, 1986, 1988; NTP, 1988, 1990). Based on this body of evidence, IARC (1995) has classified TCE as a probable human (Group 2A) carcinogen.

Recent public health concerns with exposures to TCE and PCE have extended to the appreciation and prediction of their toxicokinetics (TK) with the application of PB-TK (physiologically-based toxicokinetics) modeling. TCE and PCE are among the few environmental toxicants that their TK parameters have been studied extensively and rather successfully using PB-TK modeling. One reason for such a high modeling potential is that TCE and PCE are two of the few lipophilic solvents rapidly absorbed and metabolized to a variety of metabolites, including those that are toxic to the liver and kidneys. As alluded to in Chapter 7, PB-TK modeling may be used to help discern the quantitative distribution of both the parent compound and its metabolites within an organism's body. Accordingly, many human and animal PB-TK (i.e., PB-PK) models have been developed and updated for TCE to further appreciate its quantitative disposition and that of some of its prominent metabolites in the human and animal bodies (e.g., Evans *et al.*, 2009; Isaacs *et al.*, 2004; Simmons *et al.*, 2002; WHO, 2000c).

As for any toxicant, a well-designed PB-TK model can be used to help unfold the relationship between the internal dose of TCE measured and its toxic effects observed. Available PB-TK human models for TCE have been applied specifically for cancer risk assessment by utilizing results observed in animal studies (WHO, 2000c). Animal results utilized in the human models included tumor incidence in mouse liver (Bogen, 1988; Fisher and Allen, 1993), tumor incidence in rat kidneys (Bogen, 1988), and kinetics data in rats (Koizumi, 1989). Some of the human and animal PB-TK models developed for PCE can be found in the guidance document published by WHO (2000b). Apparently, the models discussed in that guidance document can easily be extended for use on TCE.

References

ATSDR (Agency for Toxic Substances and Disease Registry), 1996. Toxicological Profile for Methyl *tert*-Butyl Ether. U.S. Department of Health and Human Services, Atlanta, Georgia, USA.

ATSDR (Agency for Toxic Substances and Disease Registry), 1997a. Toxicological Profile for Tetrachloroethylene (PERC). U.S. Department of Health and Human Services, Atlanta, Georgia, USA.

ATSDR (Agency for Toxic Substances and Disease Registry), 1997b. Toxicological Profile for Trichloroethylene (TCE). U.S. Department of Health and Human Services, Atlanta, Georgia, USA.

ATSDR (Agency for Toxic Substances and Disease Registry), 1999. Toxicological Profile for Formaldehyde. U.S. Department of Health and Human Services, Atlanta, Georgia, USA.

ATSDR (Agency for Toxic Substances and Disease Registry), 2000. Toxicological Profile for Methylene Chloride. U.S. Department of Health and Human Services, Atlanta, Georgia, USA.

ATSDR (Agency for Toxic Substances and Disease Registry), 2007. Toxicological Profile for Benzene. U.S. Department of Health and Human Services, Atlanta, Georgia, USA.

Balek B, 2009. New VOC Limits for Cleaning Products Effective Beginning of 2009. ISSA (International Sanitary Supply Association – The Worldwide Cleaning Industry Association): News Release issued on 21 January. ISSA Headquarters, 7373 N. Lincoln Avenue, Lincolnwood, Illinois, USA.

Bogen KT, 1988. Pharmacokinetics for Regulatory Risk Analysis: The Case of Trichloroethylene. *Regul. Toxicol. Pharmacol.* 8:447-466.

Carpenter CP, 1937. The Chronic Toxicity of Tetrachloroethylene. *J. Ind. Hyg. Toxicol.* 19:323-336.

Cordes DH, Brown WD, Quinn KM, 1988. Chemically Induced Hepatitis after Inhaling Organic Solvents. *West J. Med.* 148:458-460.

Environment Canada, 2013. *Consultation Document*: Revisions to the Proposed Volatile Organic Compound (VOC) Concentration Limits for Certain Products Regulations. 10 Wellington, 23rd Floor, Gatineau QC, K1A 0H3, Canada.

European Parliament, 2009. Decision No 455/2009/EC of the European Parliament and the Council of 6 May 2009 – Amending Council Directive 76/769/EEC as Regards Restrictions on the Marketing and Use of Dichloromethane. *Off. J. Eur. Un.* L137(3 June):3-6.

Evans MV, Chiu WA, Okino MS, Caldwell JC, 2009. Development of an Updated PBPK Model for Trichloroethylene and Metabolites in Mice, and Its Application to Discern the Role of Oxidative Metabolism in TCE-Induced Hepatomegaly. *Toxicol. Appl. Pharmacol.* 236:329-340.

Fisher JW, Allen BC, 1993. Evaluating the Risk of Liver Cancer in Humans Exposed to Trichloroethylene Using Physiological Models. *Risk Anal.* 13:87-95.

Fukuda K, Takemoto K, Tsuruta H, 1983. Inhalation Carcinogenicity of Trichloroethylene in Mice and Rats. *Ind. Health* 21:243-254.

Goldman S, 2010. Parkinson's Disease Risk Is Increased in Discordant Twins Exposed to Specific Solvents. Presented at the American Academy of Neurology's 62nd Annual Meeting in Toronto 10-17 April.

GWPC (Groundwater Protection Council), 2007. *Groundwater Report to the Nation: A Call to Action – Groundwater and Underground Storage Tanks*. GWPC, 13308 N. MacArthur Boulevard, Oklahoma City, Oklahoma, USA.

IARC (International Agency for Research on Cancer), 1987. IARC Monographs on the Evaluation of Carcinogenic Risks to Humans, Supplement 7: Overall Evaluations of Carcinogenicity – An Updating of IARC Monographs Volumes 1 to 42. Lyon, France: WHO Press.

IARC (International Agency for Research on Cancer), 1995. IARC Monographs on the Evaluation of Carcinogenic Risks to Humans, Volume 63: Dry-Cleaning, Some Chlorinated Solvents and Other Industrial Chemicals. Lyon, France: WHO Press.

IARC (International Agency for Research on Cancer), 1999a. IARC Monographs on the Evaluation of Carcinogenic Risks to Humans, Volume 73: Some Chemicals That Cause Tumours of the Kidney or Urinary Bladder in Rodents and Some Other Substances. Lyon, France: WHO Press.

IARC (International Agency for Research on Cancer), 1999b. IARC Monographs on the Evaluation of Carcinogenic Risks to Humans, Volume 71: Re-evaluation of Some Organic Chemicals, Hydrazine and Hydrogen Peroxide (Part One, Part Two, Part Three). Lyon, France: WHO Press.

IARC (International Agency for Research on Cancer), 2006. IARC Monographs on the Evaluation of Carcinogenic Risks to Humans, Volume 88: Formaldehyde, 2-Butoxy-Ethanol and 1-tert-Butoxy-2-Propanol. Lyon, France: WHO Press.

IPCS (International Programme on Chemical Safety), 1997. INCHEM Poisons Information Monographs (PIM) 343 – Methylene Chloride. IPCS World Health Organization, 20 Avenue Appia, 1211, Geneva, Switzerland.

Isaacs KK, Evans MV, Harris TR, 2004. Visualization-Based Analysis for a Mixed-Inhibition Binary PBPK Model: Determination of Inhibition Mechanism. *J. Pharmacokin. Pharmacodyn.* 31: 215-242.

Kobayashi A, Ando A, Tagami N, Kitagawa M, Kawai E, Akioka M, Arai E, Nakatani T, Nakano S, Matsui Y, Matsumura M, 2008. Severe Optic Neuropathy Caused by Dichloromethane Inhalation. *J. Ocular Pharmacol. Therap.* 24:607-612.

Koizumi A, 1989. Potential of Physiologically Based Pharmacokinetics to Amalgamate Kinetic Data of Trichloroethylene and Tetrachloroethylene Obtained in Rats and Man. *Br. J. Ind. Med.* 46:239-249.

Lacson J, Toki G, 2006. C2 Chlorinated Solvents (CEH Marketing Research Report Abstract). *Chemical Industrial Newsletter* by SRI Consulting, February issue (http://chemical.ihs.com/nl/Public/2006Feb.pdf).

Maltoni C, Lefemine G, Cotti G, 1986. Experimental Research on Trichloroethylene Carcinogenesis. In *Archives of Research on Industrial Carcinogenesis* (Maltoni C, Mehlman MA, Eds.), Volume 5. Princeton, New Jersey, USA: Princeton Scientific Publishing, p.393.

Maltoni C, Lefemine G, Cotti G, Perino G, 1988. Long-Term Carcinogenicity Bioassays on Trichloroethylene Administered by Inhalation to Sprague-Dawley Rats and Swiss and B6C3F1 Mice. *Ann. NY Acad. Sci.* 534:316-342.

Melnick RL, White MC, Davis JM, Hartle RW, Ghanayem B, Ashley DL, Harry GJ, Zeiger E, Shelby M, Ris CH, 1997. Potential Health Effects of Oxygenated Gasoline. In *Interagency Assessment of Oxygenated Fuels*, National Science and Technology Council (Committee on Environment and Natural Resources Fuels), Washington DC, USA.

Morris JB, Smith FA, Garman RH, 1979. Studies on Methylene Chloride-Induced Fatty Liver. *Exp. Mol. Path.* 30:386-393.

Narotsky MG, Hamby BT, Mitchell DS, Kavlock RJ, 1992. Full-Litter Resorptions Caused by Low-Molecular Weight Halocarbons in F-344 Rats (Abstract 67). *Teratology* 45:472-473.

NCI (U.S. National Cancer Institute), 2009. Formaldehyde and Cancer Risk. NCI FactSheet, issued 20 November. U.S. National Institutes of Health, NCI Public Inquiries Office, 6116 Executive Boulevard, Rm 3036A, Bethesda, Maryland, USA.

Nishio A, Yajema S, Yahogi M, Sasaki Y, Sawano Y, Miyao N, 1984. Studies on the Teratogenicity of Dichloromethane in Rats. *Gakujutsu Hikoku-Kagoshima Daigaku Nogakubu* 34:95-103 (in Japanese).

NRC (U.S. National Research Council), 1996, Toxicological and Performance Aspects of Oxygenated Motor Vehicle Fuels. Washington DC, USA: National Academy Press.

NTP (U.S. National Toxicology Program), 1986. Toxicology and Carcinogenesis Studies of Dichloromethane (Methylene Chloride) (CAS No. 75-09-2) in F344/N Rats and B6C3F1 Mice (Inhalation Studies). TR-306. U.S. Department of Health and Human Services, Research Triangle Park, North Carolina, USA.

NTP (U.S. National Toxicology Program), 1988. Toxicology and Carcinogenesis Studies of Trichloroethylene (CAS No. 79-01-6) in Four Strains of Rats (ACI, August, Marshall, Osborne-Mendel) (Gavage Studies). TR-273. U.S. Department of Health and Human Services, Research Triangle Park, North Carolina, USA.

NTP (U.S. National Toxicology Program), 1990. Carcinogenesis Studies of Trichloroethylene (without Epichlorohydrin) (CAS No. 79-01-6) in F344/N Rats and B6C3F1 Mice (Gavage Studies). TR-243. U.S. Department of Health and Human Services, Research Triangle Park, North Carolina, USA.

Rowe VK, McCollister DD, Spencer HC, Adams EM, Irish DD, 1952. Vapor Toxicity of Tetrachloroethylene for Laboratory Animals and Human Subjects. *AMA Arch. Ind. Hyg. Occup. Med.* 5:566-579.

Seinfeld JH, Pankow JF, 2003. Organic Atmospheric Particulate Material. *Ann. Rev. Phys. Chem.* 54:121-140.

Simmons JE, Boyes WK, Bushnell PJ, Raymer JH, Limsakun T, McDonald A, Sey YM, Evans MV, 2002. A Physiologically Based Pharmacokinetic Model for Trichloroethylene in the Male Long-Evans Rat. *Toxicol. Sci.* 69:3-15.

Ubrich E, Jeuland N, 2007. Panorama 2008: Perspectives for Post-Euro 4 Standards for Passenger and Light Commercial Vehicles (Euro 5, Euro 5+, Euro 6). IFP Headquarters, 1 & 4, Avenue de Bois-Préau, 92852 Rueil-Malmaison, Cedex, France.

UNEP (United Nations Environment Programme), 2005. The Songhua River Spill, China, December 2005: Field Mission Report. United Nations Avenue, Gigiri, PO Box 30552, 00100, Nairobi, Kenya.

U.S. EPA (U.S. Environmental Protection Agency), 1985. Occupational Exposure and Environmental Release Assessment of Methylene Chloride. Office of Pesticides and Toxic Substances, Washington DC, USA.

U.S. EPA (U.S. Environmental Protection Agency), 1997. Drinking Water Advisory: Consumer Acceptability Advice and Health Effects Analysis on Methyl Tertiary-Butyl Ether (MtBE). EPA-822-F-97-009. Office of Water, Washington DC, USA.

U.S. EPA (U.S. Environmental Protection Agency), 2006. Control of Hazardous Air Pollutants from Mobile Sources. *Federal Register* 71:15804-15963.

U.S. EPA (U.S. Environmental Protection Agency), 2009. 2009 Edition of the Drinking Water Standards and Health Advisories. EPA 822-R-09-011. Office of Water, Washington DC, USA.

U.S. EPA (U.S. Environmental Protection Agency), 2010. IRIS Toxicological Review of Dichloromethane (Methylene Chloride) (External Review Draft). EPA/635/R-10/-003A. Office of Research and Development, Washington DC, USA.

Watson RE, Jacobson CF, Williams AL, Howard WB, DeSesso JM, 2006. Trichloroethylene-Contaminated Drinking Water and Congenital Heart Defects: A Critical Analysis of the Literature. *Reprod. Toxicol.* 21:117-147.

Wells GG, Waldron HA, 1984. Methylene Chloride Burns. *Br. J. Ind. Med.* 41:420.

WHO (World Health Organization), 2000a. *Air Quality Guidelines for Europe*, Second Edition, Chapter 5.7: Dichloromethane. WHO Regional Publication, European Series, No. 91, Copenhagen, Denmark.

WHO (World Health Organization), 2000b. *Air Quality Guidelines for Europe*, Second Edition, Chapter 5.13: Tetrachloroethylene. WHO Regional Publication, European Series, No. 91, Copenhagen, Denmark.

WHO (World Health Organization), 2000c. *Air Quality Guidelines for Europe*, Second Edition, Chapter 5.15: Trichloroethylene. WHO Regional Publication, European Series, No. 91, Copenhagen, Denmark.

Yauck JS, Malloy ME, Blair K, Simpson PM, McCarver DG, 2004. Proximity of Residence to Trichloroethylene-Emitting Sites and Increased Risk of Offspring Congenital Heart Defects among Older Women. *Birth Defects Res.* 70(A):808-814.

Zahm SH, Stewart ZP, Blair A, 1987. A Study of Mortality among Workers Exposed to Methylene Chloride. Feasibility Report. U.S. National Cancer Institute, Bethesda, Maryland, USA.

Review Questions

1. Briefly distinguish the definition of VOCs in general terms from that of VOCs of regulatory concern.

2. List the two series of chemical reactions through each of which VOCs can serve as precursors for ozone formation.

3. What is the general mechanism whereby VOCs can serve as precursors for the formation of secondary organic aerosols?

4. What are the three main sources of occupational exposure to formaldehyde?

5. How may formaldehyde become a major component of photochemical smog?

6. What happened to the health of those victims of Hurricane Katrina and Hurricane Rita that lived in trailers and mobile homes provided by the U.S. federal government?

7. Name three chemicals that are simple derivatives of benzene, and the one regarded as being among the most widely produced.

8. What happened to the greater city of Harbin in China following the Songhua River pollution in 2005?

9. What are the main sources for environmental release of benzene into the atmosphere?

10. Explain why toluene is less toxic than benzene under normal conditions.

11. What may be the one main health concern regarding benzene exposure?

12. What may be the metabolic fate of benzene in the human body?

13. What is the major industrial use of MTBE? And why is this VOC considered more as a water contaminant than as an air pollutant?

14. What are the major uses and health effects of MTBE?

15. What are the major uses and health effects of methylene chloride?

16. What are the major health effects of PERC vapors when inhaled at high concentrations?

17. Which of the following VOCs is best known as *the* dry-cleaning fluid? a) benzene; b) formic acid; c) MTBE; d) dichloromethane; e) perchloroethylene; f) trichloroethene.

18. Give an example for vapor intrusion as a potential source of indoor air exposure to VOCs.

19. What are the major uses and health effects of TCE?

20. Which of the following VOCs is (are) classified by IARC as a: I) Group 1 human carcinogen; II) Group 2A probable human carcinogen; III) Group 2B possible human carcinogen?

    a) formaldehyde; b) benzene; c) MTBE; d) methylene chloride; e) PERC; f) TCE.

21. Name the following VOCs whose degradation in the atmosphere is mostly through reaction with hydroxyl radical? a) methylene chloride; b) MTBE; c) TCE; d) PERC; e) formaldehyde; f) benzene.

CHAPTER 14

Toxic and Radioactive Metals

14.1. Introduction

The history of metals dates back to 6000 BC, beginning with gold (Au). Chemically, metals can be defined as all the non-hydrogen (H) elements in the periodic table (Figure 14.1) appearing on the left of the line bordered by boron (B), silicon (Si), germanium (Ge), antimony (Sb), and polonium (Po). That is, as many as 88 (75%) of the 118 elements (or so) can be treated as metals. Even the five elements forming the stairstep line, along with arsenic (As) and tellurium (Te), may be chemically considered as metals since they are metalloids having some of the chemical properties of a metal. Those metals in the cation state (i.e., ion with positive charge) can form salts with acids, basic oxides with oxygen, and alloys with one another. To many people, metals are nonetheless more commonly known as electropositive elements that generally have a shiny surface, tend to be competent thermal and electrical conductors; and they can be hammered, melted, or otherwise processed into thin sheets or wires.

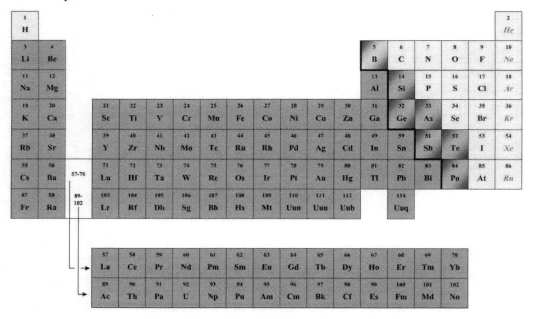

Figure 14.1. Simplified Version of the Periodic Table (*primarily for illustration of metals vs. nonmetals: solid background = metal; two-tone = metalloid; light background = nonmetal; italicized letters = noble gas*)

14.1.1. Concepts of Minerals and Heavy Metals

In the literature, the terms *mineral* and *heavy metal* are generally ill defined when discussing metal chemistry or toxicology. The term *mineral* is commonly used to refer to chemical elements including metals. Yet in many references, a mineral is specifically defined as a naturally occurring *solid* formed through geological processes ending with a characteristic chemical composition, a highly ordered atomic structure, and certain physical properties. Therefore, at least about 20 chemical elements (mainly elements No. 93 through 113) in the periodic table may not be treated as minerals since they are *synthetic* in origin. The statement that metals are minerals neither *created* nor destroyed by humans is thus somewhat misleading. Moreover, at room temperature a few elements (e.g., mercury, bromine) occur in *liquid* form. A close analogy for the taxonomic relationship between minerals and elements or metals is that between animals and humans.

Likewise, the so-called *heavy* metals are at best members of an ill-defined subset of chemical elements that exhibit certain *user-defined* metallic properties. It appears that the elements in this subset can be defined per any of the various combinations of their density, atomic number, chemical properties, and toxicity that a scientific sector prefers.

14.1.2. Metals of Environmental Health Concern

Not all metals are toxic to humans, wildlife, or the ecosystem. Copper (Cu), calcium (Ca), magnesium (Mg), zinc (Zn), chromium III (Cr^{3+}), and iron (Fe) are some examples that are essential to human health as long as they are not excessively accumulated in the human body. Regardless of how they are defined, in environmental toxicology the main concerns with metals are their health threats, sources of pollution, and frequency of occurrence in the environment. In this chapter, the 11 metals selected from four categories are thereby discussed along this line of concern. The selection made here does not suggest in any way that those metals not discussed are harmless. At most, it means that their toxicity receives relatively less public health attention. It is also important to note that many metals discussed here (as well as many not discussed here) are also toxic to plants or lower order animals at high levels of exposure. For example, as discussed in Chapter 10, cadmium (Cd) and arsenic are phytotoxic metals known to retard plant growth. Additional examples for this kind can be found in other chapters of this book.

14.2. The Three Heavy Metals

Whether defined by density, atomic number, toxicity, or any other criterion, lead (Pb), mercury (Hg), and Cd (cadmium) are in the small group so-called the (three) most toxic heavy metals. These three elements are treated as the metal pollutants of most concern to environmental health, both in terms of their toxicity and ubiquity. There is no known biological need in humans for any of these three metals. In fact, these three and many of the other so-called heavy metals all have a strong affinity for sulfhydryl (-SH) groups which many proteins and enzymes are rich in. In most cases, the binding of foreign molecules to these sulfhydryl (a.k.a. thiol) groups can interfere with the normal functions of enzymes in the body to ultimately result in very severe health consequences (Section 9.4.2).

14.2.1. Lead

Lead (Pb) is a soft, malleable metal with a bluish-gray color when freshly cut. It will tarnish to a dull grayish color on exposure to air, and to a shiny silver luster when melted into a liquid. Since its discovery some 9,000 years ago, lead has been used in artwork, plumbing, gasoline, batteries, paints, and manufacturing of metal products. Today, it can be found everywhere in the environment, owing to the vast variety of human activities involving its processing and use, such as mining, burning fossil fuel, and manufacturing. Due to its ubiquity in the air and the concerns over its health effects and persistence in the environment, lead is designated as one of the six criteria air pollutants in the United States (along with the four inorganic gases discussed in Chapter 11 and particular matter discussed in Chapter 12). In recent years, lead exposure from paints and ceramic products, caulking, and pipe solder has been dramatically reduced. In 1996, the use of lead as an additive to gasoline was banned in the United States.

Like many other metals, lead as a free element does not break down; only its compounds are changed by sunlight, air, and water. Therefore, when lead is released into the atmosphere, it may travel long distances prior to settling onto the ground or water. Once it falls onto the soil, lead generally sticks to the particles there. Food plants thereby can be contaminated with lead through uptake from the soil.

Transport of lead from the soil into groundwater depends on the type of lead compounds and the characteristics of the soil involved. Water pipes in some older homes may contain lead solder from which lead can leach out into the drinking water. Some people may inhale lead dust from deteriorating lead-based paint. Some others may be exposed to lead when working in a job where the metal is used, or when engaging in hobbies that involve its use, such as in making stained glass. Still some other people may be exposed to lead from using health care products or folk remedies that contain lead.

Of all metals, lead is specifically known as a *systemic* poison, as it can affect virtually every organ and system in the (human) body. The adverse health effects of lead are the same whether it enters the body through inhalation or ingestion. The main organ target for lead toxicity is the nervous system in both adults and children, despite the fact that well over 90% of its content in the body eventually ends up in the bone. Recent cases continue to show that acute lead poisoning (a.k.a. plumbism) in children, such as from lead on children's jewelry and toys, often gets misdiagnosed initially as viral gastroenteritis (Berg *et al.*, 2006; VanArsdale *et al.*, 2004; Section 21.4.2).

Lead exposure can cause anemia, weakness in ankles, fingers, or wrists, and a small increase in blood pressure, particularly in middle-aged and older people. Exposure to high levels of lead can cause severe damage to the kidneys and brain in adults or children and ultimately death. In pregnant women, high levels of exposure to lead can cause miscarriage. In men, exposure to high levels of lead can cause damage in those body tissues and organs responsible for sperm production (ATSDR, 2007a; U.S. EPA, 2004). Long-term exposure to lead can decrease a person's ability to perform certain nervous system functions.

Due to its strong affinity for the thiol (-SH) group, lead can inhibit the enzymatic activity of δ-ALAD (δ-aminolevulinic acid dehydratase) at very low blood concentrations (<10 µg/dL) in adults and children. Accordingly, the activity of δ-ALAD has been treated as a sensitive indicator of lead poisoning (e.g., Berny *et al.*, 1992; Gurer-Orhan *et al.*, 2004; Pattee and Pain, 2003). As part of the second step in the porphyrin and heme biosynthetic pathway, the δ-ALAD enzyme is responsible for catalyzing the conversion of δ-aminolevulinic acid (δ-ALA) to porphobilinogen, a precursor of heme. Heme is not only a component of the oxygen-carrying hemoglobin, but also the building block of many other hemoproteins that are likewise essential to a number of other biological functions. When the enzymatic activity of δ-ALAD is inhibited, such as by lead, the acid δ-ALA is accumulated in the body and thereby can be monitored in the urine.

There is no conclusive evidence that elemental lead can cause cancer in humans. However, laboratory studies evaluated by U.S. EPA (2004) showed a significant increase in the incidences of renal carcinoma and some other tumors in rats and mice when given large doses of lead acetate ($Pb[C_2H_3O_2]_2$) or lead phosphate ($Pb_3[PO_4]_2$). IARC (2006) has classified inorganic lead compounds as probable human (Group 2A) carcinogens. (IARC's classification for carcinogenicity potential is summarized in Box 18.1.)

14.2.2. Mercury

Mercury (Hg) occurs naturally in several forms. The metallic (i.e., elemental) form at ambient temperature is a shiny, silver-white, odorless liquid. If this elemental liquid or a compound of mercury is heated, it can give off a colorless, odorless vapor. When the metal combines with chlorine (Cl), sulfur (S), or other elements to form mercury salts, these inorganic compounds usually appear as white powders or crystals. Mercury also combines with carbon to form organic compounds, of which some like methylmercury (e.g., CH_3Hg^+) are colorless. While methylmercury is produced primarily by bacteria in water and soil and is regarded as the most toxic form of mercury compounds, it is also the form most easily bioaccumulated in many living organisms.

Elemental mercury is used in electrolytic process to synthesize chlorine gas (Cl_2), with caustic soda (NaOH) formed as a co-product. In some countries, the metal is widely used in amalgams (for dental fillings), barometers, batteries, and thermometers. Mercury and its compounds have been used in medicine as a preservative in vaccine, in topical antiseptic, and for treatment of syphilis.

Mercury and its inorganic compounds can enter the atmosphere from mining of ores, manufacturing plants, and waste incineration. From natural deposits, waste disposal, and volcanic activity, these compounds can contaminate the nearby waters and soils.

One major source of human exposure to mercury is via consumption of seafood contaminated with organic mercury compounds, especially at levels when bioaccumulation can become a phenomenon of concern. Other major sources include inhalation of and dermal contact with mercury vapors in various occupational or environmental settings, such as the air from chemical spills, incinerators, and industries burning fuel that contains mercury compounds. Mercury can also be released from dental work and medical treatments (e.g., from treatment with some Chinese herbal medicines).

The various forms of mercury collectively can cause a wide array of untoward health effects in humans (ATSDR, 1999; U.S. EPA, 1997), including neurotoxicity (CH_3Hg^+, Hg^0), teratogenicity (CH_3Hg^+), nephrotoxicity (Hg^0, $HgCl_2$), and death (Hg^0, CH_3Hg^+). To this date, the most widespread mercury poisoning (a.k.a. mercurialism) has been the epidemic occurring in rural Iraq in winter 1971, when farmers there used a seed grain mistreated with a CH_3Hg^+-based fungicide to make bread. In that epidemic, more than 6,000 cases of food poisoning and at least 459 deaths were reportedly caused by consumption of bread made from the contaminated grain (Bakir *et al.*, 1973).

Short-term exposure to high levels of metallic mercury vapors can cause lung damage, nausea, vomiting, diarrhea, hypertension, and tachycardia, in addition to irritation to the skin, the eyes, and the respiratory tract. The nervous system is particularly sensitive to elemental (Hg^0) and organic (e.g., CH_3Hg^+) mercury, since in these forms more mercury can enter the brain. In any event, exposure to high levels of mercury in any form can be very harmful, such as causing permanent damage to the brain, kidneys, and the fetus. Effects on brain functioning may result in irritability, tremors, shyness, poor vision, poor hearing, and memory difficulties, which are all signs and symptoms that first became evident from the mercury poisoning disaster occurring in the mid-1950s in a Japanese village named Minamata (e.g., Ishimure, 1990; Smith and Smith, 1975).

The Minamata incident was caused by the release of methylmercury from the industrial wastewater beginning in the 1930s from a chemical factory located in Kumamoto, Japan. Over the years, this highly toxic metal had bioaccumulated considerably in fish and shellfish in the nearby Minamata Bay, which is part of the Shiranui Sea. After consuming the contaminated seafood for many years, in the mid-1950s more than 3,000 villagers in Minamata reportedly had suffered from a degeneration of their nervous system, with symptoms being largely those described in the preceding paragraph.

The data on human and animal cancers are considered as insufficient for most forms of mercury. However, studies (ATSDR, 1999) have linked a significant increase in kidney tumors in male mice to methylmercuric chloride (CH_3HgCl) and a considerable increase in several types of tumors in rats and mice to mercuric chloride ($HgCl_2$). Accordingly, IARC (1997) has classified CH_3Hg^+ compounds as possible human (Group 2B) carcinogens but considered other mercury compounds, including metallic mercury, as Group 3 carcinogens (i.e., agents not classifiable as to their carcinogenicity to humans).

14.2.3. Cadmium

Cadmium (Cd) is a soft, silver-white metal with high resistance to corrosion. As such, the metal has many commercial and industrial applications including electroplating and manufacture of metal coatings. It is widely used in batteries, pigments, plastics, solders, and jewelry. Cadmium is commonly found as a mineral containing other elements such as oxygen (as in CdO), chlorine ($CdCl_2$), or sulfur (CdS, $CdSO_4$). It can be extracted during the production of zinc (Zn) and some other metals.

Like mercury, cadmium enters the atmosphere, water, and soil mostly from mining of ores, industrial facilities, and waste incineration. Its airborne residues can travel long distances prior to settling onto the ground or water. Although cadmium residues in some forms may dissolve in water, in most cases they bind strongly to soil particles. The metal in the environment can build up in plants, fish, and other animal tissues.

Low levels of cadmium are found in most foods, with the liver, shellfish, and kidney meats having the highest. There is usually less cadmium found in tobacco smoke than in foods. However, because the lungs absorb cadmium more efficiently than the stomach does, tobacco smoke is frequently regarded as the single most significant source of cadmium exposure to humans. Despite the common observation that plants in non-industrial areas contain only small amounts of cadmium, yet owing to its great propensity for long-term buildup in the animal body's tissues, high levels of this metal can still be found in the liver and kidneys of adult herbivorous animals including humans.

Other sources of human exposure include inhalation of air and consumption of water contaminated with the metal. Buildup of cadmium levels in the air, water, and soil is not uncommon in industrial areas. People are therefore at a greater risk if they live near or work in facilities that discharge cadmium into the environment.

Exposure to cadmium can result in various health effects, including emphysema, renal failure, cardiovascular diseases, and cancer. The kidney is considered as the most vulnerable organ. Eating food or drinking water with very high levels of cadmium can severely irritate the stomach, leading to vomiting, diarrhea, and other symptoms.

Chronic exposure to low levels of cadmium in the air, foods, or water can lead to a buildup of cadmium in the kidneys at levels that can cause severe renal diseases, such as proteinuria and increased formation of kidney stone (ATSDR, 1997, 2008a). Other long-term effects include bone fracture and lung damage. Data from human and animal studies suggested that exposure to high, or sometimes even low, levels of cadmium would cause osteopenia and osteoporosis (Bhattacharyya, 2009; Brzóska and Moniuszko-Jakoniuk, 2004; Gallagher *et al.*, 2008; Satarug *et al.*, 2010). Osteoporosis is the major cause of bone fractures in elderly women, a common occurrence worldwide.

Historically, the largest outbreak involving cadmium-induced osteoporosis and renal failure occurred also in Japan and likewise around the 1950s. The syndrome experienced from that incident led to a chemically-induced disorder known as *itai-itai byo* in Japanese (meaning *ouch-ouch pain* or *sickness* in English). The term *itai-itai* (*byo*) was coined by Japanese locals living in the Jinzu river basin region, where most of the consumed rice was grown in fields irrigated with river water. Unfortunately, starting in 1910 and continuing through 1945, the rivers in the basin were constantly contaminated with cadmium discharged in significant quantities by mining companies operating up in the mountains.

The water in these rivers was also used for drinking, washing, and fishing by the down-stream residents. Many of these local residents, particularly the postmenopausal older women, suffered from several pains induced in the joints and spine. Their pains and sufferings were not linked to cadmium exposure until the mid-1950s (Kobayashi, 1978; Kogawa, 1981).

As seen in victims in the *itai-itai* incident, one of the main health effects of long-term cadmium poisoning is a painful skeletal condition resulting from weak, brittle, or deformed bones. Spinal and leg pains are generally the first complaints, eventually accompanied by a waddling gait due to bone deformities. These symptoms typically progress for several years until the patient is eventually unable to walk. The pain then becomes debilitating, with fractures becoming more common as the bone weakens. Other complications include coughing, anemia, renal failure, and even death.

The adverse health effects of cadmium in humans are somewhat special even among the toxic heavy metals. Owing to its long half-life (>30 years) within the human body, chronic exposure of even very low levels of cadmium can result in the buildup to levels that can lead to severe health problems. The human body can store cadmium in the liver, kidneys, and other tissues by first binding the metal to a low-molecular-weight, cysteine-rich protein named metallothionein (MT) which is present in virtually all forms of life and normally binds to certain essential metals such as zinc. Due to its higher affinity for thiol groups, cadmium can competitively displace these essential metals and bind to MT more tightly. Therefore, to some extent, the Cd-MT binding may be treated as a way of reducing the bioavailability and hence the toxicity of cadmium in the body. However, certain other essential metals such as copper have an even stronger affinity for thiol groups and thus can replace cadmium on these binding sites. A more serious concern with the Cd-MT binding is that when transported to and retained in the kidney, the protein portion of the complex is rapidly degraded. This then leaves the free cadmium to accumulate in the kidney, which is the metal's notorious site of toxic action.

Laboratory studies showed low fetal weight, skeletal malformations, impaired neurological development, and other developmental effects linking to cadmium exposure in animals, amidst inconclusive evidence from human studies (ATSDR, 1997). Several animal and occupational studies demonstrated an increase in lung cancer from long-term inhalation exposure to cadmium (ATSDR, 1997, U.S. EPA, 1999a), although the evidence from the occupational data was not treated as strong due to several confounding factors inherent in the study designs (U.S. EPA, 1999a). IARC (1997) nonetheless has classified the metal and its compounds as human (Group 1) carcinogens; and U.S. EPA (1999a) has classified cadmium as a probably human (Group B1) carcinogen.

14.3. Select Secondary/Pseudo Heavy Metals

The term *secondary* or *pseudo heavy metal* used here is even more ill defined than the term *heavy metal*. However, in environmental toxicology, the term (or another term with a similar notion) is needed to distinguish metals in this group from the three heavy metals discussed above. The reality is that there are other "heavy" metals also ubiquitous in the environment and abundant in the Earth's crust, although their health impacts are not as devastating as those of lead, mercury, or cadmium. Yet like the few toxic trace and radioactive metals discussed in Sections 14.4 and 14.5 below, some of the so-called pseudo or secondary heavy metals are still important to environmental toxicology.

Aluminum is considered in this section owing to the controversy over its toxicity, particularly in relation to Alzheimer's disease. Arsenic is included because it has an ancient and villainous history for being "heavy", with its name being coined to king of poisons. And beryllium, as with aluminum, is one of the least dense elements and therefore may not be qualified as a heavy metal by *density* criterion. Yet this second lightest element is included here because it is one of the few highly toxic *industrial* metals around.

14.3.1. Aluminum

Aluminum (Al) is the most abundant metal in the Earth's crust, followed by silicon (Si). Pure aluminum is highly malleable and ductile, with a silvery-white appearance. It is commonly found as a trivalent cation (Al^{3+}) in natural waters and in the tissues of most living organisms. The metal is most available as a mineral or an alloy that contains also silicon, oxygen, fluorine, and some other elements, as from such it can be extracted. In the air, aluminum can stay attached as a component of small particulate matter for days. Under most conditions, only a small fraction of the aluminum in water will get dissolved. Some plants can take up much of the metal from contaminated soils.

Compounds of aluminum have many different uses and applications, such as aluminum sulfate ($Al_2[SO_4]_3$) in treatment of drinking water and aluminum oxide (Al_2O_3) in extraction of the metal as well as in abrasives and polishing applications. Aluminum compounds are also used for beverage cans, cooking utensils, aircrafts, siding, roofing, foil, and in many consumer products such as antacids, buffered aspirin, food additives, cosmetics, and antiperspirants. Although aluminum is ubiquitous in the diet, it does not accumulate in persons with normal physiological functions. In the United States, the average dietary intake of aluminum for adults is less than 10 mg per day. Urban water supplies may contain a higher level of aluminum since water of this kind is usually treated with aluminum sulfate or certain other aluminum compounds.

People at the greatest risk of aluminum exposure are those staying in or near areas where the air is dusty, where ore deposits are mined or processed into the metal, or where certain toxic waste sites are located. Children and adults may be exposed to small amounts of aluminum from vaccinations, or from consumption of substances containing high levels of aluminum (e.g., antacids). However, under normal physiological conditions, only a small fraction of the absorbed doses will enter the bloodstream.

To this date, much of the toxicity of aluminum to humans has been controversial. Exposure to aluminum generally is not considered harmful, despite the fact that at high levels it may cause skeletal and neuromuscular problems, digestive disorders, coughing, and minor pulmonary effects. As with exposure to lead, in some instances inhalation of aluminum dusts or fumes by workers can cause a decrease in their ability to perform certain nervous system functions (ATSDR, 2008b).

People with renal failure will usually retain excess amounts of aluminum in their body, a condition that allegedly caused certain bone and brain diseases in some cases. Laboratory studies showed that the nervous system is a sensitive target of aluminum toxicity in animals. Yet obvious signs and symptoms of neurological damage have not been observed in test animals treated with aluminum even at high oral doses. A few studies in the 1970s implicated that exposure to high levels of the metal would cause Alzheimer's disease after finding traces of aluminum in the brains of patients with the disease (e.g., Crapper *et al.*, 1973, 1976). Subsequent studies had either offered supportive results (e.g., Peri, 1985) or failed to confirm a similar positive correlation (e.g., Markesbury *et al.*, 1981; McDermott *et al.*, 1979; Trapp *et al.*, 1978). It does not appear that aluminum can cause cancer in animals or humans (ATSDR, 2008b).

14.3.2. Arsenic

Arsenic (As) is found primarily in three crystalline forms. Its most predominant form is a brittle, metallic gray solid. The other two forms are a black solid structurally similar to red phosphorus and a yellow solid produced from abrupt cooling of arsenic vapors. Arsenic compounds, which collectively are termed *arsenicals*, are each present in one of several oxidation states which offer strikingly different toxicological properties. Most arsenicals occur in the +3, +5, or -3 oxidation state, referred to as arsenites (e.g., $NaAsO_2$), arsenates (e.g., KH_2AsO_4), and arsenides (e.g., Na_3As), respectively.

The metalloid is widely distributed in the Earth's crust. In the environment, arsenic is commonly found to be combined with oxygen, chlorine, sulfur, or some other elements to form inorganic compounds. Some inorganic arsenical compounds such as chromated copper arsenate (CCA) are used as heavy duty wood preservatives. In the United States, CCA is no longer used for residential outdoor structures, although it is still being used in industrial applications. In the tissues of living organisms, arsenic combines with hydrogen and carbon to form organic compounds. Both organic and inorganic compounds of arsenic have been used as pesticides, such as lead arsenate ($PbHAsO_4$), arsenic pentoxide (As_2O_5), and monosodium methyl arsenate (CH_4AsNaO_3). Arsenic has long been used as an antiseptic to treat syphilis (Lockhart and Atkinson, 1919).

Arsenic present in minerals may enter the air, water, and soil from wind-blown dust and may enter groundwater from runoff and leaching. In the air, arsenic dust particles get dropped onto lands or into waters through wet depositions by rain and snow. In water, many common arsenicals get dissolved and then ultimately end up in soils or sediments. Fish and shellfish can accumulate arsenic which occurs mostly in a less harmful, organic form named arsenobetaine. Certain bacterial species can use their own enzymes known as glutaredoxin (a.k.a. arsenate reductase) to derive energy for growth by catalyzing the reduction of arsenates to form arsenites.

Although arsenate may be the more common form found in humans, it can be readily reduced to the more toxic arsenite (Kingston *et al.*, 1993). Arsenite is more toxic largely owing to its strong affinity for thiol groups. More specifically, it can inhibit an essential metabolic enzyme named pyruvate dehydrogenase which is responsible for the conversion of pyruvate to acetyl CoA. With the enzyme's activity being inhibited, acetyl CoA can no longer be available for use in the citric acid cycle (Figure 9.3) to carry out the critical function of cellular respiration.

People are at the greatest risk when working in or living near places where there are high levels of arsenic minerals found in rocks, or where large arsenic production or use is involved (e.g., pesticide application, copper smelting, wood treatment). Small amounts of arsenic are almost always present in the diet and drinking water.

Arsenic has had its nefarious name as king of poisons since the Renaissance days, when the Spanish-Italian noble family Borgias frequently used the metalloid as poison of choice for political assassinations. Acute exposure of inorganic arsenic at high levels can cause irritation in the throat and lungs, and even death. Chronic or subchronic exposure to low levels can cause various systemic effects including nausea, vomiting, decrease in red and white blood cell counts, irregular heartbeat, damage to blood vessels, and a tingling sensation in hands and feet. Long-term exposure can also cause a darkening of the skin as well as the development of small warts on the palms, soles, and torso. Skin contact with inorganic arsenic can cause redness and swelling (ATSDR, 2007b).

Arsine (AsH_3) is a flammable, highly toxic gaseous arsenic compound. Acute inhalation exposure to the gas by people, even at 25 to 50 ppm (parts per million) for half an hour, can result in death (U.S. EPA, 1999b). A chelating agent known as British anti-Lewisite (BAL) was developed by a group of British biochemists during World War II as the antidote to an arsine-based chemical warfare agent named Lewisite.

Little information is available regarding the untoward health effects of organic arsenic compounds in humans. However, ingestion of methyl and dimethyl arsenic compounds was found to cause diarrhea and damage to the hepatic and renal systems in animals (ATSDR, 2007b). Animal studies also showed that several simple organic arsenic compounds were less toxic than most inorganic arsenicals known today.

Several human studies showed that ingestion of inorganic arsenic had a higher risk of cancer in the skin, liver, bladder, and lungs. Inhalation of inorganic arsenic was also found to cause an increased risk of lung cancer in humans. U.S. EPA (1999b) and IARC (1987) thereby have classified inorganic arsenic as a human (Group A and Group 1, respectively) carcinogen.

14.3.3. Beryllium

Beryllium (Be) is a brittle, steel-grayish metal commonly found in volcanic dusts, coal, petroleum, soils, and certain rock minerals. While beryllium is the second lightest chemical element, it has one of the highest melting points (>1,200° C) and as such offers an ideal material in the aerospace and manufacturing industries. Owing to its relatively high transparency to X-rays, the metal has made good uses in the fields of nuclear medicine and radiation physics.

Alloys and ores of beryllium are commonly used in microcircuits, dental plates, golf club, thermal castings, and more. The metal itself, which can be extracted from the beryllium minerals mined, has many desirable properties. In particular, the metal is more elastic than steel and is nonmagnetic with an excellent thermal conductivity.

Beryllium dust particles are released into the atmosphere from burning coal and oil and will eventually settle onto the land and water. It can get into natural waters from erosion of rocks and soils as well as from industrial wastes. Although some beryllium compounds will get dissolved in water, most will adsorb to the sediments. Like lead, beryllium tends to stick to soil particles and thus, under normal conditions, is not taken up by plants in any large amount. Beryllium rarely accumulates in any food chain.

Individuals at the greatest risk to beryllium exposure are those working in industries where beryllium ores are mined, processed, extracted into the metal, or converted into its alloys. Residents living near these places or around uncontrolled hazardous waste dumps may also inhale higher than normal levels of beryllium.

Depending on their atmospheric levels, beryllium dusts or fumes may or may not be harmful to people inhaling them. At sufficiently high levels (>1 mg/m^3) for even a short interval, a condition resembling acute chemical pneumonitis can result. Acute chemical pneumonitis is an inflammation of the lungs confined to the walls in the air sac (i.e., the alveolar) region. This acute condition is more specifically termed *acute beryllium disease*. This condition varies in severity, but including death. The less severe form of this acute disease can result from dermal contact with beryllium dusts or fumes, ending with signs and symptoms similar to those of contact dermatitis.

For some ($<15\%$) people sensitive to beryllium, they may later develop an inflammatory reaction in the respiratory system long (10-15 years) after termination of their months- or years-long exposure to the metal at sufficient levels (>0.5 µg/m^3). This chronic lung disorder, characterized by noncancerous nodular lesions, is called chronic beryllium disease, or *berylliosis* in medical terms. Such exposure may also affect other organs as beryllium can be transported to other body parts via the bloodstream. In fact, the advanced cases may involve formation of kidney stones as well as enlargement of the liver, spleen, and right heart. However, the common symptoms of berylliosis usually include only irritation of the mucous membranes, reduced lung capacity, breathing difficulties, coughing, chest pain, and fatigue (ATSDR, 2002; U.S. EPA, 1998, 1999c).

Both berylliosis and the acute condition are treated as industrial diseases. This is because the ambient air levels of beryllium are typically very low, normally at the nanogram (<0.2 ng/m^3) levels (ATSDR, 2002). Several epidemiological and animal studies implicated chronic exposure to beryllium as a cause that would increase the risk of lung cancer (ATSDR, 2002; U.S. EPA, 1998, 1999c). Although U.S. EPA (1999c) has classified beryllium alone and only as a probable human (Group B1) carcinogen, IARC (1997) has classified the metal and its compounds as human (Group 1) carcinogens.

14.4. Select Toxic Trace Metals

In addition to the metals discussed thus far in this chapter, there are many that could still be regarded as "heavy metals" by different criteria. However, a considerable number of these and other metals are essential to human health and thereby are expected to be available in the body at least in trace amounts. As with all other substances, regardless of their importance, these metals are harmful to humans if they are too much in excess in the body. Some sources (e.g., Goyer and Clarkson, 2001; Reilly, 2004) have suggested that the list of chemical elements essential to human health should include (but might not be limited to) calcium (Ca), sodium (Na), potassium (K), magnesium (Mg), iron (Fe), manganese (Mn), copper (Cu), nickel (Ni), molybdenum (Mo), cobalt (Co), zinc (Zn), chromium (Cr), and selenium (Se). Among these dozen metals or elements essential to biological functions, the first four are generally available to the human body in large quantities and hence are not regarded as truly essential or in trace amounts.

Among the remaining nine elements on the above list, nickel, copper, and chromium appear to be of greater concern to environmental health and are thus discussed below. After all, even though iron overdose has been a leading cause of death among children for swallowing large amounts of iron-supplemented pills (e.g., vitamins), a common human health problem with iron is actually its deficiency generally seen in adults and children. Iron deficiency can cause notably anemia and hence fatigue.

14.4.1. Chromium

Chromium (Cr) is a steely-gray, lustrous, hard metal naturally occurring in rocks, and can be found in animals, plants, and soil. Although the metal exists in several oxidation states, its most commonly encountered forms are elemental Cr(0), trivalent Cr(III), and hexavalent Cr(VI). Elemental chromium is used mostly for steel production whereas Cr(III) and Cr(VI) are used primarily for chrome plating, dyes, pigments, leather tanning, and wood preserving. Chromium compounds are odorless and tasteless.

Chromium enters the atmosphere, water, and soil predominately in its trivalent (Cr^{3+}) or hexavalent (Cr^{6+}) form. In the air, chromium compounds are present mostly as fine dust particles which eventually settle onto the land and water. Chromium can attach firmly to soil particles. Only a small fraction of soil chromium can dissolve in water to be able to seep into the underground water layer. No significant amount of the metal from the water has been found to accumulate in fish.

Trivalent chromium, denoted by Cr(III) or Cr^{3+}, in trace amounts is an essential nutrient required for metabolism of sugar, fat, and protein molecules in humans and animals. Insufficient dietary intake of Cr(III) can actually lead to increase in certain hematological disorders and hyperinsulinemia (Anderson, 1994; Pechova and Pavlata, 2007).

In contrast, acute inhalation of Cr(VI) at high levels can cause irritation to the respiratory tract including predominately the nose. The symptoms typically include shortness of breath, coughing, and wheezing. Perforations and ulcerations of the septum, bronchitis, decreased lung function, asthma, and pneumonia are commonly seen as associated with chronic inhalation. Exposure to large amounts of Cr(VI) from ingestion can lead to gastrointestinal (GI) disorders, neurological effects, convulsions, liver and kidney damages, or even death (ATSDR, 2008c). In addition, dermal contact with certain Cr(VI) compounds can cause skin ulcers and contact dermatitis. The human body can detoxify some fraction of Cr(VI) to form Cr(III). Some people are extremely sensitive to Cr(VI) or even Cr(III), frequently with allergic reactions resulting in severe redness and swelling of the skin. Damage to sperms and the male reproductive system have been observed in laboratory animals exposed to Cr(VI).

The more important industrial sources of airborne chromium are those related to the production of ferrochrome (FeCr) alloy. Other industrial sources include: ore mining and refining; chemical and refractory processing; brake lining and catalytic converters for automobiles; leather tanneries; and chrome pigments (ATSDR, 2008c). Individuals may be exposed to chromium via dermal contact during the use or processing of the metal in the workplace. People in the general population are usually exposed to chromium by ingestion of foods and drinking water containing the metal or its compounds. Other potential sources of exposure for the general population are living around uncontrolled hazardous waste sites or near industries that use or process chromium compounds.

Several occupational and laboratory studies have implicated Cr(VI) as a carcinogen of the human lung (ATSDR, 2008c; U.S. EPA, 1999d). An increase in stomach tumor was observed in humans and animals exposed to Cr(VI) in drinking water. The mechanism of Cr(VI) carcinogenicity in the lung is thought to be via its reduction to Cr(III) which will lead to the generation of a number of reactive intermediates. Due to these findings, U.S. EPA (1999d) and IARC (1990) have both classified airborne Cr(VI) as a human (Group A and Group 1, respectively) carcinogen. The human carcinogenicity of Cr(VI) in drinking water was publicized in 2000 in the American movie *Erin Brockovich*.

14.4.2. Nickel

Nickel (Ni) is a silvery white, lustrous metal with a slight tinge of gold color. It is an abundant element occurring predominately in the form of nickel sulfide (NiS), nickel oxide (NiO), and nickel silicate (known as garnierite, $[Ni, Mg]_3Si_2O_5[OH]$) minerals in the Earth's crust. Small amounts of this metal are commonly found in the air, soil, water, and foods as a result of its widespread use. The use of nickel dates back to around 3500 BC. Nickel can be combined with other metals, such as iron, copper, chromium, and zinc, to form alloys. These alloys in turn are used to make coins, jewelry, and other items such as valves, spark plugs, catalysts, batteries, and heat exchangers. Most elemental nickel is used to make stainless steel, particularly in the early days. Nickel and its compounds have no characteristic odor or taste.

Small amounts of nickel are found in the ambient air as a result of releases from oil-burning power plants, sewage sludge incineration, and metal refining as well as other manufacturing facilities involving the use or application of nickel (ATSDR, 2005; IPCS, 1991). In the atmosphere, nickel often attaches to small dust particles which will settle onto the ground or get removed out of the air through precipitation. From industrial wastewater, nickel usually ends up in the soil or sediment where the metal will attach strongly to particles that contain iron or manganese. Nickel does not appear to accumulate in food chains in any considerable amount.

According to ATSDR (2005), inhalation is the major route of occupational exposure to nickel and its compounds. Food and drinking water are the main sources of exposure for the general population, with an average daily intake of 100 to 300 μg estimated for adults. Individuals may also be exposed to nickel from tobacco smoking and via contact with jewelry containing or stainless steel utensils made of this metal.

In humans, the most common health effect from chronic dermal exposure to nickel is allergic dermatitis, with skin eczema (rash and itching of the hands and forearms) being the most characteristic symptom. Despite the metal's possible essentiality to human health, it has been estimated that around 15% of American people are sensitive (allergic) to nickel. People can become sensitive to nickel when their skin comes in contact for a sufficiently long time with jewelry (e.g., earrings) or other items containing the metal. Once a person is sensitized to nickel, further contact with the metal may cause the allergic reaction to flare up. Some people sensitive to nickel may also have the allergic reaction when they consume foods and water contaminated by the metal or inhale dust containing the metal. Less frequently, certain other sensitized individuals could have asthma attacks following exposure to nickel by whatever route (ATSDR, 2005).

As implicated by a number of animal studies, chronic exposure to nickel or its compounds would cause GI distress (e.g., vomiting, nausea, diarrhea) as well as adverse effects on the blood, liver, kidneys, central nervous system, and immunological system. Long-term exposure to nickel via inhalation can specifically result in adverse respiratory effects, including bronchitis, decrease in lung functions, and a type of asthma specific to nickel exposure. Laboratory studies showed that soluble nickel compounds tended to be more toxic, (though not necessarily more carcinogenic) than nickel compounds that are less soluble, particularly from inhalation exposure (ATSDR, 2005).

Along with a handful of animal experiments, several epidemiological studies implicated an increase in the risks of lung and nasal cancers from exposure to nickel subsulfide (Ni_3S_2) and nickel refinery dusts (ATSDR, 2005). Lung cancer was also implicated in studies where animals were dosed with nickel carbonyl ($Ni[CO]_4$), which is a highly toxic soluble compound. Headaches, GI distress, and chest pain are commonly observed in patients of nickel carbonyl poisoning, followed by coughing, cyanosis, hyperpnoea (i.e., increase in the depth or rate of breathing), and weakness. The symptoms may be accompanied by fever and leukocytosis, with the more severe cases progressing to pneumonia, respiratory failure, cerebral edema, and ultimately death (IPCS, 1991).

Risks of lung and nasal cancers were found highest among workers exposed to metallic nickel over a long period of time or to high levels of the more soluble nickel sulfide and nickel oxide. IARC (1990) has classified nickel compounds as human (Group 1) carcinogens and metallic nickel as a possible human (Group 2B) carcinogen. And U.S. EPA

(1999e, 1999f) has classified nickel refinery dust and nickel subsulfide as human (Group A) carcinogens and nickel carbonyl as a probable human (Group B2) carcinogen.

14.4.3. Copper

Copper (Cu) is a highly malleable and ductile metal with a very high electrical and thermal conductivity. Pure copper has a freshly exposed surface in pinkish or peachy color. The metal occurs naturally in the environment and is one of the few metals occurring naturally as an uncompounded mineral. Copper is one of the oldest civilizations in humankind history, with a use history dating back to at least 10,000 years ago when the era then was known as the Copper Age.

Copper is an essential nutrient in humans, animals, and higher order plants. In mammals including humans, copper deficiency can cause neurodegeneration and a form of anemia specifically related to pancytopenia (i.e., reduction in red and white blood cell counts). The neurological disease can be seen most commonly in human infants with Menkes (kinky hair) syndrome, which is a genetic recessive disorder affecting copper levels in the body to eventually cause its deficiency. Copper is involved in the incorporation of iron into the heme group in hemoglobin.

Owing largely to its high thermal and electrical conductivity, copper is used extensively as a thermal or an electrical conductor to make various kinds of wiring products. Other products made with copper include plumbing fittings, sheet metal, roofing, rainspouts, cookware, doorknobs, and other fixtures in the house. Copper is also combined with other metals (e.g., zinc, tin) to make brass and bronze products. Some other copper compounds have been used as fungicides to treat plant diseases, for water treatment, and as preservatives for leather and wood.

Like many other metals, copper is released into the environment largely from mining and manufacturing operations or through wastewater discharging into rivers and lakes. Copper is also released from natural sources such as volcanoes, wind-blown dusts, decaying vegetation, farming, and forest fires. Copper released into the environment usually attaches to the clay, soil, sand, or organic matter particles. As with lead, copper itself does not break down in the environment. However, its compounds can break down easily to release free copper into the air, water, soil, or foods.

People may be exposed to copper from various common sources, such as by inhaling contaminated air, drinking contaminated water, and ingesting contaminated foods. They may also be exposed to copper via skin contact with the metal as well as with particulates or compounds containing the metal. High levels of copper can be found in drinking water when the house has copper pipes filled with acidic water or in lakes and rivers that have been treated with copper compounds to control algae. Soils located near copper smelting plants may also contain high levels of copper. In addition, people may be exposed to copper by ingesting vegetation treated with fungicides containing the metal as an ingredient, or if they reside close to or work in copper mines or facilities where the metal is processed into alloys or other products.

Ingestion of large amounts of copper sulfate ($CuSO_4$) can cause hepatic necrosis and even death. Even at moderate levels, inhalation of copper can induce irritation of the nose and throat. Experimental studies on humans showed that ingestion of drinking water containing copper at 3 mg or higher per liter produced GI symptoms such as nausea, vomiting, and diarrhea (Pizaro *et al.*, 1999). Studies also implicated that individuals with deficiency in the enzyme glucose-6-phosphate dehydrogenase would have a greater risk for the hematological effects of copper, even though the magnitude of the risk remained largely unknown (Goldstein *et al.*, 1985).

Available epidemiological studies have not indicated any link between copper exposure and cancer risk (IPCS, 1998). To this date, neither IARC nor U.S. EPA has classified copper or its compounds as potential human or animal carcinogens.

By most standards, the health effects of copper are not as severe as those of nickel or chromium VI. Copper is included in this section all because of the rising concerns over the recent dramatic increase of environmental exposure to the metal. There is rising indication that the widely used oral contraceptives by women can promote copper absorption and thereby can increase the level of copper in their blood (Berg at al., 1998; Liukko *et al.*, 1988). Studies also revealed that copper released from the equally widely used copper IUDs (i.e., intrauterine devices) could increase menstrual blood loss and pain in women (Cox and Blacksell, 2000; Hubacher *et al.*, 2006). Still another rising concern is that copper, along with iron and zinc, can act as a pro-oxidant to promote the generation of free radicals such as ROS (reactive oxygen species) which have been implicated in the pathogenesis of a few degenerative disorders such as Alzheimer's disease (Brewer, 2007; Christen, 2000) and the cardiovascular disease atherosclerosis (Brewer, 2007).

There is nonetheless also the prevailing issue that copper is one of the few best examples showing how an essential nutrient can become harmful to individuals with certain hereditary disorders. As a case in point, Wilson's disease (a.k.a. hepatolenticular degeneration) is an autosomal recessive genetic disorder that can result in a buildup of excess copper in tissues to cause damage in the eyes, kidneys, brain, and notably liver. Individuals with this genetic disorder thereby may suffer from severe neurological or psychiatric symptoms as well as liver disease. Severe cases need to be treated with chelation therapy or other medications to either remove the excess copper from the body or reduce its absorption into the body. In all cases, where the liver is severely damaged, a liver transplant may become necessary (Kaler, 2007).

14.5. Select Radioactive Metals

Radioactive metals are each a metallic element with an unstable nucleus that can spontaneously emit its protons, neutrons, or photons to generate the so-termed *alpha* (α), *beta* (ß), or *gamma* (γ) radiation. These types of radiation are capable of penetrating, to some degree, matter impervious to ordinary light. When two protons and two neutrons in the unstable nucleus are bound together as a particle, the emission (i.e., the release) of such is referred to as an α-radiation, α-ray, or the radiation of an α particle. On the other hand, a ß-radiation involves the emission of one electron converted from an excess neutron, or the emission of one positron converted from an excess proton, all in a nucleus containing an unbalanced number of protons and neutrons. When a nucleus emits an α or a ß particle, the nucleus is sometimes left in an excited state. Gamma decay occurs whenever a highly excited nucleus, as a result of falling down to a lower energy state, emits an electromagnetic type high energy photon known as γ particle.

Rays of α and ß particles are relatively non-penetrating. In fact, a thin sheet of aluminum is sufficient to halt their penetration. Yet sufficient external exposure to these particles can still cause localized damage (e.g., radiation burns to the exposed skin). In contrast, γ rays are more penetrating to the skin as they have the shortest wavelengths and hence the most energy in the electromagnetic spectrum. As such, γ rays can cause *diffuse* damage throughout the body, and have been used clinically to destroy cancer cells.

To this date, a total of 38 radioactive metals have been identified, including technetium (Tc), promethium (Pm), and all those above bismuth (Bi) in the periodic table (Figure 14.1). Actually, the last nine elements from 100 through 118 (i.e., those between darmstadtium [Ds] and ununoctium [Uuo], inclusively) should be classified as *suspected* radioactive elements only because their chemical and radioactive properties have yet to be (further) unfolded. Radium (Ra) and radon (Rn) are discussed here not only because they are ubiquitous in the environment, but also because they are highly carcinogenic.

14.5.1. Radium

Radium (Ra), with a silvery-white appearance, is both the *most* heaviest alkaline earth element (i.e., the heaviest in the heaviest series) and an extremely radioactive metal. It can exist in more than 20 atomic forms, each with a nucleus containing the same number of protons (thus the same atomic number) but a variable number of neutrons (thus resulting in a different atomic mass number). Each of these atomic forms is chemically referred to as an isotope, or loosely as a progeny particularly when it has a relatively short half-life. Radium is formed as a decay product of uranium (U) or thorium (Th) in the environment. Uranium and thorium are found in trace amounts in most rocks and soils. ^{226}Ra (that with 88 protons and 138 neutrons and hence the atomic mass of 226) and ^{228}Ra are two principal radium isotopes found in the environment.

As with any other radioactive metal, when radium undergoes radioactive decay, it divides into two parts. One part is the radiation and the other, a daughter nucleus. The daughter nucleus *per se*, like that of radium, may be highly radioactive and thereby may continue to undergo radioactive decay until a stable, nonradioactive daughter is born. The most stable isotope of radium is ^{226}Ra, with a half-life of about 1,600 years.

Radium was formerly used as a component of self-luminous paint for watch and clock dials, for instrument panels, and for compasses. It was added to some household products (e.g., toothpastes) or foods for taste or as a preservative until the late 1950s. Radium (mostly in the form of radium chloride [$RaCl_2$]) has been used in medicine as a radiation source for treatment of cancer and certain non-neoplastic diseases, such as the chronic inflammatory rheumatic disease termed *ankylosing spondylitis* involving primarily arthritis of the spine (Alberding *et al.*, 2006; Lassmann *et al.*, 2002). Radium has been used in radiography of other metals and as a neutron source for laboratory research.

Aside from being present in trace amounts in most rocks and soils, radium may be found in the air and water in certain areas, such as near uranium and thorium mines. The radioactive metal may therefore be found in plants through uptake from contaminated soils or in fish and other aquatic creatures through uptake from contaminated water. Consequently, humans can be exposed to at least a trace amount of the metal in the air, water, or foods. Uranium miners and those engaging in uranium grinding are expected to have the greatest risk of occupational as well as environmental exposure to radium.

No information on health effects is available for short-term exposure to radium, especially at low levels. However, as noted by ATSDR (1990), (subchronic) exposure to high levels of radium can cause anemia, teeth fracture, cataracts, necrosis of the jaw, abscess in the brain, and terminal bronchopneumonia. German patients who were injected with radium between 1946 and 1950 for treatment of certain diseases (e.g., tuberculosis) were found significantly shorter as adults than those not treated with the metal.

Long-term exposure to high levels of radium by the oral route is known to cause cancer in the lungs, bone, head, and nasal passage (ATSDR, 1990). IARC (2001) has classified ^{224}Ra, ^{226}Ra, ^{228}Ra, and their progenies as human (Group 1) carcinogens.

14.5.2. Radon

Radon (Rn) is a colorless, odorless, and tasteless radioactive noble gas. It occurs naturally as the decay product of radium and, as such, is said to be formed somewhat midway via the radioactive decay chain beginning with uranium or thorium. Therefore, inasmuch as uranium has been around since the Earth was formed and its most common isotope has a half-life of 4.5 billion years, both radium and radon likewise continue to be around for billions of years. Radon is one of the densest elements that remain a gas under normal conditions. Its most stable isotope is ^{222}Rn, with a half-life of ~4 days. Strictly speaking, radon is not a metal. However, its parent ^{226}Ra is indeed a true metal; radon is therefore treated in this section as if it were a metal, for the sake of simplicity.

Radon accounts for the majority of exposure to ionizing radiation by the general population. It is frequently the single largest source of a person's background radiation dose. This noble gas from natural sources can accumulate in buildings, predominately in confined areas such as cracks in a basement. Since radon is a *noble* gas with thereby *low* chemical reactivity, it can release itself easily from almost any type or form of chemical binding. As a gas it can travel freely and far enough to reach the air, water, and soil. Like radium, radon in high concentrations is typically found near uranium or thorium mines where milling operations of these grandparent radioactive metals occur.

When radon or its isotope undergoes radioactive decay, some of the decays expel α particles which become the main cause of human health concerns. Many epidemiological studies have implicated that this type of radiation from long-term residential exposure would increase the risk of developing lung cancer (Darby *et al.*, 2005; Krewski *et al.*, 2005). Accordingly, radon is now regarded as a significant indoor pollutant worldwide. In the United States, radon is treated as the second most frequent cause of lung cancer, only after cigarette smoking, and accounts for about 21,000 lung cancer deaths each year (U.S. EPA, 2003). IARC (2001) has likewise classified radon as a human (Group 1) carcinogen. Health effects other than lung cancer caused by acute or chronic exposure to radon, if any, are not known or not well documented at this moment.

References

Alberding A, Stierle H, Brandt J, Braun J, 2006. Effectiveness and Safety of Radium Chloride in the Treatment of Ankylosing Spondylitis. Results of an Observational Study. *Z. Rheumatol.* 65: 245-251 (in German).

Andersen RA, 1994. Stress Effects on Chromium Nutrition of Humans and Farm Animals. In *Proceedings of Alltech's 10th Annual Symposium, Biotechnology in Feed Industry* (Lyons TP, Jacques KA, Eds.). Loughborough, Leics, U.K: Nottingham University Press, pp.267-274.

ATSDR (Agency for Toxic Substances and Disease Registry), 1990. Toxicological Profile for Radium. U.S. Department of Health and Human Services Atlanta, Georgia, USA.

ATSDR (Agency for Toxic Substances and Disease Registry), 1997. Toxicological Profile for Cadmium. U.S. Department of Health and Human Services, Atlanta, Georgia, USA.

ATSDR (Agency for Toxic Substances and Disease Registry), 1999. Toxicological Profile for Mercury. U.S. Department of Health and Human Services, Atlanta, Georgia, USA.

ATSDR (Agency for Toxic Substances and Disease Registry), 2002. Toxicological Profile for Beryllium. U.S. Department of Health and Human Services, Atlanta, Georgia, USA.

ATSDR (Agency for Toxic Substances and Disease Registry), 2007a. Toxicological Profile for Lead. U.S. Department of Health and Human Services, Atlanta, Georgia, USA.

ATSDR (Agency for Toxic Substances and Disease Registry), 2007b. Toxicological Profile for Arsenic. U.S. Department of Health and Human Services, Atlanta, Georgia, USA.

ATSDR (Agency for Toxic Substances and Disease Registry), 2008a. Toxicological Profile for Cadmium (*Draft*). ATSDR, U.S. Department of Health and Human Services, Atlanta, Georgia, USA.

ATSDR (Agency for Toxic Substances and Disease Registry), 2008b. Toxicological Profile for Aluminum. U.S. Department of Health and Human Services, Atlanta, Georgia, USA.

ATSDR (Agency for Toxic Substances and Disease Registry), 2008c. Toxicological Profile for Chromium (*Draft*). U.S. Department of Health and Human Services, Atlanta, Georgia, USA.

Bakir F, Damluji SF, Amin-Zaki L, Murtadha M, Khalidi A, Al-Rawi NY, Tikriti S, Dahahir HI, Clarkson TW, Smith JC, Doherty RA, 1973. MethylHg Poisoning in Iraq. *Science* 181:230-241.

Berg G, Kohlmeier L, Brenner H, 1998. Effect of Oral Contraceptive Progestins on Serum Copper Concentration. *Eur. J. Clin. Nutr.* 52:711-715.

Berg KK, Hull HF, Zabel EW, Staley PK, Brown MJ, Homa DM, 2006. Death of a Child after Ingestion of a Metallic Charm – Minnesota, 2006. *MMWR* (*Morbidity and Mortality Weekly Report,* published by the U.S. Centers for Disease Control and Prevention) 55(23 March):1-2.

Berny PJ, Côté LM, Buck WB, 1992. Erythrocyte δ-Aminolevulinic Acid Dehydratase (ALAD) Activity as an Indicator of Lead Exposure in Dogs and Cats: Optimal Test Conditions. *Toxicol. Mech. Mthds.* 2:57-68.

Bhattacharyya MH, 2009. Cd Osteotoxicity in Experimental Animals: Mechanisms and Relationship to Human Exposures. *Toxicol. Appl. Pharmacol.* 238:258-265.

Brewer GJ, 2007. Iron and Copper Toxicity in Diseases of Aging, Particularly Atherosclerosis and Alzheimer's Disease. *Exp. Biol. Med.* 232:323-335.

Brzóska MM, Moniuszko-Jakoniuk J, 2004. Low-Level Lifetime Exposure to Cadmium Decreases Skeletal Mineralization and Enhances Bone Loss in Aged Rats. *Bone* 35:1180-1191.

Christen Y, 2000. Oxidative Stress and Alzheimer Disease. *Am. J. Clin. Nutr.* 71 (suppl):621-629.

Cox M, Blacksell SE, 2000. Clinical Performance of the Nova-T380 IUD in Routine Use by the UK Family Planning and Reproductive Health Research Network: 2-Month Report. *Br. J. Fam. Plann.* 26:148-151.

Crapper DR, Krishnan SS, Dalton AJ, 1973. Brain Aluminum Distribution in Alzheimer's Disease and Experimental Neurofibrillary Degeneration. *Science* 180:511-513.

Crapper DR, Krishnan SS, Quittkat S, 1976. Aluminum, Neurofibrillary Degeneration and Alzheimer's Disease. *Brain* 99:67-80.

Darby S, Hill D, Auvinen A, Barros-Dios JM, Baysson H, Bochicchio F, Deo H, Falk R, Forastiere F, Hakama M, Heid I, Kreienbrock L, Kreuzer M, Lagarde F, Mäke-läinen I, Muirhead C, Oberaigner W, Pershagen G, Ruano-Ravina A, Ruosteenoja E, Schaffrath Rosario A, Tirmarche M, Tomáek L, Whitley E, Wichmann H-E, Doll R, 2005. Radon in Homes and Risk of Lung Cancer: Collaborative Analysis of Individual Data from 13 European Case-Control Studies. *Brit. Med. J.* 330:223-227.

Gallagher CM, Kovach JS, Meliker JR, 2008. Urinary Cd and Osteoporosis in U.S. Women ≥50 Years of Age: NHANES 1988-1994 and 1999-2004. *Environ. Health Perspect.* 116:1338-1343.

Goldstein BD, Amoruso MA, Witz G, 1985. Erythrocyte Glucose-6-Phosphate Dehydrogenase Deficiency Does Not Pose an Increased Risk for Black Americans Exposed to Oxidant Gases in the Workplace or General Environment. *Toxicol. Ind. Health* 1:7-80.

Goyer RA, Clarkson TW, 2001. Toxic Effects of Metals. In *Casarett and Doull's Toxicology: The Basic Science of Poisons* (Klaassen CD, Ed.). New York, New York, USA: McGraw-Hill, Chapter 23.

Gurer-Orhan H, Sabırb HU, Özgüne H, 2004. Correlation between Clinical Indicators of Lead Poisoning and Oxidative Stress Parameters in Controls and Lead-Exposed Workers. *Toxicology* 195:147-154.

Hubacher D, Reyes V, Lillo S, Pierre-Louis B, Zepeda A, Chen P-L, Croxatto H, 2006. Preventing Copper Intrauterine Device Removals due to Side Effects among First-Time Users: Randomized Trial to Study the Effect of Prophylactic Ibuprofen. *Hum. Reprod.* 21:1467-1472.

IARC (International Agency for Research on Cancer), 1987. IARC Monographs on the Evaluation of Carcinogenic Risks to Humans, Supplement 7: Arsenic and Arsenic Compounds. Lyon, France: WHO Press.

IARC (International Agency for Research on Cancer), 1990. IARC Monographs on the Evaluation of Carcinogenic Risks to Humans, Volume 49: Chromium, Nickel and Welding. Lyon, France: WHO Press.

IARC (International Agency for Research on Cancer), 1997. IARC Monographs on the Evaluation of Carcinogenic Risks to Humans, Volume 58: Beryllium, Cd, Hg, and Exposures in the Glass Manufacturing Industry. Lyon, France: WHO Press.

IARC (International Agency for Research on Cancer), 2001. IARC Monographs on the Evaluation of Carcinogenic Risks to Humans, Volume 78: Ionizing Radiation, Part 2: Some Internally Deposited Radionuclides. Lyon, France: WHO Press.

IARC (International Agency for Research on Cancer), 2006. IARC Monographs on the Evaluation of Carcinogenic Risks to Humans, Volume 87: Inorganic and Organic Lead Compounds. Lyon, France: WHO Press.

IPCS (International Programme on Chemical Safety), 1991. Environmental Health Criteria 108 – Nickel. World Health Organization, Geneva, Switzerland.

IPCS (International Programme on Chemical Safety), 1998. Environmental Health Criteria 200 – Copper. World Health Organization, Geneva, Switzerland.

Ishimure M, 1990. *Paradise in the Sea of Sorrow: Our Minamata Disease.* Kyoto, Honshū, Japan: Yagamuchi Publishing House (translated by L. Monnet).

Kaler SG, 2007. Wilson's Disease. In *Cecil (Textbook of) Medicine.* (Goldman L, Asiello D, Eds.), Twenty-Third Edition. Philadelphia, Pennsylvania, USA: Saunders Elsevier, Chapter 230.

Kingston RL, Hall S, Sioris L, 1993. Clinical Observations and Medical Outcome in 149 Cases of Arsenate Ant Killer Ingestion. *J. Toxicol. Clin. Toxicol.* 31:581-591.

Krewski D, Lubin JH, Zielinski JM, Alavanja M, Catalan VS, William FR, Klotz JB, Létourneau EG, Lynch CF, Lyon JI, Sandler DP, Schoenberg JB, Steck DJ, Stolwijk JA, Weinberg C, Wilcox HB, 2005. Residential Radon and Risk of Lung Cancer: A Combined Analysis of 7 North American Case-Control Studies. *Epidemiology* 16:137-145.

Lassmann M, Nosske D, Reiners C, 2002. Therapy of Ankylosing Spondylitis with 224Ra-Radium Chloride: Dosimetry and Risk Considerations. *Rad. Environ. Biophys.* 41:173-178.

Liukko P, Erkkola R, Pakarinen P, Järnström S, Näntö V, Grönroos M, 1988. Trace Elements during 2 Years' Oral Contraception with Low-Estrogen Preparations. *Gynecol. Obstet. Invest.* 25: 113-117.

Lockhart WT, Atkinson JR, 1919. Administration of Arsenic in Syphilis. *Can. Med. Assoc. J.* 9: 129-135.

Markesbury WR, Ehmann WD, Hossain TI, Allauddin M, Goodin DT, 1981. Instrumental Neutron Activation Analysis of Brain Aluminum in Alzheimer Disease and Aging. *Ann. Neurol.* 10: 511-516.

McDermott JR, Smith AI, Iqbal K, Wisniewski HM, 1979. Brain Aluminum in Aging and Alzheimer Disease. *Neurology* 29:809-814.

Pattee OH, Pain DJ, 2003. Lead in the Environment. In *Handbook of Ecotoxicology* (Hoffman DJ, Rattner BA, Burton GA Jr, Cairns J Jr, Eds.). Boca Raton, Florida USA: Lewis Publishers, Chapter 15.

Pechova A, Pavlata L, 2007. Chromium as an Essential Nutrient: A Review. *Veterinarni Medicina* 52:1-18.

Peri DP, 1985. Relationship of Aluminum to Alzheimer's Disease. *Environ. Health Perspect.* 63: 149-153.

Pizarro F, Olivares M, Uauy R, Contreras P, Rebelo A, Gidi V, 1999. Acute Gastrointestinal Effects of Graded Levels of Copper in Drinking Water. *Environ. Health Perspect.* 107:117-121.

Reilly C, 2004. *The Nutritional Trace Metals.* Oxford, UK: Blackwell Publishing, Chapter 1.

Satarug S, Garrett SH, Sens MA, Sens DA, 2010. Cd, Environmental Exposure, and Health Outcomes. *Environ. Health Perspect.* 118:182-190.

Smith WE, Smith AM, 1975. *Minamata.* New York, New York, USA: Holt, Rinehart & Winston.

Trapp GA, Miner GD, Zimmerman RL, Mastri AR, Heston LL, 1978. Aluminum Levels in Brain in Alzheimer's Disease. *Biol. Psychiatry* 13:709-718.

U.S. EPA (U.S. Environmental Protection Agency), 1986. Health Assessment Document for Nickel. EPA/600/8-83/012F. National Center for Environmental Assessment, Office of Research and Development, Washington DC, USA.

U.S. EPA (U.S. Environmental Protection Agency), 1997. Hg Study Report to Congress – Volume V: Health Effects of Hg and Hg Compounds. EPA-452/R-97-007. Office of Air Quality Planning & Standards and Office of Research and Development, Washington DC, USA.

U.S. EPA (U.S. Environmental Protection Agency), 1998. Toxicological Review of Beryllium and Compounds (in support of summary information on IRIS). National Center for Environmental Assessment, Washington DC, USA.

U.S. EPA (U.S. Environmental Protection Agency), 1999a. Integrated Risk Information System (IRIS) on Cd. National Center for Environmental Assessment, Washington DC, USA.

U.S. EPA (U.S. Environmental Protection Agency), 1999b. Integrated Risk Information System (IRIS) on Arsine. National Center for Environmental Assessment, Washington DC, USA.

U.S. EPA (U.S. Environmental Protection Agency), 1999c. Integrated Risk Information System (IRIS) on Beryllium. National Center for Environmental Assessment, Washington, DC, USA.

U.S. EPA (U.S. Environmental Protection Agency), 1999d. Integrated Risk Information System (IRIS) on Chromium VI. National Center for Environmental Assessment, Washington DC, USA.

U.S. EPA (U.S. Environmental Protection Agency), 1999e. Integrated Risk Information System (IRIS) on Nickel Refinery Dust. National Center for Environmental Assessment, Washington DC, USA.

U.S. EPA (U.S. Environmental Protection Agency), 1999f. Integrated Risk Information System (IRIS) on Nickel Subsulfide. National Center for Environmental Assessment, Washington DC, USA.

U.S. EPA (U.S. Environmental Protection Agency), 2003. EPA Assessment of Risks of Radon in Homes. EPA-402-R-2003. Office of Radiation and Indoor Air, Washington DC, USA.

U.S. EPA (U.S. Environmental Protection Agency), 2004. Integrated Risk Information System (IRIS) on Lead and Compounds (Inorganic). National Center for Environmental Assessment, Washington DC, USA.

VanArsdale JL, Leiker D, Kohn M, Merritt TA, Horowitz BZ, 2004. Lead Poisoning from a Toy Necklace. *Pediatrics* 114:1096-1099.

Review Questions

1. How many elements in the periodic table may be classified as having metallic properties?

2. What are metalloids? List the elements in the periodic table that are considered as metalloids.

3. What are the three most toxic heavy metals? And what do they have in common in terms of their interference with the normal functions of enzymes in the human body?

4. Briefly describe the relationship between blood lead levels and the enzymatic activity of δ-ALAD in the human body.

5. What is a systemic poison? And which metal is most commonly referred to as such?

6. What is the most toxic form of Hg? And what are the likely adverse human health effects caused by this form (as evident from the Minamata disaster)?

7. What are the adverse human health effects commonly caused by the metal responsible for the *itai-itai* disease?

8. What appears to be the main controversy over the toxicity of aluminum in humans?

9. Which metal has its nefarious name as king of poisons? And in what oxidation state is this metal most toxic to humans?

10. Name a metal that, like lead, tends to stick to soil particles and at high levels can cause acute chemical pneumonitis.

11. Name the elements that are commonly regarded as essential trace metals.

12. Briefly describe the adverse human health effects caused by hexavalent chromium.

13. What is likely to happen to individuals sensitized to nickel who now have come in contact with foods or jewelry containing the metal?

14. What may happen to people exposed to high levels of copper, particularly when they have Wilson's disease?

15. What may be a potential major health problem for women who use oral contraceptives *and* engage in copper smelting operations?

16. What are radioactive metals? And how do they emit alpha, beta, or gamma radiation?

17. Which of the following types of radiation is most penetrating to the human skin? a) alpha; b) beta; c) gamma; d) non-ionizing.

18. What is a radon progeny? And what human health effects may be caused from long-term exposure to radon or its progeny?

19. List all the metals (whether or not due to their compounds only) discussed in this chapter that have been classified by IARC as a human (Group 1) carcinogen.

20. What human health effects may be caused from long-term exposure to radium?

21. Which of the metals in the periodic table are radioactive? And which are synthetic in origin?

CHAPTER 15

Pesticides and Pesticide Residues

15.1. Introduction

Pests of agricultural and public health concerns are defined as nonhuman organisms that are destructive or troublesome or living where they are not wanted. They thus represent a wide variety of nuisances including insects, weeds, fungi, bacteria, viruses, ticks, fleas, and rodents (or other unwanted small animals). Pesticides are active ingredients of products used to prevent, destroy, repel, mitigate, or otherwise control these pests. Most of these active ingredients are synthetic chemicals while many are highly toxic, carcinogenic, and capable of disrupting the endocrine system (Chapter 19) in humans and animals. The term *pesticide residues* refers to those *applied* pesticide particles remaining in the environment, especially in foods or food crops and on the workers. In practice, it is the pesticide residues, not pesticides, that are most relevant to environmental toxicology.

15.1.1. Health Impacts and Concerns

As estimated by WHO (1990), during the early 1990s there were around 3 million cases of acute, severe pesticide poisoning worldwide per year, of which about one-third were non-suicidal. This estimate did not include the many cases of chronic effects, those not reported, or those poisoned in a nonagricultural setting. In fact, it was estimated that the under-reporting rate of pesticide poisoning in Central America was up to 98% in those years, all due to poor access to hospitals and other health care facilities (Murray *et al.*, 2002). The acute toxicity of many pesticides to humans, as well as their excessive use, was emphasized by Rachel Carson (1962) in her classic *Silent Spring*. It was largely due to such concerns that the U.S. Federal Insecticide, Fungicide, and Rodenticide Act (FIFRA) was rewritten in 1972 to regulate not only the efficacy of pesticides, but also their sale and use, in an effort to protect human health and preserve the natural environment. This federal law has since been amended numerous times, including some significant changes in the form of the Food Quality Protection Act (FQPA) of 1996.

The FIFRA provides U.S. EPA with the specific authority to: (1) strengthen the pesticide registration process by shifting the burden of proof to the pesticide registrants; (2) enforce regulatory compliance against unregistered pesticide products; and (3) promulgate the regulatory framework missing from the original version of the law. The FQPA then amended both the U.S. Federal Food, Drug, and Cosmetic Act (Chapter 21) and the FIFRA by changing the way in which U.S. EPA assesses and regulates pesticide safety. The FQPA specifically mandates U.S. EPA to consider cumulative exposures (Chapter

23) to all pesticides that share a common mechanism of toxicity, particularly for young children who most health scientists believe are generally more sensitive or vulnerable to chemical exposure when compared to adults.

15.1.2. Pesticide Residues as Pollutants

Many pesticides used today can be treated not only as soil but also as water pollutants. As hinted in Chapter 5 (and a couple of other chapters as well), many environmental pollutants from a variety of natural and anthropogenic sources are subject to frequent mobilization and distribution across environmental compartments via various biological and chemical processes. The pesticides discussed in this chapter for the most part are no exceptions. Many pesticides are used on or for agricultural commodities in the form of pellet, powder, dust, and predominately spray solution. By convention, these pesticide residues are perceived more as soil- or land-borne than as water-borne pollutants due to their major uses or disposal sites being on land or soil properties (e.g., farmlands, landfills). Otherwise, the more persistent members of pesticides can be found eventually at substantial levels in ground waters, estuaries, rivers, or other water bodies, as through leaching and runoff. In fact, one of the most alarming effects of pesticide contamination of drinking water came to light around 2002, when the residues of many organochlorine (OC) and organophosphate (OP) pesticides were detected in bottled water sold in the Delhi region in India (Mathur *et al.*, 2003).

Some pesticides, particularly those of the soil fumigant kind, can also be detected in the air if they are persistent (and volatile) enough to evaporate off the soil, land properties, or water. Methyl bromide (CH_3Br), for example, was once widely applied as a soil or structural fumigant in many countries. A global full phase-out of this fumigant was scheduled for 2005 under the international treaty *Montreal Protocol on Substances That Deplete the Ozone Layer*. The major global concern with methyl bromide is that the fumigant is readily photolyzed in the air to release elemental bromine (Br) which is highly destructive to stratospheric ozone (O_3). Ozone in the stratosphere has the function to protect life on the Earth by absorbing over 95% of the sun's harmful ultraviolet light.

15.2. Use and Classification of Pesticides

Literally well over 800 different pesticide active ingredients are currently available in the market worldwide (e.g., Tomlin, 2011). While a few pesticide active ingredients are inorganics or from natural products such as sulfur (S), chlorine (Cl), mercury (Hg), copper (Cu), rotenone, and neem, most are synthetic organic compounds.

15.2.1. Statistics on Pesticide Use

As summarized in Table 15.1, the pesticide active ingredients used in the United States between 1982 and 2001 were consistently around 1.2 billion pounds per year (U.S. EPA, 2004a). For some uninformed reasons, the agency has stopped providing pesticide

Table 15.1. Estimates of Annual Amounts, in Million Pounds, of Pesticide Active Ingredients Used in the World, the United States, and the state of California (from 1989 to 2008), in All Market Sectors

Year	United States[a]					World[b]					California[c]
	Herbicide	Insecticide	Fungicide	Others	Total	Herbicide	Insecticide	Fungicide	Others	Total	Total
1989	567	123	98	405	1,193						113
1990	564	121	91	425	1,201						181
1991	546	114	86	408	1,154						161
1992	554	116	81	435	1,186						192
1993	527	115	80	440	1,162						200
1994	583	124	79	443	1,229						191
1995	556	125	77	452	1,210	2,210	1,500	550	1,450	5,710	205
1996	578	116	79	456	1,229						198
1997	568	112	81	467	1,228	2,254	1,470	539	1,421	5,684	208
1998	555	103	86	462	1,206	2,148	1,427	553	1,522	5,650	217
1999	534	126	79	505	1,244	2,040	1,417	556	1,666	5,679	204
2000	542	122	74	496	1,234	1,944	1,355	516	1,536	5,351	189
2001	553	105	98	472	1,203	1,870	1,232	475	1,469	5,046	153
2002											170
2003											176
2004											180
2005											195
2006											188
2007											172
2008											162

Sources: [a]U.S. EPA (2004a); [b]U.S. EPA (1997a, 1999, 2002, 2004a); [c]California Department of Pesticide Regulation (CDPR, 2008), which did (and still does) not provide the public with use statistics by target pest type or pesticide category.

use statistics to the public since 2001. There is nonetheless a strong belief that the annual usage in the nation has remained around 1 billion pounds in recent years. Supporting this speculation is the notion that the annual usage in the state of California has not reduced significantly in recent years (e.g., Table 15.1); and California is regarded as having one of the most extensive databases on pesticide usage in the world.

Another supporting fact is that the California usage contributes close to 20% of the total pesticide usage in the United States. This is a startling statistic as the state's cropland represents less than 4% of the total planted acreage in the nation. The estimates provided by U.S. EPA in the earlier years indicated that the pesticide active ingredients used in the United States represented nearly a quarter of the world's usage (i.e., around 5 billion pounds per year). U.S. EPA's data also showed that the largest uses of herbicides, insecticides, and fungicides, in that order, collectively accounted for 60% or more of all pesticide active ingredients used in the United States and worldwide (e.g., Table 15.1). The agricultural market sector was reportedly responsible for roughly 75% of each year's pesticide usage in the United States and worldwide. The home/garden, commercial, industrial, and government were (and still are) the major nonagricultural market sectors.

15.2.2. Classification of Pesticides

A common way in which pesticides are classified is according to the specific type(s) of pests that they each control or destroy. Pesticides thereby are commonly referred to as insecticides, rodenticides, herbicides, fungicides, nematocides, miticides, tickicides, algaecides, piscicides, avicides, bactericides, and so forth. There are however pesticides either belonging to a common product group or having unique biological functions that can (more effectively) be classified as such. These pesticides include, but are not limited to, fumigants, antibiotics, botanicals, anticoagulants, petroleum oils, plant growth regulators, and pheromones (e.g., Ware and Whitacre, 2004).

In environmental toxicology, however, pesticides may be best classified or characterized according to the chemical group(s) that they belong to. This is because pesticides in the same chemical family tend to share more similar pesticidal and toxicological properties. Of the numerous chemical groups involved (e.g., Ware and Whitacre, 2004), several are most often implicated in symptomatic illnesses (NEETF, 2002; Reigart and Roberts, 1999) and are hence considered to have greater public health concerns. The more prominent pesticides in these special chemical families are therefore discussed in the sections that follow, with a focus on their uses, pesticidal actions, and health effects.

15.3. Organochlorine Pesticides

Until the beginning of World War II, when organochlorines (OCs) and organophosphates (OPs) were first used as insecticides, chemicals used to control insects were limited to a few from the so-called multipurpose group consisting of primarily arsenicals, sulfur, nicotine, rotenone, and hydrogen cyanide gas. The OC pesticides are chlorinated hydrocarbon (i.e., organic) compounds. Because of their strong covalent chlorine-carbon (Cl-C) bonds and high lipophilicity, these compounds break down very slowly in the environment and tend to accumulate in the fatty tissues of humans and animals. Consequently, they tend to stay in the environment and the food web long after they have been applied. Most OCs were used as insecticides, with all being used rather extensively from the 1940s through the 1960s in agriculture or for mosquito control. DDT was the first OC insecticide used on a large scale in the United States, until it was banned in 1973 after reconsideration of its harm to the health of wildlife and humankind. Many OC insecticides are determined or suspected as capable of disrupting the endocrine system in the body (Chapter 19). Although most of these compounds are no longer used in the United States as many are treated as potent neurotoxicants, some are still being produced by American companies for use elsewhere, mostly in the developing countries.

As with many pesticides in other chemical classes, the OCs collectively are used on a wide variety of crops in various formulations. Whether in the form of spray, dust, or pellet, some OCs are applied to foliar surfaces to get rid of insects settling there. Some others are used to preserve wood from insect damage; and still some others are applied to control insects found in grain storage facilities. Structurally and broadly, the OC pesticides can fall into the following three subclasses: (1) the dichlorodiphenylethane-related; (2) the chlorinated cyclodiene-related; and (3) the chlorinated cyclohexane-related.

15.3.1. The Dichlorodiphenylethane-Related

The most prominent member in this diphenyl subclass is dichlorodiphenyltrichloro-ethane ($C_{14}H_9Cl_5$), known most commonly by its acronym DDT. Some other members are ethylan, methlochlor, methoxychlor, chlorobenzilate, and dicofol. The last two are examples of OC pesticides used more specifically as acaricides or miticides than as (general) insecticides. Some of the compounds noted above, such as dicofol and ethylan, do not contain exactly the bare bone structure *dichlorodiphenylethane* found in DDT (Figure 15.1), but only with the bulk of their structure looking similar to this nucleus. They are put in this subclass largely for their sharing similar toxicological properties with DDT.

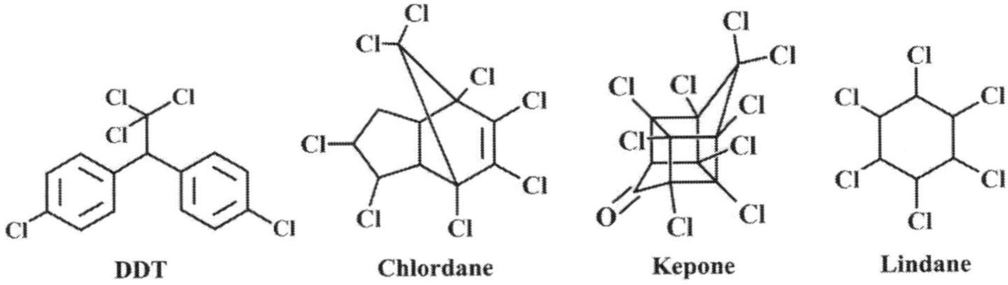

Figure 15.1. Chemical Structures of Four Select Organochlorine Pesticides

Of all the OC members in this subclass, DDT is the most widely known and the most notorious chemical in modern pesticide history. Nearly 1.4 billion pounds of DDT were applied in the United States for insect control between 1940 and 1970, with the peak annual use reaching nearly 80 million pounds in the year 1959 (U.S. EPA, 1975). DDT proved to be extremely effective against flies and mosquitoes. It works by binding to the voltage-gated sodium channel in the insect's nerve cell, thereby locking the channel in the open state to allow prolonged influx of sodium ions (Section 9.2.3). Such an "ion leakage" in turn will cause the nerve to fire repeatedly the electrical impulses expressed as muscle tremors, with the ultimate consequence being the insect's death. DDT is considered as a practical and powerful insecticide all due to its high specificity of binding to the sodium channel proteins in *insects*, but not in higher order animals.

This species-specific binding property that DDT possesses may explain in part why this and some other diphenyl OCs are found to be less toxic to mammalians from acute exposure when compared to OPs and pesticides in many other chemical groups. Nonetheless, due to their greater chemical stability and tendency to accumulate in animals, these diphenyl compounds tend to cause more severe *chronic* effects compared to OPs and pesticides in many other chemical groups. In general, exposure to the diphenyl OCs at high doses can affect the nervous system in humans, with acute signs of excitability, tremors, and seizures. Even at low doses, chronic exposure to OCs in this subclass, especially to DDT, can affect the liver (ATSDR, 2002a).

DDT is remarkably stable in the environment except when in the air under sunlight, where it will be broken down quickly (with a half-life of 2 or 3 days) to TDE = DDD (dichlorodiphenyldichloroethane, $C_{14}H_{10}Cl_4$) and DDE (dichlorodiphenyldichloroethylene, $C_{14}H_8Cl_4$). Both metabolites are equally persistent in the environment with physicochemical and toxicological properties similar to those of DDT. A study with limited data indicated a possible link between DDE exposure and Parkinson's disease (Koldkjaer *et al.*, 2004). Due to the way in which the two chlorides on their two benzene rings can be positioned, DDT, DDD, and DDE each have isomers in the *o,p'*- and *p,p'*-forms. The term *total DDTs* (*products*) refers to all the isomers of DDT, DDD, and DDE in a mixture. IARC (1991) has classified all DDT isomers as possible human (Group 2B) carcinogens.

15.3.2. The Chlorinated Cyclodiene-Related

This subclass (commonly referred to as *cyclodienes* for short) includes aldrin, chlordane, chlordecone (more known by its trade name kepone), dieldrin, endosulfan, endrin, heptachlor, mirex, and toxaphene. The nucleus of this subclass is a chlorinated methylene group forming a bridge across a six-member carbon ring (Figure 15.1). Cyclodienes are fairly stable in soils and moderately stable to sunlight in the air. As such, they have been widely used for control of termites and soil-borne insect larvae that feed on plant roots. Due to their persistence often resulting in a large amount of residues present beyond the time for harvest, many cyclodienes were restricted from use on most crops.

Cyclodienes are prominent blockers of *gamma*-aminobutyric acid (GABA)-activated chloride channels found in insects, in that these OCs have the ability to antagonize the inhibitory neurotransmitter GABA's action which otherwise helps increase the uptake of chloride ions when binding to GABA's specific receptor. GABA receptors are found in the brains of vertebrates and invertebrates, as well as in insect muscles. These receptors possess chloride channels that, if not open as in the absence of GABA, would reduce the chloride ion intake leading to hyperexcitation, convulsions, and ultimately death. This is because the influx of chloride ions has the effect of significantly lowering the transmembrane potential and thus the effect of dampening the firing of nerve impulses.

The cyclodienes produced in the greatest quantity were aldrin ($C_{12}H_8Cl_6$), its metabolite dieldrin ($C_{12}H_8Cl_6O$), and chlordane ($C_{10}H_6Cl_8$). Chlordane (Figure 15.1) is a broad-spectrum contact insecticide once widely used for nonagricultural purposes and on select field crops (e.g., maize, potatoes) and livestock. In the mid-1970s, about a third of this OC's use in the United States was on agricultural crops, with the rest being used in or around homes and by structural pest control operators (ATSDR, 1994). In 1974, over 20 million pounds of chlordane were produced in the United States (IARC, 1979). In 1986, two years prior to the cancellation of almost all of its uses, only about 4 million pounds of chlordane were distributed in the United States (ATSDR, 1994). Today, the use of chlordane in the United States is limited to the control of fire ants. Chlordane affects the nervous system, the digestive system, and the liver in humans and animals. People exposed to high doses of chlordane experienced headaches, irritability, confusion, gastrointestinal (GI) disorders, weakness, vision problems, and even convulsions or death. Some metabolites or by-products of chlordane, such as oxychlordane, heptachlor, and heptachlor epoxide, are known to be more toxic than the parent compound (ATSDR, 1994). Chlordane and heptachlor are also regarded as among the most potent cyclodiene carcinogens tested in animal models. IARC (1991, 2001) has thus classified both of these cyclodiene compounds as possible human (Group 2B) carcinogens.

In the United States, aldrin use reached a peak in 1966, close to 20 million pounds (ATSDR, 2002b). Environmental exposure to aldrin is mostly from eating contaminated root crops or seafood. This is equally true for dieldrin, inasmuch as aldrin can rapidly break down to dieldrin in the environment or within the animal body. Convulsions and deaths were seen in people ingesting large amounts of either cyclodiene. The health effects caused by these two cyclodienes, including those on the nervous system, may occur from exposure to even very small amounts if for a long period, since their residues will build up in the host's body for years. Some workers exposed to moderate levels of aldrin or dieldrin for a long period experienced headaches, irritability, and uncontrolled muscle movements (ATSDR, 2002b). Although both cyclodienes are shown to cause liver cancer in mice, IARC (1987) has not classified either as a potential human carcinogen.

Historically, the cyclodiene member most notorious for causing environmental pollution was chlordecone ($C_{10}Cl_{10}O$), known also by its trade name kepone (Figure 15.1). Kepone, structurally a cousin of aldrin, chlordane, and dieldrin, is chemically similar to mirex. It is a carcinogen and can cause damage to the liver, the kidneys, and the reproductive organs, in addition to the acute signs of headaches, tremors, and irritability if exposed at sufficiently high doses. From 1966 to 1973, each year about 400,000 pounds of kepone were produced by a U.S. manufacturing facility located in the state of Virginia (for use primarily as ant and roach baits). In late 1975, it was discovered that the manufacturer not only had its workers exposed to considerable amounts of this cyclodiene, but also had the wastes illegally dumped into the nearby James River (which flows into the Chesapeake Bay). Due to the pollution concern, the river from around the state capital Richmond to the Chesapeake Bay was then shut down for commercial fishing; and many businesses and restaurants along the river thereby suffered considerably. As of 2002, kepone (chlordecone) was still detected in the majority of white perch and striped bass samples taken from the James River (Luellen *et al.*, 2006).

15.3.3. The Chlorinated Cyclohexane-Related

This subclass includes the single hexachlorobenzene (HCB), also known as benzene hexachloride (BHC), and eight (theoretically possible) isomers of hexachlorocyclohexane (HCH). As their names imply, the only structural difference between HCB (C_6Cl_6) and HCH ($C_6H_6Cl_6$) is that the former has all its six chlorine atoms on a benzene ring and hence without any hydrogen possible, whereas the latter contains a non-double bond cyclohexane ring instead (*see*, e.g., lindane in Figure 15.1).

Hexachlorobenzene is a chemical once widely used to manufacture fireworks, rubbers, and ammunitions. It was also used extensively as a fungicide to protect onion seeds, sorghum seeds, wheat, and other grains until 1965. In the United States, no HCB has been manufactured for commercial use since the late 1970s. Chronic oral exposure to HCB in humans was linked to skin lesions with discoloration, ulceration, thyroid effects, photosensitivity, bone effects, loss of hair, and a liver disease termed *porphyria cutanea tarda*. Studies showed that HCB was capable of crossing the human placenta to accumulate in fetal tissues, transferring itself in human breast milk, and causing teratogenic effects, neurological changes, as well as embryolethality in animals (ATSDR, 2002c). Laboratory data revealed an increase in the incidences of liver, kidney, and thyroid cancers in animals (ATSDR, 2002c). IARC (2001) has thus classified HCB as a possible human (Group 2B) carcinogen. Hexachlorobenzene is highly toxic to aquatic organisms.

The predominate form of the cyclohexane HCH is its γ-isomer known commercially as lindane (Figure 15.1). In the United States, lindane has been used in various ways from protecting crop seeds against insects to controlling household pests. It is also the active ingredient in many shampoos and soaps medicated for control of head lice and scabies. Over 200,000 pounds of lindane were used annually in the United States, mostly on corn and wheat seeds (ATSDR, 2005). The γ-isomer is now banned or severely restricted in over 50 nations. In the United States, it is now restricted to seed treatment for a few grain crops, but still used for control of head lice and scabies except in California.

Lindane is a neurotoxicant that, like (most of) the cyclodienes, interferes with the action of GABA neurotransmitter by blocking the GABA receptor-chloride channel complex at the binding site specific to picrotoxin (a phytochemical known for its ability to block GABA receptors). All HCH isomers, including specifically lindane, can affect the nervous system, liver, and kidneys. Prenatal exposure to *beta*-HCH, another isomer frequently available as a by-product of lindane production, can affect brain development and has been linked to altered thyroid hormone levels (ATSDR, 2005). IARC (1987) has classified all HCH isomers as possible human (Group 2B) carcinogens.

15.4. Organophosphate Pesticides

As a chemical class of now ending with about 40 active members, OPs (organophosphorus compounds, or organophosphates for short) are still among the most widely used insecticides in the world. As the family name implies, each OP member contains the nucleus *phosphate* or a core component resembling a phosphoric salt (*see*, e.g., parathion in Figure 15.2). More specifically, each member is an ester of phosphoric acid (H_3PO_4) or a related acid (e.g., phosphonic acid C-PO[OH]$_2$; for further examples, *see* Corbett *et al.*, 1984). Many important macromolecules are structurally of the OP kind, including DNA (Chapter 18). OPs are also the basis of many herbicides and nerve agents. In addition, they are widely used as solvents, as plasticizers, and as extreme pressure additives for lubricants.

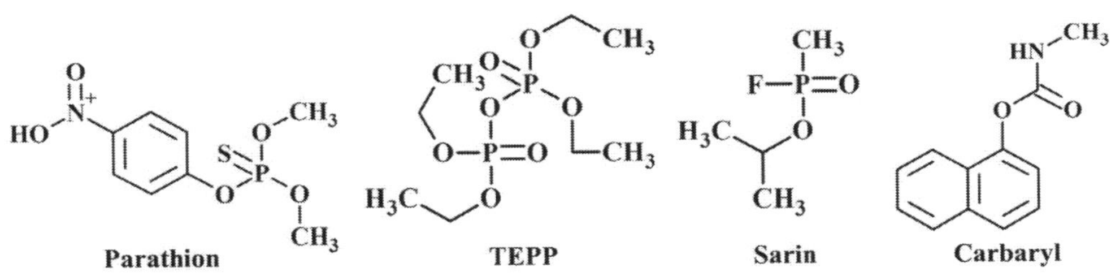

Figure 15.2. Chemical Structures of Three Select Organophosphates and One Carbamate

To many entomologists and environmental toxicologists, the term *OPs* usually refers to the group of insecticides or nerve agents that can affect the nerve function in humans, other mammalians, but primarily insects. As noted in Section 9.2.4, the notorious effects of these insecticides come about through their ability of binding to the active site of the enzyme AChE (acetylcholinesterase) at the brain synapses and neuromuscular junctions, where the enzyme's substrate acetylcholine (ACh) acts as a neurotransmitter. Biochemically, the inhibition of AChE by an OP is via an attack by the OP's relatively positive phosphorus (P) atom on the hydroxyl group (OH) of the amino acid serine ($C_3H_7NO_3$) residue. After an OP binds to this OH active site on the AChE's serine residue, the enzyme may be reactivated by a strong nucleophile such as pralidoxime (2-PAM), which along with atropine (otherwise a poisonous alkaloid) is the mainstay of treatment for OP poisoning. Another possible fate is that the OP may undergo endogenous hydrolysis by the enzymes paraoxonase or esterase. Yet in most cases, the affected AChE will "age or wear out" to become functionless inasmuch as the binding tends to be *irreversible*.

15.4.1. Delayed Neurotoxic Agents

Historically, the first OP used as an insecticide was the extremely potent AChE inhibitor tetraethyl pyrophosphate (TEPP, $C_8H_{20}O_7P_2$; Figure 15.2) developed in Germany in 1942. Other some 200 OP esters available at one time included the now commonly used insecticides malathion ($C_{10}H_{19}O_6PS_2$) and diazinon ($C_{12}H_{21}N_2O_3PS$), and the once widely used liquid plasticizer tri-*ortho*-cresyl phosphate (TOCP, $C_{21}H_{21}O_4P$). TOCP has never been knowingly used as a pesticide, but is discussed here to illustrate the importance of its delayed neuropathy effect shared by certain OP insecticides such as chlorpyrifos ($C_9H_{11}Cl_3NO_3PS$) and dichlorvos ($C_4H_7Cl_2O_4P$) when ingested at near lethal doses. TOCP was reportedly responsible for the infamous ginger Jake paralysis episode occurring in the United States in the early 1930s. This paralysis, nicknamed Jake leg, is characterized by unsteady gait, ataxia, muscular weakness, and flaccid paralysis of the limbs. Through its metabolic products formed one to two weeks later thereby resulting in a *delayed* onset, TOCP is then capable of inhibiting AChE. The delayed paralysis is typically manifested by wrist and foot drops. One of TOCP's neurotoxic metabolites observed as conclusively linked to the ginger Jake syndrome was tri-*ortho*-tolyl phosphate.

Before the year 1930, TOCP was widely used in the United States as an adulterant to boost the potability of Jamaica ginger extract (the so-called "Jake", which contains ~75% alcohol by weight) that was made available to circumvent the Prohibition laws. Early in the year 1930, thousands of American consumers began to lose the use of their hands and feet. The toxicity of TOCP was studied extensively soon after its use was linked to the episode. TOCP, along with some OP insecticides, can induce a delayed neuropathy after a single high dose. This is especially the case in chickens of about 60 days old, which are the species and the age that are now used by default as the standard animal model for assuring the negative *organo*phosphate-*i*nduced *d*elayed *n*europathy (OPIDN) potential of those OP compounds intended to be registered for use as insecticides. The initial effects of OPIDN do not seem to involve AChE inhibition, but rather the inhibition of the neurotoxic esterase (NTE) enzyme (Johnson, 1975, 1976). The exact role of NTE inhibition in the initiation of OPIDN remains unknown, although its enzymatic activity is known to be highest in nervous tissue (e.g., Hodgson *et al.*, 1998).

15.4.2. Acetylcholinesterase Inhibitors

Many OPs not involved in delayed neuropathy induction are still regarded as the most *acutely* toxic pesticides owing to their ability to inhibit AChE directly, rapidly, and effectively. They affect the enzyme in various ways and thus in their potential for poisoning. For example, parathion ($C_{10}H_{14}NO_5PS$; Figure 15.2) is one of the first OPs commercialized and is many times more potent than malathion, the latter being commonly used in combating the Mediterranean fruit flies and the mosquitoes that transmit West Nile virus. Signs and symptoms of OP poisoning include tremors, muscle twitching, and myosis, as well as the mnemonic acronym SLUDGE: *s*alivation, *l*acrimation, *u*rinary incontinence, *d*efecation, *G*I upset/diarrhea, and *e*mesis.

The popularity of OP insecticides increased after many of the OC (organochlorine) in-secticides were banned (worldwide) in the 1970s. Chlorpyrifos has been one of the few largest selling OP insecticides worldwide in the past decade. Some other commonly used OP pesticides (mainly as insecticides) are acephate, azinphos-methyl, diazinon, dichlor-vos, ethion, fenthion, fonofos, malathion, and terbufos. OP-based nerve agents include sarin ($C_4H_{10}FO_2P$; Figure 15.2), soman, tabun, and VX. Some of these nerve (gas) agents were not simply mass destruction weapons of the long (and recent, as in 2013 in Syria) past. In 1995, for instance, the Japanese domestic perpetrators named the Aum Shinrikyo cult terrorized their local communities by releasing sarin gas on several train lines of the Tokyo Metro subway, killing 13 people and injuring some 6,000 others.

Studies recently linked chlorpyrifos with delays in learning rates, reduced physical coordination, and behavioral problems in children, including particularly *attention deficit hyperactivity disorder* (ADHD) and pervasive developmental disorder problems (Rauh *et al.*, 2006). Although chlorpyrifos was banned from residential use in the United States in 2001, it is still applied intensively on some field crops such as corn and soy. In California alone, over 1 million pounds of chlorpyrifos were applied on crops each year between 1998 and 2008 (CDPR, 2008). Newer studies also showed that exposures to OP and OC pesticides were linked to an increased risk of Alzheimer's disease (Hayden *et al.*, 2010). In part because OPs degrade rapidly in both the environment and the animal body, not many members in this chemical group have been found to profoundly cause cancer or other severe chronic effects.

15.5. Major Carbamate Pesticides

Carbamates (CBs) are esters of one of the simplest amino acids named carbamic acid (NH_2COOH; *see*, e.g., that in carbaryl in Figure 15.2). Carbamate insecticides are said to interact with AChE in the same manner as OPs do, with the carbamate moiety attacking the same hydroxyl group in the serine residue at the enzyme's active site. Yet unlike the binding of OPs to the AChE's active site, that of CBs is generally *reversible*.

15.5.1. Carbaryl

Carbaryl (1-naphthyl methylcarbamate, $C_{12}H_{11}NO_2$; Figure 15.2), the first successful insecticide in the CB family, was introduced in 1956. Worldwide it has been used more than all the other CBs combined. In the United States, nearly 4 million pounds of car-baryl are used annually, with about half for agricultural use (U.S. EPA, 2004b). Carbaryl, also known by its trade name sevin, is registered for use on over 400 different sites in-cluding fruit and nut trees, vegetable and grain crops, nurseries, landscapes, lawns, golf courses, home gardens, and pet collars. Although carbaryl is readily absorbed through the human skin, it has low to moderate toxicity in humans other than its moderate ability to inhibit AChE. U.S. EPA (2007a) has classified carbaryl as a possible (Group C) carcino-gen based on vascular cancer observed in mice. Since its initial, inconclusive evaluation performed more than 30 years ago, IARC (1976) has not reached any decision regarding the carcinogenicity of carbaryl in humans or animals.

15.5.2. Propoxur and Several Others

Examples of CB insecticides that are used less frequently but commonly referenced include aldicarb, carbofuran, carbosulfan, ethiofencarb, methomyl, propoxur, alanycarb, pirimicarb, and indoxacarb. Of these, the last three are newer CBs; and the very last one has been designated by U.S. EPA (2000) as a "reduced-risk" pesticide. Propoxur, on the other hand, is perhaps the most toxic insecticide in the CB family, as well as one of the most widely used home and garden pesticides in the United States (Grossman, 1995). Propoxur is a non-systemic insecticide used to control a broad-spectrum of pests including fleas, ticks, mosquitoes, flies, cockroaches, and insects on lawns and turfs. Although U.S. EPA (1997b) has long classified propoxur as a probable human (Group B2) carcinogen, IARC (e.g., 1987) has not classified the CB as a potential human or animal carcinogen for lack of acceptable carcinogenicity data.

15.6. Pyrethrin and Pyrethroid Pesticides

As with the above three major chemical classes, all known pyrethroids have been used mostly as insecticides. This newer class accounts for a large percentage of the pesticide market today. Pesticides in this class are *synthetic* compounds with basic structure and chemical as well as toxicological properties very similar to pyrethrin. Pyrethrin is a *naturally occurring* compound found in certain species of the flowering plant *chrysanthemum*. The word *pyrethrum* generally refers to any of these plant species but sometimes is used synonymously with pyrethrin. Both pyrethrin and pyrethroid insecticides act by altering the nerve function of insects to ultimately cause their death.

When rats are exposed to pyrethroids at high doses, one of two symptom patterns is generally observed, depending on the chemical configuration of these modified pyrethrins. The Type I pyrethroids, which each *lack* a cyano group (C≡N), would produce the so-called T syndrome: *t*remors; aggressive sparring; and enhanced startle response. In contrast, the Type II variants, which each *contain* a cyano group, would produce the so-called CS syndrome: *c*horeoathetosis; *s*alivation; and seizures. Like DDT, both types of pyrethroids interact with the sodium channel on neuronal cell membranes, delaying closure of these channels. In addition, like the cyclodienes, Type II pyrethroids are capable of blocking the inhibitory effect of the neurotransmitter GABA.

15.6.1. Pyrethrins

The natural pyrethrum extract that possesses insecticidal activity is actually a mixture of six esters: three closely related esters of chrysanthemic acid named Pyrethrins I or chrysanthemates; and three corresponding esters of pyrethrin acid named Pyrethrins II or pyrethrates (WHO, 2009). The three Pyrethrins I esters are called pyrethrin I ($C_{21}H_{28}O_3$), cinerin I ($C_{20}H_{28}O_3$), and jasmolin I ($C_{21}H_{30}O_3$), whereas the three Pyrethrins II esters are named pyrethrin II ($C_{22}H_{28}O_5$), cinerin II ($C_{21}H_{28}O_5$), and jasmolin II ($C_{22}H_{30}O_5$).

All six botanical active ingredient esters degrade rapidly in sunlight (typically within 24 hours) and therefore are not economical to be used extensively for control of agricultural pests due to the high cost of reapplying them. When made available as insecticides, pyrethrin products are therefore likely formulated with synergists, such as with piperonyl butoxide or MGK-264, to extend or enhance their insecticidal properties. Piperonyl butoxide is a known inhibitor of several key microsomal oxidase enzymes. As such, it is used in the pyrethrin products to prevent these enzymes from clearing the pyrethrin off the insect's body, thereby prolonging the botanical compound's activity for acting as an insect neurotoxicant. MGK-264 (*N*-octyl bicycloheptene dicarboximide), which is an esterase inhibitor used as a mosquito repellent, has been found to be a very successful synergist (or more correctly, potentiator) of pyrethrins.

15.6.2. Pyrethroids

Pyrethroids have been synthesized to be very similar in structure to, but more stable in the environment than, pyrethrins. These synthetic compounds, especially when formulated with synergists (or potentiators), such as again with piperonyl butoxide or MGK-264, are comparatively more toxic to insects and inadvertently to mammals as well. Even though more than 1,000 pyrethroids have been synthesized, only about two dozens of them are actively used in the United States. Some of the active ones include the allethrin stereoisomers, bifenthrin, *beta*-cyfluthrin, *cis*-permethrin, cyfluthrin, cypermethrin, cyphenothrin, *delta*-methrin, esfenvalerate, fenpropathrin, *gamma*-cyhalothrin, imiprothrin, *lambda*-cyhalothrin, permethrin, prallethrin, resmethrin, sumithrin, *tau*-fluvalinate, tefluthrin, tetramethrin, tralomethrin, and *zeta*-cypermethrin.

The history of pyrethroids involves three or four periods over some 60 years. However, in terms of efficacy, they may be classified into two generations. The first generation began with allethrin in 1949, the first and only pyrethroid at that time, to several more effective ones used in agriculture in the early 1970s. The newer ones of this first generation included fenvalerate and permethrin, with highly effective (i.e., highly potent) insecticidal activity of around 0.1 lb of active ingredient per acre treated. They were relatively unaffected by sunlight, lasting about 1 week as efficacious foliar residues.

The current, second generation appears to be even more promising to the agricultural sector for at least two reasons. First, the photostability of the pyrethroids in this second group is up to 10 days. Second and the more important, their insecticidal efficacy is in the range of 0.01 to 0.05 lb of active ingredient per acre treated. Some of the pyrethroids in this generation include bifenthrin, cypermethrin, *lambda*-cyhalothrin, cyfluthrin, *delta*-methrin, and esfenvalerate.

Among all the pyrethroids available, permethrin ($C_{21}H_{20}Cl_2O_3$; Figure 15.3) is by far the most widely used. In agriculture, permethrin is used mainly on maize, cotton, wheat, and alfalfa crops, and to kill parasites on chicken and other poultry. It is used extensively in Europe as a timber treatment against wood-boring beetles. This pyrethroid is also used in health care to eradicate head lice and mites responsible for scabies, and in homes and industrial settings to control ants and termites. Permethrin is highly toxic to fish and particularly to cats, inasmuch as many cats died either after being given flea treatments with permethrin intended for dogs, or by coming in contact with dogs that had been recently treated with the pyrethroid (Dymond and Swift, 2008; Linnett, 2008; Sutton *et al.*, 2007). U.S. EPA (2007b) has classified permethrin as a likely (i.e., possible) human carcinogen on the basis of two reproducible benign tumor types (lung and liver) observed in mice along with equivocal evidence of carcinogenicity observed in rats. This classification is different from the decision made by IARC (1991), which has not considered the pyrethroid as a potential human or animal carcinogen for lack of sufficient evidence.

Contrary to the common health effect of the naturally occurring pyrethrins, very few cases of allergic contact dermatitis have been reported for exposure to pyrethroids. The most documented adverse effect of pyrethroids to humans appears to be paresthesia (ATSDR, 2003; O'Malley, 2007). Unlike allergic contact dermatitis (evidenced by skin rash, itching, and sometimes blisters), paresthesia is an abnormal cutaneous sensation involving feelings of pins and needles on the exposed skin.

Pyrethroids are regarded as among the least acutely toxic of all insecticides to mammals, as they are applied at very low rates and are quickly detoxified by metabolic processes. However, they are an excitatory nerve poison that still can cause convulsions and even death to animals when exposed to at sufficiently high doses for a long period of time. Animal studies showed that certain pyrethroids were carcinogenic (U.S. EPA, 2007b), able to cause liver damage (Hayes, 1982), and capable of inducing adverse effects on the endocrine or immunological system (ATSDR, 2003). In addition to insects, many pyrethroids have been found toxic to fish, other aquatic organisms, and birds.

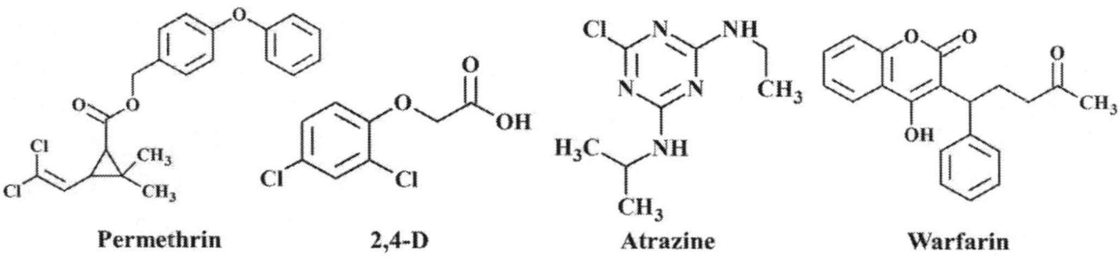

Figure 15.3. Chemical Structures of Four Select Pesticides, with One from
Each of the Pyrethroid, Phenoxy, Triazine, and Coumarin Families

15.7. Major Phenoxy Pesticides

The number of chemical classes involved in getting rid of weeds or undesired plants is greater than those involved in controlling any other type of pests. Of all the herbicides available, the *phenoxy* ($C_6H_5O^-$) compounds are among the most studied largely due to the environmental health concerns with their two prominent members, which are more commonly known by their acronyms 2,4-D (2,4-dichlorophenoxyacetic acid, $C_8H_6Cl_2O_3$) and 2,4,5-T (2,4,5-trichlorophenoxyacetic acid, $C_8H_5Cl_3O_3$). The only structural difference between 2,4-D (Figure 15.3) and 2,4,5-T is that the latter has an additional chlorine (and hereby 1 hydrogen fewer) attaching to its benzene ring in the number 5 position and accordingly is named 2,4,*5-trichloro*phenoxyacetic acid. Most phenoxy herbicides have some phytohormone or plant growth regulator properties as they all have some resemblance to the natural growth hormone indoleacetic acid. All members in the indoleacetic acid class act by inducing rapid, uncontrolled growth of treated broadleaf weeds, ultimately killing them. Some less familiar representatives of phenoxy herbicides include MCPA (2-methyl-4-chlorophenoxyacetic acid), 2,4-DB (4-[2,4-dichlorophenoxybutyric acid), and silvex (2-[2,4,5-trichlorophenoxy]propionic acid).

15.7.1. Dichlorophenoxyacetic Acid (2,4-D)

2,4-D (dichlorophenoxyacetic acid) is one of the most widely used herbicides in the world, with approximately 46 million pounds being used annually in the United States alone (U.S. EPA, 2005a). In nonagricultural settings, it is widely used on lawns, rangelands, and rights-of-way for control of unwanted broadleaf plants. In agriculture, it is used mainly in fields where cereal, grain, sugarcane, and other row crops are planted or to be planted. No alarming acute adverse effects to human or animal health have been associated with the widespread use of 2,4-D (or of most other phenoxy herbicides including 2,4,5-T). However, increased risks of non-Hodgkin lymphoma and amyotrophic lateral sclerosis have been linked to long-term exposure to 2,4-D. At one time and *as a group*, several phenoxy members including 2,4-D and 2,4,5-T were classified as possible human (Group 2B) carcinogens (IARC, 1987). Both 2,4-D and 2,4,5-T recently have become the subject of extended investigation for two subtle reasons.

One subtle reason is that both 2,4-D and 2,4,5-T were widely used as a mixture coded Agent Orange between 1962 and 1971 during the Vietnam War. During that period, the U.S. military there sprayed millions of gallons of the mixture and other herbicides to remove leaves from trees that would otherwise provide cover for enemy forces. Following exposure to these herbicides, a group of U.S. Vietnam veterans subsequently reported to have suffered a number of diseases including chloracne, acute and subacute peripheral neuropathy, chronic lymphocytic leukemia, non-Hodgkin lymphoma, and prostate cancers (e.g., IOM, 2010). A government report stated that for some 5 million Vietnamese exposed to Agent Orange, as many as 400,000 were later found to have early death or disabilities, along with some 500,000 children born with certain birth defects (York and Mick, 2008). Some samples from Agent Orange production were detected to contain excessive amounts of a highly toxic impurity known as 2,3,7,8-tetrachlorodibenzo-*p*-dioxin (2,3,7,8-TCDD, or dioxin for short). The potency and environmental health impacts of dioxin and other persistent organic pollutants are discussed in Chapter 16.

Another subtle reason for the extended investigation of 2,4-D is due to its widespread use on home lawns and golf courses. Due to the increasing concern with children health, especially in the United States as evident from the passage of the FQPA in 1996, more attention is now given to assess the health risk for children playing on lawns treated with herbicides. Increased efforts have also been made to ensure that golfers are free from significant exposure to harmful pesticides since these clients are often charged a high fee for playing on a golf course which is repeatedly used by many players and is frequently treated with herbicides at high rates. Yet more importantly, herbicide contamination on golf courses can easily extend to the nearby groundwater through runoff and leaching.

15.7.2. Trichlorophenoxyacetic Acid (2,4,5-T)

The reality that 2,4,5-T was phased out completely in the United States by 1985 suggested that it was determined as more toxic and problematic than 2,4-D. In fact, it was 2,4,5-T and its salts and esters, not 2,4-D, that were among the substances restricted for international trade by the global treaty *Rotterdam Convention (on the Prior Informed Consent Procedure for Certain Hazardous Chemicals and Pesticides in International Trade)*, which entered into force in 2004. These cancellation and trade restriction actions had the implication that the contamination of Agent Orange by 2,3,7,8-TCDD was more from the production of 2,4,5-T than from that of 2,4-D.

The global use of 2,4,5-T was phased out or restricted not only due to its production tending to be contaminated with 2,3,7,8-TCDD, but also due to its potent teratogenicity found in mice at the time (Courtney *et al.*, 1970). Otherwise, like 2,4-D, 2,4,5-T may not be considered to have high toxicity in mammals at low doses, despite the fact that IARC (1987) once classified both herbicides as possible human (Group 2B) carcinogens.

15.8. Major Triazine Pesticides

Like the phenoxies, the triazine compounds are a widely known group of herbicides but with fewer members. Herbicides in this group recently have received increasing attention all due to the heavy use and notoriety of its member atrazine ($C_8H_{14}ClN_5$; Figure 15.3). All triazines contain a "pseudo-benzene" ring nucleus, with three of the carbons in the benzene ring replaced with nitrogen atoms (and thus with the prefix "tri" added to the part "azine" which refers to the nitrogen-containing ring). All triazines are strong inhibitors of photosynthesis at photosystem II site A, where they block the transport of electrons and light energy. Some less notorious triazine members are simazine, propazine, prometon, prometryn, ametryn, and terbutryne, with the first two being closer to atrazine in terms of chemical and toxicological properties. Actually, several years ago U.S. EPA (2006a) performed a cumulative risk assessment for atrazine, simazine, and propazine on the decision that the three chlorinated triazines share a common mechanism of toxicity.

15.8.1. Atrazine

Even though the use of atrazine is now prohibited in the European Union (EU) states (nations), it is one of the most heavily used herbicides in some 80 other nations including the United States. Around 80 million pounds of atrazine were applied in the United States in 2003, primarily in cornfields. Its use remains controversial due to its adverse effects on nontarget species, such as amphibians, and to its widespread contamination of waterways and drinking water supplies. Yet as noted in a U.S. EPA (2003) document, the total national economic impact in the United States would exceed $2 billion a year if atrazine were banned from use as a weed killer in corn and other row crop fields.

Atrazine was banned in EU in 2004 not only because of the concern for its persistent groundwater contamination, but also due to a number of significant findings on its adverse health effects. The herbicide has been alleged to be a strong endocrine disruptor. Although it has not been classified as a potential human or animal carcinogen (IARC, 1999), studies showed that atrazine increased the risk of testicular cancer and the aromatase levels in animal cells (Fan *et al.*, 2007). Aromatase is an enzyme that converts testosterone to estrogen; its excessive elevation thus increases the risk of feminization in animals (e.g., amphibians, fish). Atrazine was also linked to low sperm counts in men. Other epidemiological studies suggested that even when atrazine's water concentrations came to near the U.S. federal MCL (maximum contaminant level) of 3 ppb (parts per billion), they would still be harmful, with implications for birth defects or low birth weights in humans (e.g., Ochoa-Acuña *et al.*, 2009; Munger *et al.*, 1977). Meanwhile, U.S. EPA (2003, 2006a) has maintained that atrazine poses no harm to the American public including young children, and does not adversely affect amphibian gonadal development.

15.8.2. Simazine and Propazine

Simazine ($C_7H_{12}ClN_5$) is predominately a pre-emergence pesticide applied to control annual grasses and broadleaf weeds in soils where almonds, apples, avocados, corn, established Christmas trees, grapes, and other crops are or will be planted, and in non-cropped areas such as around buildings, lawns, and rights-of-way. Its major use is in cornfields where it is often applied as a mixture with atrazine. Some people who drank water that contained simazine exceeding the MCL of 4 ppb were found to have problems with their blood (U.S. CFR, 2010). Skin rashes and dermatitis were also observed in workers exposed to simazine (Stevens and Summer, 1991). Like atrazine, simazine has not been classified as a potential human or animal carcinogen (IARC, 1999).

Propazine ($C_9H_{16}ClN_5$) is used as a post-emergence selective herbicide in fields where carrots, celery, and fennel are planted. It is also used as a pre-emergence herbicide for control of broadleaf weeds and annual grasses but largely in the sweet sorghum field. Propazine is less toxic to mammals compared to atrazine or simazine. There is some evidence though linking the three triazines to neuroendocrine disruption (U.S. EPA, 2006b). IARC has not yet evaluated propazine's carcinogenicity to humans or animals.

15.9. Coumarin and Indandione Pesticides

Both of these two classes are anticoagulants used to control rodent pests by inhibiting prothrombin formation, the process in blood responsible for clotting (Section 9.4.1). Vitamin K is commonly used as the choice of antidote for accidental poisoning by most anticoagulants belonging to these two classes. Anticoagulant poisoning is a major safety and health problem in the United States. In 2007 alone, over 10,000 cases were reported to the various poison control centers. Of these cases, over 95% involved accidental ingestion and over 85% occurred in children less than 6 years old (Bronstein *et al.*, 2007). To protect children from accidental ingestion of these anticoagulants, registered labels require that the treated baits be placed in tamper-proof boxes or in stations inaccessible to children. There are rodenticides available without anticoagulant properties, such as DDT, bromethalin, thallium sulfate, red squill, strychnine, and zinc phosphide. Bromethalin is a new lethal rodenticide acting on the CNS (central nervous system) by uncoupling of oxidative phosphorylation (as defined in Section 9.5.2.F). Red squill is a compound of the glycoside family extracted from the bulb of the Mediterranean squill plant *Urginea maritima*. Strychnine is a highly toxic alkaloid from the Asiatic tree *Strychnos nux vomica*.

15.9.1. Coumarins

Warfarin (named after the acronym WARF for the U.S. *W*isconsin *A*lumni *R*esearch *F*oundation; $C_{19}H_{16}O_4$; Figure 15.3) is the most successful of all known coumarin rodenticides in that rats do not develop bait shyness to it. Other known coumarin rodenticides include coumachlor, coumatetralyl, coumafuryl, dicumarol, and the two newer members brodifacoum and bromadiolone. The structures of these rodenticides all bear the nucleus coumarin ($C_9H_6O_2$) which can be found in many plants and *per se* has no anticoagulant activity until after its transformation to the anticoagulant species by fungi or other means. While coumarin has medical value, the phytocompound is moderately toxic to the liver and kidneys. Rats and other rodents have the specific and extra ability to oxidize coumarin to 3,4-coumarin epoxide, a metabolite that can cause internal hemorrhage and death.

15.9.2. Indandiones

This subgroup refers to all the synthetic anticoagulants derived from 1,3-indandione which is an isomer of coumarin and hence has the same molecular formula ($C_9H_6O_2$) as coumarin. The more prominent indandione anticoagulants include pindone, chlorophacinone, and diphacinone. The last two have the ability to uncouple oxidative phosphorylation. This additional ability partially explains the success of the two as a single-dose rodenticide capable of causing lethal neurological and cardiopulmonary injuries in the rat before hemorrhage can take place. Neither of the two non-anticoagulant injuries mentioned here has been reportedly associated with human poisoning.

15.10. Select Novel/Specialty Pesticides

There are many more novel, loner, and specialty pesticides available in the market today than can be accounted for in this section. Only a very few of the more prominent and more intriguing are introduced here as a reminder that many more pesticides or pesticide classes are available than those covered in this chapter. Neonicotinoids are a class of newer insecticides worth considering here because of their widespread use and low toxicity to mammals. In this section, glyphosate, paraquat, and sodium monofluoroacetate (a.k.a. Compound 1080) are treated as among the loner or specialty group, for lack of a better term. They are included here likewise due to their current or once widespread use, but more to their unique toxicological properties.

15.10.1. Neonicotinoids

The mode of pesticidal action of neonicotinoid compounds, which are produced by the tobacco plants, is similar to that of the natural insecticide nicotine. They all act on the target insect's CNS by causing excitation of its nerves and eventually paralysis which can lead to death. Because these compounds bind at a different site called the postsynaptic *nicotinic* acetylcholine receptor, they are not cross-resistant to the CB (carbamate), OP (organophosphate), or pyrethroid insecticides. As a group, neonicotinoids are effective against sucking insects and the chewing ones, such as beetles, some Lepidoptera, and particularly cutworms. All neonicotinoid compounds have been classified as for general use and registered under U.S. EPA's Conventional Reduced Risk Program mainly due to their favorable toxicological profiles.

Imidacloprid ($C_9H_{10}ClN_5O_2$; Figure 15.4) was first marketed in the United States in 1992 and is currently the most widely used insecticide in the neonicotinoid group. It has a wide range of target pests and sites including soils, seeds, pets, and foliar applications to a variety of crops (e.g., field crops, vegetables, pome fruits, pecans, turf). It has a long residual activity and is effective against a wide range of insects (e.g., sucking insects, whiteflies, turf insects, and Colorado potato beetle). U.S. EPA (2005b) has qualified the insecticide as a "Group E" carcinogen (i.e., one with no evidence of carcinogenicity). In animals and humans, imidacloprid is quickly and almost completely absorbed from the GI tract and eliminated via urine and feces within 48 hours. Among all the neonicotinoids available, imidacloprid is the most toxic to birds and fish. Both imidacloprid and another neonicotinoid called thiamethoxam are highly toxic to honeybees and have been linked to the abrupt disappearance of honeybee colonies across the United States, a phenomenon known as colony collapse disorder (CCD) or honeybee depopulation syndrome. CCD has allegedly jeopardized the production of crops that rely on bees for pollination.

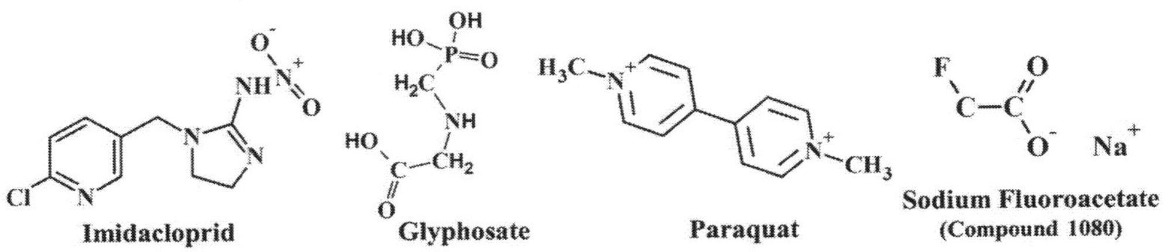

Figure 15.4. Chemical Structures of Four Select Novel/Specialty Pesticides

15.10.2. Glyphosate, Paraquat, and Compound 1080

Glyphosate ($C_3H_8NO_5P$; Figure 15.4) is the common name for N-[phosphonomethyl]-glycine, a nonselective systemic herbicide used to kill weeds, especially perennials. It is among the most used herbicides in the United States. Its most common uses include control of broadleaf weeds and grasses grown in hay/pasture, soybeans, field corn, lawns, turf, rights-of-way, forest plantings, and greenhouses, with about 85 to 90 million pounds being used in the agricultural sector (U.S. EPA, 2004a). The American public is perhaps more familiar with glyphosate under the trade name Roundup, which is readily available in stores where gardening products and equipment are sold. As with another herbicide named sulfosate, glyphosate acts by inhibiting the enzyme EPSP synthase responsible for catalyzing the synthesis of the aromatic amino acids phenylalanine, tryptophan, and tyrosine. The herbicide's use is limited to foliar applications as it will be rapidly and firmly bound to soil particles. Glyphosate, though having a Toxicity Category I (i.e., so classified due to being either severely irritating or highly toxic) for eye irritation, is rated least dangerous in comparison to other herbicides or pesticides. Nonetheless, a recent *in vitro* study showed that, even at low doses, various formulations of glyphosate and its metabolic products could induce apoptosis (programmed cell death) as well as necrosis in the umbilical, embryonic, and placental cells (Benachour and Sralini, 2009).

Paraquat (trade name of N,N'-dimethyl-4,4'-bipyridinium dichloride, $C_{12}H_{14}Cl_2N_2$; Figure 15.4) is a quaternary nitrogen herbicide widely used in the world until recently overtaken by glyphosate. It is a potent, fast-acting, and nonselective photosynthesis inhibitor, killing green plant tissue on contact. The herbicide is also highly toxic to humans when swallowed, often leading to acute respiratory distress syndrome with no specific antidotes. Even a single gulp can cause death from fibrous tissue developing in the lungs, leading to asphyxiation. The actual mechanism by which paraquat damages the lungs remains unknown. After the herbicide enters the body, even via the oral or dermal route, it will be distributed to all parts of the body including the liver, the kidneys, and particularly the lungs. Long-term exposure to low levels of paraquat may cause chronic pneumonitis. IARC has not evaluated paraquat for carcinogenicity. U.S. EPA (1997c) on the other hand has qualified the herbicide as a Group E carcinogen (i.e., no carcinogenicity to humans) for lack of evidence of carcinogenicity in two animal studies.

Sodium (mono)fluoroacetate ($FCH_2CO_2^-Na^+$; Figure 15.4) occurs naturally as an anti-herbivore metabolite in several species of Australian and African plants that have been implicated for the poisoning of livestock grazing on them (U.S. EPA, 1995). The compound can also be produced as a derivative of fluoroacetic acid. This organofluorine derivative is known commonly as Compound 1080, with the number reportedly coming from an invoice number that the material was assigned during its investigation in the U.S. government laboratories (U.S. EPA, 1995). Compound 1080 is especially toxic to warm-blooded animals, including humans, and is used mainly as a rodenticide. Dogs and cats appear to be most susceptible to poisoning by fluoroacetate, a compound similar to acetate ($CH_3CO_2^-$) which plays a key role in cellular metabolism. Fluoroacetate disrupts the Krebs cycle by combining with coenzyme A to form fluoroacetyl CoA which reacts with the enzyme citrate synthase to produce fluorocitrate (Section 9.4.2). The resultant fluorocitrate is a lethal metabolite in that it will bind tightly to the enzyme aconitase, thereby halting all other reactions in the Krebs cycle (while at the same time causing the accumulation of a substantial amount of citric acid in the blood) to deprive the affected cells of energy. Such a radical energy deprivation can lead to convulsions and death from cardiac failure or respiratory arrest. Many invertebrates (e.g., cockroaches, aphids, moth, fleas, ants) are also thought to be susceptible to fluoroacetate poisoning (Notman, 1989).

References

ATSDR (Agency for Toxic Substances and Disease Registry), 1994. Toxicological Profile for Chlordane. U.S. Department of Health and Human Services, Atlanta, Georgia, USA.

ATSDR (Agency for Toxic Substances and Disease Registry), 2002a. Toxicological Profile for DDT, DDE, and DDD. U.S. Department of Health and Human Services, Atlanta, Georgia, USA.

ATSDR (Agency for Toxic Substances and Disease Registry), 2002b. Toxicological Profile for Aldrin/Dieldrin. U.S. Department of Health and Human Services, Atlanta, Georgia, USA.

ATSDR (Agency for Toxic Substances and Disease Registry), 2002c. Toxicological Profile for Hexachlorobenzene. U.S. Department of Health and Human Services, Atlanta, Georgia, USA.

ATSDR (Agency for Toxic Substances and Disease Registry), 2003. Toxicological Profile for Pyrethrins and Pyrethroids. U.S. Department of Health and Human Services, Atlanta, Georgia, USA.

ATSDR (Agency for Toxic Substances and Disease Registry), 2005. Toxicological Profile for Hexachlorocyclohexane. U.S. Department of Health and Human Services, Atlanta, Georgia, USA.

Benachour N, Séralini GE, 2009. Glyphosate Formulations Induce Apoptosis and Necrosis in Human Umbilical, Embryonic, and Placental Cells. *Chem. Res. Toxicol.* 22:97-105.

Bronstein AC, Spyker DA, Cantilena LR Jr, Green JL, Rumack BH, Heard SE, 2008. Annual Report of the American Association of Poison Control Centers' National Poison Data System (NPDS): 25th Annual Report. *Clin. Toxicol. (Phila)* 46:927-1057.

Carlson LR, 1962. *Silent Spring*. Boston, Massachusetts, USA: Houghton Mifflin.

CDPR (California Department of Pesticide Regulation), 2008. Summary of Pesticide Use Report Data, 2008, Indexed by Chemical. Cal/EPA Department of Pesticide Regulation, Sacramento, California, USA.

Corbett JR, Wright K, Baillie RC, 1984. *The Biochemical Mode of Action of Pesticides*. London, UK: Academic Press.

Courtney KD, Gaylor DW, Hogan MD, Falk HL, Bates RR, Mitchell I, 1970. Teratogenic Evaluation of 2,4,5-T. *Science* 168:864-866.

Dymond NL, Swift IM, 2008. Permethrin Toxicity in Cats: A Retrospective Study of 20 Cases. *Aust. Vet. J.* 86:219-223.

Fan WQ, Yanase T, Morinaga H, Gondo S, Okabe T, Nomura M, Komatsu T, Morohashi K-I, Hayes TB, Takayanagi R, Nawata H, 2007. Atrazine-Induced Aromatase Expression Is SF-1 Dependent: Implications for Endocrine Disruption in Wildlife and Reproductive Cancers in Humans. *Environ. Health Perspect.* 115:720-727.

Grossman J, 1995. What's Hiding under the Sink: Dangers of Household Pesticides. *Environ. Health Perspect.* 103:550-554.

Hayden KM, Norton MC, Darcey D, Østbye T, Zandi PP, Breitner JCS, Welsh-Bohmer KA, 2010. Occupational Exposure to Pesticides Increases the Risk of Incident AD: The Cache County Study. *Neurology* 74:1524-1530.

Hayes WJ Jr, 1982. *Pesticides Studied in Man*. Baltimore, Maryland, USA: Williams and Wilkins.

Hodgson E, Mailman RB, Chambers JE (Eds.), 1998. *Dictionary of Toxicology*. New York, New York, USA: Grove's Dictionaries Inc.

IARC (International Agency for Research on Cancer), 1976. IARC Monographs on the Evaluation of Carcinogenic Risks to Humans, Volume 12: Some Carbamates, Thicarbamates and Carbazides. Lyon, France: WHO Press.

IARC (International Agency for Research on Cancer), 1979. IARC Monographs on the Evaluation of Carcinogenic Risks to Humans, Volume 20: Some Halogenated Hydrocarbons. Lyon, France: WHO Press.

IARC (International Agency for Research on Cancer), 1987. IARC Monographs on the Evaluation of Carcinogenic Risks to Humans, Supplement 7: Overall Evaluations of Carcinogenicity – An Updating of IARC Monographs Volumes 1 to 42. Lyon, France: WHO Press.

IARC (International Agency for Research on Cancer), 1991. IARC Monographs on the Evaluation of Carcinogenic Risks to Humans, Volume 53: Occupational Exposures in Insecticide Application, and Some Pesticides. Lyon, France: WHO Press.

IARC (International Agency for Research on Cancer), 1999. IARC Monographs on the Evaluation of Carcinogenic Risks to Humans, Volume 73: Some Chemicals That Cause Tumours of the Kidney or Urinary Bladder in Rodents and Some Other Substances. Lyon, France: WHO Press.

IARC (International Agency for Research on Cancer), 2001. IARC Monographs on the Evaluation of Carcinogenic Risks to Humans, Volume 79: Some Thyrotropic Agents. Lyon, France: WHO Press.

IOM (Institute of Medicine), 2011. *Veterans and Agent Orange: Update 2010*. Washington DC, USA: The National Academies Press.

Johnson MK, 1975. Organophosphorus Esters Causing Delayed Neurotoxic Effects. Mechanism of Action and Structure/Activity Studies. *Arch. Toxicol.* 34:259-288.

Johnson MK, 1976. Mechanism of Protection Against the Delayed Neurotoxic Effect of Organophosphorus Esters. *Fed. Proc.* 35:73-74.

Koldkjaer OG, Wermuth L, Bjerregaard P, 2004. Parkinson's Disease among Inuit in Greenland: Organochlorines as Risk Factors. *Int. J. Circumpolar Health* 63(Suppl 2):366-368.

Linnett PJ, 2008. Permethrin Toxicosis in Cats. *Aust. Vet. J.* 86:32-35.

Luellen DR, Vadas GG, Unger MA, 2006. Kepone in James River Fish: 1976-2002. *Sci. Total Environ.* 358:286-297.

Mathur HB, Johnson S, Mishra R, Kumar A, Singh B, 2003. Analysis of Pesticide Residues in Bottled Water – Delhi Region. CSE/PML-6/2002. Centre for Science and Environment, 41, Tughtakabad Institutional Area, New Delhi, India.

Munger R, Isacson P, Hu S, Burns T, Hanson J, Cherryholmes K, Van Dorpe P, Hausler WJ Jr, 1997. Intrauterine Growth Retardation in Iowa Communities with Herbicide-Contaminated Drinking Water Supplies. *Environ. Health Perspect.* 105:308-314.

Murray D, Wesseling C, Keifer M, Corriols M, Henao S, 2002. Surveillance of Pesticide-Related Illness in the Developing World: Putting the Data to Work. *J. Int. Occ. Environ. Health* 8:243-248.

NEETF (The National Environmental Education & Training Foundation), 2002. Implementation Plan – National Strategies for Health Care Providers: Pesticide Initiative. NEETF, 1707 H Street, NW, Suite 900, Washington DC, USA.

Notman P, 1989. A Review of Invertebrate Poisoning by Compound 1080. *N. Zeal. Entomologist* 12:67-71.

Ochoa-Acuña H, Frankenberger J, Hahn L, Carbajo C, 2009. Drinking-Water Herbicide Exposure in Indiana and Prevalence of Small-for-Gestational-Age and Preterm Delivery. *Environ. Health Perspect.* 117:1619-1624.

O'Malley M, 2007. Pesticides. In *Current Occupational and Environmental Medicine,* (Ladou J, Ed.), Fourth Edition. New York, New York, USA: McGraw-Hill, Chapter 31.

Rauh VA, Garfinkel R, Perera FP, Andrews HF, Hoepner L, Barr DB, Whitehead R, Tang D, Whyatt RW, 2006. Impact of Prenatal Chlorpyrifos Exposure on Neurodevelopment in the First 3 Years of Life among Inner-City Children. *Pediatrics* 118:e1845-1859.

Reigart JR, Roberts JR (Eds.), 1999. *Recognition and Management of Pesticide Poisonings*, Fifth Edition. EPA #735-R-98-003. Office of Pesticide Programs, Washington DC, USA.

Stevens JT, Sumner DD, 1991. Herbicides. In *Handbook of Pesticide Toxicology* (Hayes WJ Jr, Laws ER Jr, Eds.), Volume 3. San Diego, California, USA: Academic Press, pp.1317-1408.

Sutton NM, Bates N, Campbell A, 2007. Clinical Effects and Outcome of Feline Permethrin Spot-on Poisonings Reported to the Veterinary Poisons Information Service (VPIS), London. *J. Feline Med. Surg.* 9:335-339.

Tomlin C (Ed.), 2011. *The Pesticide Manual, a World Compendium: Incorporating the Agrochemicals Handbook*, Fifteenth Edition. British Crop Protection Council, Bath, UK: The Bath Press.

U.S. CFR (U.S. Code of Federal Regulation), 2010. Title 40 (Protection of Environment), Part 141 (National Primary Drinking Water Regulations), Appendix A to Subpart O of Part 141.

U.S. EPA (U.S. Environmental Protection Agency), 1975. A Review of Scientific and Economic Aspects of the Decision to Ban Its Use as a Pesticide. EPA-540/1-75-022. Office of Pesticide Programs, Washington DC, USA.

U.S. EPA (U.S. Environmental Protection Agency), 1995. Reregistration of Eligibility Decision (RED) – Sodium Fluoroacetate. EPA-738-R-95-025. Office of Prevention, Pesticides and Toxic Substances, Washington DC, USA.

U.S. EPA (U.S. Environmental Protection Agency), 1997a. Pesticides Industry Sales and Usage – 1994 and 1995 Market Estimates. EPA-733-R-97-002. Office of Prevention, Pesticides and Toxic Substances, Washington DC, USA.

U.S. EPA (U.S. Environmental Protection Agency), 1997b. Reregistration of Eligibility Decision (RED) – Propoxur. EPA-738-F-97-009. Office of Prevention, Pesticides and Toxic Substances, Washington DC, USA.

U.S. EPA (U.S. Environmental Protection Agency), 1997c. Reregistration of Eligibility Decision (RED) – Paraquat Dichloride. EPA-738-F-96-018. Office of Prevention, Pesticides and Toxic Substances, Washington DC, USA.

U.S. EPA (U.S. Environmental Protection Agency), 1999. Pesticides Industry Sales and Usage – 1996 and 1997 Market Estimates. EPA-733-R-99-001. Office of Prevention, Pesticides and Toxic Substances, Washington DC, USA.

U.S. EPA (U.S. Environmental Protection Agency), 2000. Pesticide Fact Sheet (New Chemicals) – Indoxacarb. Office of Prevention, Pesticides and Toxic Substances, Washington DC, USA.

U.S. EPA (U.S. Environmental Protection Agency), 2002. Pesticides Industry Sales and Usage – 1998 and 1999 Market Estimates. EPA-733-R-02-001. Office of Prevention, Pesticides and Toxic Substances, Washington DC, USA.

U.S. EPA (U.S. Environmental Protection Agency), 2003. Interim Reregistration of Eligibility Decision (IRED) for Atrazine. Office of Prevention, Pesticides and Toxic Substances, Washington DC, USA.

U.S. EPA (U.S. Environmental Protection Agency), 2004a. Pesticides Industry Sales and Usage – 2000 and 2001 Market Estimates. EPA-733-R-04-001. Office of Prevention, Pesticides and Toxic Substances, Washington DC, USA.

U.S. EPA (U.S. Environmental Protection Agency), 2004b. Carbaryl IRED Facts [Revised 10/22/04]. Office of Prevention, Pesticides and Toxic Substances, Washington DC, USA.

U.S. EPA (U.S. Environmental Protection Agency), 2005a. Reregistration of Eligibility Decision (RED) for 2,4-D. EPA-738-R05-002. Office of Prevention, Pesticides and Toxic Substances, Washington DC, USA.

U.S. EPA (U.S. Environmental Protection Agency), 2005b. Imidacloprid; Pesticide Tolerances for Emergency Exemptions. *Federal Register* 70:59268-59276.

U.S. EPA (U.S. Environmental Protection Agency), 2006a. Cumulative Risk from Triazine Pesticides. Office of Prevention, Pesticides and Toxic Substances, Washington DC, USA.

U.S. EPA (U.S. Environmental Protection Agency), 2006b. Report of the Food Quality Protection Act (FQPA) Tolerance Reassessment Progress and Risk Management Decision (TRED) for Propazine. EPA-738-R-06-009. Office of Prevention, Pesticides and Toxic Substances, Washington DC, USA.

U.S. EPA (U.S. Environmental Protection Agency), 2007a. Reregistration of Eligibility Decision (RED) for Carbaryl. EPA-738-R07-018. Office of Prevention, Pesticides and Toxic Substances, Washington DC, USA.

U.S. EPA (U.S. Environmental Protection Agency), 2007b. Permethrin Facts. EPA-738-F-09-001. Office of Prevention, Pesticides and Toxic Substances, Washington DC, USA.

Ware GW, Whitacre DM, 2004. *The Pesticide Book*, Sixth Edition. Willoughby, Ohio, USA: MeisterPro Information Resources.

WHO (World Health Organization), 1990. Public Health Impact of Pesticides Used in Agriculture, WHO in Collaboration with UN Environment Programme, Geneva, Switzerland.

WHO (World Health Organization), 2009. WHO Specifications and Evaluations for Public Health Pesticides: Pyrethrum (Pyrethrins). Evaluation Report 32/2009. Geneva, Switzerland.

York G, Mick H, 2008. Last Ghost' of the Vietnam War. *The Globe & Mail*, 12 July.

Review Questions

1. Define the terms *pesticide*, *pest*, and *pesticide residues*.
2. What is the regulatory mandate of Food Quality Protection Act of 1996 to U.S. EPA regarding pesticide risk assessment in the United States?
3. What are the annual estimates of pesticide use in the United States and in the world?
4. Name four chemical classes of pesticides used predominately or exclusively as insecticides.

5. How many cases of *non*-suicidal, acute severe type pesticide poisoning were estimated to occur around the world each year during the early 1990s?

6. Which member in the organochlorines is the most notorious pesticide in the world? Briefly describe its mode of pesticidal action.

7. Briefly describe the mode of pesticidal action of the chlorinated *cyclodiene* insecticides.

8. Which organochlorine pesticide was associated with the James River pollution?

9. Which HCH (hexachlorocyclohexane) isomer has been used not only to protect crop seeds against pests, but also as an active ingredient in shampoos and soaps medicated for control of head lice and scabies?

10. What are the common signs and symptoms of *acute* OP poisoning? Name the member in the OP family that was responsible for the Jake leg episode occurring in the early 1930s.

11. What is the mechanism of insecticidal action of carbamates? And how does this mechanism differ from that of OP insecticides?

12. What are the most documented health effects of pyrethrins, and of pyrethroids? And what are the Type I and Type II symptoms from significant exposure to pyrethroids?

13. Which of the pyrethroids is considered the most widely used insecticide worldwide?

14. What are the subtle reasons for which 2,4-D and 2,4,5-T have recently become the subject of extended investigation?

15. What are some of the potential health effects of atrazine? Briefly explain why the herbicide has not been banned from use in cornfields in the United States.

16. Briefly describe the mode of pesticidal action and toxicity of neonicotinoids.

17. What is commonly used as the antidote for accidental poisoning by coumarin and indandione rodenticides? And briefly explain why or how it can be used biochemically as the antidote.

18. Briefly describe the use and toxicity of the three loner or specialty pesticides covered in this chapter.

CHAPTER 16

Persistent Toxic Substances

16.1. Introduction

In environmental toxicology, persistent toxic substance (PTS) means any toxic material that has an alarming half-life in an environmental medium (e.g., air, water, sediment, soil, foods). These substances collectively represent a huge group of environmental pollutants. Half-life, conventionally denoted by $t_{1/2}$, refers to the time t required for the quantity or concentration of a substance in a medium to diminish to half of its original value and thereby is highly medium-specific. The numerical criteria adopted by various health authorities for what constitutes a warning half-life in each of the common media are summarized in Table 16.1 and further highlighted in Section 16.1.2, following the clarification given below for chemical $vs.$ environmental persistence.

16.1.1. Chemical $vs.$ Environmental Persistence

Bioaccumulation is an environmental phenomenon discussed extensively in Chapter 6. It results in an increase of a pollutant's concentration in an organism's tissue that exceeds what is normally expected. On the other hand, a pollutant's persistence in an environmental medium is a measure, or at least a reflection, of its susceptibility to degradation or loss in that medium. That is, the pollutant's persistence, along with its bioaccumulation potential in the environment, is what makes it actually available for environmental exposure. Therefore, parallel to bioaccumulation, persistence is a component more crucial than toxicity in assessing the health risk of an environmental toxicant. Supporting this notion is the argument that a substance's toxicity tends to be more static in nature, whereas environmental exposure to the substance typically is more dynamic.

There are two major quantities or aspects of persistence for each substance present in the environment. The first is about its intrinsic or chemical persistence and the other, about its persistence in the environment. By definition, chemical persistence refers to a substance's ability to remain unchanged both in its natural physicochemical state and in its composition over time. This ability is still influenced considerably by the immediate environmental conditions in which the substance is present.

In contrast, environmental persistence is a concept used to imply a constant quantity of a substance in the environmental medium of concern. It can be argued that even an extremely persistent substance would pose no threat of environmental persistence if it were kept inside a durable, well-sealed, well-insulated container all the time. By convention, a substance's environmental persistence is expressed in terms of its degradation half-life.

The use of half-life implies first-order kinetic behavior in chemical concentration, a concept borrowed from radioactive decay. The problem with such a simple definition is that many pollutants are present concurrently in more than one environmental compartment.

16.1.2. Numerical Persistence Criteria

The numerical criteria used for identifying or qualifying a substance as alarmingly persistent in the environment vary somewhat among health (regulatory) entities in the western countries. As shown in Table 16.1, the Canadian Environmental Protection Act (CEPA, 1999) considers a substance to be persistent when its half-life in the air is more than 2 days (or when it is subject to atmospheric transport from its source to a remote region), or when its half-life in water or soil exceeds 180 days, or when its half-life in sediment exceeds 364 days.

Table 16.1. Numerical Screening Criteria for Qualifying Toxic Substances as Persistent and Bioaccumulative Pollutants in the Environment

Authority[a]	Persistence Half-Life (Days)[b]				Bioaccumulativity[c]	
	Air	*Water*	*Soil*	*Sediment*	*BCF(BAF)*	*Log K_{ow}*
UNEP	>2	>60	>180	>180	5,000	5
UNECE	>2	>60	>180	>180	5,000	5
Canada (CEPA)	>2	>180	>180	>180	5,000	5
U.K. DEFRA	>2	>180	>180	>180	5,000	5
European Commission	–	>40 (f); >60 (m)	–	>120 (f); >180 (m)	2,000	–
U.S. EPA	>2	>60	>60	>60	1,000	–

[a]UNEP (United Nations Environment Programme, 2001); UNECE = (United Nations Economic Commission for Europe, 2004); CEPA = (Canadian Environmental Protection Act, 1999); U.K. DEFRA (United Kingdom Department for Environmental, Food, & Rural Affairs, 2002); European Commission (2003); U.S. EPA (U.S. Environmental Protection Agency, 1999a, 1999b), particularly for chemical substances subject to the Emergency Planning and Community Right-To-Know Act of 1986.

[b]in the air, water, soil, or sediment, where applicable; f = fresh; m = marine.

[c]BAF = bio*accumulation* factor $\cong$ BCF = bio*concentration* factor, where applicable; K_{ow} = octanol-water partition coefficient (*see* Chapter 6 for estimation of BCF with this partition coefficient).

The United Kingdom government (U.K. DEFRA, 2002) has adopted a similar set of numerical criteria for qualifying a substance as a PTS. In contrast, the numerical criteria used by U.S. EPA (1999a, 1999b) are somewhat more health conservative (Table 16.1). Other nations outside of the western continents tend to follow the criteria set forth by the European Commission. What is certain today is that many health and regulatory authorities focus more on water, soil, and sediment than on air as the environmental medium of concern. Such a bias is not surprising in that atmospheric compartments *per se* are less likely an ideal *direct* environment for long-term bioaccumulation or long-range transport for most pollutants unless some grasshopper effect is involved (Chapter 5).

16.1.3. Relevance to Long-Range Transport

The issues on bioaccumulation and environmental persistence are closely related to the concern with long-range transport (LRT) of environmental pollutants. Both the relevance and the importance of this environmental concern are on the international level, as evident from the well-publicized workshop held about a decade ago addressing the LRT of air toxics into and out of the Great Lakes basin (Ann Arbor Statement, 2003). Another indication is the editorial comments by Matthies and Scheringer (2001), who were specifically concerned with the occurrence of certain pesticides and industrial chemicals in the arctic. As they put it, "*These substances have never been emitted in such regions and, thus, must have been transported over long distances from moderate or even tropical climatic zones.*"

Contrary to the classic belief, the mode of LRT is no longer restricted to atmospheric. There are ample data (AMAP, 1997) showing that nuclear wastes and certain POPs (persistent organic pollutants) can be transported in ocean currents over long distances, such as from reprocessing plants in Europe to the Arctic Ocean. Furthermore, as discussed in Chapter 6 on bioaccumulation, at least one case study (Ewald *et al.* 1998) revealed the Pacific salmon's capability of transporting PCBs (polychlorinated biphenyls) and other POPs over a long distance from the ocean back to their spawning lakes. Another study also indicated that with the aid of storms or cyclone activities, even soil dust particles emitted from the Mongolian and Chinese arid regions could be transported over the North Pacific Ocean, all the way to North America (Takemura *et al.*, 2002).

16.2. The Stockholm Convention of 2001

Many PTS, including those of special global health concern, tend to bioaccumulate in living organisms. This explains why PTS are frequently treated as synonymous with the group of environmental pollutants termed *persistent, bioaccumulative, and toxic substances* (PBTs). To this date, the PTS or PBTs of global concern have been predominately POPs, the chemical group that has been the subject of increasing international attention since the adoption of the global treaty *Stockholm Convention on POPs* in 2001. Section 16.2.1 below gives a brief account of the Convention's current list of POPs of global concern, followed by Section 16.2.2 highlighting the Convention's specific actions aiming to contain the persistent pollutants on its priority list.

16.2.1. Persistent Pollutants of Global Concern

From the brief discussion above (Section 16.1.3) on the LRT potential for PTS, it is apparent that global efforts are required in order to minimize the distribution and thereby the presence of these pollutants in the global environment. Such efforts require global consensus which is never an easy task due to the complex political issues involved and the limited resources available across nations. Yet some efforts of such have been proven successful by the United Nations Environment Programme, when delegates from 127 nations in May 2001 approved the convention on POPs held in Stockholm, Sweden. As anticipated, the approval underwent a great deal of negotiations and disputes over numerous diverse economic interests and political concerns.

By law, a global agreement must be ratified by 50 nations or more in order for it to become a legal international treaty. Accordingly, following the approval of the agreement at the Convention, the parties needed to obtain the required ratification from their own governments, a task expected to take at least a couple of years to accomplish. For example, in the United States, the treaty was submitted by then President George W. Bush to the U.S. Senate for ratification about a year later in April 2002. In any event, as soon as the treaty finally entered into force in 2004, it banned outright the use of eight OC (organochlorine) pesticides (aldrin, chlordane, dieldrin, endrin, heptachlor, hexachlorobenzene, mirex, and toxaphene). The Convention has since taken various initiatives to restrict the use of DDT, PCBs, and the unintentional by-products PCDDs (polychlorinated dibenzo-*p*-dioxins) and PCDFs (polychlorinated dibenzofurans), all of which are also OC compounds. This initial group is collectively nicknamed *the dirty dozen*.

By May 2011, the amendments to the Stockholm Convention included 10 new POPs on its list either for elimination of their production or for restriction of their use. The 10 additional POPs represent four chemical groups: (1) six pesticide-related OCs, including chlordecone (a.k.a. kepone), pentachlorobenzene, endosulfan (plus its isomers), and three (α-, β-, γ-) isomers of hexachlorocyclohexane (HCH); (2) one polybrominated biphenyl (PBB) named *hexa*brominated biphenyl (*hexa*BB); (3) two *commercial* polybrominated diphenyl ethers (PBDEs) named *penta-* and *octa*-brominated diphenyl ether (*penta*BDE and *octa*BDE); and (4) perfluorooctane sulfonate (PFOS) plus its salts.

There is high speculation that members of several other chemical groups, such as certain organotin compounds, certain phthalates, and certain alkylphenols, may soon be added to the Convention's POPs action list. This is because in recent years, there have been increasing global concerns over the environmental persistence and toxic nature of these other chemicals (e.g., Albaigés, 2005; Lind, 2004; Peters, 2006).

The OC pesticides on the Convention's POPs list are discussed in some detail in Chapter 15. Overviews of the remaining five groups of non-pesticide POPs are given in their own sections below following a brief account of the Convention's practical actions aiming to contain the POPs on its priority list. Again, the five groups not used as pesticides but placed on the Convention's action list are PFOS, PBBs, PBDEs, PCBs, and PCDDs/PCDFs. The dioxins PCDDs and the furans PCDFs are discussed together in the same section because they are exceptionally similar in chemical structure and properties.

16.2.2. The Convention's Aims and Actions

The Stockholm Convention is a global treaty with the aims to protect human health and the environment from POPs, of which many are considered as carcinogenic or capable of disrupting the endocrine system or suppressing the immunological system in humans. The Convention's practical actions and programs dealing with the POPs on its priority list include, where applicable as by party consensus: planning, coordinating, and implementing the reduction or elimination of the POPs releases from intentional as well as unintentional production and from stockpiles or wastes. The Convention has the additional obligation of decreasing the environmental levels of the POPs over time.

According to the treaty, once any of the POPs becomes a waste, all relevant parties to the Convention are obligated to develop and implement appropriate strategies for identifying stockpiles, products, and articles in use that contain or are contaminated by the pollutant at issue. These parties must then manage the stockpiles and wastes in an environmentally sound manner to the extent that the POP content is destroyed or irreversibly transformed. The parties must also develop strategies for identifying contaminated sites and perform eventual remediation in an environmentally sound manner.

Another global treaty named *The Basel Convention (on the Control of Transboundary Movements of Hazardous Wastes and Their Disposal)* has developed the technical guidelines on waste management for POPs. The Basel Convention, which went into force in 1992, is considered as the most comprehensive global environmental agreement on hazardous and other wastes. Under these guidelines as part of the cooperative agreement, the Stockholm Convention is responsible for setting levels of destruction and irreversible transformation necessary to ensure the absence of any POPs characteristics.

The Stockholm Convention has yet another responsibility to coordinate as well as to implement the Global Monitoring Plan (GMP) for the POPs on its priority list. As part of the treaty, parties to the Convention are each required to prepare their own plan on how they are going to implement the obligations under the agreement and to make efforts to put their own plan into operation. Their GMP thereby represents and requires a collective effort, in the sense that the plan aims to provide a harmonized organizational framework for the collection of comparable monitoring data on the presence of the POPs from all relevant regions. The data obtained are necessary for identifying changes in levels over time, as well as for providing information on the regional and global environmental transport of POPs. The GMP is therefore a key component of the evaluation on the treaty's own effectiveness and success in reducing the adverse health effects of POPs to humans and the environment. The first monitoring report for the effectiveness evaluation was presented at the fourth meeting of the Conference of the Parties in May 2009, and served as a baseline for subsequent evaluations. The second report, for which all regional monitoring data were due by October 2010, is not yet available to the public at this time.

16.3. Perfluorooctane Sulfonate

Perfluorooctane sulfonate (PFOS) is a fully fluorinated anion and as such a member of perfluoroalkyls (i.e., a group also broadly called perfluorinated compounds). Due to its ability to lower the surface tension of water and some other liquids allowing easier spreading, PFOS is used in a wide variety of applications such as its inclusion as a component in surfactants, lubricants, food packaging, floor polishes, leather products, paper and textile coatings, and fire retardant foams. This fluorosurfactant is also used in large quantities in the photographic and photolithographic industries (as a component in aqueous film forming foam) and in the aviation industry (as a component in hydraulic fluids). Unlike the other four groups of POPs discussed below, PFOS and its salts structurally are not a family member of polyhalogenated aromatic hydrocarbons (known commonly by its acronym PHAHs), as they do not contain any benzene ring (Figure 16.1).

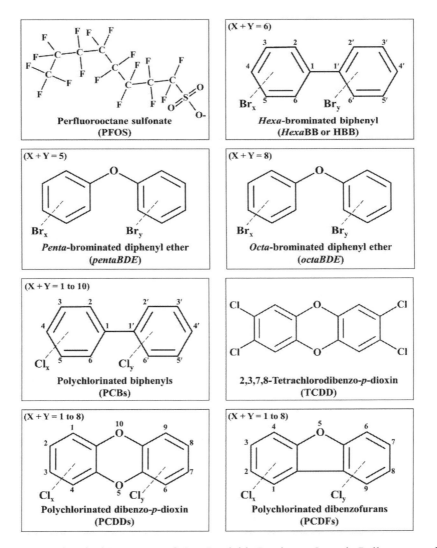

Figure 16.1. Chemical Structures of Non-Pesticide Persistent Organic Pollutants on the Stockholm Convention's Action List, as of May 2011

16.3.1. Use and Pollution Sources

PFOS is a highly stable compound both in industrial applications and in the environment, owing to the chemical effects of its aggregate strong carbon-fluorine bonds. The fluorosurfactant was once the principal ingredient in numerous stain repellents including notably Scotchgard®, a fabric as well as an upholstery protector manufactured by the 3M company in the United States. Along with perfluorooctanoic acid (PFOA), PFOS is one of the most common contaminants found in foods and water. PFOA is also a synthetic, persistent perfluoroalkyl. It structurally differs from PFOS only in having a carboxylic acid (COOH) group instead of the sulfonic acid (SO$_3$H) group (Figure 16.1).

PFOS can be produced from industrial processes or through the degradation of its precursors. It has been detected worldwide in wildlife including bald eagle (in the midwestern region of the United States), carrion crow (in Tokyo Bay, Japan), harbor seal (in the Wadden Sea, Denmark), and common dolphin (in Mediterranean Sea, Italy). In some of these wildlife, the PFOS levels detected in the liver, egg, serum, kidney, and plasma samples collected were found high enough to cause human health concern.

PFOS persists in both the human body and the environment. The anion has not shown any degradation in tests of hydrolysis, photolysis, or biodegradation under any environmental condition assayed. The only known condition whereby PFOS can be degraded is via high temperature incineration. The fluorosurfactant fulfills the criteria for bioaccumulation due to its significantly higher concentrations observed in predators on higher trophic levels (e.g., polar bears, seals, bald eagles, and minks in the arctic, Sweden, and the United States) than in those on lower trophic levels.

Unlike the other POPs discussed below, PFOS has a unique bioaccumulation property in that it binds to (tissue) proteins, instead of accumulating in fatty tissues. Like most other fluorocarbons, the longer C$_8$F$_{17}$ subunit of PFOS is both hydrophobic and lipophobic, with its shorter sulfonate subunit tending to increase water solubility. PFOlS meets the criteria for having the potential of atmospheric LRT. This is evident from monitoring data showing higher levels of PFOS in various remote parts of the northern hemisphere.

16.3.2. Environmental Health Concerns

PFOS fulfills the general criteria for being a toxic substance. It has shown toxicity on mammals in subchronic studies. It has also displayed maternal toxicity with mortality of pups occurring shortly after birth. PFOS is toxic to aquatic organisms, with the lowest *no observed effect concentration* (NOEC) of 0.25 mg/L being detected in small shrimp-like creatures.

Epidemiological studies revealed that workers in certain occupational settings had serum levels of PFOS exceeding 1,000 ppb (parts per billion), while a small segment in the general population had over 90 ppb (Betts, 2008). Yet studies on male mice implicated that PFOS at the serum level of ~90 ppb would affect the immunological system, thus raising the concern that highly exposed people and wildlife are immunocompromised (Betts, 2008). Furthermore, in studies where chicken eggs were dosed at 1 ppb of egg weight, some eggs were found to have developed into chickens with serum PFOS at 150 ppb or higher. Effects such as brain asymmetry and decreased immunoglobulin levels were observed in some of these chickens (Peden-Adams *et al.*, 2009). To this date, IARC has not determined the human or animal carcinogenicity of PFOS or PFOA.

The voluntary phase-out of PFOS production by the 3M company has led to a substantial reduction in the production and use of PFOS-related substances. However, it is likely that the fluorosurfactant is still being produced in some other countries, inasmuch as the Stockholm Convention has data showing that some other countries continue to use considerable amounts of the perfluorinated compound. Since PFOS-related substances can be transported in the atmosphere to regions far away from their sources, measures taken by single or a few nations are not sufficient to abate the pollution caused by these persistent substances. The Convention thereby decided that regional action against PFOS was warranted, and thus in August 2010 added the pollutant to the POPs priority list.

16.4. Polybrominated Biphenyls

Polybrominated biphenyls (PBBs), known also as polybromobiphenyls, are a family of structurally similar brominated hydrocarbons with 2 to 10 bromine (Br) atoms attaching to the biphenyl nucleus ($C_{12}H_{10}$). For completeness, the *mono*-brominated congeners (i.e., those with one Br atom attaching to the biphenyl) are frequently included when characterizing the PBBs. The chemical structure of *hexa*-brominated biphenyl (*hexa*BB or HBB) is selectively depicted in Figure 16.1 because this PBB congener has been specifically added to the Stockholm Convention's POPs action list since August 2010. The biphenyl core molecule is simply the bulk portion of the PBB structure without the attachment of any Br atom. Note that the chemical structure of HBB depicted in Figure 16.1 can be used to represent any member in the PBB family, simply by attaching the desired number of Br atoms to the core molecule (i.e., by allowing the *sum* of the *x* and the *y* number of Br atoms to be between 1 and 10).

16.4.1. Use and Pollution Sources

From the structure shown in Figure 16.1, and with some computation, it can be seen that up to 209 compounds (including the *mono*brominated) are theoretically possible as congeners (or less technically, members) of the PBB family. Considering the *number* of bromine substituents alone (i.e., regardless of their positions), there are 10 homologous subgroups (i.e., homologs) of PBBs in total, ranging from *mono-* to *deca*-brominated. The *mono-*, *di-*, *tri-*, *tetra-*, *penta-*, *hexa-*, *hepta-*, *octa-*, *nona-*, and *deca*-homologs each can have 3, 12, 24, 42, 46, 42, 24, 12, 3, and 1 possible stereoisomer(s), respectively, thus yielding in total 209 possible PBB congeners.

Following the numbering scheme illustrated in Table 16.2, which also reveals the possible sites for halogenation, each of the 209 possible congeners can be identified with a unique number from 1 to 209. The 209 possible PBB congeners are different from one

Table 16.2. Chemical Identities of *Poly*brominated Biphenyls (*P*BBs), of *Poly*brominated Diphenyl Ethers (*P*BDEs), and of *Poly*chlorinated Biphenyls (*P*CBs)[a]

No.	Position of Halogenation	No.	Position of Halogenation	No.	Position of Halogenation	No.	Position of Halogenation
mono-BB, -BDE, -CB		52	2,2',5,5'	106	2,3,3',4,5	160	2,3,3',4,5,6
1	2	53	2,2',5,6'	107	2,3,3',4',5	161	2,3,3',4,5',6
2	3	54	2,2',6,6'	108	2,3,3',4,5'	162	2,3,3',4',5,5'
3	4	55	2,3,3',4	109	2,3,3',4,6	163	2,3,3',4',5,6
di-BB, -BDE, -CB		56	2,3,3',4'	110	2,3,3',4',6	164	2,3,3',4',5',6
4	2,2'	57	2,3,3',5	111	2,3,3',5,5'	165	2,3,3',5,5',6
5	2,3	58	2,3,3',5'	112	2,3,3',5,6	166	2,3,4,4',5,6
6	2,3'	59	2,3,3',6	113	2,3,3',5',6	167	2,3',4,4',5,5'
7	2,4	60	2,3,4,4'	114	2,3,4,4',5	168	2,3',4,4',5',6
8	2,4'	61	2,3,4,5	115	2,3,4,4',6	169	3,3',4,4',5,5'
9	2,5	62	2,3,4,6	116	2,3,4,5,6	*hepta-BB, -BDE, -CB*	
10	2,6	63	2,3,4',5	117	2,3,4',5,6	170	2,2',3,3',4,4',5
11	3,3'	64	2,3,4',6	118	2,3',4,4',5	171	2,2',3,3',4,4',6
12	3,4	65	2,3,5,6	119	2,3',4,4',6	172	2,2',3,3',4,5,5'
13	3,4'	66	2,3',4,4'	120	2,3',4,5,5'	173	2,2',3,3',4,5,6
14	3,5	67	2,3',4,5	121	2,3',4,5',6	174	2,2',3,3',4,5,6'
15	4,4'	68	2,3',4,5'	122	2,3,3',4',5'	175	2,2',3,3',4,5',6
tri-BB, -BDE, -CB		69	2,3',4,6	123	2,3',4,4',5	176	2,2',3,3',4,6,6'
16	2,2',3	70	2,3',4',5	124	2,3',4',5,5'	177	2,2',3,3',4',5,6'
17	2,2',4	71	2,3',4',6	125	2,3',4',5',6	178	2,2',3,3',5,5',6
18	2,2',5	72	2,3',5,5'	126	3,3',4,4',5	179	2,2',3,3',5,6,6'
19	2,2',6	73	2,3',5',6	127	3,3',4,5,5'	180	2,2',3,4,4',5,5'
20	2,3,3'	74	2,4,4',5	*hexa-BB, -BDE, -CB*		181	2,2',3,4,4',5,6
21	2,3,4	75	2,4,4',6	128	2,2',3,3',4,4'	182	2,2',3,4,4',5,6'
22	2,3,4'	76	2,3',4',5'	129	2,2',3,3',4,5	183	2,2',3,4,4',5',6
23	2,3,5	77	3,3',4,4'	130	2,2',3,3',4,5'	184	2,2',3,4,4',6,6'
24	2,3,6	78	3,3',4,5	131	2,2',3,3',4,6	185	2,2',3,4,5,5',6
25	2,3',4	79	3,3',4,5'	132	2,2',3,3',4,6'	186	2,2',3,4,5,6,6'
26	2,3',5	80	3,3',5,5'	133	2,2',3,3',5,5'	187	2,2',3,4',5,5',6
27	2,3',6	81	3,4,4',5	134	2,2',3,3',5,6	188	2,2',3,4',5,6,6'
28	2,4,4'	*penta-BB, -BDE, -CB*		135	2,2',3,3',5,6'	189	2,3,3',4,4',5,5'
29	2,4,5	82	2,2',3,3',4	136	2,2',3,3',6,6'	190	2,3,3',4,4',5,6
30	2,4,6	83	2,2',3,3',5	137	2,2',3,4,4',5	191	2,3,3',4,4',5',6
31	2,4',5	84	2,2',3,3',6	138	2,2',3,4,4',5'	192	2,3,3',4,5,5',6
32	2,4',6	85	2,2',3,4,4'	139	2,2',3,4,4',6	193	2,3,3',4',5,5',6
33	2,3',4'	86	2,2',3,4,5	140	2,2',3,4,4',6'	*octa-BB, -BDE, -CB*	
34	2,3',5'	87	2,2',3,4,5'	141	2,2',3,4,5,5'	194	2,2',3,3',4,4',5,5'
35	3,3',4	88	2,2',3,4,6	142	2,2',3,4,5,6	195	2,2',3,3',4,4',5,6
36	3,3',5	89	2,2',3,4,6'	143	2,2',3,4,5,6'	196	2,2',3,3',4,4',5,6'
37	3,4,4'	90	2,2',3,4',5	144	2,2',3,4,5',6	197	2,2',3,3',4,4',6,6'
38	3,4,5	91	2,2',3,4',6	145	2,2',3,4,6,6'	198	2,2',3,3',4,5,5',6
39	3,4',5	92	2,2',3,5,5'	146	2,2',3,4',5,5'	199	2,2',3,3',4,5,5',6'
tetra-BB, -BDE, -CB		93	2,2',3,5,6	147	2,2',3,4',5,6	200	2,2',3,3',4,5,6,6'
40	2,2',3,3'	94	2,2',3,5,6'	148	2,2',3,4',5,6'	201	2,2',3,3',4,5',6,6'
41	2,2',3,4	95	2,2',3,5',6	149	2,2',3,4',5',6	202	2,2',3,3',5,5',6,6'
42	2,2',3,4'	96	2,2',3,6,6'	150	2,2',3,4',6,6'	203	2,2',3,4,4',5,5',6
43	2,2',3,5	97	2,2',3,4',5'	151	2,2',3,5,5',6	204	2,2',3,4,4',5,6,6'
44	2,2',3,5'	98	2,2',3,4',6'	152	2,2',3,5,6,6'	205	2,3,3',4,4',5,5',6
45	2,2',3,6	99	2,2',4,4',5	153	2,2',4,4',5,5'	*nona-BB, BDE, -CB*	
46	2,2',3,6'	100	2,2',4,4',6	154	2,2',4,4',5,6'	206	2,2',3,3',4,4',5,5',6
47	2,2',4,4'	101	2,2',4,5,5'	155	2,2',4,4',6,6'	207	2,2',3,3',4,4',5,6,6'
48	2,2',4,5	102	2,2',4,5,6'	156	2,3,3',4,4',5	208	2,2',3,3',4,5,5',6,6'
49	2,2',4,5'	103	2,2',4,5',6	157	2,3,3',4,4',5'	*deca-BB, -BDE, -CB*	
50	2,2',4,6	104	2,2',4,6,6'	158	2,3,3',4,4',6	209	2,2',3,3',4,4',5,5',6,6'
51	2,2',4,6'	105	2,3,3',4,4'	159	2,3,3',4,5,5'		

[a] *see*, e.g., ATSDR (2004) and Mills *et al.* (2007) for further discussion, which are also the primary sources for this table.

another only in the number of Br atoms as well as in their positions on the biphenyl nucleus. There are no known natural sources for any of these congeners. And the number of these congeners found in commercial PBB mixtures is much smaller than 209.

The commercial PBB mixtures were widely used in plastics, textiles, electronic substances, electrical equipment, and other materials in the early 1970s, primarily as flame retardants. In the United States, both the production and the use of *hexa*brominated biphenyl (*hexa*BB) were banned shortly after a major agricultural contamination episode took place in the state of Michigan during 1973-1974. This disaster also led to the discontinued production and use of the *octa*brominated biphenyl (*octa*BB) and the *deca*brominated biphenyl (*deca*BB) formulation in 1979.

The massive PBB contamination in Michigan began in September 1973, when a farmer in the southern region started noticing his herd of 400 dairy cattle suffering from hair loss, hematomas, and abnormalities in hoof growth, along with significant reductions in milk production and appetite. Exposure of the cattle to PBBs was not identified as the cause until about a year later, after several thousand pounds of PBB powder (consisting of mainly *hexa*BB) in mislabeled bags were distributed to and used by many farms in the state as the livestock feed additive magnesium oxide (MgO). The MgO additive was supposed to be mixed with the feed to increase milk production.

16.4.2. Environmental Health Concerns

The health and economic impacts of the PBB contamination in Michigan went far beyond the loss of a herd of 400 cattle. Many farm animals consumed the contaminated feed before the mistake was discovered, including more than a million of chickens, tens of thousands of other cattle, and thousands of pigs and sheep (e.g., Fries, 1985). Over 4,000 people in Michigan were also found to have been exposed to PBBs in 1973 as a result of this disaster. Those dairy farmers exposed to the PBB contaminants were found to have significant abnormalities with their immunological system, including decreases in the number and percentage of peripheral blood lymphocytes and in functional response to specific test antigens (Bekesi *et al.*, 1978). A cohort study following 327 girls aged 5 to 24 years for two decades found that, even after adjustment for potential confounding factors, the breastfed daughters exposed to PBBs *in utero* at or above 7 ppb had an earlier age at menarche, when compared to both the breastfed girls exposed to lower levels of PBBs *in utero* and those girls not breastfed (Blanck *et al.*, 2000). IARC (1987) has classified all PBB congeners as possible human (Group 2B) carcinogens.

When used as additives, certain PBB congeners are physically and selectively mixed into electronic products (e.g., computer monitors), instead of chemically bonded to them. Therefore, under normal conditions, these compounds will be more readily released (leached) into the local environment. There is a rising concern over the export of e-waste (electronic waste) to developing nations for fear of widespread releases of *hexa*BB during recycling operations (Zhao *et al.*, 2008). PBB homologs that were manufactured for commercial use typically consisted of the highly-brominated congeners such as *hexa*BBs and up. Based on a use-life expectancy of 5 to 10 years for most electrical and electronic products, it is expected that many of the PBB-containing products now have already been disposed of or are still being disposed of. It is also very likely that the *hexa*BB congeners are still being applied to electrical and electronic products in some developing countries. Highly-brominated PBBs hence are expected to be detected in the e-waste and around the affected local environments. It was partly due to such public health concerns that in 2006, many parties to the Stockholm Convention proposed that commercial *hexa*BB, along with commercial *octa*brominated diphenyl ether (*octa*BDE), be added to its POPs action list. In August 2010, that proposal became a reality.

16.5. Polybrominated Diphenyl Ethers

Polybrominated diphenyl ethers (PBDEs) are also brominated hydrocarbons but each with a diphenyl ether molecule ($C_{12}H_{10}O$), instead of a biphenyl, as their nucleus (Figure 16.1). Otherwise, they are structurally identical to PBBs and hence also have a possible total of 209 congeners as well as 10 homologs. As summarized in Table 16.2 and implicit in the PBDE structure in Figure 16.1, the 209 congeners each can also be referred to by a unique number between 1 and 209. Note that even though each of the 10 homologs refers to the isomers within it, its *commercial* term means a mixture of isomers from certain homologs. For example, commercial *penta*BDE is a mixture of mostly PBDE 99 (a *penta*BDE congener) but also with some PBDE 47 (a *tetra*BDE congener); and commercial *octa*BDE is a mixture of mostly *octa*-homolog congeners (e.g., PBDE 203) with some *hexa*-homolog (e.g., PBDE 153) and some *hepta*-homolog (e.g., PBDE 180) congeners.

16.5.1. Use and Pollution Sources

Like the PBB congeners, the PBDE members are part of the group called brominated flame retardants (BFRs). Of the 10 homologs, *penta*-, *octa*-, and *deca*-BDEs are the most used. Collectively. the three PBDE homologs are used widely as important flame retardants contained in a variety of plastics, fabrics, and foams that are components of many consumer products. In particular, *penta*BDEs are commonly used in flexible polyurethane (e.g., furniture) foams; and *deca*BDEs are frequently used in plastics for television (TV) cabinets, consumer electronics, and wire insulation, as well as in back coatings for draperies and upholstery. And the *octa*BDE congeners are used widely in plastics for small appliances and personal computers. Inasmuch as PBDEs are often used in high-impact polystyrene, epoxy resins, and rubber, they can be found in many e-waste products such as obsolete circuit boards, cables, and TV sets (Zhao *et al.*, 2008).

The annual global production of PBDEs as flame retardants (and for other minor purposes) is well over 67,000 tons (BSEF, 2000), of which PBDE 209 (the only *deca*BDE isomer) accounts for as much as 70% and is predominately used in North America. Many PBDE-containing plastics and polyurethane foams were once widely used in electrical and electronic products that now are referred to as end-of-life e-waste. Unlike some other

PBDE congeners, PBDE 209 can be degraded rapidly through exposure to light (e.g., ultraviolet radiation, sunlight) or through biological activity in the environment, in that case with a short half-life being in days (Zhao *et al.*, 2008).

PBDEs are mixed with polymers during the production of plastics. Because like PBBs they are not chemically bonded with the plastic, they too tend to leach out of the final consumer product easily. Accordingly, PBDEs can be found in many homes due to the ubiquity of plastics present in today's modern world. They are also different from most other POPs in that their main source is consumer products, whereas those for most other POPs that people are exposed to are foods and drinking water.

16.5.2. Environmental Health Concerns

Although the application of flame retardant chemicals preserves lives and properties, it comes with undesired consequences. There is growing evidence that PBDEs persist in the environment and bioaccumulate in living organisms. Studies showed that these retardants caused liver and thyroid toxicities (ATSDR, 2004). Data on mice also indicated that neonatal exposure to certain PBDE congeners (e.g., PBDE 47, PBDE 99) resulted in adverse effects on learning and memory functions, spontaneous motor behavior, and habituation capability that worsened with age (Eriksson *et al.*, 2001, 2002). To this date, IARC has not determined the human or animal carcinogenicity of PBDEs.

There is evidence that PBDE 71 is an endocrine disruptor in rats during their development (Zhou *et al.*, 2002). A more recent fertility study demonstrated that women with high blood levels of PBDEs (especially the *penta-* and *octa*-homologs) took much longer to get pregnant than women with lower levels (Harley *et al.*, 2010).

Environmental monitoring programs in various global regions (e.g., Asia, Europe, the arctic) found trace amounts of several PBDEs in human breast milk, fish, aquatic birds, and elsewhere in the environment. Homologs such as *tetra-* to *hexa*-BDEs were those most commonly detected in wildlife and humans. While the exact mechanisms or pathways through which PBDEs got into humans and the environment remain unknown, it is more certain that the main sources of environmental exposure to PBDEs include releases from processing of these chemicals into such products as plastics or textiles, and from wear and tear of the consumer products that are being used.

Workers engaging in the production of PBDE-containing materials are likely exposed to highest levels of these compounds. These POPs tend to accumulate in blood, breast milk, and fatty tissues. Bioaccumulation is therefore of high concern in such instances, especially for workers in e-waste recycling sites and electronics repair shops. The general public is likely exposed to low levels of PBDEs through dietary intake and inhalation. In the United States, near universal exposure to PBDEs was found in the general population, with 97% of the adults sampled in the comprehensive National Health and Nutrition Examination Survey (more known by its acronym NHANES) having detectable levels of PBDEs in their blood (Sjödin *et al.*, 2008). As alluded to earlier, exposure to PBDEs is (more) common in residential areas due to the ubiquity of consumer products in homes.

Under their Restriction of Hazardous Substances Directive coming into force in 2006, the European Union restricted the uses of PBDEs and PBBs in electrical and electronic devices, with an upper limit of 1 g/kg for the sum of the two chemical groups. In the United States, *penta-* and *octa-*BDEs are no longer produced. However, millions of pounds of these homologs are expected to remain in American homes and their environment owing to the continuous extensive use in PBDE-based consumer products.

The *deca*BDE congener is still widely used today, largely due to its relatively shorter half-life. In the United States, around 50 million pounds of this homolog (with only one congener) are used each year, mostly in TV casings. The use of *deca*-BDE is expected to grow in this country, since the congener is now approved for use to meet new federal fire safety standards for residential furniture and mattresses. It is of note that *deca*BDE can break down into *penta-* and *octa*-BDEs easily; yet the commercial *penta-* and *octa*-BDEs have been added to the Stockholm Convention's POPs list since August 2010.

16.6. Polychlorinated Biphenyls

As with PBBs and PBDEs, PCBs (polychlorinated biphenyls) are a group of up to 209 theoretically possible hydrocarbon congeners (Figure 16.1), for which there is no known natural source. Similarly, these 209 possible congeners differ from one another only in the number of chlorine (Cl) atoms as well as their positions on the biphenyl nucleus (as reflected in Figure 16.1 and Table 16.2). About 60% of these congeners can be found in some of the PCB mixtures once widely used in electrical equipment or as plasticizers.

16.6.1. Use and Pollution Sources

Monsanto Corporation was the principal U.S. manufacturer of PCBs from 1929 until the ban of their production in 1977. The company marketed mixtures of PCBs under the trade name Aroclor followed by a four-digit code to signify the number of carbons and the mass of chlorines contained in each mixture. Due to the widespread application of these congeners in the past and to their notorious persistence, PCBs can still be found in many places including particularly the e-waste sites. Most transformers and capacitors manufactured prior to 1977 contain considerable amounts of PCBs. As estimated by the International Programme on Chemical Safety (IPCS, 2003), about 2 million tons of PCBs were produced worldwide between 1929 and their global ban in 2001; and as of 2003, about 10% of this production remained in mobile environmental reservoirs.

As can be seen in Figure 16.1, PCBs are structurally (and hence usually chemically as well) very akin to the dioxin (as discussed in Section 16.7 below) and PBB compounds. Twelve of the PCB congeners are known to have toxic effects very similar to those of dioxins and by convention are referred to as *dioxin-like* PCB congeners. In particular, like dioxins, the dioxin-like PCB congeners can bind to the aryl hydrocarbon (Ah) receptors (Section 9.2.3) to cause toxic effects very similar to those induced by dioxins. Therefore, PCBs are frequently classified into the "dioxin-like" and "nondioxin-like" subgroups.

PCBs can also be classified into the two subgroups known as *nonplanar* and *coplanar* congeners to align with their dioxin-like properties. This classification practice is influenced by the observation that a PCB congener can cause more health effects when the entire chemical molecule is situated in the same plane (i.e., coplanar). The degree of planarity is determined largely by the number of chlorine substitutions in the *ortho* positions. Note that sites 2, 2', 6, and 6' (Figure 16.1) are called *ortho* positions, as they are closest to the *other* benzene ring; sites 3, 3', 5, and 5' are called the *meta* positions; and sites 4 and 4' are called the *para* positions. The two benzene rings can rotate around the bond connecting them and hence can yield two extreme configurations with one being (*co*)*planar* (i.e., in which the two rings are in the same plane) and the other being *nonplanar* (i.e., in which the rings are at a 90° angle to each other).

The substitution of the smaller-size hydrogen atoms in the *ortho* positions with the larger-size chlorine atoms forces the benzene rings to rotate out of the planar configuration. In essence, the benzene rings of non*ortho* substituted PCBs, along with the mono-*ortho* substituted PCBs, may assume a planar configuration. These PCBs are thereby referred to as non*ortho* or non*ortho*-substituted PCBs. The rest of the PCB congeners with the two benzene rings not capable of assuming a coplanar configuration are referred to as nonplanar congeners. Coplanar PCBs (e.g., PCB 77, PCB 126, PCB 169) tend to have dioxin-like properties and generally are among the most toxic PCB congeners.

16.6.2. Environmental Health Concerns

Despite the notion that dioxin-like PCBs are generally more potent in causing toxic effects, they usually account for only a small portion of the mass of PCBs found in the environment or in biological samples. The use of the term *nondioxin-like PCBs* is therefore not necessarily useful. While the congeners in this larger subgroup are not included in the toxic equivalency factors (TEF) scheme (as described in Section 16.8 below), they are not truly a single subclass of compounds but rather collectively have multiple toxicities with multiple structure-activity relationships (Barnes *et al.*, 1991). There simply has not enough congener-specific research performed to fully characterize the compounds in this larger subgroup. For instance, the "neurotoxic" PCBs have been defined by structure-activity relationships, rather than by the degree of their planarity, for analysis of their effects on cell dopamine content (Shain *et al.*, 1991) and on microsomal as well as mitochondrial Ca^{2+}-sequestration in rat cerebellum (Kodavanti *et al.*, 1996).

PCBs have been linked to neurological and behavioral problems in children, and to other adverse health effects including cancer, immunological dysfunction, as well as liver and skin disorders. These chlorinated hydrocarbons as a group have been classified as a probable human (Group 2A) carcinogen (IARC, 1987). They can disrupt hormonal functions and cause developmental and thyroid effects. PCBs were found to have metabolites with hormonal activities more potent comparing to those of themselves the parents. Studies supporting this claim included the experiment conducted by Andersson *et al.* (1999), in which the estrogenic activities of four structurally diverse PCB congeners and five of their hydroxylated derivatives (OH-PCBs) were investigated. That experiment involved a series of *in vitro* assays in which the PCB compounds were tested for their ability to induce the proliferation of MCF-7 human breast cancer cells and for their ability to express the vitellogenin (VTG) gene in rainbow trout hepatocytes. In both cell species, the OH-PCB metabolites were shown as more hormonally active than their parent PCBs were, with one being almost as potent as the natural estrogen. Another study in human cells showed that, in examining PCBs and several other OCs for their binding affinity to the thyroid hormone receptors (and to the thyroid hormone transport proteins), only the OH-PCBs were bound to the thyroid hormone receptors (Cheek *et al.*, 1999).

Note that the VTG mentioned above is an egg yolk precursor protein expressed only in the females of almost all oviparous species (e.g., fish) and is normally dormant in the males. However, when the males are exposed to estrogen mimickers, the VTG gene will be expressed in a dose-dependent manner, thus making the protein expression in a male oviparous a highly effective biomarker of exposure to estrogenic disruptors.

16.7. Polychlorinated Dibenzo-*p*-Dioxins/Dibenzofurans

Dioxins is a general term referring to the family of polychlorinated dibenzo-*p(ara)*-dioxins (PCDDs), and frequently including the family of polychlorinated dibenzofurans (PCDFs). This practice is owing to the fact that the congeners in the two families are exceptionally similar in structure as well as in chemical and toxicological properties. The PCDD and PCDF congeners, along with the dioxin-like PCB congeners, all share a certain common cellular mechanism of action (i.e., activation of the AhR, as illustrated in Figure 9.2) and induce comparable biological and toxic responses. As depicted in Figure 16.1, the nucleus or skeletal structure of PCDDs is a dioxin ($C_4H_4O_2$), having one more oxygen atom than the nucleus of furan (C_4H_4O) in PCDFs. Unlike the two benzene rings in PCBs, PBBs, or PBDEs, those in PCDDs and PCDFs each have 4, instead of 5, carbons that chlorine atoms can bond to. As such, PCDDs and PCDFs each have 75 and 135 possible congeners, respectively, together yielding a total of 210 possible congeners. PCDDs have 60 fewer possible congeners than PCDFs have because, unlike the furan nucleus, the dioxin nucleus is in a symmetric shape leading to fewer distinct stereoisomers. For the purpose of the discussion in this section, except where necessary to make the distinction, the term *dioxins* includes furans and at times also the dioxin-like PCBs.

16.7.1. Use and Pollution Sources

Dioxins (i.e., both the PCDDs and PCDFs) are generally considered as unintentional by-products of chemicals that are used to manufacture certain pesticides and wood preservatives, such as 2,4-D and 2,4,5-T (Chapter 15). Yet even prior to industrialization, low levels of naturally occurring dioxins were found in the environment as a result of natural combustion (e.g., forest fires) and geological processes. Today, the major environmental source of dioxins is incineration, although various levels of these chlorinated hydrocarbons have been detected in different environmental media (e.g., animal tissues, plants, foods, water, sediment, soil).

Dioxins are highly persistent in the environment with half-lives in the soil and sediment reportedly ranging from months to years. Because these hydrocarbons are practically neither volatile nor water-soluble, most are contained in soils and sediments serving as environmental reservoirs from which they may be released over a long period of time. Volatilization and particle re-suspension from these environmental reservoirs are therefore major potential sources for the global distribution of dioxins.

Dietary intake is the principal source of exposure to dioxins for the general population, with meat, dairy products, fish, and other seafood accounting for over 90% of the total daily toll. Dioxins are absorbed through the gastrointestinal (GI) tract, skin, and respiratory tract, and then distributed throughout the body via the bloodstream. Absorption is congener-specific, with the highly-chlorinated homologs having higher absorption rate compared to those containing fewer chlorines. Because of their lipophilic nature, dioxins tend to accumulate in the fatty tissues and the liver. Dioxins are slowly metabolized by oxidation or reductive dechlorination and conjugation. The major routes of their excretion in the human body are via the bile and feces, with small amounts being eliminated in the urine. Their half-lives in the human body reportedly range from 5 to 15 years.

16.7.2. Environmental Health Concerns

Dioxins can induce the enzymatic activity of Ah (acryl hydrocarbon) hydroxylase in the liver. They can bind to a cytosolic Ah receptor which is capable of regulating the synthesis of a variety of proteins. This receptor is present in many human tissues including the lungs, placenta, liver, and lymphocytes. Although there is evidence that the receptor is involved in many biological responses to dioxins, the general notion is that its characteristics alone are not sufficient to account for the complexity and broad spectrum of the biological effects that dioxins have reportedly induced (e.g., ATSDR, 1998).

In animal studies, of which many involved oral exposure, numerous types of adverse health effects were observed as induced by dioxins, including hepatic, GI, hematological, neurological, hormonal, skin, immunological, reproductive, and developmental. Several studies in humans suggested that exposure to dioxins would cause harm to children and the developing fetuses. There were data linking dioxin exposure to adverse developmental effects in fish, mammals, and birds at low exposure levels (ATSDR, 1998).

IARC (1997) and U.S. EPA (ATSDR, 1998) have classified 2,3,7,8-tetrachlorodibenzo-*p(ara)*-dioxin (2,3,7,8-TCDD, TCDD, or the dioxin for short) as a human (Group 1) and a probable human (Group B2) carcinogen, respectively, but have not determined extensively or conclusively the human or animal carcinogenicity of all of the other dioxins (including furans). Several epidemiological studies showed a link between exposure to TCDD and an increase in the mortalities from all types of cancers combined as well as from certain specific cancers (e.g., soft-tissue sarcoma, non-Hodgkin's lymphoma, respiratory tract, GI tract). There is some evidence that TCDD can act as a tumor promoter.

As many environmental toxicologists would concur and advise, the most toxic of all dioxins is TCDD. This PCDD congener is also called Seveso dioxin, named after the largest dioxins accident ever occurring in the world's history. This disaster took place on 10 July 1976, involving an explosion in a chemical plant located in a northern Italian town named Seveso. Following the explosion, a huge cloud of dioxins containing TCDD and some other congeners drifted well over 100 feet into the sky. Even though Seveso was the area most affected by the explosion, other neighboring towns including Cesano Maderno, Desio, and Meda were also affected, collectively amounting to over 100,000 residents affected. The most evident adverse health effect, ascertained some 14 years after the accident (Bertazzi, 1991), was 193 cases of chloracne. Other reversible, early adverse effects included peripheral neuropathy and excess liver enzyme induction.

16.8. Toxic Equivalency Factors

Many dioxin mixtures were each found to include some furan and dioxin-like PCB congeners. These compounds reportedly all share the common mechanism of toxicity involving activation of the Ah receptor, though with each having its own toxicity level. To express such a mixture's overall potential for inducing the same adverse effect, the World Health Organization (WHO) through the assistance of two expert groups (van den Berg *et al.*, 1998, 2006) has developed a toxic equivalency (TEQ) concept for dioxins.

16.8.1. Concepts of Toxic Equivalency

The TEQ concept weighs the toxicity of each of the less potent congeners in the dioxin mixture as a fraction of the toxicity of the most potent 2,3,7,8-TCDD in humans or other mammalians, with the latter given a reference value of 1 by WHO. Each of these other congeners is thereby attributed a specific *Toxic Equivalency Factor* (TEF) equal to or less than 1. The TEF values that WHO has established for the individual relevant dioxins and dioxin-like congeners are presented in Table 16.3 below.

To calculate the *total* TCDD-toxic equivalent concentration of a dioxin mixture containing a total of n dioxins and dioxin-like compounds, the concentrations of the individual dioxins and dioxin-like congeners are multiplied by their own specific TEF value, and then *added* together as follows:

$$\text{(total TCDD-based) TEQ} = \Sigma\ C_i \times \text{TEF}_i \qquad (16.1)$$

where C_i is the concentration of the ith congener in the mixture. Note that this method is for quantifying specifically the toxic effects mediated by activation of the cellular AhR; other types of adverse effects induced by dioxins are not intended to be so quantified.

16.8.2. Application of Toxic Equivalency Factor

The TEF approach developed by WHO offers a methodology in which the potential

Table 16.3. Toxic Equivalency Factors Developed by the World Health Organization (WHO) in 1998 and Updated in 2005 for Dioxins and Dioxin-like Compounds[a]

Dioxin or Dioxin-like Compound	WHO 1998	WHO 2005
Polychlorinated Dibenzo-p(ara)-Dioxins (PCDDs)		
2,3,7,8-tetraCDD (-TCDD)	1.0	1.0
1,2,3,7,8-pentaCDD	1.0	1.0
1,2,3,4,7,8-hexaCDD	0.1	0.1
1,2,3,6,7,8-hexaCDD	0.1	0.1
1,2,3,7,8,9-hexaCDD	0.1	0.1
1,2,3,4,6,7,8-heptaCDD	0.01	0.01
1,2,3,4,6,7,8,9-octaCDD	0.0001	0.0003
Polychlorinated Dibenzofurans (PCDFs)		
2,3,7,8-tetraCDF (-TCDF)	0.1	0.1
1,2,3,7,8-pentaCDF	0.05	0.03
2,3,4,7,8-pentaCDF	0.5	0.3
1,2,3,4,7,8-hexaCDF	0.1	0.1
1,2,3,6,7,8-hexaCDF	0.1	0.1
1,2,3,7,8,9-hexaCDF	0.1	0.1
2,3,4,6,7,8-hexaCDF	0.1	0.1
1,2,3,4,6,7,8-heptaCDF	0.01	0.01
1,2,3,4,7,8,9-heptaCDF	0.01	0.01
1,2,3,4,6,7,8,9-octaCDF	0.0001	0.0003
Nonortho-Substituted Polychlorinated Biphenyls (PCBs)		
PCB 77 (3,3′,4,4′-tetraCB)	0.0001	0.0001
PCB 81 (3,4,4′,5-tetraCB)	0.0001	0.0003
PCB 126 (3,3′,4,4′,5-pentaCB)	0.1	0.1
PCB 169 (3,3′,4,4′,5,5′-hexaCB)	0.01	0.03
Monoortho-Substituted Polychlorinated Biphenyls (PCBs)		
PCB 105 (2,3,3′,4,4′-pentaCB)	0.0001	0.00003
PCB 114 (2,3,4,4′,5-pentaCB)	0.0005	0.00003
PCB 118 (2,3′,4,4′,5-pentaCB)	0.0001	0.00003
PCB 123 (2,3',4,4',5'-pentaCB)	0.0001	0.00003
PCB 156 (2,3,3′,4,4′,5-hexaCB)	0.0005	0.00003
PCB 157 (2,3,3′,4,4′,5′-hexaCB)	0.0005	0.00003
PCB 167 (2,3′,4,4′,5,5′-hexaCB)	0.00001	0.00003
PCB 189 (2,3,3′,4,4′,5,5′-heptaCB)	0.0001	0.00003

[a]for humans and other mammalians; adapted from WHO (van den Berg *et al.*, 1998, 2006).

health or ecological effects can be quantified for exposure to a complex mixture of dioxins and dioxin-like compounds. However, this approach should be used with caution. The WHO methodology estimates the dioxin-based effects of a mixture by assuming dose-additivity and characterizes the mixture in terms of an equivalent mass of TCDD. The reality is that although the mixture may have the toxicological potential of TCDD, neither it as a single entity nor its non-TCDD constituent congeners can be assumed to undergo the same environmental fate as TCDD does, even for exposure assessment purposes. The fate of a mixture in its environment is supposed to be the resultant totality of the fates of all its constituent congeners in their own individual environments. Yet different congeners typically have different physicochemical properties (e.g., octanol-water partition coefficient, vapor pressure, photolysis rate, binding affinity to organic matter). Therefore, it is likely that a mixture's absolute concentration for environmental exposure would be different from the calculated sum of the relative concentrations of its constituent congeners making up the emission entity that travels through an environmental medium while subject to the effects of various meteorological conditions.

In June 2005, an expert meeting was held by the WHO/International Programme on Chemical Safety in Geneva, Switzerland, during which the TEF values were reassessed for dioxins and dioxin-like compounds. As a result of the reassessment (van den Berg *et al.*, 2006), WHO advised that the 2005 TEF values be used from here on to replace the 1998 values. The real consequence of these TEF changes on the TEQ for biotic or abiotic samples of dioxin mixtures has not been looked into seriously. One such evaluation study (Hong *et al.*, 2009) was conducted not too long ago, nonetheless, using the data from a major exposure study in which serum, household dust, and soil levels of dioxins and dioxin-like compounds were measured in several regions of Michigan. The mean total TEQ was found to reduce significantly by 26%, 12%, and 14% for the serum, household dust, and soil samples, respectively, when the TEFs used in the evaluation study were based on the 2005 values instead of those available in 1998. The resultant reductions were apparently all due to the down-weighting of the newer TEF values used.

References

Albaigés J, 2005. Persistent Organic Pollutants in the Mediterranean Sea. In *The Handbook of Environmental Chemistry, Volume 5, Part K: The Mediterranean Sea* (Saliot A, Ed.). New York, New York, USA: Springer Berlin Heidelberg, pp.89-149.

AMAP (Arctic Monitoring and Assessment Programme), 1997. Arctic Pollution Issues: A State of the Arctic Environment Report. AMAP, Oslo, Norway.

Andersson PL, Blom A, Johannisson A, Pesonen M, Tysklind M, Berg AH, Olsson PE, Norrgren L, 1999. Assessment of PCBs and Hydroxylated PCBs as Potential Xenoestrogens: *In vitro* Studies Based on MCF-7 Cell Proliferation and Induction of Vitellogenin in Primary Culture of Rainbow Trout Hepatocytes. *Arch. Environ. Contam. Toxicol.* 37:145-150.

Ann Arbor Statement, 2003. *Long-Range Transport of Toxic Substances into the Great Lakes Basin.* The International Joint Commission's 2003 Great Lakes Conference Workshop, 16-17 September, Ann Arbor, Michigan, USA.

ATSDR (Agency for Toxic Substances and Disease Registry), 1998. Toxicological Profile for Chlorinated Dibenzo-*p*-dioxins (CDDs). U.S. Department of Health and Human Services, Atlanta, Georgia, USA.

ATSDR (Agency for Toxic Substances and Disease Registry), 2004. Toxicological Profile for Polybrominated Biphenyls and Polybrominated Diphenyl Ethers (PBBs and PBDEs). U.S. Department of Health and Human Services, Atlanta, Georgia, USA.

Barnes D, Alford-Stevens A, Birnbaum L, Kutz FW, Wood W, Patton D, 1991. Toxicity Equivalency Factors for PCBs? *Qual. Assur.* 1:70-81.

Bekesi JG, Holland JF, Anderson HA, Fischbein AS, Rom W, Wolff MS, Selikoff IJ, 1978. Lymphocyte Function of Michigan Dairy Farmers Exposed to Polybrominated Biphenyls. *Science* 199:1207-1209.

Bertazzi PA, 1991. Long-Term Effects of Chemical Disasters: Lessons and Results from Seveso. *Sci. Total Environ.* 106:5-20.

Betts KS, 2008. Chemical Exposures: Not Immune to PFOS Effects? *Environ. Health Perspect.* 116:A290-A290.

Blanck HM, Marcus M, Tolbert PE, Rubin C, Henderson AK, Hertzberg VS, Zhang RH, Cameron L, 2000. Age at Menarche and Tanner Stage in Girls Exposed *in utero* and Postnatally to Polybrominated Biphenyl. *Epidemiology* 11:641-647.

BSEF (Bromine Science and Environmental Forum), 2000. *An Introduction to Brominated Flame Retardants.* 37 Square de Meeûs, 1000 Brussels, Belgium.

CEPA (Canadian Environmental Protection Act), 1999. Persistence and Bioaccumulation Regulations (SOR/2000-107;23 March 2000). *Canada Gazette* Part II,134(7):607-612.

Cheek AO, Kow K, Chen J, McLachlan JA, 1999. Potential Mechanisms of Thyroid Disruption in Humans: Interaction of Organochlorine Compounds with Thyroid Receptor, Transthyretin, and Thyroid-Binding Globulin. *Environ. Health Perspect.* 107:273-278.

Eriksson P, Jakobsson E, Fredriksson A, 2001. Brominated Flame Retardants: A Novel Class of Developmental Neurotoxicants in Our Environment? *Environ. Health Perspect.* 109:903-908.

Eriksson P, Viberg H, Jakobsson E, Örn U, Fredriksson A, 2002. A Brominated Flame Retardant, 2,2′,4,4′,5-Pentabromodiphenyl Ether: Uptake, Retention, and Induction of Neurobehavioral Alterations in Mice during a Critical Phase of Neonatal Brain Development. *Toxicol. Sci.* 67:98-103.

European Commission, 2003. *Technical Guidance Document on Risk Assessment.* EUR 20418 EN/2. Joint Research Centre, Institute for Health and Consumer Protection, European Chemical Bureau, Ispra, Italy.

Ewald G, Larsson P, Linge H, Okla L, Szarzi N, 1998. Biotransport of Organic Pollutants to an Inland Alaska Lake by Migrating Sockeye Salmon (*Onchorhynchus nerka*). *Arctic* 51:478-485.

Fries GF, 1985. The PBB Episode in Michigan: An Overall Appraisal. *Crit. Rev. Toxicol.* 16:105-56

Harley KG, Marks AR, Chevrier J, Bradman A, Sjödin A, Eskenazi B, 2010. PBDE Concentrations in Women's Serum and Fecundability. *Environ. Health Perspect.* 118:699-704.

Hong B, Garabrant D, Hedgeman E, Demond A, Gillespie B, Chen Q, Chang CW, Towey T, Knutson K, Franzblau A, Lepkowski J, Adriaens P, 2009. Impact of WHO 2005 Revised Toxic Equivalency Factors for Dioxins on the TEQs in Serum, Household Dust and Soil. *Chemosphere* 76: 723-733.

IARC (International Agency for Research on Cancer), 1987. IARC Monographs on the Evaluation of Carcinogenic Risks to Humans, Supplement 7: Overall Evaluations of Carcinogenicity – An Updating of IARC Monographs Volumes 1 to 42. Lyon, France: WHO Press.

IARC (International Agency for Research on Cancer), 1997. IARC Monographs on the Evaluation of Carcinogenic Risks to Humans, Volume 69: Polychlorinated Dibenzo-*para*-Dioxins and Polychlorinated Dibenzofurans. Lyon, France: WHO Press.

IPCS (International Programme on Chemical Safety), 2003. Polychlorinated Biphenyls: Human Health Aspects. CICAD 55, (published under the joint sponsorship of the United Nations Environment Programme, the International Labour Organization, and the World Health Organization). Geneva, Switzerland.

Kodavanti PR, Ward TR, McKinney JD, Tilson HA, 1996. Inhibition of Microsomal and Mitochondrial Ca^{2+}-Sequestration in Rat Cerebellum by Polychlorinated Biphenyl Mixtures and Congeners: Structure-Activity Relationships. *Arch. Toxicol.* 70:150-157.

Lind G, 2004. *REACH – What Happened and Why? The Only Planet Guide to the Secrets of Chemicals Policy in the EU.* Affärstryckeriet, Nortälje, Sweden: Inger Schörling (Greens/European Free Alliance, European Parliament).

Matthies M, Scheringer M, 2001. *Editorial*: Long-Range Transport in the Environment. *Environ. Sci. Pollut. Res.* 8:149-149.

Mills SA 3rd, Thal DI, Barney J, 2007. A Summary of the 209 PCB Congener Nomenclature. *Chemosphere* 68:1603-1612.

Peden-Adams MM, Stuckey JE, Gaworecki KM, Berger-Ritchie J, Bryant K, Jodice PG, Scott TR, Ferrario JB, Guan B, Vigo C, Boone JS, McGuinn WD, DeWitt JC, Keil DE, 2009. Developmental Toxicity in White Leghorn Chickens Following *in ovo* Exposure to Perfluorooctane Sulfonate (PFOS). *Reprod. Toxicol.* 27:307-318.

Peters RJB, 2006. *Man-Made Chemicals in Food Products.* TNO Report 2006-A-R0095/B (Version 2). TNO, Laan van Westenenk 501, P.O. Box 342, 7300 AH Apeldoom, The Netherlands.

Shain W, Bush B, Seegal R, 1991. Neurotoxicity of Polychlorinated Biphenyls: Structure-Activity Relationship of Individual Congeners. *Toxicol. Appl. Pharmacol.* 111:33-42.

Sjödin A, Wong LY, Jones RS, Park A, Zhang Y, Hodge C, DiPietro E, McClure C, Turner W, Needham LL, Patterson DG Jr, 2008. Serum Concentrations of Polybrominated Diphenyl Ethers (PBDEs) and Polybrominated Biphenyl (PBB) in the United States Population: 2003-2004. *Environ. Sci. Technol.* 42:1377-1384.

Takemura T, Uno I, Nakajima T, Higurashi A, Sano I, 2002. Modeling Study of Long-Range Transport of Asian Dust and Anthropogenic Aerosols from East Asia. *Geophy. Res. Letters.* 29:2158-2161.

U.K. DEFRA (U.K. Department for Environmental, Food, and Rural Affairs), 2002. Chemicals Stakeholder Forum Meetings – First Meeting of the UK Chemicals Stakeholders Forum: 2nd October 2000 Criteria for Concern CSF/00/7. London, UK.

UNECE (United Nations Economic Commission for Europe), 2004. *Handbook for the 1979 Convention on Long-Range Transboundary Air Pollution and Its Protocols.* Section XI (Recent Decisions of the Executive Body), Decision 1998/2 (ECE/EB.Air/60). Geneva, Switzerland, p.299.

UNEP (United Nations Environmental Programme), 2001. *Final Act of the Conference of Plenipotentiaries on the Stockholm Convention on Persistent Organic Pollutants.* UNEP/POPS/CONF4. UNEP, Geneva, Switzerland, p.41, dated 5 June.

U.S. EPA (U.S. Environmental Protection Agency), 1999a. Persistent Bioaccumulative Toxic (PBT) Chemicals; Lowering of Reporting Thresholds for Certain PBT Chemicals; Addition of Certain PBT Chemicals; Community Right-to-Know Toxic Chemical Reporting. *Federal Register* 64: 58666-58753.

U.S. EPA (U.S. Environmental Protection Agency), 1999b. Category for Persistent, Bioaccumulative, and Toxic New Chemical Substances. *Federal Register* 64:60194-60204.

van den Berg M, Birnbaum L, Bosveld AT, Brunstrom B, Cook P, Feeley M, Giesy JP, Hanberg A, Hasegawa R, Kennedy SW, Kubiak T, Larsen JC, van Leeuwen FX, Liem AK, Nolt C, Peterson RE, Poellinger L, Safe S, Schrenk D, Tillitt D, Tysklind M, Younes M, Waern F, Zacharewski T, 1998. Toxic Equivalency Factors (TEFs) for PCBs, PCDDs, PCDFs for Humans and Wildlife. *Environ. Health Perspect.* 106:775-792.

van den Berg M, Birnbaum LS, Denison M, De Vito M, Farland W, Feeley M, Fiedler H, Hakansson H, Hanberg A, Haws L, Rose M, Safe S, Schrenk D, Tohyama C, Tritscher A, Tuomisto J, Tysklind M, Nigel W, Peterson RE, 2006. The 2005 World Health Organization Reevaluation of Human and Mammalian Toxic Equivalency Factors for Dioxins and Dioxin-like Compounds. *Toxicol. Sci.* 93:223-241.

Zhao G, Wang Z, Dong MH, Rao K, Luo J, Wang D, Zha J, Huang S, Xu Y, Ma M, 2008. PBBs, PBDEs, and PCBs Levels in Hair of Residents around E-Waste Disassembly Sites in Zhejiang Province, China, and Their Potential Sources. *Sci. Total Environ.* 397:46-57.

Zhou T, Taylor MM, DeVito MJ, Croftonr KM, 2002. Developmental Exposure to Brominated Diphenyl Ethers Results in Thyroid Hormone Disruption. *Toxicol. Sci.* 66:105-116.

Review Questions

1. Define the term *half-life* in relation to environmental persistence.

2. What are the main differences between the two major aspects of persistence for pollutants in the environment?

3. How is long-range transport of pollutants related to their persistence and bioaccumulation potential in the environment?

4. What are the main differences among PTS, PBTs, POPs, and POCs?

5. Which of the following authorities appear(s) to be more health conservative with respect to their prevention and control of PTS? a) UNEP; b) CEPA; c) European Commission; d) U.S. EPA; (e) UNECE; f) U.K. DEFRA.

6. Name the so-called *dirty dozen* POPs on the Stockholm Convention's *initial* priority list, and those added to the list between 2004 and 2011.

7. Briefly describe the practical actions being taken by the Stockholm Convention of 2001 on those POPs placed on its priority action list.

8. Name the international treaty that has *provided* the technical guidelines on waste management for POPs.

9. What are the likely sources of environmental exposure to PFOS?

10. How is PFOS structurally different from PFOA? And how is it biochemically different from the other POPs in terms of bioaccumulation?

11. What may be the major types of toxic effects of PFOS in humans?

12. How many congeners of PBBs, of PBDEs, and of PCBs are theoretically possible, and why? Also, why do the *deca*BB, *deca*BDE, and *deca*CB homologs each have only one congener?

13. What are the likely sources of environmental exposure to PBBs worldwide?

14. What may be the major adverse health effects of PBBs on humans, as evident from the massive PBB contamination of livestock feed in Michigan during 1973-1974?

15. What may be the major adverse health effects of PBDEs on humans?

16. What is *commercial pentaBDE* commonly used for? And which of the following congeners are typically contained in this mixture? a) PBDE 180, PBDE 203; b) PBDE 47, PBDE 99; c) PBDE 47, PBDE 153; d) PBDE 99, PBDE 180; e) PBDE 153, PBDE 203.

17. Which of the following PBDE homologs is still widely produced in the United States today? a) *tetra*BDE; b) *penta*BDE; c) *hexa*BDE; d) *octa*BDE; e) *deca*BDE.

18. What are the main differences between *coplanar* and *nonplanar* PCB congeners, and between *ortho*-substituted and non*ortho*-substituted PCB congeners?

19. What is the widely accepted common mechanism of toxicity shared by both the dioxin and the dioxin-like PCB congeners?

20. What may be the major adverse health effects of OH-PCBs on humans?

21. Why does the PCDD family have fewer possible congeners than the PCDF family has?

22. What is the one major environmental source of dioxins found in these days? And where in today's environment can dioxins be detected?

23. What is the main source of exposure to dioxins for the general population?

24. Which congener in the dioxin family is considered as the most potent? Briefly describe this congener's major adverse health effects on humans.

25. Which of the following POPs are *least likely* to be found in e-waste? a) PCDDs, PFOS; b) PBBs, PBDEs; c) PBBs, PCBs; d) PBDEs, PCBs; e) PCBs, PCDFs.

26. What is the *total* TCDD-toxic *equivalent* concentration of a dioxin *mixture* in fish tissue containing (ppt = parts per trillion): 10 ppt of TCDD; 20 ppt of PCB 81; 30 ppt of PCB 118; and 40 ppt of 1,2,3,6,7,8-*hexa*CDF?

CHAPTER 17

Biological and Physical Toxic Agents

17.1. Introduction

This chapter serves as a reminder that in some parts of the world, there are as many biological and physical toxic agents as there are chemical toxicants in the environment. Fortunately or not, nowadays many of these "nonchemical" toxic agents such as malaria and guinea worm parasites are seldom found in the well-developed regions where environmental toxicology practice is more active. Perhaps as some form of trade-off, certain nonchemical toxic agents such as traffic congestion and noise pollution have been causing environmental health problems predominately in the advanced countries as well as in many developing regions.

In this chapter, biological and special physical toxic agents of general environmental health concern are discussed categorically following the clarifications below on several terms, concepts, and definitions deemed crucial to the discussion on biological agents. The first clarification is that, as to be consistent with legal (U.S. Code, 2013) and proper (e.g., Gillard, 2001; Section 1.1.1) usage, the term *toxin* will refer to a poisonous, mostly proteinaceous product of the metabolic activities of a *living* organism. Further, when the toxin is delivered by an organism to its victim by means of a bite or sting, it is commonly termed *venom*. In contrast, the term *toxicant* is defined as just about any toxic agent including toxin. Yet there are still people, particularly in nonscientific sectors, who would include mercury (Hg) and other chemical agents as toxins found in living organisms.

17.1.1. Concepts of Biological Agents

The term "*nonchemical agent*", as implicated in this chapter, also needs clarification. For one thing, the most critical constituents in snake venoms are proteolytic enzymes (Section 17.6.1), which literally are all (bio)*chemical* substances. Yet the agent to which the *exposure* is of immediate concern is the snake or its bite, not so much its proteinaceous toxins which are nevertheless biological in origin if not in nature.

It is also important to recognize that biological toxic agents refer to all living organisms that cause harm, not only the natural toxins that they produce. Although some microbes can produce fatal toxins in humans or other organisms, they or some others can be even more toxic on their own. Research (e.g., HHMI, 2002) has shown that overgrowth of certain types of bacteria (e.g., *Lactobacillus*) in a body tissue could lead to the development of cancer or other serious disorders (e.g., stomach ulcers) at that very site, potentially signifying the toxic mechanism of direct (bacterial) damage (Section 9.1.2).

To avoid confusion, those superficially comparable terms such as *toxins from fish* and *fish toxins* are not used interchangeably in this chapter, as they may mean different things to different people. For instance, many tribal hunters use various fish toxins, such as fish stupefying plants, to paralyze fish so that their captives become easier to be caught by hand. In contrast, some highly potent toxins, such as tetrodotoxin and ciguatoxin (Section 17.4.1), can be found *in* (or *on*) certain types of fish or shellfish.

17.1.2. Infection *vs.* Infectious Disease

As another confusion to avoid, some people may argue that a pandemic of infectious disease is more of a concern to public health practitioners than to environmental toxicologists. Yet the declaration of a disease pandemic is almost always based on some form of health risk assessment which, as stated in Chapter 3, has preoccupied the field of environmental toxicology for the past several decades. As also noted in Chapter 3, for this type of pandemics, both the laboratory confirmation of the infecting microbial agent (or known commonly as pathogen) and the development of a vaccine are more related to toxicity testing, the role of a toxicologist with the appropriate training.

Still another important point for clarification is that infection and infectious disease do not mean exactly the same thing, but are often loosely used interchangeably to facilitate discussion. Actually, infection takes place when a pathogen enters a host's body to start colonizing. In contrast, the disease as a result of the infection occurs only if the microbe starts to multiply aggressively to the level that certain symptoms manifest. The body of most any mammalian host, including that of a human, has high capacity to fight off microbial invasion. Diseases result only when these protective mechanisms are compromised. An infection is thus the invasion and the colonization by a microbial agent in the host organism; and an infectious disease occurs only when the colonization becomes aggressive. In an infection, the pathogen seeks to utilize the resources in the host to multiply. The pathogen can interfere with the normal functioning of the host leading to acute or chronic symptoms, tissue death, loss of an infected limb, or even death.

17.2. Pathogenic Microbial Agents

Infectious diseases as a single entity kill far more people worldwide than any other cause. The microbial agents responsible for diseases of this type are tiny living things that are found everywhere in the environment. Infectious diseases are also called communicable or transmissible diseases owing to their potential for transmission from one person or one species to another by a replicating agent (as opposed to a toxin produced by a specific microbe). People can get infected by touching, drinking, eating, or inhaling something that contains the microbes which are known more commonly as germs to the general public. Germs can also spread through kissing, sexual contact, and animal or insect bites. Most pathogenic agents can be classified into the following four microbe groups: bacteria, viruses, fungi, and protozoa. Examples of pathogenic (microbial) agents of some special or uncommon groups include viroids and prions. Viroids are each composed exclusively of a single piece of circular single-stranded RNA which may contain some double-stranded regions. These RNA strands (Chapter 18) cause mostly plant diseases but recently have been found also to cause disease in humans. Prions are misfolded proteins; they have been implicated for causing BSE (bovine spongiform encephalopathy), which is known commonly as mad-cow disease (Chapter 1). Due to their simplified structures, both prions and viroids are often called subviral particles.

In medical microbiology, the causal relationship between a pathogen and a disease is supposed to be confirmed by a set of widely accepted criteria known as the Henle-Koch postulates which specify certain conditions that must be fulfilled (e.g., Evans, 1976). These conditions are: (1) The agent (i.e., the pathogen) must be present in all cases suffering from the disease, but not (sufficiently) in subjects without the disease; (2) the agent must be isolated from the infected host and grown in pure culture *in vitro*; (3) when such a culture is inoculated into a healthy susceptible host, the disease must be reproducible; and (4) the agent must be recoverable from the experimentally infected host.

17.2.1. Pathogenic Bacteria

Bacteria are microscopic, single-celled organisms having a shape like a ball, rod, or spiral. Thousands of different bacterial species are living in virtually every conceivable environment around the world, with some found living even in radioactive wastes. For diagnostic identification purposes and where appropriate, bacterial species are differentiated into two main groups termed *Gram-positive* and *Gram-negative* on the basis of their cell wall's stainability into violet-like color or not, respectively, by means of a procedure known as the Gram method (e.g., Holt, 1994). The predominant symptoms of bacterial infection are localized redness, swelling, pain, and discharge in the affected area.

Although a vast majority of the bacteria are harmless to humans (and animals), some are highly pathogenic. One bacterial infection with the most disease burden today is tuberculosis, caused by the species *Mycobacterium tuberculosis*. According to the World Health Organization (WHO, 2009), this disease in 2008 alone killed about 1.5 million people worldwide who were tested negative with human immunodeficiency virus (HIV). Other bacterial diseases of global concern include pneumonia caused by the genera *Streptococcus* and *Pseudomonas*, and foodborne illnesses by the genera *Campylobacter*, *Shigella*, and *Salmonella*. Botulism, tetanus, typhoid fever, syphilis, and diphtheria are examples of serious diseases that are now limited to local or regional concerns.

The common pathogenic species of regional concerns include: *Escherichia coli (E. coli); Helicobacter pylori (H. pylori); Haemophilus influenzae (H. influenzae)*; and those in the *Staphylococci* (Staph), *Streptococci* (Strep), and *Salmonella* genera. In particular, *E. coli* tends to cause gastrointestinal (GI) dysfunctions as it is inclined to colonize the GI tract in the human or animal body. This species can also cause food poisoning when transmitted through contaminated food products (e.g., hamburger). *H. pylori* is the main culprit responsible for stomach ulcers. *H. influenzae* is one of the most common bacterial species affecting the body. The associated symptoms include several types of meningitis and infection of the ear as well as the respiratory tract (without the flu). Children are now immunized against one of its strains named *H. influenzae* type b.

Many Staph bacteria live harmlessly in or on the human body. However, some others can cause infection and eventually disease. Symptoms from this type of infection include skin rash, boil, abscess, eczema, and impetigo. Some Staph varieties can cause inflammation of the breasts known as mastitis (that releasing the bacteria to the mother's milk) to cause thereby complications for the infant's health. Methicillin-resistant *Staphylococcus aureus*, known also by its acronym MRSA, gets its name because this Staph species has mutated over time to a different strain ending with a resistance to most antibiotics (but mainly methicillin) used to treat it. MRSA can cause serious skin infection that becomes difficult to treat. Many *Salmonella* species are foodborne pathogens causing diarrhea and other common symptoms of food poisoning. Undercooked poultry, eggs, and ground beef are common causes (as well as sources) of *Salmonella* infection. Also commonly found in a local or regional environment are several Strep species that can cause the more familiar Strep throat infection or other common respiratory infections (e.g., pneumonia).

17.2.2. Pathogenic Viruses

Most viruses are each about one hundred times smaller than an average bacterium, thus being too small to be seen even with a light microscope. They each consist of two or three parts known collectively as virion or viral particle: (1) the genetic material made from either DNA (Chapter 18) or RNA (Chapter 18); (2) a protein coat that protects this genetic material; and (3) in some cases a lipid-like envelope surrounding the protein coat when the latter is outside a cell. While viruses can replicate only inside the living cells of the body of an organism, they are able to infect all forms of organisms, from animals and plants of high order to bacteria and archaea. There are millions of different viral species, of which roughly 5,000 have been investigated in some detail.

Viruses spread in many ways. Plant viruses are typically transmitted from plant to plant by insects such as aphids that feed on sap, whereas animal viruses can be carried by blood-sucking insects commonly referred to as vectors. Influenza viruses in humans are spread largely by sneezes and coughs. The norovirus and rotavirus, which are common causes of viral gastroenteritis (a.k.a. stomach flu, characterized by vomiting and watery diarrhea for up to 7 days), are found in the stool or the vomit of infected people and in contaminated foods or drinks. HIV is one of several viruses transmitted through sexual contact and by exposure to contaminated blood.

Viral infections in humans can cause illnesses as mild as the common cold and as severe as AIDS (acquired immune deficiency syndrome) or encephalitis. In general, viral diseases are systemic, in that they eventually involve many different parts of the body at the same time. Many viral infections provoke an immunological response capable of eliminating the infecting virus. Immunological responses can also be produced by vaccines which confer an artificially acquired immunity to the specific viral invasion. Some viral pathogens such as those causing AIDS and hepatitis unfortunately can sidestep the immunological response to result in chronic or fatal infectious diseases.

Some viruses do not kill the host cell but alter its biochemical functions instead. Sometimes the infected cell loses control over normal cell division and becomes cancerous. Some viruses leave their genetic material in the host cell where the material remains dormant for an extended time (to result potentially in a latent infection). When the cell is sufficiently disturbed, the dormant viral material may begin replicating again and cause disease. Most viruses initially infect one particular type of cells, such as cold viruses infecting predominately cells of the upper respiratory tract. Most viruses also infect a few species of plants or animals only, whereas some infect only people.

The most common viral infections are those of the nose, throat, and upper airways, with symptoms including sore throat, sinusitis, and the common cold. Influenza is a viral respiratory infection tending to cause severe symptoms in infants, older people, and people with other health problems.

Viruses that infect the human nervous system include those causing rabies, St. Louis, Japanese, and several other types of encephalitis. Viral infections can also occur around the skin, sometimes resulting in warts or other blemishes. Other common viral infections in humans are caused by the various types of human herpesviruses (HHVs) that normally remain within a host cell in a dormant state. During the host's lifetime, any of these viruses can become reactivated to cause disease (again).

17.2.3. Pathogenic Fungi

Fungi are a large collection of eukaryotic organisms (i.e., those whose cells contain complex structures enclosed within their membrane) that live in the air, soil, water, or on plants or other moist and humid surfaces. They can be carried by pets and inanimate objects (e.g., combs, brushes, pillows, shoes, towels). Some fungi reproduce via spores (i.e., tiny, usually single-celled reproductive body) in the air. People hence can be exposed by inhaling the spores; or these spores can land on them. As a result, fungal infections often start in the lung or on the skin. Fungi can be difficult to kill. Their major phyla include yeasts, molds, and mushrooms. Most yeasts (e.g., the genus *Candida*) and some molds (e.g., the genus *Aspergillums*) can be seen only through a light microscope.

While usually progressing slowly, fungal infections are rarely serious unless the immunological system is sufficiently weakened, as by disorders (e.g., AIDS) or drugs. In those cases, they may end in serious bacterial infections. Most fungal infections seen in humans are caused by a type of fungi called dermophyte that tends to infect the top layer of the skin, hair, or nail. The clinical condition induced by fungal infections of the skin is known as ringworm (*tinea*). There are many types of ringworms, including body ringworm (*tinea corporis*), jock itch (*tinea cruris*) around the groin, scalp ringworm (*tinea capitis*), athlete's foot (*tinea pedis*), and nail ringworm (*tinea unguium*). The ringworm typically resembles a rash that forms ring-shaped patches each in pink or red with a clear center and about one inch in diameter. The rash may itch from slightly to unnerving.

Mycosis is the medical term for any infection or disease caused by a fungus. Some of the more serious fungal infections found in humans include blastomycosis, coccidioidomycosis, paracoccidioidomycosis, and histoplasmycosis. Blastomycosis, caused by the species *Blastomyces dermatitidis* found in wood and soil, is endemic to portions of North America. Its symptoms include flu-like illness with fever, chills, myalgia, headaches, and a nonproductive cough resolving in days. Coccidioidomycosis, caused by *Coccidioides immitis* or *posadasii*, is also known as California disease or San Joaquin valley fever in the United States. It is endemic to certain parts of Arizona, California, Nevada, New Mexico, Texas, and Utah. The disease is usually mild, with flu-like symptoms and rashes. Paracoccidioidomycosis, caused by *Paracoccidioides brasiliensis*, is known commonly as Brazilian or South American blastomycosis. Its symptoms include pulmonary infection and skin ulcer. As its nicknames imply, it is endemic to South and Central America. Histoplasmycosis, caused by *Histoplasma capsulatum*, is also known as Cave disease, Darling's disease, Ohio valley disease, or reticuloendotheliosis. It is common among AIDS patients due to their lowered immunological system, and has symptoms similar to those of blastomycosis. Further characteristics of these various types of fungal infections can be found in the volume by Bologna *et al.* (2007) or by Ryan and Ray (2004).

17.2.4. Pathogenic Parasites

Parasites are organisms that live on or inside another organism with the potential to harm the host organism. They count on the materials, including cells and tissues, in their host for survival and reproduction, as they are not capable of producing energy or food on their own. The waste products that some parasites release can be highly toxic to their host. Parasitic infections are more common in rural and underdeveloped regions than in industrialized areas. In industrialized areas, this type of infections may still occur in places with poor sanitation or unhygienic practices, such as in some mental institutions and daycare centers. They may also occur in people with a weakened immunological system and in frequent overseas travelers. According to news reports, some U.S. soldiers returning from overseas service brought with them a number of parasites.

Parasites that infect humans include two prominent subgroups called helminthes and protozoa. Examples of protozoa include those that cause mosquito-borne malaria. Like bacteria, protozoa are microscopic, single-celled organisms. In contrast, helminthes are larvae-producing worms with internal organs consisting of many cells. Members in this second subgroup include the water flea-borne guinea worm (*Dracunculiasis medinensis*), which is among the longest roundworms (technically termed *nematodes*) infecting humans. It is in this sense that helminthes might not be qualified as *micro*organisms.

The most common infectious protozoa in the world are the genus *Cryptosporidium* and the species *Giardia lamblia, Toxoplasma gondii,* and *Entamoeba histolytica.* These tiny parasites can be transmitted through contaminated foods and water or from person to person, and subsequently throughout the affected body to cause abscesses in the lungs, liver, kidneys, heart, brain, or other tissues. On rare occasions, they can be transmitted through blood transfusions, through injections with a contaminated needle, or from a pregnant woman to her fetus.

The most common helminthes found in humans and their pets are pinworms, round-worms, tapeworms, hookworms, and liver fluke. Pinworms (e.g., *Enterobius folliculars*) are among the most common human helminthes found in the United States. They make their home in the host's colon, but lay their eggs outside the host's body. Their transmission can occur through unclean hands and inanimate objects (e.g., bed sheet). The associated symptoms include irritation and scratching in the anal area.

17.3. Toxins from Microorganisms

Covering a subject matter as broad as toxins from microorganisms makes selectivity a necessity here. At any rate, there are more toxins from bacteria studied, followed by toxins from fungi, than toxins from all other microbes combined. Saxitoxin, brevetoxin, and domoic acid are nonetheless three familiar toxins produced by algae, not by bacteria or fungi. These three potent toxins are responsible for, specifically and respectively, the symptoms of neurotoxic, paralytic, and amnestic shellfish poisoning. Moreover, as noted in Section 17.2.4, parasites are known to excrete waste products which can be very toxic or allergic to their host, although the characteristics of these waste products are not well documented except for a few cases. One exception case is malaria toxin, a glycolipid named glycosylphosphatidylinositol produced by the protozoan *Plasmodium falciparum*. Malaria toxin is capable of stimulating the production of tumor necrosis factor (TNF) in host cells (e.g., Caro *et al.*, 1996). TNF is a cytokine as well as a term referring to a superfamily of cytokines (i.e., small proteins secreted by specific cells of the immunological system) capable of causing death of tumor cells and systemic inflammation. Overproduction of TNF is reportedly responsible for the severe, at times life-threatening, pathologies associated with cerebral or complicated malaria (Schofield *et al.*, 1993).

Toxins produced by viruses are not uncommon, inasmuch as many viral components and their by-products can accumulate in the host cell during the course of virus replication. Nonetheless, viral toxin can be a confusing or loose term. There are scholars who would consider any double-stranded RNA (dsRNA) as a viral toxin (e.g., DeWitte-Orr and Mossman, 2011). The dsRNA genomes are known to encode a diverse group of viruses including the families *totiviridae* and *reoviridae*. Virus L-A in the *Saccharomyces cerevisiae* yeast cells is a dsRNA of the totiviridae family. This virus has the ability to encode the cytotoxic proteins called killer toxins K1, K2, K28, and zygocin (Reiter *et al.*, 2005; Schmitt and Breinig, 2002; Schmitt and Reiter, 2008). In general, the dsRNA genomes, the viruses encoded by these genomes, and the toxic proteins that the dsRNA encoded may all be referred to as viral toxins.

Under most circumstances, the toxins produced by any type of microorganisms should be regarded as significant virulence determinants of microbial pathogenicity, even though some of them also play a key role in medicine. Potential applications of toxins in medical research include their use in the development of novel anti-cancer drugs and as tools in neurobiology and cellular biology. In the two (sub)sections that follow, as due to space limitation, only certain toxins produced by bacteria and certain toxins produced by fungi are highlighted.

17.3.1. Toxins from Bacteria

Toxins from bacteria can be broadly divided into two subclasses: *exotoxins* and *endotoxins*. Exotoxins are toxins actively secreted by the bacteria either inside the host cell or in the host cell's external environment. In contrast, *endo*toxins are part of the bacteria themselves, usually located on their outer membranes, and are not released until the microbes are destroyed by the host's immunological system or by antibiotics. The groups called *enterotoxins*, *neurotoxins*, and *leukocidins* all refer to toxins whose primary adverse action is on that implicit target site (i.e., mucous membrane of the intestine, nervous system, white blood cells, respectively). Some of the toxins from bacteria, such as tetanus toxin and botulin, are the most potent known. The toxicological profiles of tetanus and botulinum toxins, together with those of several prominent ones from other bacteria species, are summarized in Table 17.1.

It is noteworthy here that tetanus toxin and botulin are both neurotoxins produced by the Gram-positive bacteria genus *Clostridium*. Naturally, the bacterial species *botulinum* and *tetani* are producers of the botulinum toxin and the tetanus toxin, respectively. *C. botulinum* is an anaerobic bacterium widely distributed in soils, ponds, lake and pond sediments, and decaying vegetation. Accordingly, the intestinal tracts of birds, mammals, and fish may occasionally contain the bacteria as a transient. Foodborne botulism, which resembles Staphylococcal food poisoning, is not an infection but an intoxication, in that it results from the ingestion of foods containing the preformed *botulinum* toxin. On absorption in the duodenum and jejunum, the toxin passes into the bloodstream by which it reaches the peripheral neuromuscular synapses and there blocks the release of the neurotransmitter ACh (acetylcholine); the neurotransmitter is required for a nerve to stimulate a muscle (Section 9.2.4). *C. tetani* is commonly found in soils, especially where manure is heavily used, and in the intestinal tracts and feces of various animals. The tetani bacteria produce terminal spores which can get into the human body via a skin wound loaded with the contaminated soil, dust, or animal waste. Despite the fact that these bacteria each have a typical Gram-positive cell wall, they may still stain Gram-negative or Gram-variable. Like botulism, tetanus is a fatal human disease.

17.3.2. Toxins from Fungi

Many toxic (secondary) metabolites produced by *micro*fungi tend to colonizing crops. These metabolites are termed *mycotoxins*. That is, toxins found in the macroscopic mushrooms are not referred to as such, but are simply called toxins from mushrooms. The toxins found in mushrooms include *alpha*-amanitin, coprine, ergotamine, gyromitrin, muscarine, orellanine, phallotoxin, psilocybin, and more. Poisoning from ingestion of toxins

Table 17.1. Toxicological Profiles of Select Major Toxins Found in Certain Pathogenic Bacteria[a]

Toxin	Pathogenic Species	Major Toxic Effects/Specific Health Concerns
Botulinum toxin (neurotoxin)	*Clostridium botulinum* (Gram-positive, rod-shaped, anaerobic)	Neurologic: blurred vision, numbness around the mouth, weakness of skeletal muscles, respiratory paralysis; in foodborne botulism, the toxin is ingested with food in which the bacterial spores have germinated
Tetanus toxin (*tetanospasmin; neuro-toxin*)	*Clostridium tetani* (Gram-positive, rod-shaped, endospore-forming, anaerobic)	Pain in and stiffness of jaw, neck, and/or abdominal muscles, with difficulty swallowing; through a skin wound loaded with soil, dust, or animal waste that contains the pathogen as well as the toxin
Clostridium perfringens enterotoxin	*Clostridium perfringens* (Gram-positive, rod-shaped, anaerobic)	Symptoms typically including gangrene, diarrhea, dysentery; possibly hemolytic
Anthrax toxin	*Bacillus anthracis* (Gram-positive, aerobic and anaerobic)	Induction of cytokine release leading to death of target cells; a disease affecting primarily domesticated animals and wildlife
Pertussis toxin	*Bordetella pertussis* (Gram-negative aerobic coccobacillus)	Whooping cough; inhibition of phagocytosis by macrophages and neutrophils; hemolytic as well as leukolytic
Diphtheria toxin	*Corynebacterium diphtheriae* (aerobic, Gram-positive, rod-shaped, nonmotile)	Inhibition of protein synthesis leading to cell death; hemolytic
Cholera toxin	*Vibrio cholerae* (Gram-negative, straight or curved rods)	A severe contagious disease with symptoms including massive diarrhea, dehydration, and vomiting that collectively may lead to death
Staphylococcus aureus exfoliatin; exotoxin; enterotoxin	*Staphylococcus aureus* (Gram-positive, spherical)	Scalded skin syndrome by exfoliatin; toxic shock syndrome by exotoxin; food poisoning by enterotoxin; otherwise most strains of the species and most species of the genus are harmless to humans or animals
Streptolysin O (cytolysin); pyrogenic toxin	*Streptococcus pyogenes* (Gram-positive, nonmotile, nonspore-forming)	Lysis of red/white blood cells by Streptolysin O; scarlet fever/systemic toxic shock syndrome by erythrogenic (pyrogenic) toxin
Shiga toxin; shiga-like toxin	*Shigella dysenteriae* (Gram-negative rod); Shigatoxigenic group of *E. coli*	Diarrhea and dysentery, with gastrointestinal and kidney complications; inhibition of protein synthesis within target cells; apoptosis
E. coli heat-labile enterotoxin	*Escherichia coli* (a.k.a., *E. coli*; Gram-negative, rod-shaped)	Symptoms similar to cholera; otherwise the intestine of many warm-blooded animals can be colonized by *E. coli* (head of the enterobacteriaceae family which includes *Salmonella, Shigella,* and *Yersinia*)
Cytolethal distending toxin	*Salmonella typhi* (Gram-negative, nonspore-forming); some other Gram-negative bacteria (e.g., *Haemophilus ducreyi, E. coli*)	Cell cycle arrest, cytoplasm distention, and eventually cell death by damage to the DNA strands; some species in the genus *Salmonella* may cause paratyphoid fever, typhoid fever, and the foodborne illness salmonellosis

[a] see, e.g., Brachman and Abrutyn (2009) and Henkel *et al.* (2010) for further discussion, which are also the primary sources for this table.

In mushrooms is known as mycetism, with symptoms varying from slight GI discomfort to death. On the other hand, not all mycotoxins are harmful to humans. Some of their derivatives have been used as antibiotics, growth promoters, and drugs, although some others have been tested for use as warfare agents. As reflected in Table 17.2, six groups of mycotoxins are regarded as most relevant to environmental health. Of this short list, aflatoxins, fumonisins, trichothecenes, and zearalenones are either more investigated or with more intriguing toxicity, and thus are specifically discussed below.

Aflatoxins are a subgroup of mycotoxins produced by many species of the fungal genus *Aspergillus*, including most notably *A. flavus* and *A. parasiticus*. Although about a dozen kinds of aflatoxins are produced in nature, the term *aflatoxins* usually refers to the four kinds named B_1, B_2, G_1, and G_2. Aflatoxins are largely associated with agricultural commodities produced in the tropics and subtropics, such as cotton, peanuts, spices, maize, and pistachios. Aflatoxins B_1 and B_2 are produced by *A. flavus* and *A. parasiticus*, whereas aflatoxins G_1 and G_2 are produced exclusively by *A. parasiticus*. Aflatoxins M_1 is a metabolite of B_1 found in humans and animals, whereas M_2 is a metabolite of B_2 found in milk of cattle grazing on contaminated hay.

Aflatoxins B_1, B_2, G_1, and G_2 are similar to one another in structure and toxicity, with B_1 being the most toxic and among the most potent carcinogens. Aflatoxins B_2 and G_2 are the dihydroxy derivatives of B_1 and G_1, respectively. All four kinds have been positively correlated to adverse health effects, such as liver cancer, in many animal species. After entering the body, aflatoxin B_1 may be metabolized by the liver to a highly reactive epoxide intermediate, to aflatoxicol of moderate carcinogenicity, or to the less harmful aflatoxin M_1. All five aflatoxins mentioned in this paragraph (i.e., aflatoxins B_1, B_2, G_1, G_2, M_1) have been classified by IARC (2002) as human (Group 1) carcinogens.

Fumonisins, trichothecenes, and zearalenones are other subgroups of mycotoxins produced by various species of the genus *Fusarium*. As listed in Table 17.2, other mycotoxins produced from *Fusarium* include beauvericins, enniatins, butenolides, equisetins, and fusarins (Desjardins and Proctor, 2007). These eight families of *Fusarium* toxins all have a history of infecting the grains of developing cereals (e.g., wheat, maize).

Fumonisin B_1 is the most prevalent member of the fumonisin family, produced by several species of *Fusarium* molds. The *Fusarium* molds occur mainly in maize, wheat, and certain other cereals. Contamination of maize by fumonisin B_1 has been reported worldwide on the parts per million (mg/kg) level. Human exposure occurs on levels of μg to mg per day, and is greatest in regions where maize products are the dietary staple. Fumonisin B_1, an inhibitor of the enzyme ceramide synthase, is toxic to the liver and kidneys in all animal species studied. Fumonisin B_2, produced by *F. verticillioides* and *F. moniliforme*, is a structural analog of fumonisin B_1 but is more cytotoxic. Like all other members in the fumonisin family, fumonisin B_2 tends to contaminate maize (and other crops), can affect the nervous systems of horses, and can cause cancer in rodents.

Trichothecenes are produced by various species of the fungal genera *Myrothecium*, *Cephalosporium*, *Dendrodochium*, *Stachybotrys*, *Trichothecium*, *Verticimonosporium*,

Table 17.2. Toxicological Profiles of Six Major Common Groups of Mycotoxins
Found in Certain Pathogenic Fungi[a]

Mycotoxin	Major Pathogenic Fungal Species	Associated/Affected Commodities	Major Toxic Effects/Concerns
Aflatoxins: B_1, B_2, G_1, G_2	*Aspergillus flavus* and/or *Aspergillus parasiticus*	Maize, cotton, peanuts, pistachios, spices, nuts, and more	Highly carcinogenic (to the liver); hepatic aflatoxicosis; suppression of immunological system in animals
Fusarium toxins: fumonisins; trichothecenes; zearalenones; beauvericins; enniatins; butenolides; equisetins; fusarins	Many species of *Fusarium* (e.g., *F. oxysporum, F. proliferatum, F. verticillioides*)	Distributed mainly in soil and in association with plants; grains of developing cereals (e.g., wheat, maize)	Fumonisins: nervous systems of horses; cancer in rodents. Zearalenones: highly estrogenic causing infertility and abortion in swine. Trichothecenes: potent inhibitors of protein synthesis
Citrinin	Several species of *Aspergillus* and of *Penicillium* (e.g., *P. citrinum*)	Many human foods (e.g., cheese, soy sauce, wheat, rice, corn, barley, rye, food colored with red pigments)	Yellow rice fever in Japan; nephrotoxin in many animal species
Ochratoxin (OT) including the three secondary metabolites OT_A, OT_B, OT_C	Species of *Penicillium* (e.g., *P. verrucosum*) and of *Aspergillus* (e.g., *A. ochraceus*)	Beverages (e.g., beer, wine), grain, pork products, and dried grapes	OT_A: carcinogen (e.g., in the human urinary tract); nephrotoxin
Ergot alkaloids	In the sclerotia of species of *Claviceps* (e.g., *C. purpurea*)	Various grass species, cereals, rye, and related plants (e.g., wheat, triticale, barley)	Ergotism (a.k.a. St. Anthony's Fire): vasoconstriction leading to gangrene and loss of limbs; hallucinations; convulsion; and death
Palutin	*Penicillium* (e.g., *P. expasum*), *Aspergillus, Paecilomyces*	Rotting apples, rotting figs, and a variety of moldy vegetables and fruits	Genotoxic; damage to the immunological system in many animal species

[a] *see,* e.g., Hussein and Brasel (2001) and Richard (2007) for further discussion, which are also the primary sources for this table.

Trichoderma, and most notably *Fusarium.* These mycotoxins are strong inhibitors of protein synthesis as they react with components of the cellular ribosomes (Figure 9.1) where proteins are synthesized. They are most strongly associated with fatal and chronic toxic effects in animals and humans, and can cause rapid irritation to the skin. Large outbreaks of trichothecene-related mycotoxicoses historically were linked to the consumption of Japanese rice and Russian wheat grains both infested by species of *Fusarium.*

Zearalenones are potent estrogenic metabolites produced by *F. graminearum* that are not correlated well with any fatal toxic effects in animals or humans. They are however the primary mycotoxins responsible for infertility, abortion, enlarged uterus, enlarged mammary glands, and breeding problems, all specifically in swine. As with many other mycotoxins, zearalenones are heat-stable and are found mostly in maize. They are also found in other crops (e.g., wheat, rye, sorghum) throughout the world. Zearalenone contamination has been reported in moldy hay fed to cattle, swine, and sheep.

17.4. Toxins from Fishes and Plants

One major source of food poisoning is from consumption of poisonous fishes. Another major source is from ingestion of poisonous plants (especially by herbivores). If venomous fishes (e.g., lionfish, stonefish, scorpionfish) are included, poisonous fishes will have well over a thousand species (Smith and Wheeler, 2006). As noted in Section 17.1, the distinction between venomous and poisonous animals is simply in the way their toxins are delivered to their victims or enemies. The venomous type fishes deliver their toxins to their victims or foes by means of a sting or a bite, whereas the poisonous type have their toxins consumed by their predators. This section focuses on the latter type, which are fewer in species. Worldwide, fish and shellfish poisonings occur more commonly in the South Sea, and only occasionally in the United States (e.g., primarily in the coastal states such as California, Florida, Hawaii, New York, and Washington).

The list of poisonous plants appears to be longer, and is not easy to compile in that many times one part of them is poisonous whereas another part is edible. Plants contain many groups of biologically active chemicals including alkaloids, glycosides, peptides, and amino acids. Some constituents in these various groups (e.g. atropine, digitoxin, colchicines) happen to offer great therapeutic effects in treating human and animal diseases. Yet some others (e.g., jimson weed, nightshade) can produce acute, life-threatening poisonings. Fortunately, among the thousands of plants found in the environment, not many are poisonous to humans or animals, at least not from dermal contact or inhalation.

The health effects of poisonous plants vary considerably among animals and humans. Timing of ingestion or contact can be critical. This is because the concentrations of toxic constituents in plants are seasonal, temporal, and regional. They can also vary as a result of certain environmental factors such as drought and flood by altering the soil structure nearby. As highlighted in Section 17.4.2 below, toxins from plants can be broadly divided into four or five categories according to the body organs or tissues that are affected.

17.4.1. Toxins from Fishes

Three algae-borne toxins (i.e., saxitoxin, brevetoxin, domoic acid) causing *shellfish* poisoning are mentioned in Section 17.3. There are three toxins from *fishes* that are regarded as even more relevant and more significant to public health. These are ciguatoxin, tetrodotoxin, and scombrotoxin.

Ciguatoxin is also an algae-borne toxin. It is produced by *Gambierdiscus toxicus*, a type of dinoflagellates accumulating in big coral reef fish, such as grouper, wrasse, triggerfish, and amberjack. The toxin usually accumulates in the skin, head, viscera, and roe of the fish. It cannot be destroyed by heat from cooking. The poisonous effects of ciguatoxin come from its ability to lower the threshold for opening voltage-gated sodium channels in the synapses of the nervous system. The toxic effects of opening a sodium channel include depolarization which can cause paralysis, heart contraction, and changing the senses of hearing. Because the toxin normally cannot cross the blood brain barrier (BBB), it affects the peripheral (rather than the central) nervous system.

Tetrodotoxin is a potent neurotoxin with no known antidote. It blocks action potentials in nerves by binding to the pores of the voltage-gated sodium channels in the cell membranes, thereby preventing any affected nerve cells from firing by blocking the channels used in the course of the action. The toxin has been isolated from a variety of animal species, including predominately puffer fish and occasionally some western newts of the genus *Taricha* and toads of the genus *Atelopus*. Tetrodotoxin is some 100 times more poisonous than potassium cyanide (KCN), an inorganic that has a lethal oral dose of about 200 mg for an adult of average weight. In particular, the skin and the liver of a puffer fish together contain the neurotoxin at levels generally sufficient to cause paralysis of the human diaphragm and death from respiratory failure. The symptoms typically develop within 30 minutes of ingestion, but may be delayed by up to a few hours. Nonetheless, death has reportedly occurred as fast as 15 minutes from ingestion.

Scombrotoxin, which is composed of histamine and other amines, is often implicated for the foodborne illness caused by consumption of spoiled fish. Histamine is a mediator of allergic reactions. The symptoms from the poisoning are thus similar to those seen in severe allergic responses. The illness typically begins minutes to hours after ingestion of the spoiled toxic fish and resembles a histamine reaction, with symptoms including nausea, palpitations, tingling and burning sensations around the mouth, facial flushing, vomiting, sweating, dizziness, and rash. Some patients complained that the fish had a peppery or a metallic taste. Scombrotoxic food poisoning is about the most common type of seafood poisonings, second only to ciguatera (that caused by ciguatoxin). Seafood poisonings of this type are most commonly reported with the scombridae family (e.g., skipjack, mackerel, tuna, bonito), thereby leading to the name so given to the toxin. The biogenic amine histamine responsible for the various symptoms actually comes from the histidine that is naturally available in various fishes. The conversion from histidine to histamine takes place at temperatures above 16° C (60° F) on air contact. The resultant histamine is not labile to cooking temperatures, so even properly cooked fish can be affecting.

17.4.2. Toxins from Plants

Many different kinds of substances found in plants can be responsible for GI disturbance (e.g., nausea, vomiting, diarrhea) owing to their ability to irritate the mucous membranes during the course of ingestion. Some have found even a place in medicine as mild purgatives, such as the emodin from *Himalayan rhubarb* and *Rhamnus purshiana*. Plants (e.g., beans, cereal grains, seeds, nuts) with high concentrations of the sugar-binding protein called lectin may be harmful if consumed excessively in undercooked form. The adverse effects of lectin on humans may include nutritional deficiencies and allergic reactions. Most of these effects are possibly due to GI distress (e.g., abdominal pain, purging, bloody diarrhea) via interaction of this protein with the gut epithelial cells. Ricin is another protein that can cause GI distress. The toxin is found mostly in castor beans. If ingested, it can cause symptoms that likely begin within 3 hours and include a burning sensation in the mouth and throat (along with the GI distress characterized above).

Many plant species are known to contain cardiac or cardiotonic glycosides, of which the widely known is from *Digitalis purpurea* (including foxglove of the *Plantaginaceae* family). Glycosides are molecules in which a sugar unit is bound to a non-carbohydrate moiety. In the lily family, both squill (*Scilla maritima*) and lily of the valley (*Convallaria majalis*) contain glycosides (i.e., scillaren and convallatoxin, respectively) in their bulbs with actions resembling digitalis. Cardiac glycosides are also a class of medications used to treat heart failure. Yet their overdose can cause adverse effects on the heart, stomach, intestines, and nervous system. It is largely owing to such an adverse effect potential that these glycosides as well as their plants have been used as arrow poisons.

Cyanogens (those containing the cyano group CN) are constituents of several plant species. One of the widely known cyanogenic glycosides is amygdalin. This glycoside is found in the pits of apples, cherries, and peaches, in related genera in the rose family, and in the highest amounts in the seeds of the bitter almonds *Prunus amygdalus* (which apparently gives the glycoside's name). When amygdalin is taken orally, lethal cyanide poisoning can occur because *beta*-glucosidase is one of the enzymes capable of catalyzing the breakdown of the cyanide from amygdalin. This enzyme is present in the human small intestine and in a variety of common foods.

Alkaloids are mostly amines that contain one or more nitrogen atoms on their cyclic rings. The high concentrations of pyrrolizidine alkaloids contained in many plant species (e.g., those in the genera *Crotalaria*, *Heliotropium*, and *Symphytum*) are reportedly responsible for liver damage in the form of hepatic venoocclusive disease or liver cancer (Schoental, 1968). For kidney damage, one widely known toxin from plants is oxalate. People and many animals can develop kidney stones if they consume foods (e.g., leeks, spinach, quinoa) high in oxalate. Calcium oxalate is a chemical compound that forms needle-shaped crystals. In plants, the needle-shaped crystals are known as raphides. The poisonous houseplant dumb cane (*Dieffenbachia*) contains the toxin and on ingestion can cause oral and throat irritations with excessive drooling, usually long before the toxin has an opportunity to accumulate in the body to form kidney stones.

Taxol is a neurotoxin belonging to the class of alkaloids called taxine. It is found in the western yew tree *Taxus breviofolia*. The natural pyrethrins from chrysanthemum can also act as neurotoxins to cause severe excitation of the nervous system (Section 15.6). Swainsonine is an indolizidine alkaloid found in the Australian plant *Swainsonia canescens* and in some locoweed plants in the western United States. Aside from its capacity as a neurotoxin, the indolizidine can cause abortions and fetal malformation in pregnant livestock grazing on locoweeds that contain this alkaloid (Bunch *et al.*, 1992).

Hypericum, *Dieffenbachia*, and *Rhus* are not closely related plants. Yet some species of these genera can cause similar contact dermatitis as an allergic reaction. For example, many people are familiar with dermatitis caused by poison ivy (*R. toxicodendron*) and poison sumac (*R. vernix*). Houseplants of the genus *Dieffenbachia*, such as dumb cane mentioned earlier, can cause oral irritation, excessive drooling, and localized swelling. Moreover, cases of livestock poisoning from *H. perforatum* (a.k.a., St. John's wort) have been reported in the temperate and subtropical regions of North America, Europe, India, Turkey, Russia, and China. The most common untoward effects from this type of livestock poisonings are GI disorders, dizziness, confusion, fatigue, and sedation. On rare occasions, the effects may lead to high levels of photosensitivity that can cause increases in visual sensitivity to light or in skin sensitivity to sunburns.

17.5. Venoms from Arthropods

Arthropods are invertebrates and the largest animal phylum (i.e., division) on the Earth, each with a segmented body called the thorax and abdomen, and six or more jointed legs. The body of each arthropod is covered by a shell or a hard outer skin called exoskeleton. Some familiar arthropods include ants, bees, beetles, butterflies, crabs, fleas, hornets, lobsters, mites, mosquitoes, scorpions, shrimp, spiders, ticks, and wasps.

The bites by arthropods such as fleas, mites, mosquitoes, and ticks can make people's life miserable. Certain mosquito species are very dangerous, as they may carry diseases such as malaria and dengue fever. Malaria is brought about mainly by the protozoan species *Plasmodium falciparum* parasitizing in female mosquitoes mostly of the *Anopheles* genus. After a female mosquito bites an infected person, it will inject its salvia containing the malaria parasite into the next victim's body for multiplication in that body's liver. The parasite there then starts to infect the victim's red blood cells, causing symptoms that include fever, headaches, and in severe cases hallucinations, coma, and death. Dengue fever is caused by dengue virus, characterized by a sudden onset of fever along with headaches as well as joint and muscle pains. Lyme disease and Rocky Mountain spotted fever are other infectious diseases brought about by ticks as the vector.

Despite the fact that as many as 80% of all animals on the Earth are arthropods which are found everywhere, most lack a venom sufficient or sufficiently poisonous to pose threat to human health. The few that can produce a sufficient venom of health concern are highlighted below.

17.5.1. Venoms from Arachnids

Arachnids are a class of arthropods that all have eight legs, such as scorpions and spiders. Among some 40,000 species of spiders identified, only about 200 are known to have toxic stings. The venom, when injected through a spider's hollow teeth-like small fangs, can rapidly paralyze the victims including humans. Fortunately, most of the some 200 species are not dangerous to humans because their fangs are either fragile or not long enough to penetrate the human skin. The few exceptions include species of the genera *Latrodectus* (i.e., the so-called black widow spiders), *Loxosceles* (the brown recluse spiders), *Phidippus* (the jumping spiders), *Cheiracanthium* (the yellow sac spiders), and *Pardosa* (the wolf spiders). Studies have emerged to confirm that some species of spiders and some species of bacteria share the same or similar toxins. For example, certain species in the spider genus *Loxosceles* can cause severe necrotic lesions in the human skin owing to the presence of their venom enzyme named sphingomyelinase D, which is also found in certain species of the bacterial genus *Corynebacteria* that have reportedly caused various illnesses in livestock (e.g., Cordes and Binford, 2006).

The brown recluse spiders are also known as the violin or fiddleback spiders due to their violin shape. Their venoms usually cause some pains, itching, or burning within the first 15 minutes, and extensive tissue damage over the next two weeks ending with a sunken, open, ulcerated sore to several diameters. The wound has the appearance of a bull's eye, with a center blister surrounded by a red ring and then a blanched whitish ring. Other symptoms include chills, fever, nausea, and hemolytic anemia (i.e., a condition where the red blood cells are destroyed).

The black widow spiders are timid and prefer to be in secluded locations (e.g., attics, garages, crawl spaces, sheds) to construct their tangled, crisscross webs. Their bites cause the appearance of a pale area surrounded by a red ring. Severe muscle pains and cramps may develop within the first few hours. The cramps are usually first felt around the abdomen, shoulders, thighs, and back. Other symptoms include weakness, headaches, itching, sweating, nausea, breathing difficulty, and hypertension.

The jumping spiders are the most common biting type reported across the United States, whereas the wolf spiders are commonly found in the state of California. Much like Tarantulas of the *Theraphosidae* family, both groups are large hairy spiders. Bites from a jumping spider are painful, itchy, and cause redness as well as swelling. Other symptoms may include fever, muscle and joint pains, headaches, chills, nausea, and vomiting. The symptoms last about a couple of days. Bites from a wolf spider can cause pains, swelling, and redness. The venoms of the yellow sac spiders, so-called due to the yellow to beige color of their abdomen, can cause a small lesion in humans. Recently, its link to a definitive dermonecrosis has been challenged (Vetter *et al.*, 2006).

Scorpions are predatory arthropods of the *Scorpiones* order which is within the same *Arachnida* class that spiders belong to. Their venoms are a mixture of neurotoxins and enzyme inhibitors, with each not only causing a different effect but likely also targeting a specific animal victim. Frogs and rabbits are some animals that tend to be poisoned by a scorpion's venom. Only one bark scorpion species named *Centruroides exilicauda* in the western United States and some 25 other species worldwide are known to have venoms poisonous or potent enough to humans. Most of these venoms, including chlorotoxin produced by Deathstalker scorpions, are similar in toxicity to those from snakes.

17.5.2. Venoms from Insects

Of all the venoms from thousands of the insect species, only those from a few in the *Hymenoptera* order, such as certain species of bees, hornets, and wasps, will pose some threat to humans. The venoms from these *Hymenopterous* insects are almost all proteinaceous substances (e.g., biogenic amines, peptides, small proteins, enzymes). Most people have only localized reactions to these venoms, although a few may experience serious allergic reactions. Local, nonallergic reactions range from short-term redness, tenderness, itching, and burning to massive swelling and itching that may last for two weeks. Occasionally, a victim may suffer a life-threatening, systemic allergic reaction to a wasp or bee sting, as such a reaction can result in anaphylactic shock within minutes of being stung (as in Type I hypersensitivity reaction with shortness of breath, blockage in the throat, loss of consciousness, and fainting). In the United States, each year about 40 deaths reportedly are from anaphylaxis caused by insect sting.

In most people, a wasp sting produces an immediate pain at the sting site. There will be localized reddening, swelling, and itching. Aside from the allergic reaction, the greatest risk from insect stings is the less harmful microbial infection that follows. Unlike the honeybees, the common wasps and hornets can insert and withdraw their sting with relative ease. The amount of venom delivered by a wasp sting is much less than that by a bee. Another feature unique to the wasp and hornet stings is a pheromone contained in their venoms that attracts the attack on the victim by those of the same species around. Insect stings in nonallergic people, though painful, generally do not cause serious health problems. Nonetheless, *multiple* insect stings can cause serious complications (e.g., muscle breakdown, renal failure) and, though rarely, even death in these victims.

Fire ants are wingless members also of the *Humenoptera* order. Their venoms differ from those of the bees and wasps, inasmuch as 95% of the former are non-proteinaceous and contain dialkylpiperidine hemolytic factors. These hemolytic factors can induce the release of histamine and other vasoactive amines from mast cells, resulting in a sterile pustule at the sting site. Although these alkaloids are not immunogenic, venoms from fire ants do contain allergenic proteins capable of causing anaphylaxis in allergic victims.

17.6. Venoms from Reptiles and Amphibians

Reptiles are a class of mostly cold-blooded animals called *Reptilia* in the *Chordata* phylum. This animal class includes snakes and lizards of the *Squamata* order, turtles and tortoises of the *Testudines* order, as well as crocodiles and alligators of the *Crocodilia* order. Of all the reptiles identified today, snakes are the most notorious for having potent venoms capable of killing humans and large animals. Other groups of reptiles venomous to humans and many animals are limited to a few species of lizards.

Amphibians such as frogs, toads, salamanders, newts, and caecilians are in the animal class called *Amphibia*, belonging also to the *Chordata* phylum. Animals in this group are known to metamorphose from a juvenile water-breathing form to either an adult air-breathing form or a form that retains some juvenile traits. Some species of amphibians are known to be much more poisonous to humans and animals than all the venomous lizards and snakes identified.

17.6.1. Venoms from Snakes

Many of the some 3,000 species of snakes identified are nonvenomous; and those that are, most come from the *Elapidae* and *Viperidae* families. Cobras, mambas, kraits, copperheads, and coral snakes, along with sea snakes, are venomous elapides commonly encountered by humans. Venomous viperids familiar to humans include vipers, adders, rattlesnakes, cottonmouths, and bushmasters (Freiberg and Walls, 1984).

The venoms from snakes are highly modified saliva secreted via their mostly sharp, enlarged, as well as hollow fangs. Their salivary venoms typically contain one or more of the following four distinct types of toxic enzymes: (1) proteases; (2) phosphodiesterases; (3) phospholipases (mainly the phospholipases-A_2 subtype); and (4) hyaluronidases. In addition to some of these enzymes, a snake's saliva contains a variety of other substances such as biogenic amines, lipids, carbohydrates, and metal ions. Many snake venoms also contain adenosine triphosphatases (ATPases), which are thought to be some of the agents responsible for immobilizing smaller preys by disrupting the supply and release of cellular energy in their tissues. There is some evidence that the type of AChE (acetylcholinesterase) found in elapid venoms has the specific effect of disrupting the cholinergic transmission in the prey's central nervous system as well as at its body's neuromuscular junction (Ahmed *et al.*, 2009).

The first four types of snake enzymes noted above have their own unique venomous properties. Proteases bring about the disruption of peptide and protein bonds in the body tissue, causing the tissue to deteriorate and the blood-vessel walls to rupture. Many of these enzymes thereby have their adverse effects on hemostasis and thrombosis (Matsui *et al.*, 2000). Phosphodiesterases, which can break down the 5'-phosphodiester and pyrophosphate bonds in nucleotides and nucleic acids (as defined in Chapter 18), are responsible for the adverse cardiac reactions in the prey, most notably by lowering its blood pressure. Phospholipases-A_2 account for a wide range of toxicity, including hemolytic, myotoxic, anticoagulant, procoagulant, neurotoxic, and cardiotoxic effects (Balsinde *et al.*, 2002; Davidson and Dennis, 1990; Nevalainen *et al.*, 2004). As phospholipases-A_2 are commonly found in mammalian tissues, their elevated level and activity resulting from a snakebite will cause inflammation and pain at the site of the bite. Some other subtypes of phospholipases, such as those (e.g., ß-bungarotoxin) found in the venoms from banded kraits, have a subunit capable of destroying sensory and motor neurons (Kwong *et al.*, 1995; Lewis and Gutmann, 2004). Hyaluronidases catalyze the breakdown of hyaluronic acid, an anionic compound present throughout the human body to help cushion and support joints. These enzymes have the effect of increasing tissue permeability thereby to help increase the absorption of other toxic enzymes into the prey's tissues.

17.6.2. Venoms from Lizards

There are some 5,000 species of lizards worldwide but, until several years ago, only the Gila monster (*Heloderma suspectum*) and the related Mexican beaded (*Heloderma horridum*) species were thought to be venomous. These two species are found in Mexico and in the southwestern United States. Recent studies revealed that lizards of the *Monitor* species and of the *Iguana* genus are also venomous (Fry *et al.*, 2006). Nevertheless, none of these new finds has been reported to pose serious danger to humans, likely due to the fact that their venoms are introduced too slowly by chewing, unlike those injected by snakes. In addition to the several venomous enzymes (e.g., phospholipase, protease, hyaluronidase) commonly found in snakes, a few previously unnoticed proteinaceous substances have now been identified in the venoms from these new finds.

Also intriguing and important to know is the fact that the very largest lizard species, such as the Komodo dragons, can actually pose threat of death to their preys through bacterial infection. That is, even though Komodo dragons have not been considered as venomous, the serrations along their teeth are an ideal niche for many species of pathogenic bacteria. To put it another way, if the initial bite of a Komodo dragon did not get its prey killed, the infections caused by the bacteria living in its teeth-like fangs ultimately would.

17.6.3. Venoms from Amphibians

Most of the venomous amphibians are found in the *Salamandridae* family (e.g., the crocodile and sharp-ribbed newts) and in a group of Central American toads (e.g., the harlequin frogs). These amphibians have venomous glands on their flanks positioned adjacent to their rib tips. When picked up by their predators, these animals would use their sharp ribs as poisonous spikes by protruding them outwards through their venomous glands. Many of the venomous amphibians, such as the California newt (*Taricha torosa*) and Eastern red-spotted newt (*Notophthalmus viridescens*), possess the potent neurotoxin *tetrodotoxin* found notably in puffer fish (Section 17.4.1).

The Giant toad (a.k.a. marine toad) and the Colorado River toad are the two venomous species that are most commonly found in the United States. Their venoms are highly poisonous to pets. Dogs, the pets most likely coming in contact with a toad, have a higher risk of dying from contact with a venomous toad if they are left untreated. The skins of these venomous toads together provide well over 400 toxic alkaloids including histrionicotoxins, batrachotoxins, pumiliotoxins, and epibatidines. These toxic alkaloids collectively can cause a wide array of adverse effects to humans, including irritation, hallucination, vasoconstriction, cardiac problems, convulsion, and neurotoxic damage. One of the most poisonous frog groups is called poison dart frogs from the *Dendrobatidae* family.

17.7. Underrated Harmful Physical Agents

Harmful agents not chemical or biological in nature or origin are almost always by default treated as physical. Harmful physical agents are sometimes known as physical hazards, in that to some people the latter term embraces also physical risk factors for the harm at issue. The term *harmful physical agent* is used mostly by professionals in occupational health and safety, and by individuals or agencies complying with or advocating the worker right-to-know laws. Many of these entities (e.g., MNOSHA, 1998) have limited the hazards in this category to heat, noise, non-ionizing radiation (e.g., infrared, microwaves), and ionizing radiation (e.g., gamma rays, X-rays), which all have been determined as the basic physical agents or phenomena that can cause carcinogenic, mutagenic, teratogenic, or other toxic effects in humans. Some scholars and authorities have extended this short list to include vibration, repetitive motion, and cold stress (e.g., Tweedy, 2005). Still some others have added certain environmental situations to the list, such as the case with traffic congestion discussed in Section 17.7.1 below.

Also specifically discussed in Section 17.7.2 below is noise pollution, which is an environmental as well as a physical phenomenon causing a wide array of adverse effects on human health, human or animal behavior, and the ecosystem. Another reason for its inclusion is that, as with traffic congestion, to this date noise pollution is still one of the prevalent but most underrated environmental health problems around.

The adverse health effects of ionizing and non-ionizing radiation are briefly covered in Chapters 14 and 18. For decades now, seemingly very safe low dosages of ionizing radiation have been used in medical and research facilities. Yet huge quantities of harmful radioactive materials from nuclear power plants can be released into the environment by (avoidable) accidents, such as those due to flawed reactor designs (e.g., as with the 1986 Chernobyl nuclear explosion in Pripyat, Ukraine) and serious equipment failures (e.g., resulting from earthquakes or tsunamis, as with the 2011 Fukushima nuclear crisis in Okuma, Japan). Other physical hazards noted earlier in this section are treated as among the more relevant to industrial hygiene and medical physics. Yet for completeness, these other physical hazards are still highlighted in Chapter 20 on occupational toxicology.

17.7.1. Traffic Congestion

Traffic congestion is an environmental condition where the passage of vehicles (or pedestrians) along transportation routes exceeds the available capacity provided by the transportation system in place. This condition is characterized by slower vehicular (or pedestrian) movements and thereby longer trip times. The so-called traffic jam situation occurs whenever vehicles are fully stopped for a short enough time period. Even individual incidents (e.g., car accident or the sudden braking of one car in an otherwise smooth flow) may cause a chain reaction or a riffle effect leading to a traffic jam.

The health and economic impacts of traffic congestion on a community can be substantial. In particular, traffic delays may result in late arrival for many important events such as employment, business meetings, medical appointments, and education. Idling in traffic and frequent braking may cause more wear and tear on vehicles. In addition, road rage may result with increases in frustration and stress of the drivers and riders. Yet more important, traffic situations of this type will lead to more emission of nitrogen oxides (NO_x), carbon monoxide (CO), and other air pollutants into the atmosphere.

Studies have shown that traffic congestion is a significant contributor to poor health in affected infants (Currie and Walker, 2009) and to a surge in asthma rates in a Latino community (NRDC, 2004). Another study in Germany has implicated an increase in the risk of myocardial infarction (i.e., heart attack) for every hour a person will be stuck in traffic (Peters *et al.*, 2004).

17.7.2. Noise Pollution

Noise is the term used to refer to any unpleasant or annoying sound, the intensity of which is conventionally measured in decibel (dB) units on a logarithmic scale. In general, a normal conversation between two persons measures about 60 dB; and loud singing within 3 feet measures about 75 dB. One hazard with loud noise is acoustic trauma to the human ears when they are subjected to noise at 85 dB or higher without respite. Noise around this level is equivalent to that from an automobile or a motorcycle running within about 30 feet. By noise pollution, it implies an excessive amount of environmental noise that comes with significant negative impacts on human or animal life. Vehicles and industrial engines are the main sources of noise pollution, accounting for as much as 90% of the total in an urban area worldwide. Depending largely on the efficiency in urban planning, some cities are more affected than others by the loud and rhythmical sounds generated from transportation means, construction works, and the kind.

Noise pollution has direct impacts on human health, including both physiological and psychological effects. Nuisance noise of even medium intensity can be responsible for emotional stress, anxiety, insomnia, hypertension, and panic attacks. This type of environmental pollution can lower people's sensitivity to sounds leading to the premature aging of their auditory system. Problems such as aggression, anger, frustration, and stress are some of the psychological effects that can be caused by nuisance noise. According to the U.S. National Institute on Deafness and Other Communication Disorders (NIDCD, 2008), approximately 26 million American adults at ages 20 to 69 (i.e., about 17% of the total subpopulation in this age group) have high frequency of hearing loss that may have been induced by exposure to loud noise at work or in recreational activities.

There is strong speculation, if not substantial evidence, that noise pollution increases the mortality among animal species and affects the natural occurring phenomena that govern their world. For example, with noise pollution, birds may find themselves disturbed during expression with one another for mating desires or may have navigation problems due to the unnatural sound level present.

Worldwide, the concerns with noise pollution and the needs for acoustic control have been addressed in many presentations given annually at the INTER-NOISE Congresses, oftentimes under a sensational theme such as in 2012 being *Quieting the World's Cities*.

The INTER-NOISE Congresses are the largest international conferences from various regions on noise control engineering and have been held at venues around the world since the early 1970s. In the United States, the control measures and standards for noise emission are legally and specifically justified under the Noise Control Act of 1972.

References

Ahmed M, João Rocha JBT, Morsch VM, Schetinger MRC, 2009. Snake Venom Acetylcholinesterase. In *Handbook of Venoms and Toxins of Reptiles* (Mackessy SP, Ed.). Boca Raton, Florida, USA: CRC Press.

Balsinde J, Winstead MV, Dennis EA, 2002. Phospholipase A2 Regulation of Arachidonic Acid Metabolism. *FEBS Lett*. 531:2-6.

Bolognia JL, Jorizzo, JL, Rapini RP (Eds.), 2007. *Dermatology*. Philadelphia, Pennsylvania, USA: Elsevier Health Sciences.

Brachman PS, Abrutyn E (Eds.), 2009. *Bacterial Infections of Humans – Epidemiology and Control, Fourth Edition*. New York, New York, USA: Springer Science+Business Media.

Bunch TD, Panter KD, James LK, 1992. Ultrasound Studies of the Effects of Certain Poisonous Plants on Uterine Function and Fetal Development in Livestock. *J. Anim. Sci*. 70:1639-1643.

Caro HN, Sheikh NA, Taverne J, Playfair JH, Rademacher TW, 1996. Structural Similarities among Malaria Toxins Insulin Second Messengers, and Bacterial Endotoxin. *Infect. Immun*. 64:3438-3441.

Cordes MHJ, Binford GJ, 2006. Lateral Gene Transfer of a Dermonecrotic Toxin between Spiders and Bacteria. *Bioinformatics* 22:264-268.

Currie J, Walker R, 2009. Traffic Congestion and Infant Health: Evidence from EZPass. NBER Working Paper No. 15413. National Bureau of Economic Research, Inc., 1050 Massachusetts Avenue, Cambridge, Massachusetts, USA.

Davidson FF, Dennis EA, 1990. Evolutionary Relationships and Implications for the Regulation of Phospholipase A2 from Snake Venom to Human Secreted Forms. *J. Mol. Evol*. 31:228-238.

Desjardins AE, Proctor RH, 2007 Molecular Biology of Fusarium Mycotoxins. *Int. J. Food Microbiol*. 119:47-50.

DeWitte-Orr SJ, Mossman KL, 2011. The Antiviral Effects of Extracellular dsRNA. In *Viruses and Interferon: Current Research* (Mossman K, Ed.). Norfolk, UK: Caister Academic Press, Chapter 1.

Evans AS, 1976. Causation and Disease: The Henle-Koch Postulates Revisited. *Yale J. Biol. Med*. 49:175-195.

Freiberg M, Walls JG, 1984. *The World of Venomous Animals*. Neptune, New Jersey, USA: T.F.H. Publications.

Fry BG, Vidal N, Norman JA, Vonk FJ, Scheib H, Ramjan SFR, Kuruppu S, Fung K, Hedges SB, Richardson MK, Hodgson WC, Ignjatovic V, Summerhayes R, Kochva E, 2006. Early Evolution of the Venom System in Lizards and Snakes. *Nature* 439:584-588.

Gillard J, 2001. The Definition of Toxin. *Emer. Med. News* 23:53-53.

Henkel JS, Baldwin MR, Barbieri JT, 2010. Toxins from Bacteria. In *Molecular, Clinical, and Environmental Toxicology Volume 2: Clinical Toxicology* (Luch A, Ed.). *Experientia Supplementum* 100:1-29.

HHMI (Howard Hughes Medical Institute), 2002. Research News: *Excessive Growth of Bacteria May Also Be Major Cause of Stomach Ulcers.* HHMI, 4000 Jones Bridge Road, Chevy Chase, Marlyand, USA, issued 15 January.

Holt JG (Ed.), 1994. *Bergey's Manual of Determinative Bacteriology*, Ninth Edition. Philadelphia, Pennsylvania, USA: Lippincott Williams & Wilkins.

Hussein HS, Brasel JM, 2001. Toxicity, Metabolism, and Impact of Mycotoxins on Humans and Animals. *Toxicology* 167:101-134.

IARC (International Agency for Research on Cancer), 2002. IARC Monographs on the Evaluation of Carcinogenic Risks to Humans, Volume 82: Some Traditional Herbal Medicines, Some Mycotoxins, Naphthalene and Styrene. Lyon, France: WHO Press.

Kwong PD, McDonald NQ, Sigler PB, Hendrickson WA, 1995. Structure of *beta* 2-Bungarotoxin: Potassium Channel Binding by Kunitz Modules and Targeted Phospholipase Action. *Structure* 3:1109-1119.

Lewis RL, Gutmann L, 2004. Snake Venoms and the Neuromuscular Junction. *Semin. Neurol.* 24: 175-179.

Matsui T, Fujimura Y, Titani K, 2000. Snake Venom Proteases Affecting Hemostasis and Thrombosis. *Biochem. et Biophy. Acta (BBA) – Protein Struc. & Mol. Enzym.* 1477:146-156.

MNOSHA (Minnesota State Occupational Safety and Health Administration), 1998. An Employer's Guide to Developing an Employee Right-To-Know Program. 443 Lafayette Road North, St. Paul, Minnesota, USA.

Nevalainen TJ, Peuravuori HJ, Quinn RJ, Llewellyn LE, Benzie JAH, Fenner PJ, Winkel KD, 2004. Phospholipase A2 in Cnidaria. *Comp. Biochem. Physiol.* 139 (Part B):731-735.

NIDCD (National Institute on Deafness and Other Communication Disorders), 2008. NIDCD Fact Sheet: Noise-Induced Hearing Loss. NIH Pub. No. 08-4233. NIDCD Information Clearinghouse, 1 Communication Avenue, Bethesda, Maryland, USA.

NRDC (Natural Resources Defense Council), 2004. Hidden Danger: Environmental Health Threats in the Latino Community (principal authors: Quintero-Somaini A, Quirindongo M). 40 West 20th Street, New York, New York, USA.

Peters A, von Klot S, Heier M, Trentinaglia I, Hörmann A, Wichmann HE, Löwel H, 2004. Exposure to Traffic and the Onset of Myocardial Infarction. *NEJM* 351:1721-1730.

Reiter J, Herker E, Madeo F, Schmitt MJ, 2005. Viral Killer Toxins Induce Caspase-Mediated Apoptosis in Yeast. *J. Cell Biol.* 168:353-358.

Richard JL, 2007. Some Major Mycotoxins and Their Mycotoxicoses – An Overview. *Int. J. Food Microbiol.* 119:3-10.

Ryan KJ, Ray CG (Eds.), 2004. *Sherris Medical Microbiology*, Fourth Edition. New York, New York, USA: McGraw Hill.

Schmitt MJ, Breinig F, 2002. The Viral Killer System in Yeast: From Molecular Biology to Application. *FEMS Microbiol. Rev.* 26:257-276.

Schmitt MJ, Reiter J, 2008. Viral Induced Yeast Apoptosis. *Biochim. Biophys. Acta.* 1783:1413-1417.

Schoental R, 1968. Toxicology and Carcinogenic Action of Pyrrolizidine Alkaloids. *Cancer Res.* 28:2237-2246.

Schofield L, Vivas L, Hackett F, Gerold P, Schwarz RT, Tachado S, 1993. Neutralizing Monoclonal Antibodies to Glycosylphosphatidylinositol, the Dominant TNF-Alpha-Inducing Toxin of *Plasmodium falciparum*: Prospects for the Immunotherapy of Severe Malaria. *Ann. Trop. Med. Parasitol.* 87:617-626.

Smith WL, Wheeler WC, 2006. Venom Evolution Widespread in Fishes: A Phylogenetic Road Map for the Bioprospecting of Piscine Venoms. *J. Heredity* 97:206-217.

Tweedy JT, 2005. *Healthcare Hazard Control and Safety Management*, Second Edition. Boca Raton, Florida, USA: CRC Press, Chapter 4 (p.111).

U.S. Code (United States Code), 2013. Title 18 (Crimes and Criminal Procedure), Chapter 10 (Biological Weapons), Section 178 (Definitions). Office of the Law Revision Counsel, U.S. House of Representative, http://uscode.house.gov/, (still effective as of 19 August 2013).

Vetter RS, Isbister GK, Bush SP, Boutin LJ, 2006. Verified Bites by Yellow Sac Spiders (Genus *Cheiracanthium*) in the United States and Australia: Where Is the Necrosis? *Am. J. Trop. Med. Hyg.* 74:1043-1048.

WHO (World Health Organization), 2009. *Global Tuberculosis Control: A Short Update to the 2009 Report*. WHO/HTM/TB/2009.426. Geneva, Switzerland.

Review Questions

1. What are the main technical differences between a toxicant and a toxin or a venom?

2. What are biological toxic agents?

3. Give one example of toxins harmful to fish, and three examples of toxins found in fish.

4. What are the main technical differences between microbial infection and infectious disease?

5. Name the four main groups of pathogenic microbial agents.

6. What are prions and viroids? And what is the general term used to refer them as a special pathogenic group?

7. What are the pathogenic bacteria that are currently of global (*vs.* regional or local) concern?

8. Briefly describe the characteristics of a virus.

9. Name four fungal infections that appear to be more serious than the others, and list the pathogenic fungi that are responsible for them.

10. What are some of the most common infectious protozoa found in the world?

11. What are some of the most common helminthes found in humans?

12. Briefly describe the characteristics of viral toxins.

13. Name three toxins produced by the bacterial genus *Clostridium*.

14. What are the major symptoms or toxic effects of diphtheria and of shiga toxins?

15. How are aflatoxins M_1 and M_2 produced? And is aflatoxin M_1 more or less carcinogenic than aflatoxin B_1?

16. Name four algae-borne toxins that are commonly found in seafood. What are their main toxic effects on humans?

17. Name the mycotoxin that has toxic effects specifically or unique to swine.

18. Name the one species of scorpions that is considered to have enough venom to cause harm to a person living in the western United States.

19. Briefly characterize the symptoms caused by (the venoms of) black widow spiders.

20. Which insect order is responsible for most of the venoms that pose a serious threat to humans? Give a few examples of the venomous insects from this animal order.

21. Match the toxins found in plants (left side) to their *main* toxic effects on humans (right side).

(1) taxol	(a) cardiotoxicity
(2) oxalate	(b) hepatotoxicity
(3) pyrrolizidine alkaloid	(c) nephrotoxicity
(4) toxin from *R. vernix*	(d) GI distress
(5) ricin	(e) dermatitis
(6) toxin from foxglove	(f) neurotoxicity

22. Briefly characterize the venoms commonly found in snakes.

23. What are the two species of lizards that are found venomous to people living in Mexico or in the southwestern United States?

24. Which animal family is found to have most of the venomous amphibians? And what is the specific neurotoxin that may be found in California newt or in Eastern red-spotted newt?

25. What are the four main categories of harmful physical agents that most professionals in occupational health and safety focus on?

26. What are the major adverse health effects of noise pollution?

27. What are the major economic and health impacts of traffic congestion on a community?

CHAPTER 18

Environmental Mutagenesis/Carcinogenesis

18.1. Introduction

Mutagenesis is the process involving the formation of genetic mutations (i.e., changes in the base structure or base sequence of DNA) and their development in a cell's genetic materials. Carcinogenesis is the process whereby normal cells are transformed to tumor cells which are further developed into an abnormal mass of tissue known as tumor with the potential of becoming a cancer (Section 18.1.2). The terms *mutagenicity* and *carcinogenicity* refer to the ability or tendency to induce mutation and cancer (including tumor), respectively. The common risk factors relevant to most specific mutagenic or carcinogenic effects include one or more of the following: age; gender; race; lifestyle; family medical history; diet; occupational setting; and infection. As discussed in Chapter 10, these factors are also associated with many other diseases.

The main reason why the two pathocellular processes *mutagenesis* and *carcinogenesis* are often discussed side by side, as in this chapter, is that mutagenicity and carcinogenicity are closely interrelated. Over the years, studies have shown strong positive correlations between mutagens (i.e., agents or conditions capable of causing mutation) and carcinogens (i.e., agents or conditions capable of causing cancer). One widely referenced study in this series is the work by McCann *et al.* (1975), in which 90% (156 out of 174) of the carcinogens tested were shown mutagenic when they were subjected to the sensitive, short-term *Salmonella*/microsome assay developed by Ames *et al.* (1973). The positive correlations compiled more recently ranged from over 50% to above 90%.

18.1.1. DNA, RNA, Gene, and Chromosome

The more general term for DNA (deoxyribonucleic acid) and RNA (ribonucleic acid) is nucleic acid, which generally consists of hundreds to thousands of nucleotides. Each DNA nucleotide is made of one sugar-phosphate backbone *plus* one purine (adenine = A, or guanine = G) or one pyrimidine (cytosine = C, or thymine = T) base. The purines and pyrimidines are also known as nitrogenous bases as they each contain some nitrogen (N) atoms (Figure 18.1). The sugar-phosphate backbone includes either the sugar *ribose* (as on RNA) or *deoxyribose* (as on DNA) and one or more phosphate (PO_4^{3-}) groups.

DNA is a double-helix (i.e., double-stranded) chain of units carrying the genetic information in a cell, and is responsible for self-replication and the synthesis of RNA. As illustrated in Figure 18.2, the two strands of DNA are held together by weak hydrogen bonds between the purine and pyrimidine bases. RNA is also a constituent of all cells and of many viruses, consisting of typically a single strand with the bases A, G, C, and U (= uracil, in lieu of T) bonded to the ribose. Its base sequence and base structure are determinants of protein synthesis and of the transmission of genetic data encoded by DNA.

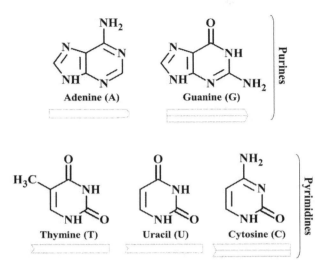

Figure 18.1. Chemical Structures of Purines and Pyrimidines on Nucleic Acids
(each dotted shape signifies the number of hydrogen bonds involved)

The term *genome* is used to denote the entire hereditary material (e.g., including the mitochondrial DNA) in a cell as well as in the organism. It is inscribed in the DNA or, for many types of viruses, in the RNA. The portion of the genome that encodes an RNA or hence a protein is referred to as a gene. The gene that encodes a protein (including enzymes) is composed of trinucleotide base units (e.g., GGA, AAC) termed *codons*, with each codon encoding a single amino acid (which is the building block of a protein).

A gene is thereby a linear sequence on the DNA molecule that encodes a certain type of RNA (and thus mostly a certain protein type) that has a specific biochemical role in the organism. An allele is a variant of this physical hereditary unit. An *onco*gene is a gene capable of transforming normal cells into tumor or cancer cells, whereas a *proto-oncogene* is a gene having the potential to become an oncogene.

Each chromosome is a single piece of long, continuous, highly coiled strand of DNA plus certain proteins. In eukaryotes (i.e., organisms whose cells contain complex structures enclosed within their membranes), chromosomes housed in the cell nucleus are packaged by the special proteins *histones* into a condensed structure termed *chromatin*, thereby allowing the very long DNA molecules to fit inside the highly crowded nucleus. The genetic materials contained in chromosomes are those that determine an organism's every trait from hair and eye color to sex and behavior. In human cells, the nuclei each contain 22 pairs of non-sex chromosomes termed *autosomes* and 1 pair of sex chromosomes known as XX chromosomes in females and XY chromosomes in males.

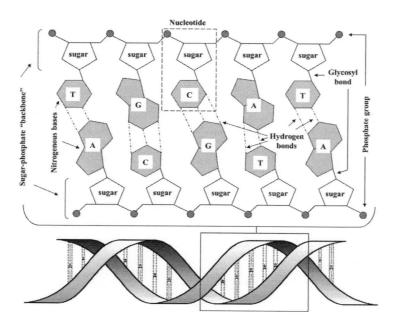

Figure 18.2. Double-Helix Structure of DNA *(Deoxyribonucleic Acid)*

Chromosomes must be replicated, divided, and passed on successfully to the daughter cells in order to ensure survival of their progeny and genetic diversity. These essential elements in cell division, or often referred to as vectors of heredity, may exist as either duplicated or unduplicated. When a chromosome replicates itself at the early stages (e.g., prophase) of cell division, the two identical pieces are termed *chromatids* and are joined together at their most condensed region termed *centromere*. Once the two chromatids have been separated from each other at the later stages (e.g., anaphase) of cell division, they each become a twin daughter chromosome. In humans, leukemias and certain solid tumors (those without cysts or liquid areas) are linked to specific chromosome alterations which, as in gene mutations, can transform certain proto-oncogenes to active oncogenes.

18.1.2. Characteristics of Cancer

To some scholars and in the medical literature, neoplasm is the more technical term for tumor; and neoplasia is the technical term for the abnormal proliferation of cells leading to an abnormal mass of tissue (i.e., tumor). Neoplasm is not synonymous with cancer. A neoplasm can be benign, premalignant, or malignant. In contrast, a cancer is supposedly always regarded as malignant and, in a few cases, does not form a solid tumor. For example, leukemia is a cancer of the blood or bone marrow characterized by an abnormal increase of blood cells, usually leukocytes (i.e., white blood cells).

Cancer is medically treated as a malignant tumor in that it is the kind characterized not only by uncontrolled cell growth, but also by its invasive property to intrude on or otherwise destruct neighboring tissues. In the more severe cases, it also has the potential to spread to more distant tissues via the bloodstream or lymphatic system. This type of cellular spread is medically termed *metastasis* (further discussed in Section 18.3.2).

18.2. Environmental Mutagenesis

Mutagenesis may either occur spontaneously *in vivo* or be induced by mutagenic factors or agents, largely by those from the environment. The mutagenicity involved may include a number of autosomal dominant disorders which are genetic diseases that can be passed down from *one* (and hence *dominant*) parent having the abnormal gene on one of the 22 pairs of autosomes. Serious consequences such as sickle-cell anemia can result if the mutation leads to the replacement of a hydro*phobic* amino acid (e.g., valine) for a hydro*philic* one (e.g., glutamic acid), or vice versa, in the affected hemoglobin. Sickle-cell anemia is a genetic blood disorder characterized by red blood cells that take on a rigid, sickle shape. It is a serious or even fatal disease in that red blood cells in sickle shape are very fragile and tend to rupture long before the end of their normal life span of about 120 days in humans. Nevertheless, it should be mindful here that not all genetic mutations are bad. Occasionally, a gene mutation can lead to a cell or a species with a greater ability to survive hardship or to cope with stress.

18.2.1. Concepts of Mutagenesis

In addition to induction by environmental mutagens (Section 18.2.4), mutagenesis can occur naturally, such as due to spontaneous lesion, integration of transposable genetic elements, or errors in DNA replication. An error in DNA replication can occur when an illegitimate nucleotide pair forms in the course of the replication. Spontaneous lesions are those damages to DNA that occur naturally, such as from the cleavage of the purine adenine (A) or guanine (G) from the DNA backbone or from the removal of an amino group (NH_2) in one of the four distinct nitrogenous bases on the DNA. The cleavage and the removal involved are referred to as depurination and deamination, respectively. There also exists a series of genetic elements that can transpose from one position on a chromosome to another position on the same or a different chromosome. These elements are called transposons if their transposition is via direct DNA transfer, or called retrotransposons if via RNA intermediates.

Although mutation rates vary considerably across species, in most cases they are very low. The more recent estimate for humans is at about one mutation in every 33 million nucleotides per generation (Xue *et al.*, 2009). Unfortunately, there exist the so-called hotspots on a DNA molecule, such as at the unusual base 5-methylcytosine (5-methyl-C), where mutations can occur up to 100 times more frequently than the norm. These hotspots are vulnerable to an array of mutagenic agents, including many of those listed in Table 18.1. The DNA (base) sequence of a gene can be altered in a number of ways. Often for simplicity, these numerous mechanisms are broadly classified into two types: (1) point or intragenic gene mutation; and (2) chromosome alteration or aberration.

18.2.2. Point Mutation and Intragenic Mutation

These two subtypes of gene mutation occur in the base sequence of a gene, which unlike chromosome aberration cannot be seen microscopically. Point mutation involves the replacement of a single base on the DNA, which can affect some vital cellular functions. For example, sickle-cell anemia is caused by a point mutation in the *beta*-hemoglobin gene that converts a GAG codon into GUG, leading to the inscription of the amino acid valine instead of glutamic acid. This type of point mutation is also called *base-pair* substitution in that the nucleotide on the opposite complementary DNA strand is also replaced accordingly. The base replacement in the opposite nucleotide becomes necessary because in the DNA nucleotide, the purine A (adenine) always forms a base pair with the pyrimidine T (thymine) by means of weak hydrogen bonding (Figure 18.2), whereas the purine G (guanine) always forms a base pair with the pyrimidine C (cytosine).

Intragenic mutation is a special form of point mutation involving *insertion* or *deletion* of a single base pair, which often produces an incorrect gene product leading to potentially a more detrimental effect on the synthesized protein (which can be an important enzyme). This form is also called frameshift mutation in that while the nucleotides are still read in triplets, they are in different frames as a result of the insertion or deletion.

18.2.3. Chromosome Aberration

Chromosome aberration brings about *structural* or *numerical* alterations of chromosomes. Numerical change that involves one or more extra or missing chromosomes is termed *aneuploidy*. For example, one of the most common aneuploidies that infants can survive with is trisomy 21, which means that these children each have an extra, third copy of autosome 21 (i.e., the 21st autosome, with the longest being named the first). These children not only suffer from mental retardation but also allegedly look like people of a certain ethnicity. This condition is also known as Down (or Down's) syndrome as it was first formally reported in 1866 by an English physician named John L. Down. Another example of aneuploidies is Turner syndrome, which attributes to a *female* human with one sex chromosome. This genetic disorder is characterized by short stature, broad chest, low hairline, low-set ears, and webbed necks. Turner syndrome is also referred to as gonadal dysgenesis in that most victims would experience gonadal dysfunction with a nonfunctional ovary that leads to sterility from absence of menstrual cycle.

The kind of toxicity leading to changes in chromosome structure is referred to as *clastogenicity*. Major types of structural changes in chromosomes include *deletion, duplication, inversion*, and (reciprocal) *translocation* of genes on chromosomes. These four subtypes occur mostly at the meiotic stage of cell division. Meiosis is a complex process in which the number of *sex* chromosomes per cell is cut in half. This process involves the sex chromosomes exchanging segments with one another via the event called crossover. If the event loses its fidelity, the structure of these chromosomes will be altered.

Chromosome deletion refers to the loss of one or more genes on a chromosome (e.g., genes A*B*CDE → ACDE), such as in children suffering from the *cri du chat* syndrome due to a missing part of autosome 5. The syndrome includes intellectual disability, microcephaly, delayed development, and weak muscle tone. It gets its name from the characteristic cry of affected infants sounding like a cat's cry due to problems with the larynx and the nervous system. Chromosome duplication (e.g., ABCDE → ABCCDDE) results from replication of one or more segments of a chromosome. An example of chromosome duplication disorders in humans is Charcot-Marie-Tooth neuropathy, characterized by loss of muscle tissue and touch sensation in the feet and legs, but in the advanced stages also in the hands and arms.

Chromosome inversion (e.g., ABCDE → ABDCE) can result from re-attachment of a chromosome segment to the original chromosome but in a reverse order, such as when caused by a mutagen or an error at the meiotic stage. As a case example, an inverted region on autosome 17 was reportedly linked to several Pick complex diseases (e.g., frontotemporal dementia) and other neurological disorders including corticobasal degeneration and progressive supranuclear palsy (e.g., Webb *et al.*, 2008). Chromosome translocation (e.g., $A_1B_1C_1D_1E_1 \rightarrow A_1B_1C_2D_2E_1$, where genes C_2 and D_2 are from *another* chromosome) can result from the attachment of a chromosomal segment to a nonhomologous chromosome. Both of the last two subtypes of chromosome aberration affect a gene's activity and regulation by altering its position on a chromosome. Accordingly, these two subtypes can lead to much more detrimental effects. Burkitt's lymphoma (Burkitt, 1958; Liu *et al.*, 2007) and Mantle cell lymphoma (Li *et al.*, 1999) are the two types of cancer reportedly caused by chromosome translocation.

18.2.4. Environmental Mutagens

Most known mutagens are environmental in origin. As expected, these mutagens can be broadly subsumed under the three main categories: physical, chemical, and biological. Examples of the various types of mutagens representing each of the three categories are given in Table 18.1, of which only certain abiological ones are elaborated on below due to space limitation. In any case, known examples of physical mutagens include mineral fibers, ultraviolet (UV) radiation, and ionizing radiation. These various types act on the DNA gene sequence via different modes. Ionizing radiation can come from X-rays or gamma rays directly and from the decay of uranium indirectly. Muller (1927) was the first to discover that X-ray could cause mutations in fruit flies. Mutagens of this type literally can pass through an organism's body to the chromosomes in its cells to directly corrupt the DNA's proper base sequence there. UV radiation (e.g., sunlight) can cause portions of DNA to be bonded together even when they should not. This will cause the DNA sequence to be misread leading to mutation. For example, UV light can cause two adjacent pyrimidine bases to form a dimer (also referred to as dimmer), such as with a T (thymine) covalently bonded to an adjacent T leading to the misreading of the true DNA base sequence. Certain natural mineral fibers, such as long-shaped asbestos, can interfere with chromosome distribution during cell division to cause genomic or chromosome aberration (Jensen *et al.*, 1996; Nelson and Kelsey, 2002).

Table 18.1. Select Agents Known or Suspected to Cause Mutation in
Human or Some Other Mammalian Cells

Subgroup/Type	Examples	Site/Mode of Mutagenic Action
Physical		
Ionizing Radiation	X-rays; gamma rays; α- or β-particles; radionuclides (e.g., isotopes of uranium)	By causing irreparable DNA damage usually from exposure at high or chronic levels
Ultraviolet Radiation	UV-A wavelength; UV-B wavelength; sunlight	By causing typically adjacent pyrimidine (thymine or cytosine) bases to covalently bond together (thereby forming pyrimidine dimers); also by inducing oxidative damage to DNA (particularly by UV-A)
Biological		
Viruses	Adenoviruses (DNA viruses); human papillomaviruses (DNA viruses); retroviruses (RNA viruses)	By inducing gene mutations much like the way mutagenic bacteriophages would; by forming gross chromosome alterations; by inducing reverse transcription by retroviruses to DNA
Bacteria	*Helicobacter pylori*	By causing inflammation-induced DNA damaging activity
Chemical		
Alkylating agents	Nitrogen mustards; cisplatin sodium azide; melphalan; nitrosoureas	Primarily by adding molecular components to DNA bases
Cross-linking agents	Melphalan; cisplatin	By creating covalent bonds with DNA bases
DNA-adductors	Benzo[α]pyrene; aflatoxin B_1	By forming stable DNA adducts (particularly with the guanine base)

Many chemical agents can alter the gene sequence by binding to the DNA in a cell. Examples of chemical mutagens include nitrogen mustards, nitrous acid, hydroxylamine, proflavine, vinyl chloride, 5-bromouracil (5-BU), benzo[α]pyrene (upon metabolic activation), aflatoxin B_1 (upon metabolic activation), and heterocyclic amines. Many of these chemical substances can be found at some level in various environments. For example, nitrogen mustards are now more used as cytotoxic chemotherapy agents in medicine. 5-BU is now frequently used as an experimental mutagen. The key precursors of nitrous acid are nitrites which are used heavily as preservatives in foods (e.g., hot dogs, luncheon meats, smoked fish). Proflavine has been used as a surface disinfectant. Vinyl chloride has been used predominately as a chemical intermediate to form PVC (polyvinyl chloride) in the plastics industry. Hydroxylamine has been used as an antioxidant for fatty acids. Aflatoxin B_1, produced by a certain genus of fungi (i.e., *Aspergillus*), tends to grow on spice, cereal, and nut type crops. Benzo[α]pyrene is a five-ring polycyclic aromatic hydrocarbon found in tobacco smoke, coal tar, and automobile exhaust fumes. Heterocyclic amines are often found in (over-)cooked meat.

Mutagens can also be divided into different categories according to their effects on DNA replication. Some of them (e.g., 5-BU) act as base analogs to replace the true nitrogenous bases on the DNA strand during replication. Some others react with DNA to cause structural changes, such as by forming adducts with DNA (e.g., as in the case with the epoxide metabolite of benzo[α]pyrene or that of aflatoxin B_1) and by intercalating (i.e., wedging) between two nitrogenous bases on the DNA (e.g., as in the case with proflavine). Both cases can lead to miscopying of the template strand when the affected DNA is replicated. Still some others work indirectly by causing the cells to synthesize chemicals that have the direct mutagenic effect. To some people, mutagens of this *synthesized* kind might not be considered as environmental in origin.

Until more recently, the mutagenicity of environmental agents was largely determined by the *Salmonella*/microsome *in vitro* assay. This relatively low-cost test utilizes several strains of the bacterium *Salmonella typhimurium* that each carry a defective gene which otherwise is responsible for encoding the essential amino acid *histidine* using the ingredients provided in the culture medium. Many agents have the ability to induce a reverse mutation on this gene so that the gene can regain its normal function to enable the bacterium strain to grow on a medium lacking histidine. Those agents that have been tested positive (i.e., to have such an ability) are qualified as (potential) mutagens.

In the *Salmonella* assay or Ames test, as named after its developer, a mixture of *hepatic* microsomes (which are rich in *liver* enzymes) is purposely added to the culture medium as an enhancer of the intended reverse (i.e., backward) mutation. This is because certain substances, such as benzo[α]pyrene and aflatoxin B_1, are not mutagenic *per se* until they have been metabolically activated. Given that *S. typhimurium* is not meant to be a perfect model for the human body as it is only a bacterium, the Ames test now is but one of several methods used to determine the mutagenicity of a suspect agent. These other testing methods include a variety of *in vitro* and *in vivo* assays using mammalian cell lines as culture media, such as the *in vitro* and *in vivo* micronucleus test, the mouse lymphoma (thymidine kinase gene mutation) assay, the bone marrow metaphase analysis, and the transgenic animal models. References and details for these other testing methods can be found in a harmonization project paper issued by the World Health Organization (WHO) on mutagenicity testing (Eastmond *et al.*, 2009).

18.3. Environmental Carcinogenesis

Carcinogenesis is a pathocellular process involving erratic cell division which otherwise under normal conditions occurs naturally in almost all tissues. A basic knowledge on cell (division) cycle is therefore considered essential to the understanding of carcinogenesis. The cell cycle represents a repeating series of biological events within a cell that leads to the cell's division and replication. In an autosomal (also called somatic) cell with a nucleus (as in the eukaryotes), the cell cycle can be broadly divided into four distinct as well as more technical phases: (1) the *first* growth G1 phase; (2) the *s*ynthesis S phase; (3) the *second* growth G2 phase; and (4) the *m*itosis M phase.

The first three (sub)phases G1, S, and G2 collectively are known as the *interphase*, during which the non-gamete (i.e., the somatic) cell grows and accumulates nutrients required for DNA replication as well as for chromatid duplication in the S phase. Further cell growth for mitosis takes place in the G2 phase which represents the last stage of the interphase. The M phase itself involves two tightly coupled events: mitosis and cytokinesis. In mitosis, the chromosomes in a somatic cell are each divided between the two identical daughter cells being formed, whereas in cytokinesis the cell's cytoplasm is divided in half to complete the formation of the two daughter cells. Initiation of each of the four phases is contingent on the proper progression and completion of the previous phase. After a cell division, each of the daughter cells begins the interphase of her own.

Meiosis is a special type of cell division involving the formation of only gamete (i.e., sperm or egg) cells. These sex cells each have to go through the *meiotic* division process twice, though with only one round of DNA replication, in order for their daughter cells each to end up having half of the number of chromosomes that they (i.e., the parent sex cells) each have. Meiosis does not lead to a cell cycle in the way that mitosis does, as fertilization of two opposite sex cells is required to extend the genetic life of each of the two sex cells. The preparatory steps that lead to meiosis include only the first two stages in the interphase (i.e., the G1 and the S phase) of the mitotic cell cycle.

Cell cycle is by no means an ever-ongoing biological process. There are a number of signal transduction pathways or systems, known commonly as *checkpoints*, in a cell cycle that play a key role in upholding the fidelity of DNA replication as well as the genetic stability in cells. For example, one checkpoint is there to prevent cells from entering mitosis if they fail to replicate all their chromosomes. Another checkpoint is there to either stall or arrest a critical stage of the cell cycle in an effort to facilitate DNA repair, whenever it senses an event leading to DNA damage or misalignment of replication structure. Typically, those checkpoints that function in response to moderate DNA damage will activate the p53 protein to block or stall the cell cycle. When the DNA damage becomes substantial enough, the p53 protein in turn will activate those genes that induce the process of programmed cell death which in more technical terms is known as *apoptosis*. Apoptosis is an important process in that it helps maintain genetic stability by destroying cells that are unlikely repairable or that represent a threat to the integrity of a multicellular organism.

18.3.1. Concepts of Carcinogenesis

A basic principle underlying most theories of carcinogenesis is the alteration of DNA sequences. Extensive alteration of the DNA sequences will lead to altered sequences of mRNA and subsequently to the synthesis of abnormal proteins, of which many are important enzymes. The functions of the synthesized abnormal enzymes consequently may become so abnormal that cell proliferation subject to their catalytic regulations or biochemical influences either becomes out of control or continues indefinitely.

The most accepted theory of carcinogenesis today is that mutations of the genetic materials in normal cells would cause an upset of the normal balance between cell proliferation and apoptosis, eventually leading to uncontrolled cell division or proliferation. The uncontrolled and often rapid proliferation of cells then lead to tumors, of which some may turn into the malignant type known as cancers.

More than one mutation is thought to be necessary for activating carcinogenesis. Only mutations in those types of genes playing a key role in the cell cycle, in DNA repair, and in cell death are likely to cause cells to lose control of their proliferation. Therefore, in general a series of mutations in at least three types of genes is required in order for cells to start dividing erratically. The three gene types are tumor suppressor genes, DNA repair genes, and proto-oncogenes. Tumor suppressor genes serve to encode proteins (largely enzymes) or anti-proliferation signals that function to suppress mitosis and cell growth. In contrast, proto-oncogenes will encode proteins that promote cell growth. And DNA repair genes will encode proteins whose normal functions are to identify and correct errors that arise when cells replicate their DNA prior to cell division. More specifically, for tumor cells to form, a mutation is needed to inactivate one or more tumor suppressor genes so that cells are allowed to proliferate beyond the normal rate. Another required mutation is one that inactivates one or more DNA repair genes to cause repair failure. Still another mutation is needed for activating proto-oncogenes into oncogenes which are more ready to produce hormones and proteins that promote uncontrollable cell proliferation. The final outcome of this series of mutations is tumor or cancer formation.

18.3.2. Mechanism of Carcinogenesis

At the mechanistic levels involving molecular as well as cellular changes, environmental carcinogenesis is currently viewed by many scholars as a multistage process involving the *initiation*, *promotion*, and *progression* phases of normal cells into tumor or cancer cells (Figure 18.3). It is thought that the transition from one of these phases to another, likely necessarily in that order, is inducible by a wide array of environmental and endogenous agents, while subject to numerous genetic regulations and various biochemical influences. Yet from a genetic perspective, carcinogenesis can still be characterized as an accumulation of mutations in the tumor suppressor genes, proto-oncogenes, and DNA repair genes, as discussed in the preceding (sub)section.

Certain endogenous and exogenous agents are known to be capable of initiating the tumorigenic (or carcinogenic) process by yielding or becoming highly reactive species that have the tendency to bind covalently to cellular DNA. These agents are referred to as procarcinogens. There are other agents that can cause DNA damage directly without their undergoing any metabolic or chemical activation. These agents are called ultimate or genotoxic carcinogens. In either case, if the DNA damage is irreparable, it will lead to irreversible genetic mutations. Other characteristics of the initiation stage include the requirement of fixation and the high likelihood of having an additive as well as a nonthreshold effect. For the *irreversible* initiation to take its full course, the damaged DNA segment needs to be placed securely (i.e., fixed) into the daughter genome throughout the DNA replication.

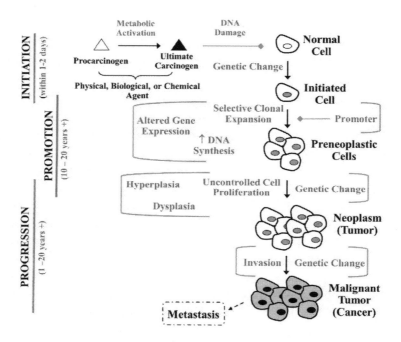

Figure 18.3. Current Conceptual Mechanism of Multistage Carcinogenesis

The promotion phase is where one or more agents or factors stimulate the proliferation and the clonal expansion of the initiated cells to yield a massive production of their daughter cells. Most of these promoting agents (e.g., tobacco smoke, alcohol), also called promoters or sometimes epigenetic carcinogens, are found extrinsic to the host. The effects that they promote often exhibit a threshold and tend to be dose-dependent and thus likely *reversible*. More specifically, these agents or factors may pose a relatively low risk for causing a tumor when the dose and the frequency of exposure are insignificantly low. An essential requirement for this phase to take its course is the setting of a mitogenic environment (i.e., that conducive of mitosis). For this second phase to have its full force and effect, the environment requires the presence of continuous stimulation which will increase the risk of inducing further genetic changes on the initiated cells.

During tumor progression, preneoplastic cells will develop into a tumor by undergoing further proliferation and expansion of the successful clones (which are each a cluster of cells derived from the same parent cell). In this final phase of carcinogenesis (or more correctly tumorigenesis), the preneoplastic cells become increasingly resistant to apoptotic stimuli and other negative regulatory controls. The progression is thought to be *irreversible*; and the proliferation and expansion involved are conceived as primarily passive and spontaneous. In a sense, the progression from a preneoplastic cell into a tumor is a chain of stepwise pathocellular changes, involving at least the hyperplastic and the dysplastic (sub)phase. In the hyperplastic phase, the preneoplastic cells in a local region of the tissue divide in an uncontrolled manner leading to an excess of cells which all still have the normal appearance. Yet further progression with the hyperplastic cells will result in a more abnormal growth not only in size but also in shape and appearance. At this point, the now dysplastic cells may become disorganized but not yet invasive to the neighboring tissues. Toward the very late progression stage, however, the tumor may become malignant if it has the ability or tendency to invade surrounding tissues and spread to regions outside of the local tissue (*see*, e.g., Weinberg, 2006).

As hinted in Section 18.1.2, the part of the progression that leads to the spread of tumor cells to more distant regions in the body is medically termed *metastasis*. This (sub)phase represents the most fearsome aspect of cancer development as it signals a very late stage disease involving highly complicated treatment with poor outcomes. Metastasis occurs most commonly by way of the bloodstream or the lymphatic system. Occasionally, it can occur by local extension from the tumor to somewhat more distant tissues. The cells in a primary tumor by nature adhere to one another as well as to a mesh of proteins that fill the space between these cells. Therefore, to begin metastasis, the (cancerous) cells must be capable of breaking away from the (nonmalignant) tumor. In most instances, the loosened cells then proceed to make their way into the bloodstream which provides them with both a means for their transport to (almost) all other parts of the body and the energy as well as nutrients required for their growth.

Not all cells in a tumor are able to metastasize (i.e., spread). For those that are able to, the extent of their dissemination is determined in part by the host's physiological conditions that may or may not be conducive for certain physiological inhibitors to kick in to suppress the invasive activity. That is, these cells must be able to fight off the host's numerous defense systems before they can re-attach themselves in a new location. Such a metastatic process also depends on the complex interaction of many factors pertaining to the nature of the primary cancer, including its type, maturity, and location.

The new cancer developed from metastasis is medically referred to as a secondary or a metastatic cancer, in that its cells all appear and behave much more like those in the primary cancer than in tissues at the invaded location. In other words, if breast cancer metastasizes to the brain, the secondary cancer is made up of abnormal breast cells, not of cells in or around the brain. In a way, metastasis is characterized by invasive activity and cell resemblance, in addition to the host's physiological conditions.

18.3.3. Environmental Carcinogens

Over the years, many chemical, physical, and biological agents found in the environment have been determined or suspected to be carcinogenic to humans or other mammalians. For some of these agents, their carcinogenicity potential has been evaluated extensively by the International Agency for Research on Cancer (IARC), which is a highly authoritative and influential extension of WHO that strives to promote intergovernmental collaboration in cancer research and prevention.

IARC's main objectives include coordinating and conducting epidemiological and laboratory studies on the causes of human cancer, as well as developing strategies for cancer control and prevention. The agency maintains a series of monographs on the carcinogenic risks to humans that are posed from exposure to various select agents. These agents are evaluated by IARC mostly on the basis of the evidence available for human exposure and carcinogenicity (e.g., IARC, 2006). After evaluation, these agents are each classified into one of the five categories of carcinogenicity potential listed in Box 18.1:

Box 18.1. Classification of Carcinogenicity Potential as Developed by the International Agency for Research on Cancer (e.g., IARC, 2006)

Group 1:	Carcinogenic to humans.
Group 2A:	Probably carcinogenic to humans.
Group 2B:	Possibly carcinogenic to humans.
Group 3:	Not classifiable as to the agent's carcinogenicity to humans.
Group 4:	Probably not carcinogenic to humans.

In their simplest terms, Group 1 in Box 18.1 is used for those agents with sufficient evidence of carcinogenicity in humans. Group 2A is used for those with limited evidence of carcinogenicity in humans but sufficient evidence of carcinogenicity in experimental animals, whereas Group 2B is used for those with limited evidence of carcinogenicity in humans and less than sufficient evidence of carcinogenicity in experimental animals. Group 3 is used for agents with *both* inadequate evidence of carcinogenicity in humans *and* inadequate or limited evidence of carcinogenicity in experimental animals. Lastly, Group 4 is used for agents with solid or sound support pointing to the lack of carcinogenicity in both humans and experimental animals.

For illustration purposes, a list of select agents covering all these five categories of carcinogenicity potential is given in Table 18.2. Note that some individual government agencies, particularly U.S. EPA, have opted to use a somewhat different scheme to rate the carcinogenicity potential for the agents under their own cancer risk assessment.

18.4. DNA Damage and Repair

DNA damage is a crucial underlying cause of genetic mutation leading to the development of tumor or cancer. Its repair thereby is a pivotal point of mutagenesis (and thus

Table 18.2. Human Carcinogenicity Potential of Select Agents or Exposures
as Determined and Classified by IARC[a]

Agent/Exposure	Carcinogenicity Potential[b]	IARC Volume[a]
Physical		
Ionizing radiation: all types	1	100D
Ultraviolet radiation: UV-A, UV-B, UV-C	1	100D
Fluorescent lighting	3	55
Biological		
Hepatitis B and C viruses (infection with)	1	59, 100B
HIV type 1 (infection with)	1	67, 100B
Human papillomavirus type 16 (infection with)	1	64, 90, 100B
Helicobacter pylori (infection with)	1	61, 100B
Salted fish, Chinese style	1	56, 100E
Human papillomavirus type 68 (infection with)	2A	100B
HIV type 2 (infection with)	2B	67
Human papillomavirus type 26 (infection with)	2B	100B
Hepatitis D virus (infection with)	3	59
Chemical		
Aflatoxins (B_1, B_2, G_1, G_2, M_1)	1	56, 82, 100F
Asbestos: all forms	1	14, Sup 7, 100C
Benzene	1	29, Sup 7, 100F
Benzo[α]pyrene	1	92, 100F
Chromium VI compounds	1	49, 100C
Diethylstilbestrol (DES)	1	21, Sup 7, 100A
Dioxin (2,3,7,8-tetrachlorodibenzo-*p*-dioxin)	1	69, 100F
Ethanol in alcoholic beverages	1	96, 100E
Formaldehyde	1	88, 100F
Vinyl chloride	1	97, 100F
Nitrogen mustards	2A	9, Sup 7
Polychlorinated biphenyls (PCBs)	2A	18, Sup 7
Carbon tetrachloride	2B	25, Sup 7, 71
DDT (4,4'-dichlorodiphenyltrichloroethane)	2B	53
Pickled vegetables (traditional in Asia)	2B	56
Dioxins other than 2,3,7,8-TCDD	3	69
Hair coloring products (personal use of)	3	57, 99
Caffeine; tea	3	51
Toluene; xylenes	3	47, 71
Vitamin K substances	3	76
Caprolactam	4	39, Sup 7, 71

[a]International Agency for Research on Cancer (*see* IARC, 2010 and the IARC website for access to and reference of each monograph volume listed); although the agents/exposures were selected arbitrarily, the attempt here is to cover all types of agents/exposures and all carcinogenicity potential categories.

[b]Group 1 = carcinogenic to humans; Group 2A = probably carcinogenic to humans; Group 2B = possibly carcinogenic to humans; Group 3 = not classifiable as to the agent's carcinogenicity to humans; Group 4 = probably not carcinogenic to humans (*see* Box 18.1).

of carcinogenesis) deserving further discussion in this chapter. Due to the enormous factors present in the environment and the high volume of metabolic processes occurring spontaneously inside a cell, DNA damage occurs very frequently in cells. It is estimated that in human cells, the spontaneous formation of DNA damage on average occurs at a rate of around 19,000 molecular lesions per cell per day (Vilenchik and Knudson, 2000). Fortunately, this still constitutes only a very small fraction of the human genome's approximately 6 billion nitrogenous bases; and in many cases, the damage can be repaired through genetic information stored in the intact, opposite strand of the double DNA helix. Moreover, most cells have a feedback system in place that, after DNA damage, several checkpoints are activated to block or stall the cell cycle in an effort to allow time for the affected cells to repair the damage before they continue to divide. Checkpoints responsive to DNA damage typically occur at the G1/S and G2/M boundaries.

18.4.1. DNA Damage

In a broad sense, DNA damage is caused either by substances produced from normal metabolic processes such as reactive oxygen species (ROS), or by external agents in the environment such as chemicals, viruses, bacteria, and UV radiation. The following types of DNA damage are found to occur commonly in cells: loss or modification of DNA base; DNA replication error; crosslinks between DNA strands, or between DNA and proteins; and DNA strand breakage.

The glycosyl bond linking a DNA base to the sugar deoxyribose (Figure 18.2) is labile under physiological conditions, thereby easily resulting in the loss of the base. All four bases on the DNA (i.e., adenine, guanine, cytosine, thymine) are susceptible to numerous modifications at various positions by UV radiation and a wide variety of chemical or biological agents. For example, the primary amino groups (NH_2) in the DNA bases are relatively unstable. They can be converted to a carbonyl group (C=O). One of the most frequent base modifications is thus the loss of an amino group (with the removal reaction being named *deamination*), such as with a cytosine being converted to a uracil. Several ROS (e.g., singlet oxygen, superoxide, peroxide radical, hydroxyl radical) can alter the DNA bases, such as in the oxidation of thymine to thymine glycol.

Other major sources of DNA damage include the generation of mismatches and the minor insertions or deletions of bases during DNA replication. Mismatches of the normal bases may occur due to a failure of proofreading during DNA replication, such as the incorporation of uracil (normally found in RNA only) in place of thymine.

Covalent linkages can be formed between bases on the same DNA strand (thus called *intrastrand* crosslink) or between bases on the opposite strand (*interstrand* crosslink). DNA topoisomerases are enzymes that facilitate DNA replication through winding and unwinding DNA's complex double helix. These proteins too can form covalent linkages between themselves and their DNA substrates during the course of their enzymatic action. These types of crosslinkage can all cause blockage of DNA replication, leading to replication arrest and cell death unless the crosslink is repaired.

Several chemotherapeutic drugs used against cancer can crosslink with DNA, such as the alkylating agents nitrogen mustards acting at the N7 position of guanine (i.e., at this base's only nitrogen atom so shown on the upper left of the molecule in Figure 18.1) on the opposite strand to form an *inter*strand crosslink. Another example is the platinum-based cisplatin which can act on the N7 position of an adjacent guanine to form an *intra*strand crosslink. Psoralen is a phytochemical used with UV-A light to treat psoriasis, eczema, and vitiligo. It has both the ability to absorb UV photons and a strong tendency to intercalate with DNA base pairs. Upon activation by UV-A radiation, this phytochemical can form covalent crosslinks between the pyrimidines of opposite strands.

Breaks in the sugar-phosphate backbone can be confined to one of the two DNA strands (i.e., a single-stranded break, SSB) or to both strands (i.e., a double-stranded break, DSB). The two kinds of strand breakage can be induced by ionizing radiation and certain chemical or antibiotic agents (e.g., bleomycin). Both SSB and DSB can also be formed during normal DNA metabolism by DNA topoisomerases and DNA nucleases, as well as during DNA repair processes though at a much lower frequency.

18.4.2. DNA Repair

DNA repair refers to an enzymatic defense system that enables a cell to enzymatically identify and correct damage to the DNA molecules. This system, present in all organisms tested today, is essential for the genetic integrity of the organism, considering that a failure to repair DNA damage can result in a severe genetic mutation. In mammalians, DNA repair is accomplished through broadly two types of defense mechanisms: (1) repair mechanisms; and (2) damage tolerance mechanisms. The repair mechanisms involve removal of DNA damage via a series of enzymatic events, whereas the damage tolerance mechanisms circumvent the damage enzymatically without fixing it.

Perhaps the most frequent cause of point mutations in humans is the spontaneous alkylation of cytosine (e.g., by addition of a methyl group CH_3^- to the base) followed by its deamination into a thymine. Fortunately, this type of base modification can be readily repaired by a series of enzymes under the so-termed *base excision repair (BER) mechanism*. First, the damaged or mismatched base is removed by the enzyme DNA glycosylase. The related phosphodiester bond (that linking two adjacent sugars via a phosphate group on the same DNA molecule) is then cut off by an enzyme named DNA AP endonuclease (where AP = *ap*urinic or *ap*yrimidinic) after recognizing the missing "tooth" (i.e., the missing base). The cleaved part is subsequently resynthesized by a DNA polymerase of the kind capable of catalyzing the polymerization of DNA into a strand. Lastly, a DNA ligase is there to perform the final nick-sealing step.

Another closely related repair mechanism is the nucleotide excision repair (NER), which recognizes and repairs various bulky helix-distorting lesions (e.g., those induced by UV radiation). A typical NER involves over 20 enzymes to recognize and excise the damage to a DNA oligonucleotide of about 30 bases in length. As with BER, NER also requires enzymes to catalyze the repair and ligation steps. A specialized form of NER known as transcription-coupled repair recognizes the DNA damage somewhat differently by deploying NER enzymes to genes that are being actively transcribed.

Mismatch repair (MMR) is an enzymatic mechanism used in DNA replication and recombination to correct errors that resulted in mispaired bases or nucleotides. In this repair, some of the enzymes involved in BER and NER may be required, in addition to those specific for recognizing and excising the mismatch.

DNA damage due to SSB, and particularly to DSB, is usually highly destructive to the cell in that such damage is more likely to cause genome rearrangements. The repair of SSB generally calls for the same enzyme systems that are used in BER or NER. For the repair of DSB, three repair submechanisms are typically involved: (1) homologous recombination (HR); (2) non-homologous end joining (NHEJ); and (3) microhomology-mediated end joining (MMEJ). Both MMEJ and NHEJ require enzymes that recognize and bind to the broken ends and bring them together for ligation. MMEJ differs from NHEJ mainly in using its *own* short (around 5 to 25) base-pair microhomologous sequences as a template for aligning the broken strands before joining. In HR, the broken ends are repaired using the genetic sequence on the intact sister chromatid or homologous chromosome as a template. Note that some cells are known to be capable of eliminating and repairing certain types of DNA damage by chemically reversing the damage without requiring a template. This process is known as direct chemical reversal.

Translesion synthesis (TLS) is a DNA damage tolerance process in which the lesion is not repaired by the usual DNA polymerases, but is bypassed by the specialized kind called DNA TLS polymerases which allow the DNA replication machinery to replicate past DNA lesions. Examples of this type of DNA lesions include *AP* sites (i.e., those *without* a purine or a pyrimidine) and thymine dimers (e.g., in response to UV radiation).

References

Ames BN, Durston WE, Yamasaki E, Lee FD, 1973. Carcinogens Are Mutagens: A Simple Test System Combining Liver Homogenates for Activation and Bacteria for Detection. *Proc. Natl. Acad. Sci. USA* 70:2281-2285.

Burkitt D, 1958. A Sarcoma Involving the Jaws in African Children. *Brit. J. Surg.* 46:218-223.

Eastmond DA, Hartwig A, Anderson D, Anwar WA, Cimino MC, Dobrev I, Douglas GR, Nohmi T, Phillips DH, Vickers C, 2009. Mutagenicity Testing for Chemical Risk Assessment: Update of the WHO/IPCS Harmonized Scheme. *Mutagenesis* 24:341-349.

IARC (International Agency for Research on Cancer), 2006. IARC Monographs on the Evaluation of Carcinogenic Risks to Humans: Preamble. Lyon, France: WHO Press.

IARC (International Agency for Research on Cancer), 2010. IARC Monographs: List of Classifications (by Alphabetical Order). Lyon, France: WHO Press.

Jensen CC, Jensen LCW, Rieder CL, Cole RW, Ault JG, 1996. Long Crocidolite Asbestos Fibers Cause Polyploidy by Sterically Blocking Cytokinesis. *Carcinogenesis* 17:2013-2021.

Li JY, Gaillard F, Moreau A, Harousseau J-L, Laboisse C, Milpied N, Bataille R, Avet-Loiseau H, 1999. Detection of Translocation t(11;14)(q13;q32) in Mantle Cell Lymphoma by Fluorescence *in situ* Hybridization. *Am. J. Pathol.* 154:1449-1452.

Liu D, Shimonov J, Primanneni S, Lai Y, Ahmed T, Seiter K, 2007. t(8;14;18): A 3-Way Chromosome Translocation in Two Patients with Burkitt's Lymphoma/Leukemia. *Mol. Cancer* 6:35 (online journal).

McCann J, Choi E, Yamasaki E, Ames BN, 1975. Detection of Carcinogens as Mutagens in the *Salmonella*/Microsome Test: Assay of 300 Chemicals. *Proc. Natl. Acad. Sci. USA* 72:5135-5139.

Muller HJ, 2007. Artificial Transmutation of the Gene. *Science* 46:84-87.

Nelson HH, Kelsey KT, 2002. The Molecular Epidemiology of Asbestos and Tobacco in Lung Cancer. *Oncogene* 21:7284-7288.

Vilenchik MM, Knudson AG Jr, 2000. Inverse Radiation Dose-Rate Effects on Somatic and Germ-Line Mutations and DNA Damage Rates. *Proc. Natl. Acad. Sci. USA* 97:5381-5386.

Webb A, Miller B, Bonasera S, Boxer A, Karydas A, Kirk C. Wilhelmsen KC, 2008. Role of the Tau Gene Region Chromosome Inversion in Progressive Supranuclear Palsy, Corticobasal, Degeneration, and Related Disorders. *Arch. Neurol.* 65:1473-1478.

Weinberg RA, 2006. *The Biology of Cancer*. New York, New York, USA: Garland Science Publishing.

Xue Y, Wang Q, Long Q, Ng BL, Swerdlow H, Burton J, Skuce C, Taylor R, Abdellah Z, Zhao Y, Asan, MacArthur DG, Quail MA, Carter NP, Yang H, Tyler-Smith C, 2009. Human Y Chromosome Base-Substitution Mutation Rate Measured by Direct Sequencing in a Deep-Rooting Pedigree. *Curr. Biol.* 19:1453-1457.

Review Questions

1. Give one good reason why the two pathocellular processes *carcinogenesis* and *mutagenesis* are commonly discussed side by side.

2. Briefly describe the main differences among DNA (deoxyribonucleic acid), codon, genome, gene, and chromosome.

3. Match *each* attribute or term listed in the left column to *only one* set of chemical substances or genetic materials listed in the right column that the attribute or term ascribes to.

(1) chromatin	(a) deoxyribose, adenine
(2) centromere	(b) sugar, sugar
(3) glycosyl bond	(c) guanine, cytosine
(4) phosphodiester bond	(d) phosphate, sugar, base
(5) nucleotide	(e) chromatid, chromatid
(6) hydrogen bond	(f) chromosome, histone

4. The five genes denoted by letters A through E and contained in a segment of a normal chromosome are present in the following order: ABCDE. Match *each* gene arrangement shown in the left column to *only one* clastogenic cause listed in the right column.

(1) $\rightarrow A_1B_1C_2D_2E_2$	(a) duplication
(2) $\rightarrow$ ABDCE	(b) deletion
(3) $\rightarrow$ ABCCDE	(c) inversion
(4) $\rightarrow$ ABCE	(d) translocation

5. Briefly describe the current concepts of mutagenesis.

6. What is a frameshift mutation? And how is it related to a point mutation?

7. What is an aneuploidy? Give two diseases from this chapter that are related to this condition.

8. What is likely to happen when a point mutation causes the conversion of the codon GAG to GUG in the *beta*-hemoglobin gene?

9. Why is the concept of reverse (i.e., backward) mutation so crucial or relevant to the *in vitro* *Salmonella* assay used for the determination of an agent's mutagenicity? And what is the purpose for this assay to add a mixture of liver microsomes to the culture medium?

10. Briefly describe the four distinct phases of a typical cell division cycle (in a eukaryote).

11. Match *each* agent listed in the left column to *only one* site/mode of mutagenic action listed in the right column (that the agent is associated with or responsible for).

(1) *Helicobacter pylori*	(a) covalent bonding with DNA bases
(2) retrovirus	(b) inflammation-induced DNA damage
(3) benzo[α]pyrene	(c) formation of stable DNA adducts
(4) *beta*-particle	(d) reverse transcription to DNA
(5) melphalan	(e) addition of molecules to DNA bases
(6) nitrogen mustard	(f) irreparable DNA damage

12. Briefly describe the main differences between mitosis and meiosis in cell division.

13. What are the current concepts of carcinogenesis?

14. Briefly describe the three main mechanistic phases (stages) that are currently accepted as involved in carcinogenesis.

15. Name five agents that are human carcinogens and another five that are *possible* human carcinogens, as classified by IARC.

16. What are the three main characteristics of metastasis? And how does it usually occur?

17. Briefly explain the importance of DNA repair and of checkpoints, both in relation to mutagenesis or carcinogenesis.

18. Briefly describe the main types of DNA damage that commonly occur.

19. How do nitrogen mustard and cisplatin normally act in terms of their capacity of crosslinking with a DNA molecule?

20. Give an example of the tolerance processes as an organism's enzymatic defense mechanism in dealing with DNA damage.

21. Briefly describe the main differences among the following DNA repair mechanisms: base excision repair (BER); nucleotide excision repair (NER); single-stranded break repair (SSBR); and mismatch repair (MMR).

22. Name three (sub)mechanisms available for repairing double-stranded breakage.

CHAPTER 19

Reproductive Toxicity and Endocrine Disruption

19.1. Introduction

The pertinence between endocrine disruption and human reproductive health is best appreciated with a review of the endocrine-reproductive system first, which hence is provided in Section 19.2 below. This physiological system is actually composed of both the endocrine system and the developmental-reproductive system. In this chapter as well as in many places in the literature, the two subsystems are treated as one in the sense that neither one can be fully appreciated without referencing the other.

The human endocrine system is also referred to as the endocrine network, as it is a network of ductless glands and the hormones that they produce. Hormones are chemical messengers that an organism's body uses to regulate or influence its many important day-to-day functions, such as those related to the body's development, growth, reproduction, and behavior. For instance, the thyroid is a crucial component of the human endocrine network in that, through its hormones, the gland affects many important daily physiological functions including body metabolism, body temperature, and heart rate.

The developmental-reproductive system, on the other hand, revolves around a process that may be regarded as a physiological cycle extremely vital on the population and species level, starting from the fertilization of an egg for the life of an individual and then back to the union of the individual's gamete (e.g., egg) with a gamete (e.g., sperm) of another individual of the opposite sex then for the life of a third individual, and so on. During this physiological cycle or process, many environmental toxicants can cause reproductive disorders by their own effects, or through their disruption on the endocrine system. Naturally, those environmental toxicants whose effects rely on endocrine disruption are called environmental endocrine disruptors (EEDs). Many EEDs tend to affect the developmental-reproductive cycle, as their effects are largely estrogenic, androgenic, or thyroidal in nature. Many of them are also natural or synthetic chemicals. For this large subgroup, they are frequently referred to as endocrine-disrupting chemicals (EDCs). Toxicants that cause birth defects are specifically termed *teratogens*.

As noted above, not all environmental reproductive toxicants or environmental teratogens have their adverse effects exerted via endocrine disruption. It is also important to understand that not all endocrine disruption effects are confined to the developmental-reproductive system, as virtually every system in the body is responsive to hormonal action. In fact, many EEDs have been linked specifically to the human nervous or immunological system, but not to the developmental-reproductive system at all.

19.1.1. Impacts and Causes of Human Birth Defects

Birth defects are congenital abnormalities of structure, function, or body metabolism present at birth and can occur in virtually any part of the fetal body. As further discussed in Section 19.4.1 below, structural malformations are those in which a specific body part is missing or malformed. In contrast, congenital metabolic defects are those in which an inborn error or disorder occurs in the fetal body's biochemical system.

Each year approximately 8 million babies are born with birth defects worldwide, of which 40% die before age 5 and another 40% are disabled for life (Christianson *et al.*, 2006). In the United States alone, each year around 120,000 babies (or about 3% of all newborns) are diagnosed with one or more birth defects (CDC, 2008). There are thousands of different kinds or forms of birth defects documented (Weinhold, 2009), ranging from minor and treatable to severe and fatal. Among the more severe kinds, many lead to permanent mental or physical disabilities and collectively are one of the leading causes of infant deaths in the United States and worldwide, particularly during their first year of life (Mathews and MacDorman, 2008; Russo and Elixhauser, 2007). The health and economic impacts of the more common and severe types of birth defects are devastating. These more severe types often cause life-long disability and require extensive medical treatment. In the United States, the estimated hospital costs for birth defects in 2004 alone amounted to $2.6 billion (Russo and Elixhauser, 2007).

Statistics also show that about two-thirds of birth defects have no apparent known cause. The remaining one-third are thought to be caused by genetic factors or environmental agents, or some interplay of the two. Environmental causes are found to take their effects mostly during pregnancy: maternal use of drugs or alcohol; maternal exposure to chemicals or physical hazards (e.g., radiation); and maternal infections (e.g., with rubella, syphilis, or Venezuelan equine encephalitis).

19.1.2. Concerns with Human Reproductive Disorders

Reproduction is the crux of every organism's survival as a species. Therefore, any massive severe effect on this physiological process can have a serious consequence to a population, including its distinction. Disorders or health problems from reproductive effects can occur at several stages during the organism's life span. In most mammalians, some of these disorders involve the reproductive system of either sex directly. Others involve a relevant body system or biochemical process, or may manifest many years after exposure to the cause or even in a later generation. Overall, the effects can manifest as abnormalities or disorders in any critical stage of reproduction, including gamete production, menstrual cycle, sexual behavior, fertilization, pregnancy, and parturition.

Aside from birth defects being treated as a distinct adverse effect category on its own, the most common reproductive disorders in humans include infertility, erectile dysfunction (ED), and ovarian cysts. Infertility means not being able to get pregnant after one year of unprotected intercourse, or six months for a woman who is over 34. Women who get pregnant but are unable to stay pregnant may also be treated as infertile. Infertility is now estimated to affect 6.1 million (10%) of American couples (e.g., APA, 2013; CDC, 2013), costing the nation about $1 billion for health care related to this problem.

A closely related problem is failure in pregnancy, which is the result of a process that involves mostly the union of a healthy ovum with a healthy sperm or the implantation (attachment) of a fertilized egg to the inside of the uterus. The failure can occur if there are problems with the above or other steps involved in the process. According to the statistics for 2006 to 2010, 6.7 million (over 10%) of American women at ages 15 to 44 reportedly had difficulty getting pregnant or staying pregnant (CDC, 2013). Ovarian cysts and ED are two major reproductive conditions that can adversely affect fertilization or pregnancy. These two reproductive disorders are specifically discussed in Section 19.4.2.

19.1.3. Concepts of Endocrine Disruption in Humans

Historically, the medical tragedy allegedly alerting some relevance of endocrine disruption to human health was the prescription of diethylstilbestrol (DES) to several million pregnant American women during the late-1930s to mid-1970s. The drug was prescribed to the women primarily as an agonist of their natural sex hormone estrogen for prevention of miscarriage. In the mid-1970s, DES was banned for such use not so much for lack of substantial efficacy data, but more for an increase in a rare vaginal clear cell carcinoma observed in 1971 in a significant number of female offspring who were exposed to the synthetic estrogen *in utero*. The DES saga however did not seem to bear as much relevance to endocrine disruption as it should, as the term *endocrine disruption* was not coined until about two decades later at a multidisciplinary conference convened in 1991. That 1991 conference, held at the Wingspread Conference Center in Racine, Wisconsin (USA), was led by Theo Colborn, Ph.D. then working for the World Wildlife Fund US. The conference's focus was primarily on issues related to transgenerational health impacts. Yet the concept consensus on endocrine disruption and its scientific discussion at the conference were found so intriguing that they were quickly turned into a journal volume (Colborn and Clement, 1992) in the following year.

Four years later, together with two new colleagues, Dr. Colborn wrote another book to give a fuller account of the issues on endocrine disruption. That book, entitled *Our Stolen Future* with a foreword by then U.S. Vice-President Al Gore, is now available in 14 languages. For many years since the book's first publication (Colborn *et al.*, 1996), the concept of endocrine disruption has been accepted amid some controversies, as some people still believe that the low ambient levels of EDCs that the public is usually exposed to are harmless (*see*, e.g., discussion in Vandenberg *et al.*, 2009). Yet in spite of such controversies, the concept on the whole has continued to gain strong support from proceedings of multiple scientific and medical conferences on the subject. A case in point is the statement published by The Endocrine Society in 2009, which elaborated a strong basis for concern regarding the health risks of endocrine disruption from even low levels of exposure (Diamanti-Kandarakis *et al.*, 2009). As discussed in Section 19.3 below, there are arising concerns about the low-threshold effects with endocrine disruption.

19.2. The Endocrine-Reproductive System

As noted at the beginning of this chapter, the human endocrine-reproductive system is composed of the endocrine system and the developmental-reproductive system. The two subsystems are highly interactive and closely interconnected. The endocrine-reproductive system is essentially a physiological cycle on the species level that becomes functional and interactive very early in both the mother and the embryo, typically by the first trimester of pregnancy. For example, in about four weeks following conception, the human embryo will produce hormones to stop the mother's menstrual cycle.

In this section, as a quick reference for further discussion, an overview is given on the developmental-reproductive cycle in humans, followed by a brief account of the endocrine system and then a summary of the hormones that this endocrine network produces.

19.2.1. The Human Developmental-Reproductive Cycle

In humans (and other mammalians), the reproductive cycle starts with gametogenesis. More specifically, the cycle starts with spermatogenesis for males and oogenesis for females. In the female, oogenesis is the process involving the formation of primary oocytes from the primordial germ cells termed *gonocytes* via mitosis, leading to the production and the development of a mature ovum. Such a developmental process takes place during the fetal period and ceases at birth (Figure 19.1). A mature oocyte is commonly called an egg or, more technically, an ovum. In the male, spermatogenesis is the parallel process leading to the production and the development of mature sperms. Like the eggs, these sperms start with gonocytes during the fetal period. After birth, these cells are transformed to spermatogonia and subsequently to spermatocytes. A mature spermatocyte is known commonly as a sperm or, more technically, a spermatozoon.

Fertilization calls for not only the availability of a healthy ovum and a healthy sperm, but also the effective delivery of the sperm and a conducive environment. The fertilized ovum (i.e., the conceptus or zygote) is then proliferated, implanted in the uterus, and later develops to full term through the embryonic and then the fetal stage. The relatively short interval from fertilization of an ovum to its implantation in the uterus is termed *the germinal stage* or *the predifferentiation period*. The embryonic stage entails four precise, sequential processes or phases, proceeding in the following order: *cell proliferation, cell differentiation, cell migration,* and *organogenesis* (Figure 19.1).

At the embryonic stage, cell proliferation is the process in which cells of the fertilized ovum that have begun to multiply during the predifferentiation period continue to do so. Cell differentiation involves the development of specialized cells to acquire specific structural, functional, and biochemical properties. Cell migration is the third substage in which cells are orchestrated to move in a specific direction to a particular location. Organogenesis is the final and critical process in the embryonic period whereby the main structures and organs are formed. This final substage is the period in which the embryo is most susceptible to the effects of environmental teratogens. In humans, this period generally begins in the fifth week and ends in the fourteenth week of the gestation period.

Not all embryonic organs or tissues are susceptible to teratogenic injuries at the same time during this period.

After organogenesis, the embryo undergoes a period of fetal development prior to parturition. The fetal stage is where the organs of the embryo, which is now more appropriately termed *fetus*, grows to full term leading to *functional* maturation. Teratogens are less likely to cause *gross structural* malformations during this fetal stage. Another likewise resistant period is the earlier germinal (predifferentiation) period, at which time teratogens tend to either cause death of the fertilized egg by killing most if not all of its cells or have no other apparent toxic effect on it. The overall developmental-reproductive cycle for humans is outlined graphically in Figure 19.1.

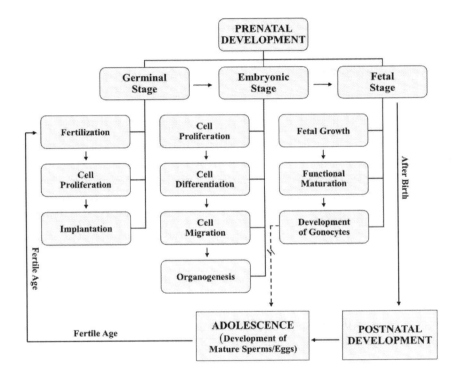

Figure 19.1. The Developmental-Reproductive Process and Cycle for Humans

19.2.2. The Human Endocrine System

Every cell, every organ, and every function of the human body are regulated or influenced practically every moment by two physiological (as well as anatomical) systems. These are the nervous system and the endocrine system. The nervous system coordinates rapid and precise responses to stimuli through action potentials. Action potential is an energy concept measuring a momentary change in electrical potential that occurs when a cell or tissue has been activated by a stimulus. The physiological functions performed by the nervous system are much more immediate, such as the control of body movement and breathing. Further discussion on this energy concept and the nervous system is beyond the purview of this chapter as well as this book. Those who have an interest in this area are referred to textbooks on general physiology or neurophysiology.

The endocrine system, in contrast, maintains homeostasis and longer-term control of body functions by means of chemical signals. It works in parallel with the nervous system to control growth and maturation along with homeostasis. The system is a collection of ductless glands that secrete hormones. The signals from these chemical messengers are passed via the bloodstream to arrive at a target organ, where there are cells possessing the proteinaceous receptors that act much like lock holes which only certain keys can fit into. Exocrine glands that secret substances that are passed outside the body are *ducted* structures, such as the familiar sweat glands, salivary glands, and digestive glands. By definition, these ducted glands are not part of the *endo*crine network.

Compared to the nervous system, the endocrine network operates in a less rapid but longer-lasting manner by synthesizing and releasing the required hormones in the proper amounts. These chemical messengers (further discussed in Section 19.2.3), via the proper transfer of information and instructions from one set of cells to another, regulate or at least influence the body's development, growth, tissue function, mood, behavior, metabolism, sexual function, and much more. In women, they support pregnancy and other reproductive processes. When either the glands in the endocrine system or the hormones that they secrete function improperly, a variety of health problems arise.

The major ductless glands that make up the human endocrine system are the *hypothalamus, pituitary, thyroid, parathyroid, adrenals, pineal body, pancreas*, and the *testes* or *ovaries* (Figure 19.2). By anatomical design, part of the pancreas is exocrine in that it is connected to the digestive system and secretes digestive enzymes into the intestine. Note that endocrine glands are not the only ones secreting hormones in the human body. Some nonendocrine organs, such as the placenta, brain, heart, lungs, liver, kidneys, thymus, and skin, are also capable of producing and releasing certain hormones.

Anatomically, the hypothalamus is a collection of specialized cells located in the lower center part of the brain. This gland is the primary link between the endocrine system and the nervous system via the pituitary gland. The pituitary gland, located at the base of the brain just beneath the hypothalamus and under the latter's control, is no bigger than a pea. These two glands together control many other endocrine functions. The pituitary is often called the "master gland", and is divided into the anterior and the posterior lobe. Nerve cells in the hypothalamus control the pituitary gland by producing chemicals that either stimulate or suppress the latter's hormone secretion.

In particular, the hypothalamus and the pituitary gland together secrete a number of hormones that are crucial to the female menstrual cycle, pregnancy, birth, and lactation. The pituitary gland-based hormones include the follicle-stimulating hormone (FSH) and the luteinizing hormone (LH). The functions of FSH include stimulating the development and maturation of a follicle in one of the woman's ovaries, whereas those of LH include bursting of that follicle (or otherwise known as undergoing ovulation) and forming a corpus luteum from the remains of the follicle. One non-sex hormone secreted by the posterior pituitary is antidiuretic hormone, which helps prevent excess water excretion by the kidneys.

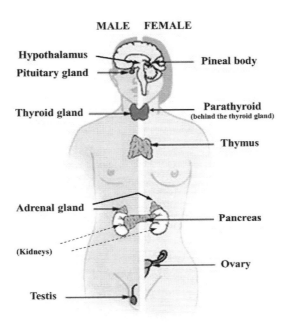

Figure 19.2. The Human Endocrine System *(image adapted from the U.S. National Cancer Institute public domain)*

The pineal body, also called the pineal gland, is located near the center of the human brain. It is stimulated by nerves from the eyes. The pineal gland secretes the hormone melatonin when the surrounding environment is dark such as at night, thereby secreting more in winter when the nights are longer. The hormone makes the individual feel sleepy and affects the individual's reproductive, thyroid, and adrenal cortex functions. Seasonal affective disorder (SAD) is a condition in which too much melatonin is released, causing profound depression, sadness, fatigue, inactiveness, over-sleeping, and thus likely weight gain as well. As expected, treatment of SAD typically consists of exposure to bright lights for several hours each day to retard melatonin production. The functions of the pineal gland have been implicated in a number of disorders including cancer, sexual dysfunction, hypertension (i.e., high blood pressure), and epilepsy.

The thyroid, located in the lower neck, is shaped like a bow tie and secretes predominately the hormones thyroxine and triiodothyronine. These two thyroid hormones together control the rate at which cells burn body fuels from food to produce energy. Accordingly, as the level of thyroid hormones increases in the bloodstream, so will the speed at which biochemical reactions occur in the body. Some other thyroid hormones like calcitonin play a key role in children in terms of their bone growth and the development of their brain and nervous system. Calcitonin is a polypeptide of 32 amino acids with the ability to decrease calcium (Ca^{2+}) levels by suppressing the release of Ca^{2+} from the huge reservoir in the bones. Locating behind the thyroid are four pea-size glands named parathyroids which function together to release the parathyroid hormone (PTH) made of 84 amino acids. PTH can counteract the effect of calcitonin by stimulating the release of Ca^{2+} from the bones into the bloodstream. It also regulates phosphate (PO_4^{3-}) homeostasis by increasing the secretion of PO_4^{3-} or its renal excretion.

The two adrenal glands are triangular in shape, with each locating on top of each kidney. Each adrenal gland has two main parts, each of which produces its own set of hormones leading to a different set of hormonal functions. The outer portion, called adrenal cortex, produces hormones such as corticosteroids which regulate the sexual function, the metabolic processes, the immunological system, the body's response to stress, and the salt and water balance in the body. Some of these corticosteroids are aldosterone, cortisol, and adrenal androgens. The inner portion of the adrenal gland, called adrenal medulla, produces epinephrine (a.k.a. adrenaline) and some other catecholamines which are a family of neurotransmitters. Epinephrine increases blood pressure and heart rate when the body experiences a sudden and substantial stress.

Again, the pancreas has two distinct functions. It serves as a ducted gland secreting digestive enzymes into the small intestine via the pancreatic duct. It also serves as a ductless gland, with its specialized cells called islets of Langerhans secreting the hormones insulin and glucagon to regulate sugar levels in the blood. The islets consist of two types of cells termed *alpha cells* and *beta cells*. The *alpha cells* secrete glucagon, which guides the liver to take carbohydrate out of storage to raise the blood sugar level when the level becomes low. The *beta cells* are responsible for the secretion of insulin. If a person's body does not make enough insulin, or if there is a reduced response of the target cells in the liver, the blood sugar may rise out of control to cause *diabetes mellitus*.

The gonads are the female's ovaries and the male's testes, and are known commonly as the sex or reproductive organs. In addition to producing gametes (i.e., sperms or ova), they secrete hormones. The secretion of these sex hormones is controlled by pituitary gland hormones including predominately FSH and LH. Although both sexes make some of each of these sex hormones, the (male) testes secrete predominately androgens, of which testosterone is the principal member. In contrast, the (female) ovaries make estrogens and progesterone in varying amounts depending on where in her menstrual cycle the woman is. In a pregnant woman, the fetus's placenta also secretes hormones to biochemically support the pregnancy.

Production of testosterone begins during fetal development, continues for a short time period after birth, nearly ceases during childhood, and then resumes at puberty. This sex hormone is responsible for several growth and sexual-related functions: growth and development of the male reproductive structures; increased skeletal and muscular growth;

enlargement of the larynx accompanied by voice change; growth and distribution of body hair; increased male sexual drive; and others.

The estrogens and progesterone contribute to the development and the functions of the female reproductive organs and sex characteristics. At the onset of puberty, the estrogens (of which estradiol is the predominant member) promote a number of crucial biological processes: development of the breasts; distribution of fat in the hips, legs, and breasts; maturation of the reproductive organs (i.e., the uterus, vagina). Progesterone, the predominant member of the subclass called progestogens, then causes the uterine lining to thicken in preparation for pregnancy.

From the short description of the endocrine system given above, it becomes clear that adverse health effects can be induced by an undesired interference with or disruption of the production, release, or use of hormones throughout the body. Also apparent is that not all endocrine disruption is necessarily detrimental, as well reflected in the intended use of the now banned DES. However, within the context of this chapter, the focus is on *unintended* or *undesired* endocrine disruption.

It is noteworthy here that the shape of each hormone molecule is specific and can be recognized by its target cells only. The binding sites on the target cells are termed *hormone receptors* which are proteinaceous in nature. Much of the hormonal regulation depends on feedback loops to maintain balance and homeostasis. *Steroids*, *peptides*, and *amines* are the three general groups of hormones classified on the basis of their chemical structure, which is the more conventional practice. Depicted in Figure 19.3 are the chemical structures of nine prominent hormones selected to represent these three groups.

19.2.3. Hormones (The Chemical Messengers)

Steroid hormones are lipids derived from cholesterols through a series of biochemical reactions. These steroids include the male sex hormones androgens and the female sex hormones estrogens. Testosterone and estradiol, which are similar in structure (Figure 19.3), are the principal member of the androgens and of the estrogens, respectively. These hormones are secreted by the gonads, adrenal cortex, and placenta. Other examples of the steroid group are androstenedione, corticosterone, glucocorticoid, and progesterone. Defects along the series of biochemical reactions often lead to hormonal imbalances with serious consequence. Once synthesized, steroid hormones are released into the bloodstream and not stored by cells.

Most hormones are *peptides* which are secreted largely by the pituitary, parathyroids, heart, stomach, liver, and kidneys. These hormones, such as insulin (Figure 19.3), are synthesized as precursor molecules and processed by the cell's endoplasmic reticulum and Golgi (Figure 9. 1) where they are stored in secretory granules. When needed, these granules are released into the blood. Different hormones can often be produced from the same precursor molecule by cleaving it with a different enzyme.

Amine hormones are derived from single amino acids, such as tyrosine and tryptophan. While secreted primarily by the thyroid and adrenal medulla, they are stored mostly as

Steroid Hormones

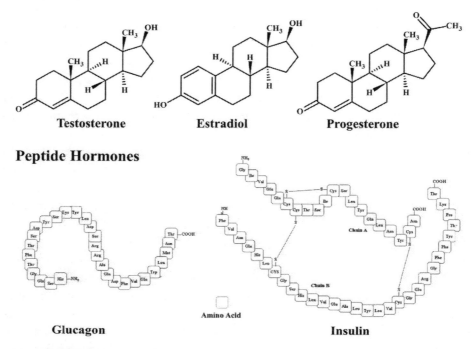

Testosterone   **Estradiol**   **Progesterone**

Peptide Hormones

Glucagon   **Insulin**

Amine Hormones

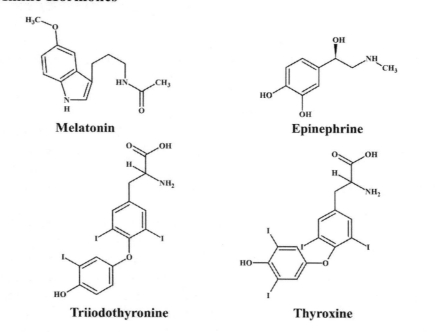

Melatonin   **Epinephrine**

Triiodothyronine   **Thyroxine**

Figure 19.3. Chemical Structures of Nine Select Hormones Found in the Human Body

granules in the cytoplasm until when needed. The notable amines included in Figure 19.3 are melatonin, thyroxine, triiodothyronine, epinephrine, and norepinephrine. Except for melatonin produced from tryptophan, the other four amines are derived from tyrosine.

19.3. Endocrine/Hormonal Disruption

In practice, the environmental health concern on endocrine disruption comes down to two pivotal points, with both revolving around its effect potential: (1) low threshold effects with ubiquitous exposure; and (2) a wide variety of persistent health effects. People are exposed to a vast number of EDCs found in many of the everyday products that they consume. Even at low doses, exposure to these chemicals can result in the disruption of the body's delicate hormonal functions leading to a wide array of untoward health outcomes. This is not an overstatement considering that even a very small alteration in hormone levels can trigger the body's endocrinal response.

There is evidence, for example, that a single low oral prepubertal exposure to the AhR (aryl hydrocarbon receptor) agonist 2,3,7,8-TCDD was sufficient to hasten a rat's reproductive senescence (Franczak *et al.*, 2006). Studies have also demonstrated that a single dose of an estrogen is sufficient to cause persistent activation of this hormone's receptors (Mackay and Lazier, 1993; Pakdel *et al.*, 1991), which can act as DNA-binding transcription factors to affect gene expression. And estrogenic chemicals such as DES have been shown able to cause carcinogenic effects that can persist into the daughter's cells to manifest only after puberty. Furthermore, as alluded to in earlier sections, the health outcomes of endocrine disruption are not limited to the numerous types of developmental-reproductive disorders discussed earlier. They include disorders involving the nervous or immunological system, the gut, the liver, the kidneys, and more, since the endocrine system also works closely with these other body organs and systems.

19.3.1. Modes of Endocrine Disruption

In toxicology, endocrine disruption may be treated as a mode of biochemical action which, when sufficient, can lead to one or more adverse health effects. In other words, endocrine disruption is not necessarily an immediate functional toxicological endpoint. There are broadly two different types of adverse endocrine disruption, each of which involves broadly two different modes of action. One type of disruption is, directly or indirectly, on the structure or the function of endocrine glands and the target cells. The other type is, directly or indirectly, on the metabolism or the function of hormones that the glands produce. In both types, the disruption can lead to either activation or inhibition of the natural hormone's normal functions. Collectively, the four modes of endocrine disruption can cause: (1) the damage to or modification of the endocrine network including the target receptors; and (2) the damage to or binding of the natural hormones.

The endocrine gland as a target organ can be impaired directly via certain toxicological actions. Alternatively, such impairment can be a secondary adverse response due to reactions or actions occurring elsewhere inside or outside of the endocrine axis. In this sense, endocrine toxicity and endocrine disruption may be regarded as two loosely interchangeable terms. Even with an endocrine gland being a toxicological target, the primary concern is still the secretion of improper amounts of hormones.

Agents that have been found to cause primary endocrine toxicity include nicotine on the adrenal, nitrogen mustards on the ovary, and estrogens on the pituitary. An example of a secondary endocrine toxicity is the development of castration cells in the pituitary as a result of direct or primary testicular toxicity (Harvey *et al.*, 1999). As another example, the DES has been banned for use by pregnant women since 1971 largely due to its carcinogenicity to the ovary of the offspring.

The biosynthesis of hormones can be impaired by the ability of an EDC to inhibit a specific enzymatic reaction during the production process, or by the intruder's ability to regulate at the DNA transcription or translation stage. The antisteroid drug aminoglutethimide, the antifungal drug ketoconazole, and the sex pheromone cyanoketone are three of the handful of chemicals found to have an inhibitory effect on the biosynthesis of steroid hormones (U.S. EPA, 1997). Overall, the EDCs collectively can exert their disruption on a natural hormone's functions in various ways. For example, some of these xenobiotics have the potential to mimic natural hormones in the body and thereby can bind to the receptors intended for the natural hormones. When the receptors mistreat the mimicker as the natural hormone, they respond as they would to the natural hormone.

In mimicking the natural hormones, some EDCs can act as inhibitors by reducing the number of target receptors, whereas some others can cause the body into over-responding to the stimulus when more receptors are activated. Still some others, such as the pesticides lindane and atrazine, can affect the metabolic pathway of certain sex steroid hormones (e.g., estradiol, testosterone, progesterone). There are also other foreign chemicals that can activate enzymes to speed up the metabolism of some hormones. For example, the testes contain enzymes specific for metabolizing estrogens (Toppari, *et al.*, 1996). These enzymes break down estrogens rapidly to a form that can no longer bind to the receptors. Either way, the metabolism and actions of some hormones can be modified by certain exogenous substances. Such a disruption can cause the natural hormone not able to bind to the target receptors at the right moment or in the proper manner.

In essence, the modes of endocrine or hormonal disruption include primarily the following: (1) binding of antagonistic and agonistic receptors; and (2) exertion of adverse effects on the biosynthesis, release, transport, storage, and clearance of natural hormones (e.g., Kavlock, *et al.*, 1996). In all cases, hormonal functions can be altered; and when the alteration is severe, some serious or even fatal health effects can result. One key mechanism of toxic action involved in endocrine disruption is the disruption of receptor functions, as discussed in some detail in this chapter and in general terms in Chapter 9.

19.3.2. Types of Endocrine Disruptors

Despite the fact that a host of chemicals are considered to have endocrine-disrupting potential, to this date there is still no global consensus on a list officially accepted as EDCs. The European Commission (2000) and U.S. EPA (2009) have published, however, their own priority list of suspected EDCs for further investigation. Some of the chemicals included in one list also appeared on the other. Many of the commonly considered EDCs are also given online by the *OurStolenFuture.org*, a website reportedly tracks the most recent scientific development in endocrine disruption.

The conception that some xenobiotics can mimic certain natural hormones is not new. The estrogenic effect of some DDT analogues was described in the ovariectomized rat by Fisher *et al.* (1952) over 50 years ago, and later confirmed by Bitman *et al.* (1968) specifically for the *o,p'*-DDT isomer. By the 1990s, two studies (Høyer *et al.*, 1998; Hunter *et al.*, 1997) were conducted to investigate the estrogenic potential of several organochlorines (e.g., DDT, DDE, PCBs, dieldrin) in breast cancer patients, as by then lifetime exposure to estrogens was already a well-known risk factor for breast cancer.

There are at least three conventional ways to categorize the EDCs considered to this date. In some documents, they are grouped according to their effects confined to a specific endocrine gland, such as regarding them as androgenic, estrogenic, or thyroidal. In some other documents, these environmental toxicants are classified according to their general use or physicochemical properties, such as putting them into the pesticide or metal group. Still in some others, they are referenced according to their specific mode of disruption, such as citing them and their actions as agonistic, antagonistic, or indirect. Considering that none of the above categorization schemes is completely effectual on its own, the select EDCs in Table 19.1 are listed by using all three schemes.

19.4. Developmental-Reproductive Effects in Humans

Reproductive toxicants are any agents that impair the reproductive capabilities in an individual or a population. As a special group being treated on their own, teratogens interfere with proper growth or health of the fetus, acting at any point from conception to birth. Agents that impair the normal growth of a child from birth to puberty are referred to commonly, if not specifically, as developmental toxicants. Some of these agents can have a beneficial effect on other occasions, such as aspirin, dental X-ray, and vitamin A. The best defense against these toxicants is therefore knowing when to avoid what. As noted earlier, not all developmental-reproductive effects are caused by endocrine disruption. Such effects from other causes can be equally or at times even more devastating. Accordingly, they are further discussed in a broader context in this section.

The sources of exposure to reproductive toxicants are broad and vary depending on the agent and the setting involved. Harmful exposures to reproductive toxicants can come from consumption of contaminated foods and water, as well as from being around workplaces and other areas where the air is contaminated. Of particular importance to newborns and infants is that they can be exposed in the womb or via breast milk. Paternal or maternal exposure prior to conception or during pregnancy can lead to adverse effects

Table 19.1. Select Common (Suspected) Endocrine Disrupting Chemicals and Their (Suspected) Endocrinal Effects[a]

Endocrine Disruptor	Endocrinal Effect[b]	Endocrine Disruptor	Endocrinal Effect[b]
Food Additives		Nonylphenol	Estrogenic
4-Hexyl resorcinol	Estrogenic	Perfluorooctane sulfonate (PFOS)	Reproductive/thyroidal
Butylated hydroxyanisole (BHA)	Estrogenic	*Pesticides*	
Propyl gallate	Estrogenic	Alachlor	Thyroidal
Metals		Aldicarb	Reproductive
Arsenic	Glucocorticoid	Aldrin, dieldrin	Estrogenic
Cadmium	Estrogenic	Atrazine	Pituitary/testosterone
Lead	Reproductive	Carbaryl	Estrogenic/progesterone
Mercury	Reproductive/thyroidal	Chlordane	Testosterone/progesterone
Persistent Organics		Cypermethrin	Reproductive
Benzene hexachloride (BHC)	Thyroidal	DDTs (dichlorodiphenyltrichloroethane)	Estrogenic/androgenic
Dioxins and furans	Reproductive	Dicofol	Estrogenic
Hydroxylated-PCBs (OH-PCBs)	Estrogenic	Endosulfan	Estrogenic
Polybrominated biphenyls (PBBs)	Estrogenic/thyroidal	Ethylene thiourea	Estrogenic
Polybrominated diphenyl ethers	Thyroidal	Heptachlor, heptachlor-epoxide	Thyroidal/reproductive
Polychlorinated biphenyls (PCBs)	Estrogenic/androgenic/thyroidal	Iprodione	Androgenic (testosterone)
Phthalates		Kepone (chlordecone)	Estrogenic
Butyl benzyl phthalate (BBP)	Estrogenic	Lindane (γ-hexachlorocyclohexane)	Estrogenic/androgenic
di-*n*-Butyl phthalate (DBP)	Estrogenic/androgenic	Malathion	Thyroidal
di-Ethylhexyl phthalate (DEHP)	Estrogenic/androgenic	Methoxychlor	Estrogenic
Diethyl phthalate (DEP)	Estrogenic	Mirex	Antiandrogenic/thyroidal
Other (Organic) Substances		Permethrin	Estrogenic
Bisphenol A	Estrogenic	Toxaphene	Estrogenic/thyroidal
Benzo[α]pyrene	Androgenic	Tributyltin	Reproductive
Isoflavones	Estrogenic	Vinclozolin	Androgenic

[a] as *suspected* or *considered* by U.S. EPA (2009), European Commission (2000), or *http://www.ourstolenfuture.org*, except for propyl gallate (Amadasi *et al.*, 2009) and 4-hexyl resorcinol (Amadasi *et al.*, 2009); the notion of commonness is largely based on their mention in the literature or in this book.

[b] glucocorticoid (i.e., a steroid hormone) may cause alteration of gene expression; reproductive effects include reduced sperm count, infertility, ovarian cyst, erectile dysfunction, or other related outcomes.

on the offspring. Overall, these various exposure sources collectively can lead to a wide range of reproductive and developmental effects from minor to life threatening. The more serious or fatal effects include fetal death, congenital abnormalities, infertility, and damage to reproductive structures. Naturally, these reproductive and developmental toxicities can be seriously affected by such critical factors as amount of exposure, timing of exposure, and sex of exposed individual.

19.4.1. Birth Defects and Environmental Teratogens

Several thousands of different kinds of birth defects have been identified or suspected (Weinhold, 2009). Of these, 45 are considered by the U.S. Centers for Disease Control and Prevention (CDC, 2006) as responsible for causing about 3% of the some 4 million babies born in the United States each year with major structural birth defects. Out of the 45 major types, CDC selected 18 that the agency considered as having greater public health concerns and thereby placed for further prevalence surveillance during the three study years from 1999 through 2001. Table 19.2 is a summary of CDC's findings on the nation's average annual prevalence (i.e., average annual number of total *existing* cases in the nation) for each of the 18 select major types of *structural* birth defects .

Table 19.2 shows that for the three years (1999-2001) under study, the most common subgroup of major structural defects at birth was chromosomal defects which affected about 6,900 newborns in each of the three years. In that subgroup, the most predominant structural defect found was Down syndrome, a condition involving some degree of mental retardation and affecting approximately 5,500 newborns in each of the three years. The subgroup with the second highest prevalence was orofacial defects, which consisted of predominately cleft palate and cleft lip and together affected about 6,800 newborns annually during those three years. Cleft palate and cleft lip are defects involving the improper formation of the lip and the mouth roof, respectively. Others among the most common subgroups of birth defects found in the three years included cardiovascular defects, musculoskeletal defects, and gastrointestinal defects.

Metabolic birth defects as a group are equally common, affecting roughly 1 in 4,000 newborns in the United States (Heese and Zori, 2009; March of Dimes, 2002), with each involving typically a missing or an improperly formed enzyme. Although most affected children show no visible abnormalities, some can suffer from a life-threatening metabolic disorder, such as the genetic conditions Tay-Sachs disease (TSD) and phenylketonuria (PKU). Newborns with TSD are without the enzyme hexosaminidase A which is responsible for the degradation of gangliosides (i.e., a subtype of glycolipids). As the fatty gangliosides accumulate in the brain, they affect the baby's sight, hearing, movement, and mental development. Babies born with PKU cannot metabolize the essential amino acid phenylalanine present in most foods. Without special diet treatment, phenylalanine will build up in the bloodstream to cause brain damage and mental retardation. All states and territories in the United States now screen for PKU in babies because if this metabolic disorder is detected early, it can be prevented by feeding the child a special diet.

Table 19.2. Average Annual National Prevalence of 18 Select Major Structural
Birth Defects in the United States, 1999-2001

Birth Defect	National Estimates[a,b]	
	Prevalence Rate	Annual Cases
Eye Defects	*2.08*	*834*
Anophthalmia or microphthalmia	2.08	834
Cardiovascular Defects	*16.25*	*6,527*
Truncus arteriosus (a.k.a. common truncus)	0.82	329
Transposition of great arteries	4.73	1,901
Tetralogy of Fallot	3.92	1,574
Atrioventricular septal defect	4.35	1,748
Hypoplastic left heart syndrome	2.43	975
Orofacial Defects	*16.87*	*6,776*
Cleft palate without cleft lip	6.39	2,567
Cleft lip with or without cleft palate	10.48	4,209
Gastrointestinal Defects	*7.18*	*2,883*
Esophageal atresia/tracheosophageal fistula	2.37	952
Rectal and large intestinal atresia or stenosis	4.81	1,931
Musculoskeletal defects	*14.45*	*5,799*
Reduction defect, upper limbs	3.79	1,521
Reduction defect, lower limbs	1.90	763
Gastroschisis	3.73	1,497
Omphalocele	2.09	839
Diaphragmatic hernia	2.94	1,179
Chromosomal Defects	*17.39*	*6,916*
Down syndrome (trisomy 21)	13.65	5,429
Trisomy 13	1.33	528
Trisomy 18	2.41	959

[a]per 10,000 live births; adapted from Table 1 in the mortality and morbidity weekly report (*MMWR*) issued by the U.S. Centers for Disease Control and Prevention (CDC, 2006).

[b]projected by CDC from the average annual prevalence rates estimated from 11 states (Alabama, Arkansas, California, Georgia, Hawaii, Iowa, Massachusetts, North Carolina, Oklahoma, Texas, Utah); adjusted for either maternal age (for chromosomal defects) or race-specific distribution (for all other birth defects) of live births in the United States during 1999-2001.

A wide variety of genetic disorders and environmental agents can cause birth defects in humans. Listed in Table 19.3 are the more specific teratogenic effects caused by some of the more prominent agents or genetic disorders, including those noted in this chapter (e.g., DES, PKU) and elsewhere in this book (e.g., methylmercury). As reflected in Table 19.3, one common birth defect shared by several of the agents and disorders listed is microcephaly, a condition in which the head or cranial capacity is abnormally small.

Table 19.3. Teratogenic Effects of Select Agents or Causes in Humans[a]

Agent/Cause	Birth Effect(s)
Alcohol	Microcephaly (abnormally small head); mental retardation
Androgen	Masculinization of external female genitalia
Cocaine	Pregnancy loss; microcephaly; neurobehavioral abnormalities
Diethylstilbestrol (DES)	*At birth*: abnormal enlargement of the clitoris in female newborns; *years later*: adenocarcinoma of the cervix/vagina of female offspring; *in general*: structural or functional disorders of the genital organs of male offspring
Diphenylhydantoin	Microcephaly; cleft palate (abnormal development of the mouth's roof); mental retardation
Lithium	Ebstein anomaly (malformation of the heart)
Metabolic imbalance *(folic acid deficiency, phenylketonuria)*	Spina bifida (incomplete development of the spinal cord or its coverings); anencephaly (abnormal formation of the brain and the skull bones); mental retardation
Methylmercury	Cerebral palsy; microcephaly; blindness; cerebellar hypoplasia (underdevelopment of the cerebellum)
Radiation	Embryonic death; leukemia; microcephaly; skeletal and genital anomalies
Retinoid *(including vitamin A)*	Malformations of brain, ears, and eyes; heart defects; mental retardation
Syphilis	Abnormal teeth and bones, mental retardation
Thalidomide	Phocomelia (reduced or absent limbs)
Trimethadione	Developmental retardation, dysmorphic facial features
Valproic acid	Spina bifida

[a]largely from those listed by OEHHA (2010).

19.4.2. Reproductive Effects and Environmental Toxicants

Examples of environmental reproductive toxicants, along with their more prominent effects, are listed in Table 19.4. Some of these agents affect specifically spermatogenesis or cause testicular atrophy in males, whereas some others damage specifically the oocytes in females. In both cases, many of their effects involve impairment of the reproductive functions and are mediated via activities of the endocrine or the nervous system.

Table 19.4. Select Environmental Reproductive Toxicants of Concern to Humans[a]

Toxicant(s)	Reproductive Effect(s)	Common Source(s) or Site(s) of Exposure
Benzo[α]pyrene	Damage to the oocytes	Charcoaled meat; tobacco smoke
Cadmium	Cause of prostate cancer	Omnipresent (a widely used metal)
Carbon Disulfide	Impotence; abnormal sperm morphology and count	Viscose rayon; fumigant; chemical production
DBCP (1,2 dibromo-3-chloropropane)	Infertility due to azoospermia and oligospermia	Pesticide application
DDT (dichlorodiphenyltrichloroethane)	Affecting the development of conceptus	Pesticide application
Ethylene oxide	Chromosome aberrations; spontaneous abortions	Health care products; food sterilization; industrial use
Glycol ethers	Spermatogenic	Omnipresent (widely used solvents)
Kepone (chlordecone)	Decreased libido; decreased sperm count, motility, and morphology	Pesticide application
Lead and lead compounds	Decreased sperm count and motility; menstrual disorders; spontaneous abortions; increased neonatal mortality	Smelting; battery; lead-based paint
Methoxychlor	Increase weight of the uterus	Pesticide application
Methylmethane sulfonate	Affecting spermatids and spermatozoa	Used widely as a research chemical and for cancer treatment
Nicotine	Affecting the development of conceptus	Cigarette smoke
Nitrogen mustards	Damage to the oocytes	As chemotherapeutic drugs
Oil Yellow AB	Testicular atrophy	As a food colorant
PCBs (polychlorinated biphenyls)	Menstrual disorders; stillbirth; low birth weight; malformations	Capacitors in telephone and electrical equipment
Vinyl chloride	Chromosome aberration; miscarriage; sperm abnormalities; stillbirth	During manufacturing and processing of polyvinyl chloride

[a]largely from those listed by OEHHA (2010).

As noted in Section 19.1.2, besides infertility, the two most common reproductive disorders found in the United States (and many other countries) are ED (erectile dysfunction) and ovarian cysts. Ovarian cysts are sacs filled with fluid on or inside the ovaries and are very common in women of childbearing age (ACOG, 2009). These cysts can rupture, resulting in significant symptoms including menstrual irregularities and pelvic pain. Fortunately or not, statistics show that many women tend to experience little or no pain or discomfort from ovarian cysts that they have in their lifetime.

The most common type of ovarian cysts is functional cysts which usually form during the menstrual cycle and consist of two kinds from two different causes: (1) follicle cysts and (2) corpus luteum cysts. Follicle cysts form when the follicle holding the egg fails to break open, as caused by the pituitary gland not releasing LH (enough) to signal the release of the egg. Corpus luteum is what is left of the follicle after the latter has ruptured to release the egg. At times, the opening of the short-lived corpus luteum is sealed off and the fluid then builds up in the sac to form a cyst. Otherwise, a healthy corpus luteum would produce the hormone progesterone which makes the lining of the uterus thick enough for implantation to ensure a healthy pregnancy.

For men, the most common reproductive disorder is ED, also known as impotence. This disorder is characterized by an inability to get an erection or sustain it long enough for sexual intercourse. In the United States, as many as 30 million men were estimated to have ED (NIH, 1993). ED can be brought about by interruption in the processes responsible for generating an erection. The causes underlying this type of interruption include the following: psychological factors such as stress, guilt, and depression; disruptions in neural activity; diseases (e.g., diabetes, alcoholism, hypertension); smoking; and exposure to toxicants that cause damage to the nerves, arteries, and other related tissues. Some of these agents or factors can reduce the health or the number of sperm cells.

Many environmental agents can exert their adverse effects on either the reproductive functions or the reproductive system of either sex. Examples of reproductive functional disorders include: ED; hypogonadism (a condition impairing the functional activity of the gonad which produces the sex hormone testosterone in males and estradiol in females); ectopic pregnancy (a condition in which a fertilized ovum is implanted on tissues other than the uterine wall); low sexual desire; and premature ejaculation.

The reproductive system of either sex *per se* can be impaired by a vast number of environmental agents. Each genital system represents a network of organs that are supposed to work together to effect reproduction. The primary (direct) function of the human male reproductive system is to provide the sperm for fertilization of a female's ovum. This male reproductive system consists of several organs located largely outside of his body around his pelvic region. His principal reproductive organs include: the testes which are housed inside the scrotum and produce sperms; the epididymis (a narrow, tightly coiled tube connecting the efferent ducts from each testicle to its vas deferens); the seminal vesicles; the prostate gland; the vas deferens which produce the ejaculatory fluid; and the penis with the urethra for copulation and deposition of the sperms.

The human female reproductive system is likewise a network of genital organs located around a female's pelvic region but primarily inside her body. The following are the principal reproductive organs found in a female's body: the vagina (a tubular tract serving as the receptacle for the sperm); the uterus (which holds the developing fetus); and the ovaries (which produce the ova). The two breasts are generally regarded as reproductive organs during the nursing stage of reproduction.

References

ACOG (American College of Obstetricians and Gynecologists), 2009. Patient Education Pamphlet AP075 – Ovarian Cysts. ACOG, 409 12th Street, SW, P.O. Box 96920, Washington, DC, USA.

Amadasi A, Mozzarelli A, Meda C, Maggi A, Cozzini P, 2009. Identification of Xenoestrogens in Food Additives by an Integrated *in silico* and *in vitro* approach. *Chem. Res. Toxicol.* 22:52-63.

APA (American Pregnancy Association), 2013. Fertility FAQ. http://americanpregnancy.org/infertility/fertilityfaq.html.

Bitman J, Cecil HC, Harris SO, Fries GF, 1968. Estrogenic Activity of o,p'-DDT in the Mammalian Uterus and Avian Oviduct. *Science* 162:371-372.

CDC (U.S. Centers for Disease Control and Prevention), 2006. Improved National Prevalence Estimates for 18 Selected Major Birth Defects – United States, 1999-2001. *MMWR* 54:1301-1305.

CDC (U.S. Centers for Disease Control and Prevention), 2008. Update on Overall Prevalence of Major Birth Defects – Atlanta, Georgia, 1978-2005. *MMWR* 57:1-5.

CDC (U.S. Centers for Disease Control and Prevention), 2013. Infertility. http://www.cdc.gov/nchs/fastats/fertile.htm.

Christianson A, Howson CP, Modell B, 2006. The March of Dimes Global Report on Birth Defects: The Hidden Toll of Dying and Disabled Children. March of Dimes Birth Defects Foundation, White Plains, New York, USA.

Colborn T, Clement C (Eds.), 1992. Chemically Induced Alterations in Sexual and Functional Development: The Wildlife/Human Connection. Princeton, New Jersey, USA: Princeton Scientific Publishing.

Colborn T, Dumanoski D, Peterson J, 1996. *Our Stolen Future: Are We Threatening Our Fertility, Intelligence, and Survival? A Scientific Detective Story.* New York, New York, USA: Penguin Books.

Diamanti-Kandarakis E, Bourguignon J-P, Giudice LC, Hauser R, Prins GS, Soto AM, Zoeller RT, Gore AC, 2009. Endocrine-Disrupting Chemicals: An Endocrine Society Scientific Statement. *Endocrine Rev.* 30:293-342.

European Commission (Environment DG, B-1049, Brussels, Belgium), 2000. Towards the Establishment of a Priority List of Substances for Further Evaluation of Their Role in Endocrine Disruption. Project M0355008/1786Q/10/11/00, prepared by BKH Consulting Engineers, P.O. Box 5094, 2600 GB Delft, The Netherlands.

Fisher AL, Keasling HH, Schueler FW, 1952. Estrogenic Action of Some DDT Analogues. *Proc. Soc. Exp. Biol. Med.* 81:439-441.

Franczak A, Nynca A, Valdez KE, Mizinga KM, Petroff BK, 2006. Effects of Acute and Chronic Exposure to the Aryl Hydrocarbon Receptor Agonist 2,3,7,8-Tetrachlorodibenzo-p-Dioxin on the Transition to Reproductive Senescence in Female Sprague-Dawley Rats. *Biol. Reprod.* 74: 125-130.

Harvey PW, Rush KC, Cockburn A, 1999. Endocrine and Hormonal Toxicology: An Integrated Mechanistic and Target Systems Approach. In *Endocrine and Hormonal Toxicology* (Harvey PW, Rush KC, Cockburn A, Eds.). New York, New York, USA: John Wiley & Sons, Chapter 1.

Heese BA, Zori RT, 2009. Molecular Biology: Genomics and Proteonomics. In *Civetta, Taylor, & Kirby's Critical Care* (Gabrielli A, Layon AJ, Yu M, Eds.), Fourth Edition. Philadelphia, Pennsylvania, USA: Lippincott Williams & Wilkins, Chapter 51.

Høyer AP, Grandjean P, Jørgensen T, Brock JW, Hartvig HB, 1998. Organochlorine Exposure and Risk of Breast Cancer. *Lancet* 352:1816-1820.

Hunter DJ, Hankinson SE, Laden F, Colditz GA, Manson JE, Willett WC, Speizer FE, Wolff MS, 1997. Plasma Organochlorine Levels and the Risk of Breast Cancer. *NEJM* 337:1253-1258.

Kavlock RJ, Daston GP, DeRosa C, Fenner-Crisp P, Gray LE, Kaattari S, Lucier G, Luster M, Mac MJ, Maczka C, Miller R, Moore J, Rolland R, Scott G, Sheehan DM, Sinks T, Tilson HA, 1996. Research Needs for the Risk Assessment of Health and Environmental Effects of Endocrine Disruptors: A Report of the U.S. EPA-Sponsored Workshop. *Environ. Health Perspect.* 104:715-740.

Mackay ME, Lazier CB, 1993. Estrogen Responsiveness of Vitellogenin Gene Expression in Rainbow Trout (*Oncorhynchus mykiss*) Kept at Different Temperatures. *Gen. Comp. Endocrinol.* 89:255-266.

March of Dimes, 2002. Birth Defects: Strategies for Prevention and Ensuring Quality of Life. Testimony Given on 26 July (by Dr. Nancy Green, Medical Director of the March of Dimes Birth Defects Foundation) before the Subcommittee on Children and Families, U.S. Senate Health, Education, Labor and Pensions Committee (U.S. Senate Hearing 107-592).

Mathews TJ, MacDorman MF, 2008. Infant Mortality Statistics from the 2005 Period Linked Birth/Infant Death Data Set. *Natl. Vital Statistics Reports* 57(2 July 30):1-32.

NIH (U.S. National Institutes of Health), 1993. Consensus Conference. NIH Consensus Development Panel on Impotence. Impotence. *JAMA* 270:83-90.

OEHHA (California Office of Environmental Health Hazard Assessment), 2010. Chemicals Known to the State to Cause Cancer or Reproductive Toxicity – 8 October 2010. California Environmental Protection Agency, Sacramento, California, USA.

Pakdel F, Féon S, Le Gac F, Le Menn F, Valotaire Y, 1991. *In vivo* Induction of Hepatic Estrogen Receptor mRNA and Correlation with Vitellogenin mRNA in Rainbow Trout. *Mol. Cell. Endocrinol.* 75:205-212.

Russo CA, Elixhauser A, 2007. Hospitalizations for Birth Defects, 2004. Statistical Brief #24. U.S. Agency for Healthcare Research and Quality, Rockville, Maryland, USA.

Toppari J, Larsen JC, Christiansen P, Giwercman A, Grandjean P, Guillette LJ Jr, Jégou B, Jensen TK, Jouannet P, Keiding N, Leffers H, McLachlan JA, Meyer O, Müller J, Rajpert-DeMeyts E, Scheike T, Sharpe R, Sumpter J, Skakkebaek NE, 1996. Male Reproductive Health and Environmental Xenoestrogens. *Environ. Health Perspect.* 104 (Suppl 4):741-803.

U.S. EPA (U.S. Environmental Protection Agency), 1997. Special Report on Environmental Endocrine Disruption: An Effects Assessment and Analysis. EPA/630/R-96/012. Risk Assessment Forum, Washington DC, USA.

U.S. EPA (U.S. Environmental Protection Agency), 2009. Final List of Initial Pesticide Active Ingredients and Pesticide Inert Ingredients to Be Screened under the Federal Food, Drug, and Cosmetic Act. *Federal Register* 74:17579-17585.

Vandenberg LN, Maffini MV, Sonnenschein C, Rubin BS, Soto AM, 2009. Bisphenol A and the Great Divide: A Review of Controversies in the Field of Endocrine Disruption. *Endocrine Rev.* 30:75-95.

Weinhold B, 2009. Environmental Factors in Birth Defects. *Environ. Health Perspect.* 117:A440-A447.

Review Questions

1. Briefly explain why thyroid is an important component of the human endocrine system.

2. What are endocrine-disrupting chemicals (EDCs)?

3. Each year about _____ babies are estimated to be born with birth defects worldwide *and* die before age 5: a) 1,000,000; b) 2,000,000; c) 3,000,000; d) 4,000,000.

4. List some of the major environmental causes of congenital abnormalities.

5. Approximately how many American couples are affected by infertility?

6. How was the use of diethylstilbestrol (DES) relevant to the concept of endocrine disruption?

7. What are the main differences between the functions of the nervous system and those of the endocrine system (in humans)?

8. Briefly describe the terms *gametogenesis*, *spermatogenesis*, and *oogenesis*.

9. In addition to infertility, what are the most common reproductive disorders occurring in the United States (and many other countries)?

10. Which of the following phases (i.e., substages) in the embryonic stage is most susceptible to the structural effects of teratogens? a) cell proliferation; b) cell differentiation; c) cell migration; d) organogenesis.

11. Which of the following is stimulated by nerves from the eyes to secrete a hormone responsible for the so-called seasonal affective disorder syndrome (SADS)? a) thyroid gland; b) hypothalamus; c) adrenal gland; d) pineal gland.

12. Which of the following regulates or influences the release of the hormones *thyroxine* and *triiodothyronine*? a) thyroid gland; b) pituitary gland; c) parathyroid; d) hypothalamus.

13. What are hormones, and what are their three main groups as classified by chemical structure?

14. Why is it important not to overlook the exposure of EDCs even at (very) low levels?

15. Briefly describe the two different types of adverse endocrine disruption in terms of biochemical action.

16. Briefly characterize the basic modes of endocrine disruption.

17. Name two common EDCs whose endocrinal effects are thyroidal and estrogenic.

18. Name the three chromosomal defects collectively having one of the highest, if not the highest, average annual national prevalence rates of congenital abnormalities in the United States.

19. What are functional cysts, as experienced by many women in their lifetime?

20. What would happen to the health of newborns with TSD (Tay-Sachs disease), or those with PKU (phenylketonuria)?

21. Which of the following is the common birth defect that several known teratogenic agents can (individually) cause? a) spina bifida; b) microcephaly; c) skeletal anomalies; d) cleft palate.

22. Give an example of a fumigant or pesticide that can cause or lead to: (a) impotence; (b) a decrease in the development of conceptus; (c) a decrease in libido *and* sperm count.

CHAPTER 20

Occupational Toxicology/Industrial Chemicals

20.1. Introduction

Occupational diseases are those resulting from work-related exposures, such as from exposures to certain metals, fibers, dusts, pesticides, and chemical solvents released during industrial processes. Diseases in this group have gained public attention since the late 18th or the early 19th century, when the Industrial Revolution Period started involving many large-scale dramatic innovations in agriculture, manufacturing, and transportation in Britain. Diseases linked to this type of exposures continue to be of great significance to this date, inasmuch as voluminous metals, inorganic compounds, and complex organic mixtures are still being utilized in industry today. It is interesting to know, however, that a few of the widely known classic occupational diseases did not occur in an industrial setting. For instance, epithelioma of the scrotum (a form of cancer located in the skin of the scrotum) was first recognized back in 1775, by a London physician named Percival Pott, as a frequent occupational hazard peculiar to chimney sweeps.

It is also important to realize that outbreaks of many infectious diseases also occur frequently in workplaces, such as the classic case with the 1976 episode of legionellosis (a.k.a. Legionnaire's disease) caused by the bacterium *Legionella pneumophila*. That episode took place in an American hotel conference held in Philadelphia, Pennsylvania being the workplace, where the source of the bacteria was never confirmed but suspected to be through the water supply or air conditioning system at the hotel.

20.1.1. Classic Industrial Diseases

Historically, lead (Pb), white phosphorus (P), and fine dust particles of silica (SiO_2) were among the handful of toxicants contributing to the classic industrial diseases that first received public attention during the Industrial Revolution Period (Cheremisinoff, 2001). Silicosis is a serious form of the restrictive lung disease known as pneumoconiosis that results from chronic exposure to silica dust particles. It was commonly observed among miners working in Britain in the 19th century. Also frequently reported around that time were cases of painful phossy jaw (i.e., exposed bone necrosis exclusively in the jaws) seen among workers exposed to white phosphorus used to manufacture matches. A third classic is potter's disease, that involving neurological disorders experienced by potters working with lead glazes in the ceramic industry. Actually, lead poisonings were observed in British miners long before 1800 (Carter, 2004). In some literature, silicosis is also known as potter's rot or potter's disease among workers in the pottery industry.

20.1.2. Uniqueness of Occupational Toxicology

Occupational toxicology, that with the objective to prevent and control occupational diseases in an effort to maintain occupational health, is unique from other subdivisions of environmental toxicology in having its focus on two distinct principles: (1) the special need for exposure limits; and (2) the reliance on workplace or worker monitoring. Industrial workplaces are engaged in the production, processing, transport, or utilization of a variety of harmful substances (e.g., pesticides, paints, metals, solvents) that people in a modern society economically cannot afford to eliminate. Therefore, it becomes more practical for such places to protect the health and safety of their workers by assessing and setting safe legal standards of occupational exposure. To ensure that the employers comply with the limits of permissible exposure, it is thereby also necessary for the laws and regulations to find ways to monitor the workplace, the workers, or both at least periodically for the exposure potential in question.

20.1.3. Occupational Health Laws

In many countries, it was the public's concerns over occupational diseases that generally prompted the passage of legislations for worker health and safety. In the United States, contrary to general misconception, the first federal legislation for worker health and safety was not the Occupational Safety and Health Act (OSH Act) passed in 1970. Rather, it was the Federal Employers Liability Act (FELA) passed during the Progressive Era being (more or less) the first. In 1908, U.S. Congress passed the FELA to help railroad workers injured on the job. Two years later in further response to a series of highly publicized tragedies of mine explosions and collapses, U.S. Congress established the U.S. Bureau of Mines with its mission being to improve safety in mining through research and training (though with no authority to regulate mine safety). At around the same time, backed by labor unions, several states passed workers compensation laws in an effort to discourage employers from letting their employees to work in an unsafe place.

Then came the mid-1960s, a time when public awareness of the pollution impacts of many notorious chemicals was at its peak leading to a politically powerful environmental movement. To address these concerns, U.S. Congress eventually passed a comprehensive occupational health and safety bill that was signed into law on 29 December 1970 by then President Richard Nixon. That legislation is known as the now widely received OSH Act of 1970.

Over the years, similar occupational health laws have been enacted in many other countries. For instance, South Australia in 1986 passed its Occupational Health, Safety and Welfare Act to protect the health, safety, and welfare of its workers. In 1993, South Africa passed its Occupational Health and Safety Act to safeguard the health and safety of its workers in connection with the use of machinery and plants. A third example is China's Occupational Disease Control Act, which came into force in May 2002.

Yet perhaps with only a few exceptions, the European Union (EU) has set the most comprehensive and stringent occupational health and safety standards in the world. EU has adopted many of its occupational health and safety laws through a series of directives, including notably the framework directive (Directive 89/391/EEC) which was brought into effect by then the Council of European Communities. The framework directive has laid down the principles of occupational health and safety as a binding commitment for the EU members. Subsequent EU directives then offer the specifics for various relevant topics such as noise, pregnancy, and the use of chemicals in various work settings.

20.2. U.S. Legislation for Occupational Health

Laws and regulations for occupational health and safety vary considerably among provinces, states, nations, and regions. Yet their central themes are similar and consistent. They all have the ultimate goal of developing standards to protect workers against injuries and illnesses from occurring in a workplace. Laws and regulations of this type are being dealt with in a number of excellent publications (e.g., DOL, 2009; Kloss, 2005; Lewis and Thornbury, 2010). It is beyond this chapter's purview to address the complexities of this type of laws and their differences across jurisdictions. Due to space limitation, this section affords only a brief account of the U.S. OSH Act of 1970 and its two main establishments, with the aims to exemplify both the scope and the level of national as well as global concerns over occupational health and safety.

20.2.1. U.S. Occupational Safety and Health Act

In the United States, the OSH Act of 1970 is the principal federal law governing occupational health and safety primarily for the private sector. As noted earlier, the federal statute was enacted by U.S. Congress in 1970 and was signed into law by then President Richard Nixon on 29 December that year. The law's main focus is on ensuring that employers provide a working environment free from recognized hazards, including those associated with mechanical dangers, excessive noise levels, heat stress, exposure to toxic chemicals, and unsanitary conditions.

The OSH Act can be found in the *U.S. Code of Federal Regulations* (CFR) in Chapter 15, Title 29. It was passed to ensure safe and healthy working conditions primarily for American nongovernment workers, by authorizing enforcement of standards developed under the act, by assisting and encouraging the states in their own efforts to assure similar safe and healthy working conditions, and by providing for research, training, information, and education in occupational health and safety or related issues.

The act established not only the U.S. Occupational Safety and Health Administration (OSHA), which is an agency component of the U.S. Department of Labor, but also the highly regarded U.S. National Institute for Occupational Safety and Health (NIOSH). NIOSH is organized as an arm to the U.S. Centers for Disease Control and Prevention (CDC) within the U.S. Department of Health and Human Services.

Many Americans appear to be familiar with OSHA's main mission being to safeguard the nation's workers from occupational hazards and injuries by promulgating safety and health standards. Yet very few of them realize that it is NIOSH that carries out the research work to develop *"information on safe levels of exposure to toxic materials and harmful physical agents and substances."* Through the joint efforts of its several functional units, such as the Biomonitoring & Health Assessment Branch and the Chemical Exposure & Monitoring Branch, NIOSH provides the nation with some of the most relevant databases for occupational toxicology.

20.2.2. U.S. Occupational Safety and Health Administration

The federal OSHA's mission is to prevent work-related injuries, illnesses, and fatality by promulgating and enforcing standards for workplace health and safety. The agency is headed by a Deputy Assistant Secretary of Labor, with its responsibility covering workplaces in mostly the private sector.

The OSH Act of 1970 permits the states to develop their own plans as long as they cover public sector employees and provide protection equivalent to that provided under federal OSHA regulations. In return, a portion of the cost of the approved state program is paid for by the federal government. As of this date, 21 states and one territory (Puerto Rico) have been operating their own (state) plans which cover both the public and the private sector. In addition, there are four states and U.S. Virgin Islands that have been operating plans for public employees only. In this latter group of five, protection of worker health and safety in the private sector remains under the federal OSHA's jurisdiction. In the year 2000, the U.S. Postal Act made the U.S. Postal Service the only quasi-governmental entity to fall under the purview of OSHA jurisdiction.

OSHA helps employers and employees reduce injuries, illnesses, and deaths in the workplace by means of three strategies as well as directions: enforcement, assistance, and cooperation. More specifically, the agency operates under the policy and direction that its regulations be followed, that outreach and training to employers and employees be provided, and partnerships as well as alliances through voluntary programs be cooperated. Below are a few of the numerous regulatory milestones that OSHA has achieved over the years in proving health and safety protection for American workers:

- Permissible exposure limits (PELs) – promulgated for protecting workers against the health effects of exposure to hazardous agents. PELs are regulatory limits on an agent's concentration in the air or its amount in a physical environment. They cover several hundreds of agents; and most are based on standards recommended by other organizations (*see* Section 20.3.1).

- Personal protective equipment (PPE) requirements – requiring that employers conduct a hazard assessment of their workplace in order to provide the appropriate PPE to their employees. The additional PPE required typically includes one or more of the following: respirator, coveralls, and gloves when handling hazardous agents; otherwise, headgear, earplugs, and goggles are required in almost all industrial and construction areas.

♦ Right-to-know standard – developed under the principle that workers have a need as well as a right to know about the hazards occurring in the workplace.

♦ Bloodborne pathogens (BBP) standard – promulgated with the intent and effort to protect health care and other workers from exposure to potentially infectious materials present in the blood (e.g., in a hospital setting).

♦ Exposure to asbestos standard – issued for worker protection from exposure to asbestos in the general industry, including a PEL and provisions for medical examinations, for appropriate PPE/engineering controls, for exposure monitoring, for hygiene facilities and practices, and for recordkeeping.

20.2.3. U.S. National Institute for Occupational Safety and Health

While with its headquarters being situated in Washington DC, NIOSH has scattered tactfully its research laboratories and regional offices in several cities across the nation, including Denver (Colorado), Anchorage (Arkansas), Spokane (Washington), Pittsburgh (Pennsylvania), Cincinnati (Ohio), and Atlanta (Georgia). This federal institute is mainly a professional organization with a diverse staff of some 1,200 scientists from a variety of disciplines including epidemiology, medicine, industrial hygiene, chemistry, engineering, safety, and biostatistics. It was established under the OSH Act of 1970 to help ensure that American people have the right to a safe and healthy workplace by providing research, information, education, and training in or related to the field of occupational health and safety. Today, with these provisions, NIOSH has become both the national and the world leader in the prevention of work-related illness, injury, disability, and death.

NIOSH has three overarching goals as well as strategies: (1) to conduct research leading to the prevention or reduction of work-related illness and injury; (2) to promote safe and healthy work conditions through interventions, recommendations, and capacity development; and (3) to foster safe and healthy work conditions at the global level via international collaborations. These strategies are supported and guided by NIOSH's program portfolio which has organized the institute's efforts into ten Sector Programs representing the various available industrial sectors (e.g., construction, transportation, services, health care and social assistance, mining). Its program portfolio further subdivides these efforts into 24 cross sectors according to adverse health outcomes, statutory programs, and global collaborations (e.g., engineering control, exposure assessment, surveillance, nanotechnology, hearing loss prevention, respiratory diseases).

Unlike its partner OSHA (or to some people, its counterpart), NIOSH is not a regulatory agency as it does not promulgate any enforceable safety or health standard. Instead, under the OSH Act of 1970, NIOSH is authorized to: (1) *"develop recommendations for health and safety standards"*; (2) *"develop information on safe levels of exposure to toxic materials and harmful physical agents and substances"*; and (3) *"conduct research on new safety and health problems."* The federal institute may also *"conduct onsite investigations (e.g., Health Hazard Evaluations) to determine the toxicity of materials used in workplaces*", and "*fund research* (conducted) *by other agencies or private organizations through grants, contracts, and other arrangements.*"

In addition, pursuant to the authority by the Mine Safety and Health Act (MSH Act) of 1977, NIOSH may provide services pertaining to worker health and safety in mining as follows: (1) to administer a medical surveillance program for miners, including chest X-rays for detection of pneumoconiosis in coal miners; (2) to develop health standard recommendations for the Mine Safety and Health Administration (MSHA); (3) to conduct onsite inspections in mines similar to those authorized for the general industry under the OSH Act of 1970; and (4) to certify PPE and hazard-measurement instruments.

Throughout the years, NIOSH has made numerous accomplishments for occupational health and safety. Among the many, two are especially noteworthy. One of these is the *Pocket Guide to Chemical Hazards* and the other, *Criteria Documents*. Each *Criteria Document* generally contains a critical review of: (1) the available technical information and scientific data relevant to the prevalence of the hazards in a workplace; (2) the existence of the safety and health risks from the occupational exposure; and (3) the adequacy of analytical methods used to identify and control the workplace hazards.

The *Pocket Guide to Chemical Hazards* is designed as an abridged source of general industrial hygiene information for workers, employers, and occupational health professionals. It details key information and data in abbreviated tabular form for collectively over 650 individual chemicals and substance groups (e.g., inorganic tin compounds, manganese compounds, tellurium compounds) found in workplaces. The industrial hygiene information contained in the pocket guide is there intended to help users recognize and control occupational chemical hazards. The chemicals and chemical groups contained in the recent revisions include those for which NIOSH has set as recommended exposure limits (RELs) and those with permissible exposure limits (PELs) found in the OSHA General Industry Air Contaminants Standard (29 CFR 1910.1000).

Historically, the pocket guide was the result of the joint effort initiated in 1974 by NIOSH and OSHA in developing a series of occupational health standards for substances with existing PELs. This joint effort was labeled the Standards Completion Program; it involved the cooperative efforts of several contractors as well as staff units from various divisions within NIOSH and OSHA. The joint program initially developed around 380 substance-specific draft standards with supporting technical information and recommendations needed for promulgating new occupational health and safety regulations. The pocket guide was developed to make the information in the draft standards more readily available to the workers, the employers, and the occupational health and safety professionals. It is now revised periodically to reflect new data on both the changes in exposure standards and the toxicities of workplace hazards.

In addition to the pocket guide and the *Criteria Documents*, NIOSH's helpful efforts can be further evident from its other publications, such as the *Alerts, Current Intelligence Bulletins (CIB), Fact Sheets*, and *Hazard IDs*. These other publications are likewise very informative and useful. For example, although not as current as its title implies, a *CIB* reports new data on a known workplace hazard, draws attention to a formerly unrecognized workplace hazard, or presents information and recommendations on hazard control. The *Alerts* are issued to request urgent assistance in preventing, solving, or controlling newly recognized workplace hazards. The *Fact Sheets* contain recommendations from research conducted in house for the prevention of work-related hazards. And the *Hazard ID* are each a brief, user-friendly document summarizing the results of the institute's studies on a specific worksite. This document also identifies current or new workplace hazards and offers the best recommendations for their control or prevention.

Another program that NIOSH takes on is developing and periodically updating RELs for hazardous substances or conditions found in workplaces. To develop these RELs, the institute reviews thoroughly all types of available information relevant to the hazards, including chemical, biological, physical, medical, engineering, and trade. It then develops proposals for appropriate preventive measures to mitigate or eliminate the adverse effects caused by these workplace hazards. Afterwards, these proposals are transmitted to OSHA or MSHA, where applicable, for use to promulgate the required standards.

20.3. Relevant Concepts for Occupational Toxicology

In response to the needs for exposure limits to workers, the PEL (permissible exposure limit) standard or its equivalent, is widely used in many countries to protect their workers. In the United States, PEL is a legal standard promulgated by OSHA for exposure to chemical substances or physical agents present in workplaces. For chemical substances, this legal standard is expressed either in parts per million (ppm) or in milligrams per cubic meter (mg/m^3). Units of measure for physical agents (e.g., lifting, noise, heat stress) are specific to the agent or exposure of concern (e.g., number of lifts per hour, sound level in decibels).

Many of the PELs promulgated by OSHA for inhalation exposure are equivalent to or based on the threshold limit values (TLVs) published (practically) every year by the American Conference of Governmental Industrial Hygienists (*see*, e.g., ACGIH, 2010), which is a nonprofit, non-governmental scientific association. In many instances, OSHA also takes into consideration the RELs published by NIOSH in promulgating some of the legally enforceable PELs. It is however somewhat ironic to find that the RELs are prepared for a 10-hour workday while the PELs are set for 8 hours as a workday.

20.3.1. Threshold Limit Values

The TLVs published by ACGIH represent non-consensus health standards asserting that *"Nearly all workers may be repeatedly exposed day after day for a working lifetime without adverse effect."* Other occupational exposure limits such as the maximum allowable concentrations (MACs) and workplace exposure limits (WELs) have been used in The Netherlands and New Zealand, respectively. Overall, the TLV concept, initially used by ACGIH in terms of MAC, tends to have wider acceptance even outside of the United

States. The TLV estimates are health-based, in that they are assessed in terms of relevant toxicity test results in experimental animals along with limited epidemiological or clinical data. Chemical substances listed in each year's TLVs booklet (since 1946) include pesticides, metals, organic solvents, fibers, dusts, and several other chemical classes. For many chemical substances, as for lack of health concerns or data, estimates are provided for only the first of the following three TLV categories established by ACGIH.

♦ TLV-TWA refers to the *t*ime-*w*eighted *a*verage (TWA) air concentration for a routine 8-hour workday and a 40-hour workweek.

♦ TLV-STEL refers to the *s*hort-*t*erm *e*xposure *l*imit (STEL) to which workers may not be exposed for more than *15 minutes* at any time during a workday; this air concentration is set with the intent to avoid workers suffering from acute irritation, narcosis, and irreversible tissue damage.

♦ TLV-C refers to the *c*eiling (namely, the maximum) air concentration that should not be exceeded during any part of the working exposure period.

20.3.2. Biological Exposure Indices

In addition to the TLVs, ACGIH (*see*, e.g., 2010) publishes an annual list of biological exposure indices (BEIs) as reference values in assessing the results of biological monitoring (a.k.a., biomonitoring) for certain chemical substances in workers. For example, included in the BEIs list is the reference value for the activity of AChE (acetylcholinesterase) in red cells for parathion, an organophosphate for which the AChE enzyme inhibition activity (e.g., Chapter 15) in whole blood or plasma is a highly sensitive indicator of exposure. Other examples include the blood concentrations of lead (Pb) and of total inorganic mercury (Hg), both of which are likewise good indicators of the extent of exposure for the two metals (whose properties are characterized in Chapter 14).

Basically, the BEIs represent the levels of biomarkers (i.e., determinants or bioindicators) that are most likely to be observed in relevant specimens (e.g., urine, blood) collected from healthy workers who have been exposed to the toxicants implicated by the biomarkers, to the same extent as workers with inhalation exposure at the TLV under normal conditions. The exceptions are for those substances for which the TLVs are based on protection against non-systemic effects (e.g., localized irritation) or when inhalation is not the only major route of exposure. By definition, BEIs are not meant for non-systemic effects. On the other hand, for *systemic* effects of those exception substances, biomonitoring should be more superior and thereby more appropriate due to the potential for significant absorption via additional routes of entry. As with environmental exposure in general, exposure in the workplace can occur via any or all of the following three major routes: inhalation; dermal contact; and ingestion (oral). Results from biomonitoring of workers thus can be used to assist in determining toxicant absorption not only via inhalation, but also through the skin and the gastrointestinal tract. More specifically, BEIs can be used to account for the exposures to a substance from all routes, whereas TLVs are limited to inhalation exposure to the same substance. Biomonitoring thereby can serve at least as a complement to exposure assessment by air sampling in the workplace.

Despite the advantages noted above, the application of BEIs and the interpretation of biomonitoring data must be treated with caution. For one thing, individuals exposed to the same working environment may not be equally affected by, or even equally exposed to, the same toxicant. The differences may be due to age, gender, body build, medication, disease state, diet, and other affecting factors (as discussed in Chapter 10). In addition, there are subtle differences in occupational exposure factors, such as work-rate intensity and duration, humidity, temperature, and concurrent exposure to other substances (e.g., ACGIH, 2010), all of which have an influence on the interpretation of biomonitoring results. Such uncertainties are less relevant to TLVs because both the interpretation and the implications of a substance's air concentration in a workplace tend to be unaffected as much by the physiological and environmental factors considered above.

20.4. Occupational Toxic Agents/Industrial Chemicals

Table 20.1 provides a representative list of TLVs and major adverse effects for the occupational toxicants that are still regarded as important today, at least in the United States and some other countries. Four major types (or classes) of toxicants are included in this list. They are pesticides, metals, organic solvents, and fibers/dusts. Of these four types, pesticides as a group appear to be most related to mild or severe *acute* poisoning from occupational exposure. According to a survey conducted in and for the Asian region (Jeyaratnam, 1990), each year as many as 25 million agricultural workers in developing countries might suffer at least one episode of mild or acute pesticide poisoning.

20.4.1. Pesticides

Each year around 1 billion pounds of pesticide active ingredients in some 16,000 pesticide products are used in the United States (e.g., Table 15.1; NIOSH, 2006). Pesticides can be highly beneficial economic poisons. When used properly, they provide significant economic benefits to a population, including increase of crop yields and preservation of produce. However, as noted in Chapter 15, pesticides also have the potential for causing harm to people (and the ecosystem). This is especially the case for workers handling pesticides or otherwise having direct contact with these chemicals. Agricultural handlers and applicators, field reentry workers, structural pest control operators, homeowner users, and other handlers are at a higher risk for exposure to various forms of pesticides that are used as fungicides, herbicides, insecticides, rodenticides, sanitizers, and more.

Each year around 15,000 of some 2.5 million agricultural workers in the United States are reported by physicians to have experienced some form of acute pesticide poisonings (Blondell, 1997; Reigart and Roberts, 1999; U.S. EPA, 2010). The observation of such a large number of annual cases is not surprising at all, considering that worker exposure

Table 20.1. Threshold Limit Values (TLVs) and Major Adverse Health Effects of Select Occupational Toxicants[a]

Toxicants		TWA[b]	STEL[b]	Major adverse effect(s)[c]
Pesticides (mg/m^3)	Aldrin (including its metabolite dieldrin)	0.25		Liver
	Carbaryl	5		AChE inhibition
	2,4-D	10		URT & skin irritation
	DDT	1		Liver
	Diazinon	0.01		AChE inhibition
	Lindane	0.5		Liver; CNS
	Parathion	0.05		AChE inhibition
	Pyrethrum	5		Liver; LRT irritation
	Sodium fluoroacetate	0.05		CNS; cardio; nausea
Metals (mg/m^3)	Arsenic (including its inorganic compounds)	0.01		Lung cancer
	Beryllium (including its compounds)	0.002	0.01	Lung cancer; berylliosis
	Cadmium	0.01		Kidney damage
	Lead (including its inorganic compounds)	0.05		CNS; PNS; hematological
	Mercury			
	alkyl	0.01		CNS; PNS; kidney
	aryl	0.1		CNS; kidney
	inorganic & elemental	0.025	0.03	CNS; kidney
	Nickel			
	elemental	1.5		Dermatitis; pneumono
	soluble compounds	0.1		Lung; nasal cancer
	insoluble compounds	0.2		Lung cancer
Organic solvents (ppm)	Benzene	0.5	2.5	Leukemia
	Carbon monoxide	25		Carboxyhemoglobinemia
	Carbon tetrachloride	5	10	Liver
	Methyl *n*-butyl ketone	5	10	PNS; testicular
	Toluene	50		URT/eye irritation; CNS
	Trichloroethylene	50	100	Liver; headaches
	Vinyl chloride	1		Lung cancer; liver
	Xylene (*o, m, p* isomers)	100	150	URT/eye irritation; CNS
Fibers/Dusts	Asbestos, all forms (f/cc)	0.1		Pneumono; cancer
	Silica (mg/m^3)	0.025		Pul fibrosis; lung cancer

[a]excerpted from ACGIH (2010); 2,4-D = 2,4-dichlorophenoxyacetic acid; DDT = dichlorodiphenyltrichloroethane.

[b]TWA = time-weighted average (Section 20.3.1); STEL = short-term exposure limit (Section 20.3.1); ppm = parts per million; f/cc = fibers per cubic meter.

[c]AChE = acetylcholinesterase; cardio = cardiovascular system; CNS = central nervous system; LRT = lower respiratory tract; PNS = peripheral nervous system (e.g., peripheral neuropathy); Pneumono = pneumoconiosis; Pul = pulmonary; URT = upper respiratory tract.

to pesticide residues can occur anytime during formulation or handling when the chemical used can contaminate the workplace due to spilling, leaking, or discharging from the processing or the mixing/loading system. Exposure to pesticide residues can also occur when fieldworkers harvest treated crops. In short, worker exposure to pesticides in agricultural applications indeed can be a common cause of acute health problem.

Surveillance for illness and injury related to worker exposure to pesticides (or any other class of toxicants) thereby becomes a critical health and safety agendum, as it can offer worker protection by analyzing the magnitude or the underlying causes of overexposure to pesticides in a workplace. The results can also be used to alert any toxic effect of the pesticide that might not have been determined during the premarket approval process. In the United States, NIOSH has been conducting surveillance for occupational pesticide-related illnesses and injuries through the Sentinel Event Notification System for Occupational Risks (SENSOR)-Pesticides program. This program involves the participation of 12 state health agencies to employ a standard set of variables along with standard case definitions to collect and analyze illness and injury data from various sources. The information is then transmitted to the program headquarters at NIOSH, where it is compiled and put into a national database. Together with U.S. EPA, NIOSH provides technical support to all and funding to some of the participating states.

Government officials and researchers both from and outside of NIOSH have been publishing findings and related implications from analyzing information compiled in the SENSOR database. Their findings have led to issues and concerns that include eradication of invasive species, pesticide poisoning in schools, and residential use of total release foggers (which are generally canister type devices used to get rid of fleas or ticks by releasing a pesticide mist).

20.4.2. Metals

As noted in Chapter 14, most metals *per se* are not synthetic elements but occur naturally in the environment. Unfortunately, many are also frequently encountered occupational toxicants, inasmuch as they have been widely utilized or processed in various industries since the early 19th century. In very small quantities, many of these metals are actually essential for or vital to human life. However, in larger quantities all will become toxic. Many metals or their compounds can also build up in the human body and thus can become a significant health hazard to workers.

In recent years, toxic metallic products are increasingly being utilized in a variety of applications, including fabrication, electroplating, smelting, and welding. Consequently, thousands of metalworkers are at risk of contracting fatal respiratory disorders from the fumes and dusts that are unavoidable by-products in a workspace. Beryllium (Be), in particular, is among the most widely used toxic industrial metals in the United States, where the nationwide workforce in this industrial sector is estimated at around 21,000 workers (ATSDR, 2002). Of this workforce, some 10 to 15% eventually will become sensitized and develop allergic type responses to the metal.

A similar health problem is that the lungs of a machinist can be severely damaged by inhalation of toxic metals other than beryllium, such as mercury (Hg), lead (Pb), cadmium (Cd), chromium (Cr), arsenic (As), manganese (Mn), cobalt (Co), and nickel (Ni). Respiratory disorders that result from chronic exposure to these metals (including beryllium) and their alloys often develop slowly. Initial symptoms may include coughing, shortness of breath, fever, fatigue, and weight loss. Over a period of time, however, this type of ongoing exposure can prove to be severe or fatal.

Metal fume fever is the most common acute respiratory illness experienced by welders and other metalworkers. This type of illness, occurring most frequently in poorly ventilated areas in a workplace, is typically caused by exposure that arises through hot metalworking processes, such as smelting and casting of zinc alloys, or welding of galvanized metals. The fumes of common worker health concern are those of zinc oxide (ZnO) and magnesium oxide (MgO), but those of copper (Cu), iron (Fe), and cadmium have also been implicated. Actually, acute exposure to high concentrations of cadmium fume can have more serious health outcomes such as severe lung irritation, pulmonary edema, or even death, before the worker will develop metal fume fever.

The symptoms associated with metal fume fever are nonspecific but are generally flu-like including fever, chills, headaches, nausea, fatigue, thirst, muscle aches, chest soreness, and joint pains. Also frequently reported by these patients are both a sweet or metallic taste in their mouth (that would distort the taste of food and cigarettes) and an irritated or a hoarse throat. The fumes of certain toxic metal compounds are also known to cause more than metal fume fever. For example, nickel carbonyl $(NiCO)_4$ is a probable carcinogen, in addition to being an irritant to the eyes and the skin.

20.4.3. Organic Solvents

As stated on the OSHA website, millions of American workers are exposed to organic solvents every day everywhere. Organic solvents are a group of liquid organic chemicals that each have the ability to dissolve certain solids, gaseous solutes, and other liquids to form a solution. Chemicals in this large group have variable lipophilicity and volatility that hence can lead to a wide array of occupational hazards, including adverse effects on the central or peripheral nervous system, impairment of reproductive or respiratory functions, damage to the liver or kidneys, and development of cancer or dermatitis.

Organic solvents are carbon-based compounds that may be divided into two subfamilies: (1) the aliphatic-chain kind, each *without* a benzene-like ring (e.g., cyclohexene, *n*-hexane); and (2) the aromatic kind, each *with* one or more benzene-like rings (e.g., benzene, naphthalene, xylene isomers). These aliphatics and aromatics each may contain one or more substituted halogens (e.g., Br, Cl, F) and accordingly may be referred to as halogenated hydrocarbons, such as chlorobenzene (C_6H_5Cl), chlorofluorocarbons (CFCs), methylene chloride (CH_2Cl_2), and trichloroethylene $(ClCH=CCl_2)$. Alcohols, aldehydes, esters, ethers, glycols, ketones, and pyridines are some of the organic solvent compounds from substitutions for one or more hydrogen atoms on the hydrocarbon chain.

Millions of workers in many countries including the United States are exposed to organic solvents because these chemicals are used every day everywhere to dissolve resins, oils, fats, rubbers, and plastics. Organic solvents are useful in a wide variety of products such as paints, varnishes, adhesives, degreasing agents, cleaning agents, glues, and lacquers, as well as in the production of dyes, plastics, textiles, printing inks, pesticides, and pharmaceuticals. The industries processing or manufacturing these various and numerous types of products collectively represent the bulk of the workforce in the United States and many other countries, likely second only to agriculture.

Organic solvents came around in the second half of the 19th century during the coal tar industry era. Their widespread and diverse applications have since grown strikingly in both the developed and developing regions. Reports of their toxicities (e.g., including predominately neurological effects) began to emerge in the early 1900s when chlorinated solvents became available. Although thousands of organic solvents are being used today, only a small number have been tested for neurotoxicity or other adverse effects.

Workers can be exposed to organic solvents from not only their workplace or being near there. They can also be exposed to these chemicals if they come in contact with contaminated water, soil, air, or foods. Ambient and indoor air, drinking and shower water, and foods are common sources of exposure to environmental toxicants in general, but to organic solvents in particular owing to their widespread use coupled with greater solubility and higher volatility as a group.

As evident from the numerous NIOSH publications noted in Section 20.2.3, organic solvents have long been recognized to cause damages to multiple body organs and systems besides the nervous system. It is well known that exposure to organic solvents can cause hematological diseases (e.g., leukemia), liver disorders (e.g., fatty liver), and kidney diseases (e.g., chronic glomerulonephritis). A number of animal and epidemiological studies have implicated that long-term exposure to certain organic solvents would cause tumors in certain body organs, including the blood, liver, and kidneys (e.g., Chapter 13).

20.4.4. Fibers/Dusts

A variety of inorganic materials are made into fine fibers for use to strengthen and insulate building and other structures. The fibrous materials used generally are from glass, rock, silica, and alumina (Al_2O_3). The resultant fibers, which are also called *m*an-*m*ade *m*ineral *f*ibers (MMMFs), are now more known as *s*ynthetic *m*ineral *f*ibers (SMFs). Some of these end products are composed of a mixture of fibers in various sizes.

In recent years, SMFs have been extensively used as alternatives to asbestos in insulation and fire-retardant products. They are recently also widely used as reinforcement materials in cement and plastic products. Worldwide, SMF products are used broadly as thermal and acoustic insulation materials in commercial and residential buildings. In the United States alone, more than 200,000 workers are exposed to SMFs in manufacturing or end-use applications (as noted on OSHA's website). SMFs are generally classified into three source/use groups as follows:

- Fiberglass (e.g., glasswool, glass filaments) – those used in automobiles, re-inforced plastics, textiles, and as electrical insulation.

- Mineral wool (e.g., rockwool, slagwool) – those used in limpet and formed insulation materials, such as acoustic insulation and fire-rating materials.

- Refractory ceramic fibers – those used for high temperature (up to $1,400°$ C) insulation applications (e.g., insulation blanket) and fire protection materials.

SMFs have been suspected to cause lung cancer and other adverse respiratory effects since the 1970s, when they became increasingly used to replace asbestos. Asbestos is a group of six naturally occurring fibrous silicate materials also used primarily for insulation applications (Chapter 4). By the mid-1900s, there were already several epidemiological studies linking elevated incidences of pulmonary fibrosis and cancer to inhalation of crocidolite and chrysotile. The amphibole-shaped crocidolite and the serpentine-shaped chrysotile are members of asbestos. The widespread use of SMFs as replacements naturally brought about similar concerns that they too might cause cancer and other adverse effects to or in the respiratory system. These concerns came about largely due to the similarities between SMFs and asbestos in both their appearance and their industrial applications. Today, a large body of data from occupational and laboratory studies is available associating a variety of adverse effects with exposure to SMFs.

In general, short-term exposure to SMFs can result in skin, eye, and/or upper respiratory tract irritation. The skin and eye cases often occur in workers having direct contact with SMF products for the first time or in those with a short lapse from exposure. The symptoms generally involve reddening, burning, itching, and inflammation around the finger nails. The respiratory tract cases largely come from inhalation to very high levels of SMFs. Long-term exposure to SMFs was linked to a slightly increased risk of lung cancer among exposed workers in early SMF industries. OSHA now recommends the use of a dust mask for persons working with fiberglass products.

Dust as a related occupational hazard consists of any tiny solid particles, not necessarily fibers, that are carried by air currents. MSHA defines dust as finely divided solids that may become airborne from the original state without any chemical or physical alteration other than fracture. These tiny particles are formed by a disintegration or fracture process, such as grinding, crushing, or impact. Agriculture, construction, and mining are the industries that contribute most to high levels of various dusts in the air.

As noted in Chapter 12, various dusts can be classified by size into the respirable and inhalable groups. Yet in terms of their composition, dusts are generally divided into the fibrogenic and the nuisance type. Fibrogenic dust particles, such as those of free crystalline silica or asbestos which have fiber-like tendencies, are biologically toxic; and if retained in the lungs, they can form fibrogenic scar tissue and impair lung functions.

In contrast, nuisance or inert dust particles can be defined as those containing less than 1% quartz. Quartz is a hard mineral composed of silica (SiO_2) in the silicon-oxygen tetrahedron (SiO_4) shape. Due to their low content of silicates, nuisance dusts have little or no history of causing any significant adverse effect on the lung. Any reaction that may occur from nuisance dusts is potentially reversible. However, excessive levels of nuisance dusts (e.g., FeO dust) in the workplace can reduce visibility, can cause unpleasant deposits in the eyes, ears, and nasal passages (e.g., Portland cement dust), and can induce injury to the skin or the mucous membranes by chemical or mechanical action.

Silicosis, that being one form of the black lung disease medically termed *pneumoconiosis*, is the most common occupational lung disease worldwide, particularly in the developing regions. According to a fact sheet published by the World Health Organization (WHO, 2000), China reported more than 24,000 deaths due to silicosis each year between 1991 and 1995, mostly among older workers. Also included in the fact sheet was WHO's projection that in the United States, among the million or so workers (e.g., sandblasters) who are occupationally exposed to free crystalline silica dusts, about 60,000 would eventually develop silicosis. On the other hand, apparently due to arising health concerns with pneumoconiosis in general, many developed countries have banned the use of asbestos in new constructions. Yet ironically, along with some developing countries (e.g., Indonesia, China, India), the United States continues to allow the use of these fibrous silicate minerals in new construction projects.

20.4.5. Other Groups of Toxic Agents

In addition to the four groups of toxicants emphasized by ACGIH as listed in Table 20.1 and discussed briefly above, there are other groups that are likewise ubiquitous in the workplace and likely as threatening to occupational health and safety. One obvious example is metalworking fluids, to which exposure can occur through inhalation or dermal contact in the workplace to result in asthma, lung disease, skin disorder, or cancer (NIOSH, 1998). Metalworking fluids are largely complex mixtures of petroleum oils used during machining and grinding to prolong a tool's life by protecting the work piece's surfaces. Approximately one million American workers engaging in machine finishing, machine tooling, and similar metalworking operations are potentially exposed to this kind of fluids (Kreiss and Cox-Ganser, 1997; Zacharisen *et al.*, 1998).

Physical and biological hazards are also commonly found in workplaces. OSHA's Hazard Communication Standard (29 CFR 1910.1020), which went into effect in 1985, is the centerpiece of a powerful common ideology in the United States known as the workplace right-to-know movement. In most literature, this regulation continues to be treated more as a requirement for *chemical* manufacturers and employers to relate information to their workers concerning the hazards of *chemical* products in their workplace. Yet as misleading as some of the terms used may seem to be, the hazard materials subject to such communication, as mandated by the federal and state laws, should also include information that concerns *physical* and *biological* hazards.

For example, the Employee Right-To-Know Act passed by the Minnesota state legislature in 1983 includes infectious agents found especially in hospitals and clinics. That state law also covers heat and noise as additional potential physical hazards. Another example is the New Jersey state law on worker health and safety, under which employees have the rights to receive monitoring records for exposures not only to chemicals, but also to noise, radiation, heat stress, cold stress, vibration, and molds.

Heat can be an occupational hazard because excessive heat from working in places like around the boilers, ovens, or furnaces can result in dehydration, heat rash, and heat stroke. Similarly, excessive cold from working in a place with air temperature below the freezing point, such as when taking inventory in a walk-in freezer, can result in frost bite, chilblains, or hypothermia. Chilblain is a general skin condition characterized by an inflammation of the skin, accompanied by burning and itching, when exposed to very cold temperatures. Hypothermia is a condition of abnormally low body temperature that can fatally affect normal metabolism and body functions. Vibration exposure too can be a physical hazard to workers engaging in jobs with vibrating machinery and equipment, such as when constantly operating a chainsaw or jackhammer. Vibration can have serious effects on the tendons, muscles, bones, joints, and other body parts including notably the nervous system, often leading to pains, tingling, and loss of sensation in the affected area. And excessive noise is not uncommon in many occupational settings. Noise can cause hearing impairment and other health problems (Chapter 17).

Ionizing radiation (e.g., X-ray, uranium isotopes) can also be found in many workplaces, such as health care facilities, research institutions, nuclear reactors, and mining areas. Non-ionizing radiation (e.g., microwave, infrared, visible light) too can be found in a wide range of occupational settings, such as when installing telephone cables, paving asphalt roadways, and working on farms. Ionizing and non-ionizing radiations collectively thus can cause a wide array of adverse health effects. Common health effects associated with ionizing radiation include cancer, damage to the eyes or the skin, sterility, cataracts, and blood disorders. Although non-ionizing radiation carries less energy and thereby less health risks compared to ionizing radiation, it can still cause severe health effects on workers from high levels of exposure. For example, persons who work outdoors constantly are most susceptible to ultraviolet radiation, to which chronic exposure can cause not only photochemical cataracts but also skin cancer (e.g., OMOL, 2009).

As noted in Section 20.1, the bacterium *Legionella pneumophila* can cause legionellosis in a workplace. To some people, it may be debatable whether or not the American Legion's 1976 convention held in Philadelphia (Pennsylvania), where the first reported episode of Legionnaire's disease took place, could be treated as a workplace. Regardless, a more recent outbreak in Norway (Nygard, 2005) is by all standards qualified as occurring in an occupational setting. In the Norway incidence, over 50 people reportedly became ill (and a few died) from Legionnaire's disease caused by the bacteria growing in a lignin spray dryer scrubber that was placed at the Borregaard plant located in Sarpsborg, a municipality near the city of Fredrikstad.

Many other infectious agents can be found in workplaces as well, especially in hospitals and clinics where health care and other workers may be exposed to these agents via inhalation or dermal contact. Health care workers may be exposed to these infectious agents not only through accidental contact with contaminated blood specimens, a concern well reflected in OSHA's BBP standard (29 CFR 1910.1030) noted earlier, but also more predominately via inhalation of contaminated air in the workplace. SARS (severe acute respiratory syndrome) may serve as a practical case of airborne infection involving a significant number of employees working in clinics and hospitals.

The principal way in which SARS spreads is by close person-to-person contact with the respiratory secretions or body fluids of a SARS patient (CDC, 2004). This respiratory disease, briefly introduced in Chapter 1, was notorious for its global pandemic occurring during the nine months from November 2002 through early July 2003. This relatively short-lived pandemic involved over 8,000 human cases, more than 700 human deaths, and some 30 nations around the world (WHO, 2003).

Among all the global SARS cases confirmed by WHO, many were health care workers. For instance, the first outbreak of SARS occurred in southern China in November 2002. When the local health authority there notified WHO about the outbreak, 105 of the 305 reported cases (and 5 deaths), or about 30%, were health care workers. A group of medical investigators (Ho *et al.*, 2003) later found that hospital workers accounted for about 25% of the cases in Hong Kong and were the first to contract SARS from a few infected patients before the disease got spread to the entire community. These investigators further noted in their study report that Canadian hospital workers had even a higher risk, accounting for 65% of all the SARS cases occurring in that nation.

References

ACGIH (American Conference of Governmental Industrial Hygienists), 2010. TLVs® and BEIs® Based on the Documentation of the Threshold Limit Values for Chemical Substance and Physical Agents & Biological Exposure Indices. 1330 Kemper Meadow Drive, Cincinnati, Ohio, USA.

ATSDR (U.S. Agency for Toxic Substances and Disease Registry), 2002. Toxicological Profile for Beryllium. U.S. Department of Health and Human Services, Atlanta, Georgia, USA.

Blondell JM, 1997. Epidemiology of Pesticide Poisonings in the United States, with Special Reference to Occupational Cases. In *Human Health Effects of Pesticides, Occupational Medicine: State of the Art Reviews* (Keifer MC, Ed.). Philadelphia, Pennsylvania, USA: Hanley & Belfus.

Carter T, 2004. British Occupational Hygiene Practice 1720-1920. *Ann. Occup. Hyg.* 48:299-307.

CDC (U.S. Centers for Disease Control and Prevention), 2004. Fact Sheet: Basic Information About SARS. U.S. Department of Health and Human Services, Atlanta, Georgia, USA.

Cheremisinoff NP, 2001. Practical Guide to Industrial Safety: Methods for Process Safety Professionals. New York, New York, USA: Marcel Dekker, Chapter 1.

DOL (U.S. Department of Labor), 2009. *Employment Law Guide: Laws, Regulations, and Technical Assistance Services.* Washington, DC, USA.

Ho AS, Sung JJY, Chan-Yeung M, 2003. An Outbreak of Severe Acute Respiratory Syndrome among Hospital Workers in a Community Hospital in Hong Kong. *Ann. Intern. Med.* 139:564-567.

Jeyaratnam J, 1990. Acute Pesticide Poisoning: A Major Global Health Problem. *World Health Stat. Q.* 43:139-144.

Kloss D, 2005. *Occupational Health Law*. Oxford, UK: Blackwell Science.

Kreiss K, Cox-Ganser J, 1997. Metalworking Fluid-Associated Hypersensitivity Pneumonitis: A Workshop Summary. *Am. J. Ind. Med.* 32:423-432.

Lewis J, Thornbury G, 2010. *Employment Law and Occupational Health – A Practical Handbook*. Oxford, UK: Wiley-Blackwell.

NIOSH (U.S. National Institute for Occupational Safety and Health), 1998. *What You Need to Know About Occupational Exposure to Metalworking Fluids*. NIOSH Pub. No. 98-116. U.S. Department of Health and Human Services, Atlanta, Georgia, USA.

NIOSH (U.S. National Institute for Occupational Safety and Health), 2006. *Pesticide-Related Illness and Injury Surveillance: A How-To Guide For State-Based Programs*. NIOSH Pub. No. 2006-102. U.S. Department of Health and Human Services, Atlanta, Georgia, USA.

Nygard K, 2005. Outbreak Investigation Collaborators. Update: Outbreak of Legionnaires' Disease in Norway Traced to Air Scrubber. *Euro. Surveill.* 10(4-6):128.

OMOL (Ontario Ministry of Labour), 2009. Ultraviolet Radiation in the Workplace. 400 University Avenue, Toronto, Ontario, Canada.

Reigart JR, Roberts JR (Eds.), 1999. Recognition and Management of Pesticide Poisonings, Fifth Edition. EPA #735-R-98-003. Office of Pesticide Program, Washington DC, USA.

U.S. EPA (U.S. Environmental Protection Agency), 2010. Funding Opportunity Announcement: Pesticide Safety Program for Agricultural Workers and Farmworker Children. Funding Opportunity No. 2010-02. Office of Pesticide Programs (Field and External Affairs Division), Washington DC, USA.

WHO (World Health Organization), 2000. Fact Sheet No. 238 (May 2000): Silicosis. Geneva, Switzerland.

WHO (World Health Organization), 2003. Summary of Probable SARS Cases with Onset of Illness from 1 November 2002 to 31 July 2003. Geneva, Switzerland.

Zacharisen MC, Kadambi AR, Schlueter DP, Kurup VP, Shack JB, Fox JL, Anderson HA, Fink JN, 1998. The Spectrum of Respiratory Disease Associated with Exposure to Metal Working Fluids. *J. Occup. Environ. Med.* 40:640-647.

Review Questions

1. Briefly describe the two unique principles as well as unique practices that occupational toxicology focuses on.

2. Name three examples of classic *industrial* diseases covered in this chapter.

3. Briefly describe the functions and organizational structure of NIOSH.

4. What was the first federal legislation on occupational health and safety in the United States?

5. Over the years, how has the European Union's Framework Directive affected the occupational health and safety regulations and standards adopted by its member states?

6. Briefly describe the different responsibilities that OSHA and NIOSH each have in protecting the health and safety of American workers.

7. How does OSHA's Hazard Communication Standard affect the health and safety of American workers?

8. Why is NIOSH's *Pocket Guide to Chemical Hazards* such an important document to both the workers and the occupational health and safety professionals in the United States?

9. In what ways is an illness surveillance program an important tool for advancing or promoting occupational health and safety?

10. How does NIOSH carry out its SENOR-Pesticides program in the United States?

11. Briefly characterize, in terms of symptoms and causes, the illness condition known as metal fume fever.

12. Briefly describe the regulatory standard referred to as *Permissible Exposure Limit*.

13. Which of the four major chemical classes or types of toxicants, as covered in the TLVs booklet, appears to be most related to acute poisoning from worker exposure?

14. What is the most common occupational lung disease worldwide?

15. Briefly describe the following concepts: TLV; TLV-C; TLV-TWA; TLV-STEL.

16. Based on the TLV-TWA values alone, rank the following pesticides from having the most to the least *potency*: a) DDT; b) parathion; c) pyrethrum; d) sodium fluoroacetate; e) 2,4-D.

17. How are the BEIs related to their corresponding TLVs provided by ACGIH for substances or compound groups that have both of these estimates?

18. Name two metals and one organic solvent that each can cause damage to the *peripheral* nervous system.

19. Briefly explain why so many workers are exposed to organic solvents each year in the United States and many other countries.

20. List and briefly characterize the three general source/use categories of SMFs.

21. Which of the following types of dust particles tend to be more toxic to humans? a) fibrogenic; b) nuisance. And why?

22. Name five types of physical hazards that are commonly found in workplaces.

23. Name four occupations as common sources of potential exposure to ionizing radiation, and another four for potential exposure to non-ionizing radiation.

24. Give two examples of infectious agents covered in this chapter that had outbreaks occurring in a workplace.

25. Why do health care workers tend to be more susceptible to SARS type infection than the general public are?

CHAPTER 21

Food Toxicants and Toxic Household Substances

21.1. Introduction

Household and food products are closer to home than any other kind of purchasable items. Household products are consumer goods that oftentimes can become a health concern to the public, especially those that can harm children and the elderly. Meantime, a large number of harmful foreign substances are frequently found in foods that people consume every day. Some of these foreign substances are added to the food intentionally or as a result of contamination. Food toxicants of lingering concern to food and environmental toxicologists may fall under three major source categories as follows: (1) direct or intentional food additives; (2) indirect or unintentional food additives; and (3) food contaminants. Note that the term *food additive* may not have the same legal connotation worldwide. However, at the minimum, the term should be used to refer to any added substance either not normally consumed as a food by itself, or not used as an ingredient of a food item (FAO/WHO, 1994).

According to the estimation by a research team (Scallan *et al.*, 2011) affiliated with the U.S. Centers for Disease Control and Prevention (CDC), each year some 48 million American people get sick, 128,000 are hospitalized, and about 3,000 die as a result of foodborne illness. For household products, the poisoning statistics are equally disturbing. The U.S. Consumer Product Safety Commission (CPSC, 2009) estimated that over 90% of suspected poison exposures occur at home with readily available household items. The Commission also reported that "*on average, each year an estimated 80,000 children (mostly younger than age 5) are treated in hospital emergency departments for unintentional poisonings.*"

The acute poisoning statistics noted above, whether for exposure to food toxicants or to toxic household substances, do not include adverse effects from chronic exposure that may lead to severe or fatal damage, such as cancer or early death. To put it another way, in terms of food or consumer product safety, the scope of health concern goes far beyond what the above statistics infer.

21.1.1. Concerns with Food Toxicants

In the United States, as authorized by the Federal Food, Drug, and Cosmetic (FD&C) Act, the federal safety regulation for most types of foods in the nation is the responsibility of the U.S. Food and Drug Administration (FDA). The federal statute was enacted in 1938 after an improperly prepared sulfanilamide antibacterial drug took the life of more than 100 people. With several amendments passed over the years, including in the form of the Food Quality Protection Act (FQPA) of 1996, the FD&C Act completely overhauled the nation's health regulatory system. Among other provisions, the law empowers FDA to promulgate food (and drug) safety standards, to conduct factory inspections, and to call for safety evidence for new food additives to be put on the market.

Foods may also be contaminated by biological agents, environmental toxicants, or toxins present within a food. Symptoms of acute food poisoning involve, at the minimum, nausea, vomiting, or diarrhea. Some foodborne toxins, such as those found in certain seafood, can affect the nervous system (and thereby are often referred to as neurotoxins). Many foreign substances are also present in foods due to environmental pollution or to faulty handling of foods. These substances are generally referred to as food contaminants, as they serve no purpose either in the food product or in its processing.

There are foreign substances that may become part of a food product as a result of their contact with or migration into the food proper due to packaging, holding, or processing. These substances are commonly referred to as *indirect* or *unintentional* food additives. There are also many substances intentionally added to foods to accomplish an intended effect, such as to increase a food's shelf life or to enhance its appeal to consumers. Still some substances are added to make a food more tractable for bountiful or consistent production. These added substances are often referred to as *intentional* or *direct* additives, amid the trend that some have been coming with questionable toxicity in recent years.

21.1.2. Concerns with Toxic Household Substances

In the United States, the federal safety regulation for most types of consumer products is the responsibility of CPSC, as authorized under the federal Consumer Product Safety Act of 1972. This federal statute empowers CPSC to promulgate health and safety standards for consumer products, including household goods, to pursue recalls for those that present unacceptable health risks to consumers, and to ban any of the more than 15,000 consumer products under its jurisdiction if there is no feasible alternative. Consumer products not under CPSC's regulations are those expressly fall within the jurisdictions of other federal agencies, such as foods, drugs, cosmetics, medical devices, pesticides, tobacco products, firearms, explosives, motor vehicles, aircrafts, and boats.

Over-the-counter (OTC) medicines, personal care products, cleaning agents, and other organic compounds are the four major source categories of toxic household substances that reportedly cause potentially more harm to young children, pregnant women, and the elderly. With toxic household substances, a particular underrated health concern is the common misconception that the OTC medicines are absolutely safe for use by the public, owing to the notion that they are all allowed by law to be sold without medical advice. Yet what remains a serious health concern, especially for long-term effects, is the potential for adverse drug (chemical) interaction between two or more OTC medicines, or between one or more OTC medicines and other prescription drugs, which are commonly taken by the same (especially elder) person at around the same time.

21.2. Toxic Substances in Food Products

As noted earlier, food toxicants can be broadly subsumed under the three major source categories: (1) intentional or direct food additives; (2) unintentional or indirect food additives; and (3) food contaminants. Figure 21.1 presents a graphic overview of the three major categories, along with their subcategories intended to highlight more specifically the sources involved. Following the graphic presentation are separate brief accounts of the general aspects of these various source (sub)categories, including the current toxicological concerns on some of the food toxicants selected as specific examples.

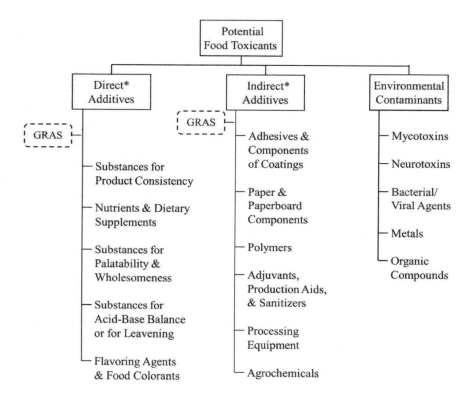

Figure 21.1. Major Source Categories of Potential Food Toxicants in the United States
(*subject to premarket review/approval by U.S. Food and Drug Administration,
except for those food additives placed on the generally recognized as safe [GRAS] list)

21.2.1. Direct Food Additives

According to an FDA (1992) document, this category includes additives that are generally referred to by their functions: emulsifiers; stabilizers; anticaking agents; thickeners; preservatives; antioxidants; bleaching and maturing agents; buffering and sequestering agents; vitamins and minerals; spices; natural and synthetic flavoring boosters; and food colorants. Many American consumers doing the cooking are familiar with the functions of these food additives and their purposes. In essence, emulsifiers are used to give foods a consistent texture and prevent them from separating. Stabilizers and thickeners are used to give foods a smooth uniform texture. Preservatives are used to retard food spoilage caused by air or microorganisms. Anticaking agents are added to foods to prevent caking or lumping. Antioxidants are a special kind of preservatives used primarily to prevent oils and fats in foods from becoming rancid. Spices and flavoring agents are used to enhance a food's taste. Food colorants are used to enhance the appearance of foods to meet consumer expectations. Vitamins and minerals are added to foods to make up for those known to be insufficient in a diet or lost in the processing.

In the United States, any *new* additive to be added to a food product must be approved by FDA as a new food ingredient. The approval is based on a premarket review of extensive scientific data on safety and toxicity. Such a premarket safety evaluation generally requires, in addition to clinical observations whenever available, animal studies that involve about eight categories related to health effects: toxicokinetics; acute toxicity; short-term toxicity; long-term toxicity; teratogenicity; reproductive toxicity; mutagenicity; and carcinogenicity. As food safety evaluation needs to rely on a benchmark (i.e., safe level) for dietary intake of the new ingredient, the safety measure *acceptable daily intake* (ADI) or its equivalent (e.g., *tolerance level*) has been adopted by food safety sectors worldwide. These ADI levels are typically determined in relation to the no observed (adverse) effect level (NO[A]EL) derived from largely animal toxicity studies. Further discussion on these health risk assessment concepts and criteria is given in Chapter 23.

It should be noted that some direct (and less so, indirect) additives have been accepted by the U.S. legislation as "generally recognized as safe" (GRAS) as far back as 1958. GRAS exemptions are granted for substances that are generally recognized or affirmed as safe by a panel of experts qualified by their scientific training and experience in evaluating the safety of these or similar substances. Currently, more than a couple thousands of substances are placed on the GRAS list, including many commonly available substances such as acetic acid, calcium carbonate, carbon dioxide, cocoa butter substitute, ethyl alcohol, hydrogen peroxide, lactic acid, malt syrup, rapeseed oil, red algae, vitamin A, vitamin D, wheat, wheat gluten, and more. The use of a number of GRAS substances is now being challenged, nonetheless, largely due to the emergence of more or new (questionable) toxicity data on these substances in recent years.

Food emulsifiers, also called food emulgents, are molecules with one water-loving (hydrophilic) and one fat-loving (hydrophobic) end. Adding molecules of this kind to a food material will make it possible for the water and oil molecules in it to become finely dispersed in each other, thereby creating a stable, homogenous, smooth emulsion (of which milk is a classic example). Egg yolk, containing the emulgent lecithin, is often applied as a food emulsifier, in spite of the fact that it is one of the common causes of food allergies in children. Some emulsifiers such as calcium and magnesium stearates (i.e., salts of a fatty acid) can also act as anticaking agents. A few other emulsifiers such as sorbitan monostearate and sorbitan tristearate can also be used as stabilizers.

The more commonly used natural raw materials for food emulsifiers include soybean lecithin and sunflower lecithin. Lecithin, a mixture of phospholipids and found in all living cells, can be used to keep oil blended with vinegar in salad dressings. The production of basic emulsifiers involves esterification of triglycerides (a type of lipids also present in the human blood) with glycerols to form monoglycerides which in turn can be esterified with other substances, such as citric acid, lactic acid, and succinic acid, to improve their emulsifying strength. Even though most food emulsifiers including the various esters of monoglyceride are of low toxicity, a significant amount of aluminum is found in them. Aluminum has been suspected to cause Alzheimer's disease (Section 14.3.1).

A nutrient is a substance that an organism's body relies on for development, growth, metabolism, or health maintenance, and must be taken in from its environment. It is used to build and repair tissues, to regulate body functions, or to provide a source for energy. Organic nutrients include carbohydrates, lipids, proteins (as well as their building blocks amino acids), and vitamins. Inorganic compounds such as dietary minerals, oxygen, and water may also be considered as nutrients.

According to the U.S. Dietary Supplement Health and Education Act (DSHEA) of 1994, a dietary supplement sold in the United States is an edible product containing an ingredient intended to supplement a diet. The ingredient may be one or any combination of the following: vitamins; minerals; herbs or other botanicals; amino acids; certain enzymes; certain organ tissues; and certain metabolites. These supplements can be extracts or concentrates and may be found in various forms such as tablets, capsules, powder, and liquid. They can be in other forms (e.g., a bar); but in that case, their label information must not represent them as a conventional food or a sole item of a diet. Whatever their form may be, DSHEA places dietary supplements in a special category under the general umbrella of foods and requires that they be labeled as a dietary supplement.

The main concern with the dietary supplements is their misuse or overuse, as such use can bring in a host of side effects. For instance, excess levels of vitamin A over 15,000 international units (IU) may lead to hepatotoxic effects and changes in vision, hair, and skin. Adverse health levels of vitamin D may result from intakes greater than 2,000 IU daily and lead to hyperkalemia or soft tissue calcification. Intakes of vitamin E over 800 IU daily may lead to untoward effects such as headaches, vomiting, fatigue, and nausea. And taking vitamin C more than the daily recommendation of 100 mg per kg of body weight may retard metabolic activities or cause stomach aches and diarrhea.

As with vitamins, minerals can also cause many side effects. For example, in large or repeated doses, calcium can cause osteoporosis. Fluorine (usually available in the form of fluoride) can lead to skeletal or dental fluorosis. Iron can cause deficiency in zinc. Excess intake of macronutrients can also cause a number of untoward health effects. At the least, the presence of a large quantity of one macronutrient (e.g., carbohydrate) as an energy source can induce adverse effects indirectly by causing a nutritional deficiency in one or more of the other macronutrients (e.g., protein, lipid) or an interference with their normal functions and utilization. In addition to vitamin and nutrient toxicities caused by overdose, dietary supplements may interact with other supplements or prescription drugs to induce adverse effects due to chemical or drug interaction.

Preservatives are substances used to maintain the palatability and wholesomeness of food. They retard food spoilage caused by air and microorganisms. Antioxidants are preservatives used primarily to prevent fats and oils in baked goods and other oily foods from becoming rancid. They also retard cut-fresh fruits such as apples and peaches from turning brownish when exposed to air. Preservatives such as butylated hydroxyanisole (BHA), butylated hydroxytoluene (BHT), sodium nitrate, sodium nitrite, and propyl gallate are commonly added to foods to maintain their palatability and wholesomeness. As listed in Table 19.1, propyl gallate and BHA are potential endocrine disruptors.

Sodium bicarbonate (baking soda) and active dry yeast are two common leavening agents that produce gas bubbles to cause biscuits, cakes, and other baked products to rise during baking. There are also leavening agents that can help modify the acidity of foods for proper flavor or taste. For example, fumaric acid, lactic acid, phosphoric acid, sodium aluminum phosphate, sodium aluminum sulfate, and tartrates may be added to adjust a baked product's acidity. Some of these agents reportedly have the potential to cause side effects. In particular, phosphoric acid, which is used in many soft drinks, has been linked to lower bone density (i.e., osteoporosis) in epidemiological studies. Sodium aluminum phosphate, commonly found in processed foods such as cheese and pickles, can be a rich source for aluminum available in the body. The toxicity of aluminum has remained controversial (Section 14.3.1), but any such excess dietary intake is certainly avoidable. Also, very high levels of lactic acid can cause a serious physiological condition with abnormally low pH in the blood and body tissues known as lactic acidosis, although dietary intake alone is not likely able to account for such a high toxicity level.

Some substances are used to simulate natural flavors, such as benzaldehyde for almond flavor even though the ADI for this flavorant might be as low as 4 mg/kg (e.g., Andersen, 2006). Some others, such as monosodium glutamate (MSG), are used to intensify food flavor and taste. One side effect of MSG ingestion is the sudden onset of an asthma-like attack, with symptoms including headaches, heart palpitations, chest pain, and shortness of breath. In the United States, the most common artificial primary colorants used in foods include allura red AC (a.k.a. FD&C red No. 40), brilliant blue FCF (FD&C blue No. 1), and tartrazine (FD&C yellow No. 5). Studies have linked excessive consumption of certain artificial colorants to a number of adverse effects, such as tartrazine yellow on the reproductive functions of male mice (Mehedi *et al.*, 2009) and allura red on the behavioral activities in young rats (Vorhees *et al.*, 1983). Note that primary colorants are those from which secondary colorants are formulated.

21.2.2. Indirect Food Additives
Unintentional or indirect food additives are substances present mostly in food-contact articles that have the potential to migrate into the food product being packaged, stored, or processed. Oftentimes, these substances are found at least in some trace amounts in the

final food product, all being part of the packaging materials or processing equipment that have migrated into the food item. Their sources thereby include the following: adhesives and components of coating; paper and paperboard components; adjuvants, production aids, or sanitizers; and polymers (e.g., mostly plastics). Also included as indirect additives are growth promoters and other drugs used during the raising of food animals; these drug residues are in a different subcategory not involving food-contact articles.

Under FDA's Threshold of Regulation program, substances that come in contact with foods are exempted from being listed as indirect food additives if they migrate into foods at levels that result in no appreciable risk to human health. FDA (1995) has outlined four "*not's*" criteria for what qualifies as the threshold of no appreciable human health risk in dealing with indirect food additives. First, migration of the food-contact substance at issue is *not* expected to result in either a dietary concentration above the threshold of 0.5 ppb (parts per billion), or a dietary intake above 1% of the ADI equivalent calculated for the additive. Second, the substance has *not* been shown or suspected to be a human or an animal carcinogen. Third, under its intended use conditions, the additive (e.g., an antioxidant residing in the packaging) must *not* produce a technical (e.g., antioxidation) effect in the food into which it migrates. The fourth and final criterion is that the additive's use must *not* have shown any significant adverse impact on the environment.

Per Title 21 of the *U.S. Code of Federal Regulations* (Section 175.105 – Adhesives), several phthalates, of which some are suspected endocrine disruptors (Table 19.1), have FDA approval for use as adhesives and components of coating in food processing and packaging materials. As a result, some phthalates may be ingested in foods (Castle *et al.* 1990; Hauser *et al.*, 2004; Page and Lacroix, 1995). Bisphenol A (BPA), which is also considered as an endocrine disruptor (Table 19.1), is a key building block of polycarbonate plastic and epoxy resins used for coating the interior surfaces of food cans, beverage cans, and plastic bottles. BPA has been found leachable from these interior surfaces, including notably those of baby bottles (e.g., Biles *et al.*, 1997; Gibson, 2007; Munguia-Lopez *et al.*, 2002). Amidst such rising concerns among authorities (e.g., Canada Gazette, 2010; FDA, 2010), Canada was the first nation to list BPA as a toxic chemical; and on 17 July 2012, FDA made it official to ban BPA-based baby bottles and sippy cups.

Paper materials are used every day for packaging or holding foods in a variety of ways. Substances in paper plates, paper cups, cartons, wrappers, and boxes can leach into foods during storage, preparation, and service activities. These substances include polystyrene and many VOCs (volatile organic compounds), such as chloroform, benzene, dichloromethane, carbon tetrachloride, and trichloroethylene. One significant source of dioxins is from chlorination (bleaching) of wood pulp which can become a large component of paper plates. Many of the above substances have been found harmful to humans when exposed to at sufficiently high levels (*see*, e.g., Chapters 13 and 16).

Polymers are long-chain giant organic molecules assembled from many smaller molecules called monomers. A common name for most synthetic polymers is plastics. Some polymers are especially ubiquitous to consumers: *polyethylene terephthalate*, as used in two-liter beverage bottles; *high-density polyethylene*, as used in milk jugs and food containers; *low-density polyethylene*, as used in film applications for meat and poultry wrapping; *polypropylene* (of normal density), as used in candy packaging; and *polystyrene*, as used in deli food containers and foam cups. Due to their relative chemical inertness and insolubility in water, plastics generally have low toxicity in their finished state; and they will pass through the gastrointestinal system without inducing any adverse effect. However, plastics frequently contain a variety of toxic additives such as BPA and phthalates. These plasticizers are often added to brittle plastics to improve the latter's flexibility for food packaging. Another concern is that plastic monomers, such as ethylene and propylene, are not harmless to humans. These monomers may remain trapped as unbound residues in the polymer plastic that they were used to build.

Per Title 21 of the *U.S. Code of Federal Regulations* (Part 178), adjuvants are agents added to a food-contact article to facilitate the action of the article's principal ingredient(s), such as toluene being utilized as a blowing agent adjuvant in the production of foamed polystyrene. Sanitizers are agents generally used to remove unpleasant or infective features by controlling microbial growth. These sanitizers include hydrogen peroxide (H_2O_2) solution, which may be used to sterilize polymeric food-contact surfaces, and lithium hypochlorite (LiClO) solution, which may be used on food processing equipment, utensils, and other food-contact articles. Production aids are agents used to offer a processing environment conducive to the production of the food-contact article. For example, both polyethylene glycol (PEG) and hydrogenated castor oil may be used in the production of articles or components of articles authorized for food-contact use. And pentachlorophenol may be used on wooden articles that are used or intended for use in packaging, transporting, or holding raw agricultural products. While the definitions of *adjuvants* and *production aids* may be overlapping, none of the examples given above (including for sanitizers) is harmless to humans at high levels of exposure.

The use of a thin dense chromium coating and a polytetrafluoroethylene (PTFE) coating can make the food-processing equipment last longer and cleaned faster. PTFE, most known by the DuPont brand name Teflon®, is a synthetic fluoropolymer with numerous applications. It is polymerized using perfluorooctanoic acid as a surfactant (Chapter 16). The supposedly nontoxic PTFE is a stable compound but begins to decompose after the cookware's temperature rises to 350° C (660° F). Its degradation by-products can cause flu-like symptoms in humans; and some of them may be carcinogenic.

Drug residues in food animals are likewise of high concern in that many food animals need to be treated with drugs during their lifetime to ensure a continuing, wholesome, and affordable food supply to the public. Although there are several hundreds of drugs used for this purpose, U.S. National Research Council (NRC, 1999) and many authorities have these drugs all subsumed under six major use categories as follows: (1) topical antiseptics, bactericides, and fungicides – e.g., those used to treat infections, wounds, and abrasions of surface skin or hoofs; (2) ionophores – e.g., those lipid-soluble molecules used to increase feed efficiency and yield; (3) steroid anabolic growth promoters – e.g., those hormones used to promote growth; (4) peptide production enhancers – e.g., those protein hormones like recombinant bovine somatotropin (rBST) used to increase milk production in dairy cattle; (5) antiparasite drugs – e.g., those used to treat parasite diseases; and (6) antibiotics – e.g., those used to treat microbial infections. The NRC report addresses not only the benefits from use of these drugs in food animals, but also the associated risks of human diseases (e.g., drug residue allergy, cancer, reproductive toxicity).

21.2.3. Food Contaminants

Food contaminants include a wide array of chemical substances and infectious agents present in various forms or types of food products. Of all the food contaminants, mycotoxins have one of the most serious consequences in terms of public health and agroeconomics. These mycotoxins can contaminate numerous various agricultural commodities before harvest or under post-harvest conditions. As noted in Chapter 17, the most notorious mycotoxins are the aflatoxins produced by the fungal species *Aspergillus flavus* and *Aspergillus parasiticus*. These microfungi tend to grow in warm and humid climates and preferentially produce aflatoxins in drought-stressed corn and groundnuts.

Food infection is caused by the presence of bacteria or other microbes in an organism's body after consumption. In contrast, food intoxication refers to the ingestion of toxins contained in the food, which can happen even when the microbes that produced the toxin (e.g., exotoxins produced by bacteria) are no longer present or able to cause infection. Despite the common term *food poisoning* being treated loosely as synonymous with food intoxication, most food poisonings are caused by a variety of pathogenic bacteria, viruses, or parasites contaminating the food, not by their toxins. *Staphylococcus*, *Salmonella*, and *Clostridium* are among the common bacterial genera causing food poisoning; and the most prominent viral contaminant found in foods is hepatitis virus.

The toxins from microbes can accumulate within certain tissues of predacious aquatic animals which may become a source of seafood poisoning for organisms on the higher trophic levels in a food web. These toxins include tetrodotoxin, saxitoxin, ciguatoxin, and domoic acid toxin, all of which affect primarily the nervous system (Chapter 17). Tetrodotoxin and saxitoxin block the sodium channels whereas ciguatoxin opens them. Domoic acid stimulates the excitatory amino acids at certain (e.g., glutamate) receptors. And ingestion of scombrotoxin in fish may cause illness resembling a histamine attack, with symptoms including facial flushing, sweating, dizziness, palpitations, tingling, and burning sensations around the mouth.

Fish and shellfish as sources actually account for a significant portion of foodborne illnesses throughout the world. In general, three types of diseases may result from seafood consumption: allergy, infection, and intoxication. These days, fish has become a popular food in the United States owing to better appreciation of their health benefits. Consequently, fishing stocks in the nation are now reportedly at an all-time low.

Examples of contaminants with less acute and more subtle symptoms are the POCs (persistent organochlorine compounds) and toxic metals (e.g., mercury, cadmium, lead) present in contaminated fish or other foods. Agrochemicals are chemicals used in agricultural practice and animal husbandry with the intent to raise farm yields at the lowest cost possible. These agents include pesticides (e.g. insecticides, herbicides, fungicides), plant growth regulators, and veterinary drugs (e.g. fluoroquinolones, malachite green, nitrofuran, chloramphenicol, rBST). Through environmental pollution, many of these contaminants can spread over a variety of media to end in the foods consumed by people. Toxic metals and pesticides as food contaminants have contributed to public's uneasiness over the pollution boom in the past half century, starting likely in the early 1960s when the publication of *Silent Spring* helped launch the environmental movement (Chapter 3). Pesticides in foods are predominantly residues from their use on growing crops, rather than from post-harvest applications on stored agricultural commodities. In contrast, toxic metals contaminate foods nearly at all stages along the food production line. The toxicological properties of toxic metals and pesticides are discussed in Chapters 14 and 15, respectively. Overall, food contaminants in these two groups, as with those in the other groups discussed earlier, contribute to a wide array of public health problems.

21.3. Toxic Substances in Household Products

Many chemical active ingredients in the household products sold in the United States are not harmless, as evident from the requirement that these chemicals all necessarily come with a Material Safety Data Sheet (MSDS) per mandate of the federal Hazard Communication Standard (Section 20.4.5). These MSDS, or their equivalents required in other countries, all contain a section on hazard identification or similar information for the material at issue. For example, cocamide diethanolamine (a.k.a. cocamide DEA) is commonly used as a foam stabilizer in hand soaps, shampoos, and other bath products. The MSDS specifies that this stabilizer can cause irritation to the skin, eyes, and respiratory tract. A study in mice showed kidney and liver cancers caused from DEA or its fatty acid derivative applied to the skin repeatedly for two years (NTP, 1999).

Of all the chemicals found in homes, about 150 were linked to asthma attacks, allergies, birth defects, tumors, and psychological abnormalities. As noted in Chapter 4, the toxic chemicals in household cleaners are three times more likely to cause cancer than outdoor air pollution. And indoor air in homes was found to have five times higher toxic chemical concentrations compared to outdoor air. According to a report cited by U.S. EPA (1989; 2013), studies from Europe and the United States showed that people in industrialized countries spent more than 90 percent of their time indoors.

Figure 21.2 presents a graphic overview of four major categories of toxic household products commonly found in homes, along with their individual subcategories intended to highlight more specifically the sources of toxic household substances. As with food toxicants, following the graphic presentation are separate brief accounts of the general aspects of these various source (sub)categories, including the current toxicological concerns on some of the toxic substances selected as specific examples.

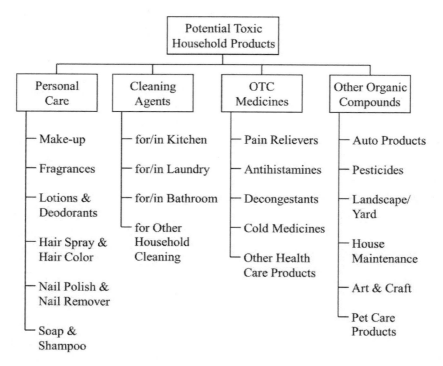

Figure 21.2. Major Categories of American Household Products in Which Potentially Toxic Substances Can Be Found *(OTC = Over-the-Counter)*

21.3.1. Substances in Personal Care Products

Products in this category represent a huge and highly diverse collection of household goods including facial tissue, cleansing pads, colognes, fragrances, cosmetics, deodorants, gloss lipsticks, eye liners, makeups, personal lubricants, mouthwashes, shampoos, skin creams, toilet papers, toothpastes, and many more. Along with cocamide DEA introduced earlier, the substances discussed here below represent only the more prominent among the numerous various ingredients in personal care products that are found to potentially pose public health concerns.

Sodium lauryl sulfate (SLS) is an anionic surfactant used in many cleaning and hygiene products, including shampoos and liquid soaps. The MSDS lists the surfactant as mutagenic for bacteria and yeast. A preliminary clinical investigation suggested that SLS in toothpastes could cause the recurrence of canker sores (Herlofson and Barkvoll, 1994). According to the *Cosmetic Ingredient Review* (CIR, 1983) issued by the U.S. Personal Care Products Council, studies showed that SLS had a high dermal absorption rate and maintained residual levels in major organs such as the liver, lungs, and brain. These findings thereby pose serious concerns regarding the surfactant's potential health threat from its use in personal care products. The review noted that when rats in a study were exposed to a formulation containing 15% ammonium lauryl sulfate (a compound identical to SLS in structure except for the cation), 4 of the 20 test animals experienced eye damage, along with depression, labored breathing, severe skin irritation, or death.

Sodium laureth sulfate (SLeS), a chemical cousin of SLS, is an inexpensive as well as a highly effective foaming agent. It is thus also commonly found in soaps, shampoos, toothpastes, and many other personal care products. Although SLeS is somewhat less irritating than SLS, it cannot be metabolized by the liver. Its toxic effects are thereby longer-lasting. Some cosmetic materials containing SLeS were found to have been contaminated with low levels of the carcinogen 1,4-dioxane (Black *et al.*, 2001).

Polyethylene glycol (PEG) and its various available forms are used in a large variety of products from cleansing (e.g., caustic spray-on oven cleaner), medical (e.g., laxative), to personal care (e.g., toothpaste). Certain PEGs of high molecular weight have been used successfully as a dietary preventive agent against colorectal cancer in test animals (Corpet *et al.*, 2000). However, many PEGs were also found to contain potential toxic impurities such as 1,4-dioxane and the neurotoxicant ethylene oxide (CIR, 1999).

Propylene glycol (PG) is a common moisturizer ingredient used in mouthwash, cosmetics, shampoo, and toothpaste, in addition to being used as a food additive and in antifreeze. It has been linked to liver and kidney damages in laboratory animals, and to common skin rashes and lesions in humans. The MSDS warns against skin contact with the chemical due to its ability to quickly penetrate the skin, as it can then cause systemic effects leading to brain, liver, and kidney problems.

Mineral oils including baby oil are produced from petroleum for use in numerous moisturizing materials. It can interfere with the skin's ability to exchange carbon dioxide for oxygen in the air, by forming an impermeable film over the skin pores. Because of this effect, it promotes acne and other skin disorders. Mineral oils have been linked to early aging. Any product containing mineral oils may be contaminated by certain PAHs (polycyclic aromatic hydrocarbons), of which many are potential carcinogens.

Isopropyl (rubbing) alcohol is a solvent and denaturant commonly found in hair color rinses, hand lotions, fragrances, and many other cosmetics. It is oxidized by alcohol dehydrogenase in the liver into acetone, a metabolite that like the alcohol is a CNS (central nervous system) depressant. Repeated inhalation of isopropyl alcohol at high levels can cause headaches, dizziness, damage to the liver and kidneys, narcosis, and coma.

Fragrances are a collection of over 3,000 mostly synthetic ingredients used in many deodorants, shampoos, sunscreens, and products for body, skin, or baby care. As many of these ingredients are petroleum by-products, some are carcinogenic whereas many others are highly toxic. Symptoms reported to the FDA to this date have included asthma attacks, headaches, dizziness, rashes, violent coughing, and skin allergic reactions. Some workers believed that the ingredients in perfumes and colognes worn by co-workers added to the chemical mixtures in indoor air that were allegedly responsible for the development or exacerbation of sick building syndrome (Fisher, 1998; FPIN, 2002).

Imidazolidinyl urea and 1,3-dimethylol-5,5-dimethylhydantoin (a.k.a. DMDM hydantoin) are two of the more common formaldehyde-releasing preservatives available today.

Nearly all brands of skin care, hair care, antiperspirants, and nail polishes found in stores contain these or other formaldehyde-releasing ingredients. Formaldehyde (CH_2O) is a colorless, pungent-smelling gas at ambient temperature (Chapter 13). It can cause watery eyes, burning sensations in the eyes, nose, and throat, as well as nausea, coughing, and breathing difficulty in some people exposed to air levels above 0.1 ppm (parts per million). At higher levels, formaldehyde can trigger asthma and allergic reactions. Formaldehyde has been found to cause cancer in humans and laboratory animals (ATSDR, 1999; CPSC, 1997; Chapter 13).

FD&C type colorants are used in many cosmetics, in addition to foods and drugs. Many of these color pigments can induce skin sensitivity and irritation. Absorption of some of these pigments can cause oxygen depletion in the body and hence even death. There is now rising controversy over their use, owing to the many inconsistent findings on their toxic effects observed in animal studies (*see* Section 21.2.1).

21.3.2. Substances in Cleaning Agents

Cleaning agents can be highly toxic if they are not handled properly. Laundry detergents and oven cleaners are the two most common examples. Other examples include carpet and upholstery shampoos, furniture polishes, toilet bowl cleaners, and dishwasher detergents. Children are at a higher risk when playing on floors contaminated by chemical residues from applications of household cleaners. These youngsters are usually the first to breathe the toxic fumes produced by these cleaning agents; and their immunological systems are not fully developed compared to those of the adults.

Laundry detergents contain phosphorus, enzymes, ammonia, phenol, and many other substances. These ingredients collectively can cause a wide array of acute (and at times also chronic) adverse health problems (e.g., rashes, itches, allergies, sinus headaches). In particular, ammonia (NH_3) is both a highly volatile inorganic gas and a very potent irritant to the skin, eyes, and respiratory tract. Phenol (C_6H_5OH) is an organic compound which in vapor form is corrosive to the skin, eyes, and respiratory tract. On prolonged contact, this organic can cause the skin to burn and break out in hives.

Oven cleaners are among the most toxic products used in homes. They contain lye and ammonia, as well as their lingering fumes that can burn the skin, eyes, and lungs. Lye's chemical name is sodium hydroxide ($NaOH$), which is also known as caustic soda and by itself is already a highly corrosive substance.

Many carpet and upholstery shampoos are designed with the additional utility of removing stains. They fulfill this added objective by including highly toxic substances such as ammonium hydroxide (NH_4OH) and PCE (perchloroethylene). As noted in Chapter 13, PCE is a carcinogenic solvent that can additionally cause damage to the kidneys, liver, and nervous system. NH_4OH, like $NaOH$, is not only a strong corrosive agent but also a potent irritant to the skin, eyes, and respiratory system.

Many dishwasher detergents contain chlorine (Cl) specifically at a high concentration. Chlorine is a potent bleaching agent and a strong disinfectant. Its harmful effects will be intensified when its fumes are heated, as in a hot shower. As per product label warning, consumers handling chlorine products are required to use goggles or face masks, protective gloves, and proper ventilation. In addition, mixing chlorine with ammonia or acid toilet bowl cleaners may easily produce fumes that can be lethal.

Air fresheners are designed to interfere with a person's sense of smell by including a nerve-deadening agent or by coating nasal passages with an oil film, such as with methoxychlor which is a toxic organochlorine (pesticide) tending to accumulate in fatty tissues. Other common toxic ingredients found in air fresheners include *p*-dichlorobenzene (e.g., the ingredient of mothball), naphthalene, and formaldehyde.

Many toilet bowl cleaners are acidic as they typically contain hydrochloric acid (HCl) and hypochlorite (ClO⁻) bleach, both of which are highly corrosive to the skin, eyes, and respiratory tract. If accidentally ingested as by naïve toddlers, these cleaner products would cause vomiting, pulmonary edema, or coma.

Furniture polishes may contain naphtha (i.e., petroleum distillates) which can cause irritation of the skin, eyes, and throat, as well as dermatitis and chronic respiratory disease. These products may also contain nitrobenzene ($C_6H_5NO_2$) which is easily absorbed through the skin and can cause fatigue, shortness of breath, cyanosis, and even coma.

21.3.3. Substances in Over-the-Counter Medicines

Over-the-counter (OTC)) medicines used in homes are mostly pain relievers, antihistamines, decongestants, and cold medicines. Pain relievers available without prescription include acetaminophen, which is the most commonly used active ingredient, and a number of anti-inflammatory drugs. These OTC drugs are supposed to be safe to use as long as they are not taken at an excess dose or for an excessive long period. Otherwise, the most common side effects from these drugs are gastritis and ulcers.

Other OTC pain-relieving compounds are largely topicals. They are predominately creams that can be rubbed on or around a painful area of the body. Some of these creams such as capsaicin (a.k.a., hot pepper) are proven helpful and can be used by patients having musculoskeletal pains. These compounds may also be used as substitutes for stronger drugs that come with more or more serious side effects.

Antihistamines are used to relieve or prevent allergy symptoms which generally include itching, sneezing, runny nose, and watery eyes. Two generations of OTC antihistamines have been made available to this date, with brompheniramine and doxylamine commonly representing the first generation whereas cetirizine and loratadine representing the second. When the body is exposed to allergens, it releases the organic nitrogen molecules known as histamines which will cause the body's cells to swell and leak fluid upon contact, leading to a sequence of allergic reactions. Antihistamines are designed to block histamines from attaching to the cells in the body and thereby from causing allergy symptoms. Some of these OTC drugs can make a patient feel drowsy, thereby affecting the patient's ability to drive safely or think clearly. In some cases, antihistamine can also cause abdominal pains and headaches.

The vast majority of (nasal) decongestants (e.g., ephedrine, pseudoephedrine) act by enhancing vasoconstriction of the blood vessels in the nose, throat, and paranasal sinuses, to result in reduced inflammation (i.e., reduced swelling) and reduced mucus formation in these areas. Common side effects with decongestants include hypertension, insomnia (sleeplessness), anxiety, dizziness, excitability, and nervousness.

In addition to nasal decongestant and antihistamine, cough suppressant and expectorant are the major types of ingredients found either alone or in combination in the OTC cold and cough medicines. Cough suppressant acts by suppressing the cough reflex in the throat and lungs, so that the mucus or irritation there will not trigger coughing. Expectorant acts by loosening thick mucus, making it easier to cough up and out. The side effects with these two types of ingredients are usually minimal.

Yet in all cases whenever possible, these OTC medicines should not be taken along with other medications or with substances such as alcohol that together can cause adverse drug interaction. Many people have heard how older folks complain about all the pills that they need to take simultaneously. There have been studies showing that a considerable number of older people are addicted to various prescription drugs and alcohol, while many others misuse them (e.g., Patterson and Jeste, 1999).

Drug-drug or drug-alcohol interaction is a biochemical reaction (Section 10.4) that indeed can result in severe health consequences. For instance, acetaminophen (e.g., the active ingredient in Tylenol®) may cause liver damage in people having excessive daily consumption of alcohol over a long period. Alcohol can aggravate CNS depression in people taking antidepressants (e.g., Prozac, Elavil, Wellbutrin) or sedatives (e.g., Valium, Phenobarbital). Drug-drug interaction can also lead to severe side effects such as fatigue, excessive sedation, coma, and even death, despite the general observation that in most cases the side effects from the individual drugs are mild or unnoticeable.

21.3.4. Substances in Other Organic Compounds

Other harmful or potentially harmful organic compounds commonly found in a home include those contained in: gasoline (e.g., for lawn mower operation); paints and paint products; floor and furniture polishes; inks; degreasers; pesticides; and (some) batteries. Paints, paint strippers, and varnishes all contain organic solvents, such as benzene, methylene chloride, or toluene. Gasoline and other fuel products also contain organic solvents, such as members of the so-called BTEX group (i.e., *b*enzene, *t*oluene, *e*thylbenzene, *xy*lene isomers), hexane, cyclohexane, and sometimes ethanol, as additives.

The following types of pesticide products are commonly found in homes: cockroach sprays and baits; insect repellents for personal use; rat and other rodent poisons; flea and tick sprays; pet collars; kitchen, laundry, or bathroom disinfectants and sanitizers; products that kill mold and mildew; some garden and lawn care products (e.g., weed killers); and swimming pool disinfectants.

Many of these (other) organic compounds found in a home are highly flammable, corrosive, or toxic (with some being discussed in some detail in Chapters 13 and 15). As so specifically urged at the CPSC and U.S. EPA websites, household products of this kind should be stored per label instructions and out of the reach of children and pets. Effective measures should include having all potentially toxic household products locked in a garden shed, in a cabinet free of food items, or in a utility area with sufficient air flow.

21.4. Learning Lessons with Food and Household Products

In addition to BPA (bisphenol A) noted above as well as in Chapter 19, in recent years at least three chemicals/chemical groups have raised public health concerns over their presence in food or household products. These include the residues of many PTS (persistent toxic substances) found in fish tissue worldwide, the lead (Pb) coated on (American) children's jewelry or toys, and the triclosan used as an antibacterial ingredient in (American) health care products. Pollution issues concerning the presence of these toxic substances are highlighted in Chapters 3, 4, 14, and 16. In this section, as part of the learning lessons of contemporary environmental health issues, further elaborations are given on specific incidences relevant to their presence in food or household products. This section as well as this chapter ends with a practical approach to the mitigation and prevention of exposure from such harmful food and household products.

21.4.1. Persistent Toxic Substances in Seafood

As noted in Chapter 16, many PTS of global concern are POCs (persistent organochlorine compounds). Between the 1990s and the early 2000s, a number of POCs were analyzed for their residue levels in fish from localities across various countries. It turned out that, as summarized in Table 6.2 (for the 1990s) and Table 6.3 (for the early 2000s), the fish samples from each of these localities had tissue residue levels far exceeding U.S. EPA's screening values for at least one of the POCs analyzed. In particular, an extensive collaboration study by Hites *et al.* (2004) showed significant residue levels of several POCs detected in farm-raised salmon from around the globe.

The collaboration study analyzed over two metric tons of farmed and wild salmon from around the world for PCBs and other POC contaminants. The analysis found significantly higher residue levels of these contaminants in farmed salmon than in their wild counterpart. The study also observed a significantly greater contaminant load in salmon raised in Europe than in North or South America. The investigators were concerned that consumption of farmed salmon might pose health risk to the point that it would detract from the basic beneficial effects of fish consumption. Their concern can be important in that, as they put it, the annual global production of farmed salmon has increased 40-fold since some 35 years ago, primarily because salmon from farms in Chile, northern Europe, and North America are now available to consumers year round at more affordable prices.

21.4.2. Lead on Children's Jewelry and Toys

In recent years, a series of acute lead poisoning cases has been linked to children's jewelry and toys sold in the United States. Many of these jewelry and toys were manufactured overseas where labor costs were more affordable. Some of these products were found to have been coated with relatively high contents of lead on their surfaces. Further investigations for these cases led to a number of nationwide product recalls.

Of particular concern at the national level were two recall cases involving two children exposed to two unsuspected objects, with both cases happening within the past decade or so. The first case occurred in the state of Oregon in 2003 (VanArsdale *et al.*, 2004). It involved a four-year-old boy with intermittent diarrhea, abdominal pain, and vomiting lingering for weeks. The boy was first misdiagnosed by his physician as having viral gastroenteritis. An abdominal radiograph performed on a later visit showed a metallic object in the boy's stomach, without evidence of obstruction. A subsequent endoscopy led to the retrieval of a U.S. coin and a medallion pendant from the patient's stomach. A venous blood lead level (BLL) measurement showed an extremely elevated content of 123 μg/dL (as currently the level of concern is typically set at 10 μg/dL).

The medallion, which the boy obtained from a toy vending machine, was reportedly made in and imported from India. It contained by weight 38.8% (388 mg/g) lead (Pb), 3.6% antimony (Sb), and 0.5% tin (Sn), as measured by the Oregon state government's Department of Environmental Quality Laboratory. Similar medallions obtained from toy vending machines shortly afterward were found containing similar high contents of lead. Oregon state health officials thus notified CPSC for a nationwide investigation, which soon resulted in a national voluntary recall of 150 million pieces of the imported metallic toy jewelry sold in vending machines (*see*, e.g., CDC, 2006).

The other recall case involved some 300,000 pieces of heart-shaped charm bracelets available during the three-month period between March and May in 2004. The bracelets were provided as a free gift with a purchase of children's footwear in certain styles manufactured by Reebok International. In 2006, Reebok received a report about a boy in Minneapolis, Minnesota dying from lead poisoning after swallowing a piece of the bracelet (*see*, e.g., CDC, 2006).

The boy, who was also four years old but with a medical history of microcephaly and developmental delay, was brought to an emergency room (ER) with a complaint of vomiting. Again, as in the previous case, the patient was misdiagnosed with a probable viral gastroenteritis, and accordingly was given an antiemetic but then released home. When the boy returned to the ER two days later with a poor oral intake and intractable vomiting, he was admitted to the hospital and received an IV (intravenous) fluid replacement. The next day, when the boy was being transferred to the radiology department, he had a seizure which led to a respiratory arrest. After resuscitation, the boy was placed on a ventilator. Different tests were then performed on the boy on the following day, including one showing a BLL of 180 μg/dL and another revealing no blood flow to the brain. The boy was pronounced dead on the fourth day of hospitalization. Abdominal radiographs revealed a foreign heart-shaped object in his stomach. When the ingested charm was measured for lead content, it was found to contain (by weight) 99.1% of lead.

In reviewing these cases where children were the victims, it is important to note again that children are more susceptible to most toxicants compared to adults. Lead is a potent neurotoxicant that can cause intellectual impairment and death particularly among children. This is because children are in the most critical phase of human development. Their frontal lobes are particularly vulnerable to the effects of lead poisoning. Lead neurotoxicity in children can result in disruption of vital functions, attention, behavioral conduct, and impulse control, all of which may not be fully appreciated until late childhood.

21.4.3. Triclosan in Antibacterial Products

Triclosan ($C_{12}H_7Cl_3O_2$) is a lipophilic polychloro phenoxy phenol commonly used as an active ingredient in many antibacterial products. Due to its widespread use in products ranging from soaps to plastics, alarming levels of this antimicrobial agent have been found in ground and surface waters (e.g., Loraine and Pettigrove, 2006; Servos *et al.*, 2007) and in the urine of nearly 1,900 (75%) of the 2,517 participants tested in a national survey (CDC, 2010). Studies showed that triclosan caused endocrine disruption in amphibians (Veldhoen *et al.*, 2006) and allergies in humans (Clayton *et al.*, 2011). A literature review (Aiello *et al.*, 2007) concluded that consumer soaps containing triclosan were no more effective than plain soaps in preventing infectious illnesses, and that this antibacterial agent could induce the development of resistant strains of bacteria.

Triclosan can promote the emergence of antibiotic-resistant bacteria because its mode of action and its target site are similar to those of many antibiotics. In other words, the bacteria that became resistant to triclosan would likely become resistant to many antibiotics as well, thereby making the latter also ineffective. Triclosan can bioaccumulate in fatty tissues due to its high lipophilicity which allows it to have an easy entry into the human body. Recent findings that triclosan might serve as a production source for several dioxin congeners also caused public health concerns (e.g., Buth *et al.*, 2010), inasmuch as some dioxins have been found carcinogenic or highly toxic to humans and animals.

21.4.4. Self-Mitigation and Self-Prevention

Most human exposures to harmful food and household products, including those such as problem toys not listed in Figure 21.2, are highly preventable. For toxic household products and many other consumer goods, the most effective mitigation measure is *self-prevention* along with common sense. It is with this notion that CPSC has urged parents and caregivers to follow the 10 poison prevention tips that the Commission (e.g., CPSC, 2003) periodically publicizes as effective prevention measures. As reproduced below, these 10 prevention tips are simply a set of common sense type housekeeping principles.

1. Keep all products locked up from children, out of sight and out of reach.
2. Use child-resistant packaging properly by closing the container securely after each use or choose child-resistant unit packaging which (that) does not need to be re-secured.

3. Call the 800 hotline immediately in case of poisoning.

4. When products are in use, keep children in sight, even if the adult must take them along when answering the phone or doorbell.

5. Keep items in original containers.

6. Leave the original labels on all products, and read the label before using.

7. Do not put decorative lamps and candles that contain lamp oil (in a place) where children can reach them. (Note: lamp oil can be highly toxic if ingested by children.)

8. Always turn the light on when giving or taking medicine so that the caregiver or patient can see what he/she is giving or taking. Check the dosage every time.

9. Avoid taking medicine in front of children.

10. Clean out the medicine cabinet periodically and safely dispose of unneeded and outdated medicines.

The manufacturers are also required to do their share. It is a law in the United States, such as under the *Federal Insecticide, Fungicide, and Rodenticide Act Section 25 (c)(3)*, that they distribute certain household products in an effective child-resistant packaging. There is also a strong appeal for them to promote more effective senior-friendly packaging of household products, along with more effective safety instructions.

For prevention of exposure to food toxicants, again by far the most effective strategy or measure would or should be the consumer's self-awareness and self-prevention. This is because in most instances, ultimate prevention of food poisoning or food intoxication is considered more practical and more effective at the individual level than either at the community level or by means of regulatory intervention.

Using the earlier case with POC-contaminated salmon as an example, the first step of self-prevention is for the consumer to make every effort to purchase younger salmon to eat since compared to older fish, younger ones have less lifetime to concentrate the POCs in their body. Prior to cleaning the younger fish thoroughly, the consumer should remove the fish's guts, since many POCs tend to concentrate not only in a fish's fat but also in its organs including especially its liver, stomach, and intestines.

Given that POCs are stored primarily in the fat, and that fat in fish is located primarily along the back, the belly, as well as the dark meat area, the consumer should trim the fat, remove the skin, and cut away the fatty dark meat. Skinning the fish will remove the thin layer of fat under the skin. The final step is for the consumer to cook the fish in a way that would allow the fat to drip away or drain off. This can be accomplished effectively with most cooking methods (e.g., baking, broiling, steaming, grilling). Data gathered by U.S. EPA (2000) showed that up to 60% of the POCs can be reduced by the way in which the fat is dripped away or drained off, although a subsequent study (Hori *et al.*, 2005) in Japan supported a reduction of only up to 31% by various cooking methods.

This lower reduction yield nonetheless might have been largely or only due to the different fish species or cooking methods used in the Japanese study.

References

Aiello AE, Larson EL, Levy SB, 2007. Consumer Antibacterial Soaps: Effective or Just Risky? *Clin. Infect. Dis.* 45(Suppl 2):137-147.

Andersen A, 2006. Final Report on the Safety Assessment of Benzaldehyde. *Int. J. Toxicol.* 25 (Suppl 1):11-27

ATSDR (Agency for Toxic Substances and Disease Registry), 1999. Toxicological Profile for Formaldehyde. U.S. Department of Health and Human Services, Atlanta, Georgia, USA.

Biles JE, McNeal TP, Begley TH, 1997. Determination of Bisphenol A Migrating from Epoxy Can Coatings to Infant Formula Liquid Concentrates. *J. Agric. Food Chem.* 45:4697-4700.

Black RE, Hurley FJ, Havery DC, 2001. Occurrence of 1,4-Dioxane in Cosmetic Raw Materials and Finished Cosmetic Products. *J. AOAC Int.* 84:666-760.

Buth JM, Steen PO, Sueper C, Blumentritt D, Vikesland PJ, Arnold WA, McNeill K, 2010. Dioxin Photoproducts of Triclosan and Its Chlorinated Derivatives in Sediment Cores. *Environ. Sci. Technol.* 44:4545-4551.

Canada Gazette, 2010. Regulatory Impact Assessment Statement. 144(Part II):3-14.

Castle L, Jickells SM, Gilbert J, Harrison N, 1990. Migration Testing of Plastics and Microwave-Active Materials for High-Temperature Food-Use Applications. *Food Addit. Contam.* 7:779-796.

CDC (U.S. Centers for Disease Control and Prevention), 2006. Death of a Child After Ingestion of a Metallic Charm – Minnesota, 2006. *MMWR* 23:1-2.

CDC (U.S. Centers for Disease Control and Prevention), 2010. National Report on Human Exposure to Environmental Chemicals – Triclosan. Fact Sheet. U.S. Department of Health and Human Services, Atlanta, Georgia.

CIR (Cosmetic Ingredient Review), 1983. Final Report on the Safety Assessment of Sodium Lauryl Sulfate. *J. Amer. College Toxicol.* 2:127-181.

CIR (Cosmetic Ingredient Review), 1999. Final Report on the Safety Assessment of PEG-2, -3, -5, -10, -15, and -20 Cocamine. *Int. J. Toxicol.* 18:43-50.

Clayton EM, Todd M, Dowd JB, Aiello AE, 2011. The Impact of Bisphenol A and Triclosan on Immune Parameters in the US Population, NHANES 2003-2006. *Environ. Health Perspect.* 119: 390-396.

Corpet DE, Parnaud G, Delverdier M, Peiffer G, Tache S, 2000. Consistent and Fast Inhibition of Colon Carcinogenesis by Polyethylene Glycol in Mice and Rats Given Various Carcinogens. *Cancer Res.* 60:3160-3164.

CPSC (U.S. Consumer Product Safety Commission), 1997. An Update on Formaldehyde, 1997 Revision. Washington DC, USA.

CPSC (U.S. Consumer Product Safety Commission), 2003. *National Poison Prevention Week Warns New Parents to Lock Up Medicines and Household Chemicals*. Release #03-092. Washington DC, USA.

CPSC (U.S. Consumer Product Safety Commission), 2009. *CPSC Warns That 9 Out of 10 Unintentional Child Poisonings Occur in the Home*. Release #09159 (dated 18 March). Washington DC, USA.

FAO/WHO (Food Agriculture Organization of the United Nations/World Health Organization), 1994. Food Additives. Codex Alimentarius, Vol. XIV. Rome, Italy.

FDA (U.S. Food and Drug Administration), 1992. Food Additives. FDA/IFIC Brochure: January 1992. Rockville, Maryland, USA.

FDA (U.S. Food and Drug Administration), 1995. Food Additives; Threshold of Regulation for Substances Used in Food-Contact Articles. *Federal Register* 60:36582-36596.

FDA (U.S. Food and Drug Administration), 2010. Update on Bisphenol A for Use in Food Contact Applications: January 2010. Silver Spring, Maryland, USA.

Fisher BE, 1998. Scents & Sensitivity. *Environ. Health Perspect.* 106:A594-A599.

FPIN (Fragranced Products Information Network), 2002. Fragrances: The Health Risks. Columbia, Missouri, USA.

Gibson RL, 2007. Toxic Baby Bottles – Scientific Study Finds Leaching Chemicals in Clear Plastic Baby Bottles. Environmental California Research & Policy Center, 3435 Wilshire Boulevard, Suite 385, Los Angeles, California, USA.

Hauser R, Duty S, Godfrey-Bailey L, Calafat AM, 2004. Medications as a Source of Human Exposure to Phthalates. *Environ. Health Perspect.* 112:751-753.

Herlofson BB, Barkvoll P, 1994. Sodium Lauryl Sulfate and Recurrent Aphthous Ulcers: A Preliminary Study. *Acta Odontol. Scand.* 52:257-259.

Hites RA, Foran JA, Carpenter DO, Hamilton MC, Knuth BA, Schwager SJ, 2004. Global Assessment of Organic Contaminants in Farmed Salmon. *Science* 303:226-229.

Hori T, Nakagawa R, Tobiishi K, Iida L, Tsutsumi T, Sasaki K, Toyoda M, 2005. Effects of Cooking on Concentrations of Polychlorinated Dibenzo-p-Dioxins and Related Compounds in Fish and Meat. *J. Agric. Food Chem.* 53:8820-8828.

Loraine GA, Pettigrove ME, 2006. Seasonal Variations in Concentrations of Pharmaceuticals and Personal Care Products in Drinking Water and Reclaimed Wastewater in Southern California. *Environ. Sci. Technol.* 40:687-695.

Mehedi N, Ainad-Tabet S, Mokrane N, Addou S, Zaoui C, Kheroua O, Saidi D, 2009. Reproductive Toxicology of Tartrazine (FD and C Yellow No. 5) in Swiss Albino Mice. *Amer. J. Pharmacol. Toxicol.* 4:130-135.

Munguia-Lopez EM, Peralta E, Gonzalez-Leon A, Vargas-Requena C, Soto-Valdez H, 2002. Migration of Bisphenol A (BPA) from Epoxy Can Coatings to Jalapeño Peppers and an Acid Food Stimulant. *J. Agric. Food Chem.* 50:7299-7302.

NRC (U.S. National Research Council), 1999. *The Use of Drugs in Food Animals – Benefits and Risks.* Committee on Drug Use in Food Animals, Board on Agriculture. Washington DC, USA: National Academy Press.

NTP (U.S. National Toxicology Program), 1999. Toxicology and Carcinogenesis Studies of Diethanolamine (CAS No. 111-42-2) in F344/N Rats and B6C3F1 Mice (Dermal Studies). Research Triangle Park, North Carolina, USA.

Page BD, Lacroix GM, 1995. The Occurrence of Phthalate Esters and Di-2-Ethylhexyl Adipate Plasticizers in Canadian Packaging and Food Samples in 1985-1989: A Survey. *Food Addit. Contam.* 12:129-151.

Patterson TL, Jeste DV, 1999. The Potential Impact of the Baby-Boom Generation on Substance Abuse among Elderly Persons. *Psychiatr. Serv.* 50:1184-1188.

Scallan E, Hoekstra RM, Angulo FJ, Tauxe RV, Widdowson MA, Roy SL, Jones JL, Griffin PM, 2011. Foodborne Illness Acquired in the United States – Major Pathogens. *Emerg. Infect. Dis.* 17:7-15.

Servos MR, Smith M, Mcinnis R, Burnison BK, Lee B-H, Seto P, Backus S, 2007. The Presence of Selected Pharmaceuticals and the Antimicrobial Triclosan in Drinking Water in Ontario, Canada. *Water Quality Res. J. Canada* 42:130-137.

U.S. EPA (U.S. Environmental Protection Agency), 1989. Report to Congress on Indoor Air Quality, Volume II: Assessment and Control of Indoor Air Pollution. EPA 400-1-89-001C. Office of Air and Radiation, Washington DC, USA.

U.S. EPA (U.S. Environmental Protection Agency), 2000. Guidance for Assessing Chemical Contaminant Data for Use in Fish Advisories: Volume 2. Risk Assessment and Fish Consumption Limits – Third Edition. EPA 823-B-00-008. Office of Water, Washington DC, USA.

U.S. EPA (U.S. Environmental Protection Agency), 2013. *Indoor Air Pollution: An Introduction for Health Professionals.* Washington DC, USA. http://www.epa.gov/iaq/pubs/hpguide.html.

VanArsdale JL, Leiker RD, Kohn M, Merritt TA, Horowitz BZ, 2004. Lead Poisoning from a Toy Necklace. *Pediatrics* 114:1096-1099.

Veldhoen N, Skirrow RC, Osachoff H, Wigmore H, Clapson DJ, Gunderson MP, Van Aggelen G, Helbing CC, 2006. The Bactericidal Agent Triclosan Modulates Thyroid Hormone-Associated Gene Expression and Disrupts Postembryonic Anuran Development. *Aquatic Toxicol.* 80:217-227.

Vorhees CV, Butcher RE, Brunner RL, Wootten V, Sobotka TJ, 1983. Developmental Toxicity and Psychotoxicity of FD and C Red Dye No. 40 (Allura Red AC) in Rats. *Toxicology* 28:207-217.

Review Questions

1. Briefly explain the major health concerns with toxic household substances.

2. Briefly explain the major health concerns with food toxicants.

3. What are the general source categories of food toxicants?

4. Are substances on the GRAS list required to undergo premarket approval by FDA? And if yes, why? And if no, why not?

5. Match *each* of the characteristics, sources, or effects in the right column to *only one* of the food additives in the left column that are potentially harmful when consumed excessively.

(1) vitamin D	(a) substance for wholesomeness
(2) lecithin	(b) on the GRAS list
(3) BHA	(c) substance for product consistency
(4) tartrazine	(d) flavoring agent
(5) vitamin C	(e) from plastic
(6) polyethylene terephthalate	(f) antioxidant
(7) monosodium glutamate	(g) food colorant

6. Briefly describe FDA's four criteria set forth in its Threshold of Regulation program for use to determine the threshold of no appreciable human health risk.

7. Name four indirect food additives commonly found in paper materials used for packaging or holding foods.

8. Name four polymers commonly found as indirect food additives.

9. Name the six major categories of drugs commonly used to treat food animals.

10. Which group of food contaminants has one of the serious consequences in terms of agroeconomics and public health? And why?

11. Name four neurotoxins commonly found in seafood.

12. What are the general source categories of toxic household substances?

13. Name eight potential toxic ingredients commonly found in personal care products.

14. What are the OTC antihistamines mostly used for? And what are their common side effects?

15. Which of the following pairs includes the two most common examples of potentially toxic cleaning agents? a) dishwasher detergents, toilet bowl cleaners; b) oven cleaners, air fresheners; c) laundry detergents, toilet bowl cleaners; d) laundry detergents, oven cleaners.

16. What are the four BTEX organic solvents commonly found in gasoline?

17. Give six use groups of pesticide products that are commonly found in a home.

18. What appears to be the understated concern with the use of OTC medicines?

19. What may be a major side effect when people take pain relievers containing acetaminophen as the active ingredient (e.g., in Tylenol®), along with excessive daily consumption of alcohol over a long period?

20. What illness or symptom would acute lead poisoning at its first stage be likely misdiagnosed with?

21. Are farm-raised salmon more or less likely to be contaminated with POCs, compared to their wild counterpart? Give a reason or justification for the answer.

22. What are the potential problems with using the antimicrobial agent triclosan?

23. For exposure to food toxicants or toxic household substances, what type of mitigation or prevention measures appears to be most effective or practical?

24. What are the basic steps that can be taken to minimize the dietary exposure to POC residues (suspected to be) present in fish?

CHAPTER 22

Human Health Aspects of Ecotoxicology

22.1. Introduction

Despite the earlier (Section 1.3.2) argument made that environmental toxicology and ecotoxicology are two separate branches of toxicology, they do have certain things in common. There are many aspects of ecotoxicology with strong implications for human health. Such strong implications from three subdivisions of ecotoxicology are introduced in this section, and further discussed in their individual sections that follow. The three select subdivisions are *aquatic toxicology, wildlife toxicology*, and *hazardous waste pollution*. They are regarded as most relevant to environmental toxicology at least in terms of their implications for human health. In each individual section, a brief account is also given about the subdivision's general development and practice in order to provide the basics for a fuller comprehension of its human health implications. It is hoped that with discussion presented in such a manner, this chapter can help attain a stronger appreciation of the significant aspects shared by the two branches of toxicology.

22.1.1. Relevance of Aquatic Toxicology

In its simplest term, aquatic toxicology is concerned with adverse effects of toxicants on aquatic organisms and on the ecosystem where these biota inhabit. Accordingly, this subdivision of ecotoxicology is largely a study of water contamination and its ecological impacts. Topics and issues covered in aquatic toxicology in general are similar to those in the toxicology for humans or other non-aquatic species: the fate and transport of major aquatic pollutants; the disposition, including toxicodynamics and toxicokinetics, of environmental toxicants in aquatic organisms; the assessment and modeling of the effects of aquatic pollution on aquatic biota; and the analysis of risks to aquatic ecosystems. As for any other types of ecosystems or other species of living organisms, the effects of toxicants on aquatic organisms may range from those at the biochemical, molecular, and cellular level to those on individuals, populations, and communities.

With respect to human health, one contribution from aquatic toxicology is the relatively simple toxicity tests developed to assure high quality of water for drinking and other uses. Water quality assurance is also crucial for supply of healthy seafood to consumers. In the United States, although the annual seafood consumption dropped slightly in 2008, it still amounted to 16 pounds per capita (NMFS, 2010). In addition, using the results from various aquatic toxicity tests developed over the years (Section 22.2.3), several health regulatory achievements have been made in the nation and worldwide.

22.1.2. Relevance of Wildlife Toxicology

For wildlife toxicology, the scope and focus are similar to those of aquatic toxicology, except for the wildlife species being broadened to include all undomesticated organisms. Wildlife toxicology thereby covers topics similar to those covered by aquatic toxicology, except for its focus being more on non-aquatic species. Pollution of concern in wildlife toxicology tends to be terrestrial in nature not only due to the plentiful terrestrial species to deal with, but also due to the notion that water pollution is by practice already covered in aquatic toxicology and to some extent also in environmental toxicology.

Although perhaps not as commonly utilized as aquatic toxicology, wildlife toxicology tends to offer a more conceivable real-life situation for human health than any other form of nonhuman models on chemical exposure or toxicity assessment. It has been argued that *in situ* exposures of pesticides to indicator species under semi-controlled, real-life conditions would offer a more realistic evaluation of effects by linking laboratory studies to observed conditions in the field (Grue *et al.*, 1982; Steffek, 1994). It thus seems unfortunate to see that much investigation into the effects of environmental pollutants in real-life situations is disregarded simply because studies of this type are exceptionally cumbersome and time-consuming to conduct with any due rigor (McBee and Lochmiller, 1996). Otherwise, field studies on wildlife and their ecosystems would offer far greater human health implications than much of the research would that has gone into investigating the toxic effects of pollutants in laboratory models (McBee and Lochmiller, 1996).

22.1.3. Relevance of Hazardous Waste Pollution

Hazardous waste is defined as any *discarded* material harmful or potentially harmful to humans or the environment. It can be a cleaning agent, fuel product, pesticide, or by-product of an industrial process. Hazardous waste thus can be in the form of a gas, liquid, solid, or sludge. The levels of various toxic wastes have been on the rise for many years, amid the public's increasing concern that individuals and industries continue to ignore this major global environmental pollution issue. Many residents and industries simply do not make a true effort either to reduce the generation of hazardous waste materials or to mitigate their toxic effects on the environment.

The reality is that most consumers tend to get rid of stuff without realizing that these waste materials would end up in a landfill or a dumpsite, and that through evaporation or leaching they could eventually come back to the residents as well as to the local or even global environment. Industries too often want to lower the high costs for the disposal of their hazardous waste. Accordingly, they prefer to have their waste materials either removed by another party or buried in landfills that they have built on site.

In any case, thousands of persistent toxic metals and chemicals can be found in hazardous waste materials. These substances can be harmful or even lethal when absorbed or ingested. When hazardous waste is landfilled, the contaminated liquid may leach and pollute groundwater used for human consumption. The implications for human health are thus much more apparent and direct with hazardous waste toxicology than with the other two subdivisions. In the United States, the Love Canal disaster is one of the most appalling environmental tragedies in the American history, and is regarded as the most tragic environmental disaster in America's history of toxic site contamination. This environmental tragedy involved the burial and subsequent discovery of some 20,000 tons of toxic waste beneath the neighborhood of Love Canal located near Niagara Falls, New York. As noted in Chapter 2, some 80 different chemicals were contained in this pile of toxic waste, of which a dozen or so were suspected or known at the time as human carcinogens.

22.2. Aquatic Toxicology and Human Health

As defined more specifically in the literature (e.g., Rand and Petrocelli, 1985; Rand *et al.*, 1995), aquatic toxicology is the qualitative as well as quantitative study of the untoward effects of toxicants on aquatic organisms. The toxic effects of concern include both lethality and sublethal toxicity. Examples of sublethal toxicity include adverse modifications in development, growth, reproduction, behavior, toxic response, and the related biochemical, physiological, or pathological functions. These detrimental effects may be expressed by quantifiable criteria such as number of organisms affected, percent of eggs hatched, percent of enzyme inhibition, change in body weight or length, incidence in skeletal abnormalities, and incidence in tumor development. In short, these adverse effects and their expressions are similar in principle to those observed and studied for wildlife and human health. Aquatic toxicology is also concerned with the concentrations and quantities of toxicants that occur or will occur in aquatic systems. Accordingly, the field necessarily includes the study of transport, distribution, biotransformation, and ultimate fate of toxicants in the aquatic environment. A brief historical account of aquatic toxicology can be found in the paper by Pritchard (1993).

22.2.1. The Basic Aquatic Environment

The aquatic environment is complex and diverse. The two principal types of aquatic ecosystems are marine and freshwater. Within each of these two distinct biomes, many different biotic (i.e., living) and abiotic (i.e., nonliving) components co-subsist.

Marine ecosystems consist of largely the open oceans, coral reefs, and estuaries. They also include salt marshes, lagoons, mangroves, the deep sea, and many other components, but to a much lesser extent in terms of academic emphasis and interest. Collectively, these components cover about 70% of the Earth's surface (e.g., Bhargava, 2001), provide over 97% of its water (e.g., UNEP, 2002), and generate about 45% of its net primary production (e.g., Geider *et al.*, 2001). The ocean region, which is the largest section of a marine biome, can be subdivided into separate zones including *oceanic* (the relatively shallow part of the ocean that lies over the continental shelf), *intertidal* (the part where the ocean meets the land), *pelagic* (where the water in the open ocean is farther from the land), *benthic* (the area below the pelagic zone), and *abyssal* (the ocean bottom). Coral reefs are considered as the rainforests of an ocean in that corals consist of predominately algae (e.g., zooxanthellae) which via photosynthesis provide a huge supply of the basic nutrients and energy for other marine lives in the food web. Estuaries are areas where freshwater streams or rivers merge with the ocean. This mixing of waters with different salt and mineral contents offers a unique aquatic ecosystem to support a highly diverse fauna, including a variety of oysters, turtles, fishes, and waterfowls.

The marine biome is home to a myriad of different species ranging from microscopic planktonic organisms, which comprise the base of the marine food chains (e.g., phytoplankton and zooplankton), to large marine mammals such as whales, dolphins, and seals. Thousands of fish species also reside in this biome, including angelfish, eel, flounder, mackerel, scup, sea bass, squid, ray, and much more. Coastal birds are likewise plentiful, including gulls, loons, pelicans, shorebirds, terns, and many more. Marine ecosystems are distinct from freshwater ecosystems due to the presence of different amounts and types of dissolved materials, especially salts, in the water. Over 80% of the dissolved materials in seawater are sodium (Na) and chlorine (Cl) molecules.

Freshwater ecosystems cover less than 1% of the Earth's surface (e.g., Likens, 1973), provide about 0.01% of its water supply or about 2.5% of its water in the form of permanent ice or snow (e.g., UNEP, 2002), and generate a negligible amount of its net primary production when compared to the marine and terrestrial ecosystems (e.g., Geider *et al.*, 2001). The freshwater biome is also home to thousands of the Earth's known fish species. There are three basic subtypes of freshwater ecosystems: *lentic* (slowly-moving water, including ponds and lakes); *lotic* (rapidly-moving water, including streams and rivers); and *wetlands* (where the soil is inundated for at least part of the time).

In both types of biomes, the biotic components consist of myriads of microorganisms, plants, and animals co-inhabiting particular niches. Also co-subsisting within each niche are abiotic components which include the physical environment (e.g., water flow, temperature, salinity). Each aquatic niche thus represents a dynamic set of complex interactions of biotic and abiotic components. The biological activities of contaminants and their impacts can be affected profoundly by such complex, dynamic interactions.

The complex, dynamic, and interactive nature of aquatic ecosystems makes it rather difficult to assess the toxic responses of these systems unless the underlying interactions have been defined and understood first. As Rand and Petrocelli (1985) put it, such an assessment is complicated by the adaptability of the biotic components, by the species diversity of the biotic components in the ecosystem, and by the differences in structural and functional responses among the biotic components.

22.2.2. Aquatic Toxicity Tests

To study the adverse responses involved in aquatic ecosystems, certain toxicity tests need to be performed. These toxicity tests are analytical tools used to quantify the toxicant amount and the exposure duration required to yield a critical or criterion effect. Due to species difference, toxicity tests employed in aquatic toxicology necessarily differ from those developed for wildlife or human health.

Algae, macroinvertebrates (e.g., clams, shrimp, oysters), and fishes are the three main groups of test organisms commonly used in aquatic toxicity tests to represent the wide range of freshwater and saltwater species that would be studied. The treated and untreated organisms can be exposed to the test water solutions and the untreated water, respectively, in a laboratory (and sometimes a field) setting, by using broadly one of the following four testing techniques (e.g., Rand and Petrocelli, 1985; Rand *et al.*, 1995):

◆ *Static test* – This involves the use of *still* water where the test organisms are exposed to the test material (e.g., the toxicant) for a fixed duration.

◆ *Re-circulation test* – In this assay, the test and control solutions are pumped or filtered through an apparatus to uphold the water quality and the concentration of the test material; it is similar to the static test in all other aspects.

◆ *Renewal test* – This is also similar to the static test in all other aspects except for the test and control solutions being renewed periodically (typically every 24 hours) by removing the test and the control organisms into chambers filled with new test and new control solutions.

◆ *Flow-through test* – In this assay, the test and the control solution flow into and out of the respective chambers housing the test subjects and the controls.

In keeping with a sound application of the above aquatic toxicity testing techniques, several protocols have been standardized by a number of public and nonprofit organizations. These include the American Public Health Association, the American Society for Testing and Materials, the International Standardization Organization, U.S. EPA, and the Organization for Economic Cooperation and Development. The testing protocols that these organizations have standardized may be categorized according to the length of exposure and the organisms to be tested. Aquatic toxicity tests thus may be separated into those with fishes, macroinvertebrates, and phytoplankton (e.g., Rand and Petrocelli, 1985; Rand *et al.*, 1995). With phytoplankton, the test is typically for a one-time event. With macroinvertebrates (e.g., *Daphnia sp.*, *Acartia sp.*, *Mysidopsis sp.*, crabs, oysters), the test is typically for acute or long-term exposure. With fishes, the various toxicity tests used are typically for bioaccumulation or for acute, early-life stage, partial chronic, or complete chronic exposure. A graphic example of the early-life stage test in fish is given in Figure 22.1 (*see*, e.g., U.S. EPA [1996] for testing guidelines). Note that the exposure duration for the newborn fish in an early-life stage test is species-dependent.

The testing protocols and techniques discussed briefly above have been used to establish the water quality criteria (WQC) recommended by U.S. EPA for approximately 150 water contaminants. Pursuant to Section 304(a) of the U.S. Clean Water Act, the WQC are published by U.S. EPA (2009) to provide guidance for states, tribes, and some other countries to use in adopting water quality standards. It is important to note that the WQC are issued not only for ecosystem quality but also (in some cases solely or mainly) for human health protection.

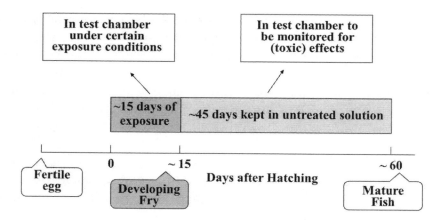

Figure 22.1. Example of an Early-Life Stage Test on Zebrafish

22.2.3. Regulatory Efforts for Water Quality

It is not surprising that in some places such as near industrial discharges, water pollution can degrade ground and surface water quality so drastically that the water there is no longer safe for drinking, swimming, crop irrigation, and other water-borne activities. In the United States, this kind of health concern has led to several regulatory efforts made to protect water quality for the public, in addition to the establishment of WQC. In particular, under the authority of the U.S. Clean Water Act, U.S. EPA established the National Pollutant Discharge Elimination System (NPDES) permit program, which controls water pollution by regulating point sources that discharge pollutants directly into aquatic systems. Point sources of pollution are defined as discrete conveyances, such as pipes or human-made ditches. In most cases, the NPDES permit program is administered by authorized states. Since its inception in 1972, the NPDES permit program has contributed many significant improvements to the nation's water quality.

Another related regulatory establishment in which U.S. EPA is obligated to implement is the Total Maximum Daily Load (TMDL) program, which aims to attain ambient water quality standards through the control of both point and non-point sources of pollution. The TMDL program also originated from the U.S. Clean Water Act. However, it was largely overlooked during the 1970s and 1980s due to the circumstance that in those years the states were very busy bringing point sources of pollution into compliance under the NPDES permit program. Several citizen lawsuits were then launched in the 1980s to eventually direct U.S. EPA into developing guidance for the TMDL program, which is now considered as equally effective in achieving the nation's water quality goals.

22.3. Wildlife Toxicology and Human Health

Wildlife toxicology has its root as early as in the late 1800s, when ingestion of spent lead shot was first brought about as the mortality factor in waterfowls (e.g., Calvert, 1876;

Holland, 1882). Over the years, the field has evolved from numerous pollution-related episodes and tragedies that undermined human health. In the United States, earlier forms of wildlife toxicology arose by much of the concerns raised on pesticide toxicity around the 1950s to 1960s, as those so publicized in the then widely read *Silent Spring* (Carson, 1962). More recently, the nation's concerns in wildlife toxicology have expanded to include critically imperiled species from extinction (e.g., bison, wild pigeon) as protected under the Endangered Species Act of 1973, and the devastating effects of oil pollution as evident from passage of the Oil Pollution Act in 1990.

The world has encountered numerous major oil spills over the past 50 years, including the more recent Deepwater Horizon BP Oil Spill in the Gulf of Mexico in 2010 and the equally largest, devastating Gulf War Oil Spill in Persian Gulf in 1991. In addition, according to U.S. EPA, each year around 14,000 oil spills are reported in the United States though each on a much smaller scale. From these oil spills, birds and other wildlife species are found to get killed in oily sludges and liquids. Birds and small mammals can be trapped by tank leaks, tank loading spills, and soils contaminated with oily liquids, often to the point that these animals will ultimately die from suffocation. Incubating embryos too can be killed by oil transferred to eggs through oily feathers. Under Section 7003 of the Resource Conservation & Recovery Act (RCRA) of 1976, U.S. EPA has the federal authority to force the cleanup for this type of soil contamination (Section 22.4.3).

While studies are still sparse concerning the health problems among workers engaging in the cleanups or among the general public, there is certainly a potential for human hazard from oil spills. The issue here is that some substances contained in crude oils have been found highly toxic to human health, such as benzene which is a known human carcinogen and mercury (Hg) which is very toxic to the human central nervous system.

22.3.1. Scope and History of Wildlife Toxicology

There are tremendous difficulties in studying wildlife toxicity, as many as those encountered in studying aquatic toxicity if not more. These study difficulties all revolve around the enormous complexities involved in determining the: definition of wildlife; species interactions; species responses to exposure; environmental components in wildlife ecosystems; and sources of stressors (e.g., pesticides, spent lead shot). In addition, there is the need to deal with a large diversity of species in wildlife ecosystems. Both the scope and the history of wildlife toxicology warrant further discussion here, as there is a general misconception that human health implications are less relevant from wildlife toxicology than from the other two subdivisions covered in this chapter.

It is of interest that the issues raised in *Silent Spring* concerning the health effects of pesticides on the environment became not only the centerpiece of today's environmental health movement, but also the momentum that helped launch the Wildlife Toxicology Working Group, which is a functional unit of The Wildlife Society (TWS). Since its foundation in 1937, TWS has maintained a mission to foster greater awareness and understanding of the adverse effects of environmental contaminants on wildlife. TWS is an international nonprofit professional association committed to excellence in wildlife stewardship through science and education. Many past, current, and special issues relevant to wildlife toxicology are well reflected in the numerous various presentations given in each year's workshops and special sessions sponsored by TWS. Two case examples that come to mind are the application of feathers as temporal bioindicators of PCB (polychlorinated biphenyl) exposure in Clapper Rails (Summers *et al.*, 2008), and the use of coastal birds as bioindicators of plastic marine debris (Nevins *et al.*, 2009).

Special interests in wildlife toxicology can also be found in research programs sponsored by other organizations. Three cases in point are the three related studies sponsored by the Contaminant Biology Program at the U.S. Geological Survey (USGS). As a series, these studies assessed the contaminant exposure and potential reproductive effects in ospreys nesting in three separate localities in the United States (Johnson *et al.*, 2009; Rattner *et al.*, 2004; Toschik *et al.*, 2005). Other similar program studies included the investigation into: the effects of sublethal dietary methylmercury exposure on American kestrels (Albers *et al.*, 2007); the levels of metal and organochlorine pesticide residues in the eggs of wading birds at the Salton Sea (Henny *et al.*, 2008); and the effects of PAHs (polycyclic aromatic hydrocarbons) on marine birds, mammals, and reptiles (Albers and Loughlin, 2003).

Meantime during the last decade, perfluorinated compounds were detected in wildlife worldwide; and the fire retardants PBDEs (polybrominated diphenyl ethers) were found doubling in bird eggs at three- to five-year intervals. Accordingly, in his paper reviewing the history of wildlife toxicology, Rattner (2009) postulated that the field had been driven considerably and inevitably by chemical use and misuse, environmental tragedies, and pollution-based events compromising human health. The reviewer further proposed that current challenges should embrace the desire to assess more thoroughly the toxic effects of chemical-related human activities on both the wildlife and their supporting habitat. These current challenges are indeed fairly consistent with the perspectives on and future trends of wildlife toxicology discussed in the recent book by Kendall *et al.* (2010).

22.3.2. The Basic Wildlife Environment

The physical (terrestrial) environment where a particular non-aquatic wildlife species inhabits is similar to the aquatic environment in principle, but different in scope and content. In both cases, the biotic and abiotic components within their own niches interrelate as well as interact to form a physical habitat (i.e., ecosystem) in dynamic equilibrium with its inputs and surroundings. In that sense, ecosystems tend to support higher biodiversity than what the human urban or agricultural environments would, given that ecosystems involve greater numbers of plant and animal (sub)species.

In addition to the aquatic systems made up of predominately oceans and freshwater bodies, wildlife ecosystems take into consideration a number of wildlife terrestrial environments. For environmental toxicologists, these terrestrial environments may be broadly subsumed under five major geographic categories as follows (e.g., Daugherty, 1998):

- *Tundra* or *arctic plain* – This region covers much of the Earth's surface north of the coniferous forest belt. It refers to an area where the tree growth is retarded by extremely cold temperatures.

- *Taiga* – This is a vast belt of coniferous forests in the northern Eurasian region. It is the Earth's largest terrestrial biome.

- *Desert* – This is a region receiving very little precipitation (e.g., <10 inches of annual rainfall), typically with a high average temperature.

- *Chaparral* – This is a shrub or heathland plant biome dominated by evergreen type vegetation with small leaves. The region has a Mediterranean-like climate of a wet, warm winter and a dry, long summer.

- *Forests* – These are subregions each with a high density of trees and other woody vegetation. Collectively, they take up an extensive portion of the Earth's terrestrial surface.

In more specific terms, a tundra region has extremely cold climate with dead organic material for energy and nutrients. It has short seasons for growth and reproduction, low or limited drainage, simple vegetation structure, low biodiversity, as well as large population fluctuations.

Taiga is the world's *largest* terrestrial biome covering most of inland Alaska, Canada, Finland, Sweden, and parts of the northern continental United States. It has a harsh continental climate with young and nutrient-poor soils while lacking the deep. Taiga is home to a number of large herbivorous mammals and small-size rodents.

In contrast, chaparral is the world's *smallest* terrestrial biome found in a little bit of most continents. Its weather is mild and moist in the winter, and dry and hot in the summer. With this type of weather, some of the plants grown in this region are likely French broom, blue oak, Lebanon cedar, and olive tree. The animal inhabitants are mainly grassland and desert types that can adapt to hot and dry weather, such as jackrabbits, mule deer, coyotes, horned toads, alligator lizards, and ladybugs.

In spite of the notorious hot and dry weather that deserts normally have, many still have fairly impressive quantities of specialized vegetation, vertebrates, and invertebrates. There are expectedly fewer large mammals found in the deserts because most large-size animals are not capable of withstanding the heat or storing sufficient water in their body. The desert biome can be separated into four general subtypes based on various meteorological and geographic features: *cold deserts*; *hot and dry deserts*; *semi-arid deserts*; and *coastal deserts*. Examples of cold deserts are those found in Greenland, Antarctic, and the Nearctic realm, with jackrabbits, kangaroo rats, and grasshoppers being some of the dominant inhabitants. Examples of hot and dry deserts include those located in the southern Asian realm, Neotropical region (South and Central America), Ethiopia (Africa), Australia, and the United States (e.g., Sonoran, Mojave), with burrowers and kangaroo rats being the dominant animals. Some semi-arid deserts are located in the United States,

Newfoundland, Russia, Europe, and northern Asia, with skunks, lizards, grasshoppers, kangaroo rats, and snakes being some of the dominant inhabitants. For coastal deserts, some can be found in the Atacama of Chile or the Neotropical realm, with amphibians, golden eagles, lizards, and snakes being some of the dominant animals.

For forests, they can be classified into at least six general subtypes according to the major kinds of climates and trees present: *tropical moist*; *tropical dry*; *temperature coniferous*; *temperate deciduous*; *sparse trees and parkland area*; and *forest plantations*. In all cases, the wildlife and the forests where they inhabit are linked closely together. Forests harbor much of the planet's biodiversity by providing it with abundant and crucial natural resources from timber to medicinal plants. In the recent decades, forests have occupies about one-third of all land areas on the Earth (Schmidt and Harbert, 2004).

22.3.3. Ecological Risk Assessment

Any in-depth characterization of a contaminant's adverse effects on wildlife requires much more than an understanding of the (terrestrial) environment involved. It necessitates some form of ecological risk assessment, which is a tool as well as a framework or construct used to develop, organize, and provide scientific information relevant to decisions given for the ecological impacts under assessment. The first influential reference on this impact assessment process was apparently the guidance document *Framework for Ecological Risk Assessment* published by U.S. EPA (1992). This guidance was updated in the agency's *Guidelines for Ecological Risk Assessment* published six years later (U.S. EPA, 1998). The two versions of the framework in the two guidance documents remained essentially the same, although the specific assessment steps involved were somewhat different due to subsequent refinement. In both documents, the emphasis was on wildlife (including fish and plants) being the ecological entities of concern.

The assessment framework developed by U.S. EPA was largely an outgrowth of the human health-based risk assessment paradigm introduced in Chapter 1 and revisited extensively in the next, final chapter. U.S. EPA's framework focuses on the evaluation of pollution impacts on wildlife, plants, and their ecosystems, not on human health. During the 1980s, the framework emerged as a prominent tool to guide policy and regulatory decision-making on ecological impacts. Its application progressed rather slowly throughout the 1980s, however, as evident from the slow-paced regulations of certain organophosphate pesticides (e.g., diazinon, malathion) concerning potential impacts on bird populations. Despite such a slow progression, the framework has gained a fair amount of global acceptance since its second release (*see*, e.g., UNEP/IPCS, 1999 [Section C]).

The ecological risk approach is distinct from the approach used for assessing (human) health risk mainly in its specific emphasis in three aspects. First, the ecological risk approach may consider effects (i.e., assessment endpoints) beyond the individual or species level to those of an entire community or ecosystem, despite the fact that data on ecological effects are generally more limited compared to those on human health endpoints. Second, the ecological values (i.e., entities and ecosystem characteristics) to be protected or upheld are selected from a wider range of possibilities based on scientific and policy concerns. Third, an ecological risk assessment may consider the effects of stressors (e.g., chemical, biological, or physical agents) on the ecological environment, not just the wild-life *per se* (U.S. EPA, 1998). Accordingly, a knowledge of comparative physiology on wildlife along with the unique habitats for them becomes beneficial, as likely more than one wildlife species niched in its own ecosystem is involved in most any ecological risk assessment. To this end, the *Wildlife Exposure Factors Handbook* published by U.S. EPA (1993) may serve as a quick and handy reference. In that handbook, exposure profiles are provided for select species of birds, mammals, amphibians, reptiles, and more, along with a brief characterization of their natural histories and ecosystems.

U.S. EPA's framework and process for ecological risk assessment includes four basic analytical steps or components: (1) problem formulation; (2) exposure analysis; (3) effects analysis; and (4) risk characterization. In practice, the four steps are intended to be carried out in three phases, as depicted in Figure 22.2, with exposure analysis and effects analysis being performed in tandem through frequent exchange of information between the two analytical components.

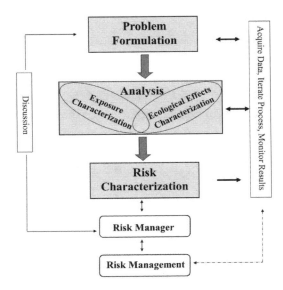

Figure 22.2. General Framework and Process for Ecological Risk Assessment
(modified from public domain image Figure 1 in U.S. EPA [1992])

The framework's *problem formulation* phase involves defining assessment goals, selecting endpoints, proposing a conceptual model, and developing an analysis plan. Assessment endpoints are each an explicit expression of the ecological values (e.g., species, ecological resource, habitat type) to be protected or preserved. These endpoints are only considered useful if they can define the ecological entity and attributes of the entity to be protected or preserved (e.g., reproductive success, age-class structure). The conceptual model describes a series of risk hypotheses used to test how the exposures to stressors may be related to the assessment endpoints. The analysis plan entails a delineation of the assessment design, measures, data needs, and methods for performing the analysis phase of the risk assessment.

The *analysis* phase or step itself engages in the generation of profiles used to characterize the exposure of ecological receptors (e.g., certain wildlife species) to stressors (e.g., pollutants) and the relationships between stressor levels and ecological effects. In *exposure* analysis, the mechanisms of contact between stressor(s) and receptor(s) are characterized; and the magnitude as well as the frequency of contact is assessed. For many ecological risk assessments, exposure characterization includes a spatially-explicit type evaluation, for which a knowledge of the wildlife environment is essential. In *effects* characterization, the adverse effects of stressors on receptors are determined, usually based on such endpoints as toxicity thresholds or exposure-response relationships. The output of effects characterization is a quantitative estimate of the severity of the (potential) harm that might occur. This subphase of the entire analysis step is thus similar in task to the toxicity assessment phase discussed in Chapter 23.

Risk characterization is the final phase of the ecological risk assessment, in which the effects and exposure analyses are integrated to obtain a *risk* estimate for making decisions on the ecological impacts assessed. This phase should also include assessment of the uncertainty and confidence in the results, the ecological significance of any risk estimated, and the data needs for future assessment. Ecological (or human health) risk is technically defined as the probability of an adverse effect on the receptor. In practice, it may be expressed in a number of ways from a simple scientific judgment to a more concrete estimate such as a *hazard quotient*. A simple hazard quotient may be estimated and interpreted as depicted in Box 22.1. Note that the effect concentration or effect dose (e.g., LD_{50}, LC_{50}, RfD) is frequently adjusted downward for the appropriate uncertainty and safety factors added due to data sparsity, interspecies variation, and such. And the site-specific exposure to the stressor is a concentration or dose typically estimated using a set of conservative assumptions to likewise err on the side of ecological protection.

The close relationship between human health and ecological risk assessments has become more apparent since the World Health Organization (IPCS, 2001) developed a perspective for performing risk analyses that would integrate the two assessment frameworks. The WHO perspective was founded on the notion that many national and international entities expressed a need for a *holistic* approach to risk analysis capable of addressing real-life complex exposure situations in which multi-chemicals, multi-media, multi-routes, and multi-species are inevitably involved. Supports for such a holistic approach have since emerged in numerous ways and places, such as in the journal *Human and Ecological Risk Assessment*, in the book with a similar title edited by Paustenbach (2002), in the journal paper by Suter *et al.* (2005) on integration of the two frameworks, and in the risk assessment projects by the U.S. Department of Agriculture (e.g., USDA, 2006) as well as by their contractors (e.g., SERA, 2008) that entail the two frameworks.

Box 22.1. Computation and Interpretation of Hazard Quotient as
Devised for and Used in Ecological Risk Assessment

$$\text{Hazard Quotient} = \frac{\text{Exposure Concentration (or Dose)}}{\text{Effect Concentration (or Dose)}}$$

Hazard Quotient	*Occurrence of Effect (Risk)*
> 1	high
~ 1	potential
< 1	low

22.4. Hazardous Wastes of Global/American Concern

As introduced earlier, hazardous waste is any *discarded* material harmful to human health or the environment when improperly disposed. These materials are generated from many sources such as by industrial facilities (e.g., chemical, electroplating, petroleum refining) and the smaller business entities which are in greater numbers (e.g., dry cleaners, automobile repair shops, clinics, exterminators). Hazardous waste pollution, along with water and air pollutions, is regarded as one of the several largest environmental health problems affecting the Earth today. In the United States, over 40 million tons of toxic waste are generated each year. Many European nations including Italy, England, and Spain are also major toxic waste generators. These countries are dumping well over half of their trash in landfills which are already near their full capacity. In particular, 14 million tons of waste materials were generated in Scotland in 1993, of which 360,000 tons were toxic or from controlled substances. Yet there are only some 900 disposal sites in that nation, with few vacant land sites being available in its northeastern region.

The global concern over hazardous waste pollution actually has reached a high point for some time, likely since the 1992 ratification of the global treaty nicknamed the Basel Convention. The official name of this global treaty is *Basel Convention on the Control and Transboundary Movements of Hazardous Wastes and their Disposal*, which is regarded as the most comprehensive global environmental treaty on toxic and other wastes. This Convention, having more than 170 parties, aims to protect human health and the environment against the harmful effects resulting from the generation, management, transboundary movements, and disposal of various hazardous wastes.

In the United States, hazardous waste pollution is regulated by a number of federal legislations, including the RCRA of 1976, the Comprehensive Environmental Response, Compensation, & Liability Act (CERCLA) of 1980, the Toxic Substances Control Act of 1976, and several other environmental health regulations pertaining specifically to water or air quality. Both the RCRA and its close cousin CERCLA are directed toward toxic waste pollution and are therefore further discussed in the two (sub)sections that follow.

22.4.1. The RCRA Definition and Implications

In the United States, regulations of various hazardous wastes began with the Solid Waste Disposal Act of 1965, which was amended in 1976 to become what is now known as RCRA (Resource Conservation & Recovery Act). The main contribution of RCRA is its mandate that the generating and operating facilities create a "cradle to grave" system of recordkeeping for all relevant hazardous wastes. In this system, all relevant hazardous wastes need to be tracked from the onset of their generation until their final disposition; that is, the system calls for monitoring every aspect of each relevant waste material's fate and transport over its life cycle. As empowered by the act, U.S. EPA has established a list of more than 500 specific kinds of hazardous wastes, and currently works closely with business entities as well as the local and state authorities for strategies and programs to ensure the proper treatment and disposal of these waste materials.

Under RCRA, which can be found in Title 40 of the *Code of Federal Regulations* (40 CFR) Parts 260 through 280, a discarded material must first be a *solid* waste to qualify as hazardous. The various specific kinds of RCRA hazardous wastes are thereby subcategories of solid waste. As misleading as the term might seem to be, a solid waste by RCRA's definition can be a gas or liquid as it only needs to be tangible. Then for an RCRA waste to be treated as hazardous, it must be one that is classifiable as a "listed" or a "characteristics" waste. A characteristics waste is one that exhibits one or more of the following characteristics factors: *ignitability* (e.g., a flammable liquid or gas); *corrosivity* (e.g., a strong acid or alkali); *reactivity* (e.g., an oxidizing agent); and *toxicity* (e.g., a pesticide with low LD_{50}). In contrast, a listed waste is one that by default is treated as hazardous owing to its generation by a specific industry or process. This type is solely based on the process or industry generating it, irrespective of any of the above four characteristics factors that the waste may or may not possess. Examples of U.S. EPA's listed wastes include: certain sludge leftovers from electroplating processes; certain wastes from steel and iron manufacturing; solvent wastes from certain cleaning or degreasing processes; and some discarded pesticides or pharmaceutical products in a *used* form.

The listed hazardous wastes determined by U.S. EPA under the authority of RCRA are organized into four specific (sub)lists under three source categories as follows:

♦ *The F-list (nonspecific source wastes)* – This group includes wastes from *common* industrial or manufacturing processes such as cleaning or degreasing operations. Because these processes are not specific to any particular sector of industry, wastes on this list are also called "*nonspecific source wastes*". Wastes included on the F-list can be found in the regulations at 40 CFR §261.31. Specific examples include spent degreasing solvents such as PCE (tetrachloroethylene) and TCE (trichloroethylene).

◆ *The K-list (source-specific wastes)* – This group includes wastes generated from *specific* industries or processes. As such, they are also referred to as *"source-specific wastes"*. Wastes included on this list can be found in the regulations at 40 CFR §261.32. To be qualified as a K-list waste, the waste must be generated from one of the following industries: organic chemicals; wood preservation; pesticides; petroleum refining; veterinary pharmaceuticals; ink formulation; inorganic chemicals; inorganic pigments; secondary lead; iron and steel; primary aluminum; coking; and explosives. For example, wastewater treatment sludge from the production of zinc yellow pigments is qualified as a K-list waste generated from the inorganic pigment industry. Another example is distillation bottoms from the production of acetaldehyde with another organic such as ethylene, which is thus qualified as from the organic chemical industry.

◆ *The P-list and the U-list (discarded commercial chemical products)* – These two sublists include specific *discarded* commercial chemical products in an *unused* form, and are hence also known as *"discarded commercial chemical products"*. Wastes on the "P" (sub)list are knowingly fatal or irreversibly damaging to humans and animals at low doses. Those on the "U" list pose a lesser hazard to humans or the environment when improperly handled. Pesticides and pharmaceuticals are included on both of these lists. Wastes included in this category can be found in the regulations at 40 CFR §261.33. Specific examples include aldicarb, parathion, and nitric oxide on the P-list, and acetone, diethylstilbestrol, formaldehyde, and kepone on the U-list.

In addition to the characteristics and listed wastes, RCRA authorizes U.S. EPA to regulate a fourth source categorized as "universal wastes". This category includes batteries, pesticides, mercury-containing equipment (e.g., thermostat), bulbs (e.g., lamps), and possibly (as of year 2013; *see* Section 4.2.3.B) pharmaceuticals, that all have been *used*. The regulations set for this fourth category are directed toward the retail stores, certain commercial sectors (including possibly clinics, hospitals, etc.), and household consumers.

22.4.2. The Superfund Law and Program

CERCLA (Comprehensive Environmental Response, Compensation, & Liability Act) was passed in 1980 by U.S. Congress initially to address the appalling tragedy of Love Canal. It authorizes U.S. EPA to compel responsible parties to clean up the toxic waste sites and, where a responsible party cannot be located, to clean up the site on the agency's own effort using a special trust fund now nicknamed "Superfund". CERCLA is hence also known as the Superfund law or program. Prior to the passage of this act, toxic wastes were disposed in regular landfills until there was evidence showing that the toxic materials in the landfills could seep deep into the ground to pollute the soils that animals and crops used, or to reach down the water table to make groundwater unsafe to consume.

In a nutshell, RCRA and CERCLA both deal specifically with toxic waste pollution. Their main difference lies in the release source that they are responsible for. RCRA protects human health and the environment by establishing a comprehensive regulatory framework for investigating and addressing releases of hazardous wastes at *present* and in some cases *future* storage, treatment, and disposal facilities. In contrast, CERCLA protects human health and the environment by establishing a similar regulatory framework for investigating and remediating uncontrolled releases of hazardous substances, but at *past* facilities instead. CERCLA has two distinct provisions for the federal government: (1) a tax on the petroleum and chemical industries as sources for the Superfund; and (2) broad federal authority to respond directly to actual or threatened releases of toxic substances at past facilities that may endanger human health or the environment. Superfund further authorizes U.S. EPA to take the two types of response actions listed below:

♦ *Short-term removals* – Regulatory actions of this type should be carried out to address actual or threatened releases requiring *prompt* response.

♦ *Long-term remedial responses* – Regulatory actions of this type involve permanent or significant remedial reduction of the hazards associated with the (threats of) releases of toxic wastes that are deemed serious, but not immediately life threatening. This type of regulatory actions can be implemented only at sites included on U.S. EPA's National Priorities List (NPL).

Both types of response actions listed above may take place at the same Superfund site, as evident in the case study presented in the next (sub)section. This case study, as introduced briefly in Section 4.2.3.C, is concerned with the uncontrolled releases of pesticide residues at the United Heckathorn (U.H.) Superfund toxic site.

22.4.3. The United Heckathorn Site (A Case Study)

The U.H. Superfund toxic site experience is selected as the case study here in part because it is a relatively recent toxic site disaster and in part because the cleanup involves years of endurance. In line with its general theme, this (sub)section has its focus primarily on events occurring at the toxic site that were deemed pertinent to the Superfund response actions or to the health implications involved.

The U.H. Superfund toxic site is located in Richmond Harbor in Contra Costa County, California (Figure 22.3). The harbor is in an industrial area dominated by petroleum and shipping terminals. The toxic site was a place used to formulate and package pesticides from 1947 to 1966, and now becomes a major source of DDT and other pesticide wastes contaminating the nearby San Francisco Bay estuary partly bounded by and southwest of the harbor. In March 1982, the U.H. site was designated as a state Superfund toxic site due to the high levels of pesticide contamination found in its soils. As authorized under CERCLA, in March 1990 U.S. EPA finally placed the site on its NPL, and in August that year took over the investigation and cleanup commitments from the state of California.

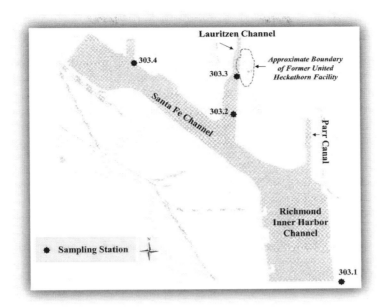

Figure 22.3. Location of the United Heckathorn Superfund Toxic Site, including Sampling Stations, in Contra Costa County, California, USA *(modified from maps.google.com)*

Chronologically as well as more specifically, from 1947 through 1966 the toxic site was used for formulating and packaging pesticides by U.H. and four other operators, with DDT accounting for approximately 95% of all pesticides handled at that time on that site. Buildings on that site were demolished from 1966 through 1970. Between 1970 and 1980, the site was used primarily for bulk storage. In 1981, Levin Metals Corp purchased the property for use as bulk shipping facilities.

U.S. EPA's efforts in cleaning up the U.H. Superfund site proceeded in two technical steps followed by three phases of investigation on release source. During the 1980s and the early 1990s, U.S. EPA with the new property owner together removed more than 3,500 cubic yards of the most highly contaminated soils, or the so-called "hot spots", from the toxic site. The actual sediment remediation did not begin until 1996, three years after completion of the *immediate* removal actions of cleaning up the hot spots.

The cleanup activity ended in 1997 after dredging the Lauritzen Channel and the Parr Canal, which are located in the harbor's north end (Figure 22.3). Approximately 107,000 tons of sediment were removed from the waterways to designated disposal facilities. Afterwards, soil samples were collected in the area to confirm the remedial results.

Step II involved setting up a drainage system to collect the potentially contaminated surface runoff, as well as capping approximately 4.5 acres of land to prevent erosion and exposure to residual levels of pesticides in the soils. The capping was achieved by a concrete cover shielding over the area where the pesticide processing facilities had been located. The capping construction began in July 1998 and ended a year later.

Upon completion of the cleanup activity in July 1997, U.S. EPA started monitoring the pesticide residues in the marine waters nearby. Water samples and mussels were collected in each of the monitoring years for analysis of pesticide levels. Mussels were the test organisms used to account for the amounts of pesticides that might accumulate in a living organism. According to the second Five-Year Review Report (U.S. EPA, 2006), the 2001 monitoring data still indicated unacceptable levels of DDT in sediments near an area excavated in the early 1990s. The 2001 results (Table 22.1) triggered U.S. EPA to undertake additional investigations to supplement data gaps and to determine the potential extent and sources of recontamination of the toxic site. The series of investigations included a Phase I Source Investigation in 2001, a Phase II Source Investigation in 2002, and a Phase III Fluid Mud and Water Quality Investigation in 2004 (U.S. EPA, 2006).

Table 22.1. Summary of Post-Remediation Concentrations (ng/L) of Dieldrin and Total DDTs in Water Samples from around the U.S. United Heckathorn Superfund Toxic Site[a]

Location[b]	Pre-Remediation	Post-Remediation[c]					
		1998 (Yr 1)	1999 (Yr 2)	2000 (Yr 3)	2001 (Yr 4)	2002 (Yr 5)	2003 (Yr 6)
Total DDTs							
Richmond	1	0.65	14.4	2.56	0.06	0.66	0.52
Lauritzen/Mouth	NS	42.6	4.61	27.9	2.88	1.70	0.65
Lauritzen/End	50	103	62.3	1,773A	142	18.4	396
Santa Fe/End	8.6	11	19,2	3.70	2.51	0.60	0.67
Parr	NS	NS	NS	NS	NS	2.57	1.8
Seep	NS	NS	NS	NS	NS	4,455	8,990
Dieldrin							
Richmond	<1	0.65	0.62	1.57	0.08	0.16	0.21
Lauritzen/Mouth	NS	8.18	0.48	8.96	0.46	0.43	0.22
Lauritzen/End	18	18	12.5	625A	8.49	2.08	15
Santa Fe/End	1.8	2.47	0.37	2.11	0.46	0.20	0.17
Parr	NS	NS	NS	NS	NS	0.98	0.88
Seep	NS	NS	NS	NS	NS	2,520	3,000

[a]adapted from Table 6.1 in the report by U.S. EPA (2006); the remediation goals for the organochlorine pesticides dieldrin and total DDTs (i.e., the various isomers of *d*ichloro*d*iphenyl*t*richloroethane and of its metabolites) were 0.14 and 0.59 ng/L, respectively.

[b]Richmond = Richmond Inner Harbor (Station 303.1, *see* Figure 22.3); Lauritzen/Mouth = at the mouth of Lauritzen Channel (Station 303.2); Lauritzen/End = at the end of Lauritzen Channel (Station 303.3); Santa Fe/End = at the end of Santa Fe Channel (Station 303.4); Parr = Parr Canal; Seep = a broken concrete outfall, located near and north of Station 303.3.

[c]A = averaged over all replicates (i.e., including an outlier replicate); NS = not sampled.

It should be noted that for cleanups of Superfund toxic sites, a five-year review of the efforts is mandated by statute first within five years of the remedial action and then every five years thereafter to ensure that the levels of hazardous wastes are below the remediation goals (e.g., those allowing for unlimited exposure). In summer 2008, U.S. EPA specifically collected fish samples of various species (e.g., California halibut, starry flounder, anchovy, walleyed perch) in an effort to supplement and update the baseline information for human health and ecological risk assessments. The highest tissue residue levels found in the fish samples were in those caught at the north end of Lauritzen Channel, ranging from 28 to 11,000 μg/kg for ΣDDTs and 10 to 550 μg/kg for dieldrin (U.S. EPA, 2008). The third Five-Year Review Report for the U.H. Superfund toxic site was released on 21 September 2011. Its overall conclusion was that the remedial action implemented at the marine area of the toxic site was not protective enough, given that the DDT concentrations in the sediments, water, and biota there were found still high enough to remain a potential exposure risk to human health and the environment (U.S. EPA, 2011).

References

Albers PH, Loughlin TR, 2003. Effects of PAHs on Marine Birds, Mammals and Reptiles. In *PAHs: An Ecotoxicological Perspective* (Douben PET, Ed.). West Sussex, England: John Wiley & Sons, Chapter 13.

Albers PH, Koterba MT, Rossmann R, Link WA, French JB, Bennett RS, Bauer WC, 2007. Effects of Methylmercury on Reproduction in American Kestrels. *Environ. Toxicol. Chem.* 26:1856-1866.

Bhargava G, 2001. *Marine Ecosystems*. New Delhi, India: Kalpaz Publications.

Calvert HS, 1876. Pheasants Poisoned by Swallowing Shot. *The Field* 47:189.

Carson LR, 1962. *Silent Spring*. Boston, Massachusetts, USA: Houghton Mifflin.

Daugherty J, 1998. *Assessment of Chemical Exposures: Calculation Methods for Environmental Professionals*. Boca Raton, Florida, USA: Lewis Publishers, Chapter 5.

Geider RJ, DeLucia EH, Falkowski PG, Finzi AC, Grime JP, Grace J, Kana TM, LaRoche J, Long SP, Osborne BA, Platt T, Prentice IC, Raven JA, Schlesinger WH, Smetacek V, Stuart V, Sathyendranath S, Thomas RB, Vogelmann TC, Williams P, Woodward FI, 2001. Primary Productivity of Planet Earth: Biological Determinants and Physical Constraints in Terrestrial and Aquatic Habitats. *Global Change Biol.* 7:849-882.

Grue CE, Powell GVN, Gorsuch CH, 1982. Assessing Effects of Organophosphates on Songbirds: Comparison of a Captive and a Free-Living Population. *J. Wildlife Magnt.* 46:766-768.

Henny CJ, Anderson T, Crayon J, 2008. Organochlorine Pesticides, Polychlorinated Biphenyls, Metals, and Trace Elements in Waterbird Eggs, Salton Sea, California, 2004. *Hydrobiologia* 604: 137-149.

Holland G, 1882. Pheasant Poisoning by Swallowing Shot. *The Field* 59:232.

IPCS (International Programme on Chemical Safety), 2001. Integrated Risk Assessment. WHO/IPCS/IRA/01/12. IPCS, World Health Organization, Geneva, Switzerland.

Johnson BL, Henny CJ, Kaiser JL, Davis JW, Schulz EP, 2009. Assessment of Contaminant Exposure and Effects on Ospreys Nesting along the Lower Duwamish River, Washington, 2006-07. U.S. Geological Survey Open-File Report 2009-1255. U.S. Geological Survey, Reston, Virginia, USA.

Kendall RJ, Lacher TE, Cobb GC, Cox SB (Eds.), 2010. *Wildlife Toxicology: Emerging Contaminant and Biodiversity Issues*. Boca Raton, Florida, USA: CRC Press.

Likens GE, 1973. Primary Production: Freshwater Ecosystems. *Hum. Ecol.* 1:347-356.

McBee K, Lochmiller RL, 1996. Wildlife Toxicology in Biomonitoring and Bioremediation: Implications for Human Health. In *Ecotoxicity and Human Health: A Biological Approach to Environmental Remediation* (de Serres FJ, Bloom AD, Eds.). Boca Raton, Florida, USA: CRC Press, Chapter 6.

Nevins H, Donnelly E, Hester M, Hyrenbach D, 2009. Seabirds as Bioindicators of Plastic Marine Debris. Session 22 (Symposium): Diseases and Toxicants Affecting Marine Wildlife: Causes, Conflicts, Solutions. The Wildlife Society 16th Annual Conference, Monterey, California, USA, 20-24 September.

NMFS (U.S. National Marine Fisheries Service), 2010. Fisheries of the United States 2009. U.S. Office of Science and Technology, Silver Spring, Maryland, USA.

Paustenbach DJ (Ed.), 2002. *Human and Ecological Risk Assessment: Theory and Practice.* New York, New York, USA: John Wiley & Sons.

Pritchard JB, 1993. Aquatic Toxicology: Past, Present, and Prospects. *Environ. Health Perspect.* 100:249-257.

Rand GM, Petrocelli SR, 1985. Introduction. In *Fundamentals of Aquatic Toxicology: Methods and Applications* (Rand GM, Petrocelli SR, Eds.). New York, New York, USA: Hemisphere Publishing, Chapter 1.

Rand GM, Wells PG, McCarty LS, 1995. Introduction to Aquatic Toxicology. In *Fundamentals of Aquatic Toxicology: Effects, Environmental Fate, and Risk Assessment* (Rand GM, Ed.), Second Edition. Washington DC, USA: Taylor & Francis, Chapter 1.

Rattner BA, 2009. History of Wildlife Toxicology. *Ecotoxicology* 18:773-783.

Rattner BA, McGowan PC, Golden NH, Hatfield JS, Toschik PC, Lukei RF Jr, Hale RC, Schmitz-Afonso I, Rice CP, 2004. Contaminant Exposure and Reproductive Success of Ospreys (*Pandion haliaetus*) Nesting in Chesapeake Bay Regions of Concern. *Arch. Environ. Contam. Toxicol.* 47:126-140.

Schmidt V, Harbert W, 2004. *Planet Earth and the New Geoscience.* Pittsburgh, Pennsylvania, USA: Metropolitan Pittsburgh Public Broadcasting, Unit 16.

SERA (Syracuse Environmental Risk Assessment), 2008. Malathion Human Health and Ecological Risk Assessment (Final Report). SERA TR-052-02-02c. USDA Forest Service Contract: AG-3187-C-06-0010. SERA, 5100 Highbridge Street, 42C, Fayetteville, New York, USA.

Steffeck DW, 1994. The Role of Monitoring in Assessing Pesticide Effects on Avian Species and Their Habitats. In *Wildlife Toxicology and Modeling: Integrative Studies of Agroecosystems* (Kendall RJ, Lacher TE, Jr, Eds.). Boca Raton, Florida, USA: CRC Press, Chapter 28.

Summers JW, Gaines KF, Garvin N, Mills GL, 2008. The Use of Feathers as Temporal Bioindicators of PCB Exposure in Clapper Rails. Session 23 (Contributed Paper): Wildlife Toxicology and Conservation and Management of Mammals. The Wildlife Society 15th Annual Conference, Miami, Florida, USA, 8-12 November.

Suter GW 2nd, Vermeire T, Munns WR Jr, Sekizawa J, 2005. An Integrated Framework for Health and Ecological Risk Assessment. *Toxicol. Appl. Pharmacol.* 207(Suppl):611-616.

Toschik PC, Rattner BA, McGowan PC, Christman MC, Carter DB, Hale RC, Matson CW, Ottinger MA, 2005. Effects of Contaminant Exposure on Reproductive Success of Ospreys (*Pandion haliaetus*) Nesting in Delaware River and Bay, USA. *Environ. Toxicol. Chem.* 24:617-628.

UNEP (United Nations Environment Programme), 2002. *Global Environment Outlook 3: Past, Present, and Future Perspectives.* London, UK: Earthscan Publications.

UNEP/IPCS (United Nations Environment Programme/International Programme on Chemical Safety), 1999. *Training Module No. 3: Chemical Risk Assessment – Human Risk Assessment, Environmental Risk Assessment and Ecological Risk Assessment.* WHO/PCS/99.2. Geneva, Switzerland.

USDA (U.S. Department of Agriculture), 2006. 2,4-D Human Health and Ecological Risk Assessment (Final Report). US Forest Service, Arlington, Virginia, USA.

U.S. EPA (U.S. Environmental Protection Agency), 1992. Framework for Ecological Risk Assessment. EPA/630/R-92/001. Risk Forum, Washington DC, USA.

U.S. EPA (U.S. Environmental Protection Agency), 1993. Wildlife Exposure Factors Handbook. EPA/600/R-93/187. Office of Research and Development, Washington DC, USA.

U.S. EPA (U.S. Environmental Protection Agency), 1996. Ecological Effects Test Guidelines: OPPTS 850.1400 – Fish Early-Life Stage Toxicity Test. EPA 712-C-96-121. Office of Prevention, Pesticides, and Toxic Substances, Washington DC, USA.

U.S. EPA (U.S. Environmental Protection Agency), 1998. Guidelines for Ecological Risk Assessment. *Federal Register* 63:26846-26924.

U.S. EPA (U.S. Environmental Protection Agency), 2006. Second Five-Year Review Report for United Heckathorn Superfund Site, Richmond, California. Contract No. 68-W-98-225/WA No. 214-FRFE-09R3. U.S. EPA Region 9, San Francisco, California, USA.

U.S. EPA (U.S. Environmental Protection Agency), 2008. Summary of Fish Tissue Sampling and Analysis, United Heckathorn Superfund Site, Richmond, California, May – June, 2008. Project No. 340138.FI.02. U.S. EPA Region 9, San Francisco, California, USA.

U.S. EPA (U.S. Environmental Protection Agency), 2009. National Recommended Water Quality Criteria. Office of Water, Washington DC, USA.

U.S. EPA (U.S. Environmental Protection Agency), 2011. Third Five-Year Review Report for United Heckathorn Superfund Site, Richmond, California. Contract No. EP-S9-08-04/WA No. 214-FRFE-09R3. U.S. EPA Region 9, San Francisco, California, USA.

Review Questions

1. Briefly discuss the relevance of aquatic toxicology, of wildlife toxicology, and of hazardous waste pollution to human health.

2. Name the two largest oil spills in the world history. And briefly explain how oil spills in general are harmful to wildlife.

3. What are the two main types of aquatic environment? And briefly explain why coral reefs are considered as the rainforests of an ocean region.

4. Which of the following aquatic toxicity test types requires the filtration of both the control and the test solution through an apparatus to maintain the water quality and the concentration of the test material? a) static; b) re-circulation; c) renewal; d) flow-through.

5. Name and give two examples for each of the three basic types of freshwater ecosystems.

6. In a *typical* early-life stage test, how long should the newborn fish be exposed to a test material? a) 5 days; b) 10 days; c) 15 days; d) species-dependent; e) for the entire study period.

7. What are the main differences between U.S. EPA's National Pollutant Discharge Elimination System permit program and the agency's Total Maximum Daily Load program?

8. Which of the following pairs includes both the largest and the smallest type of terrestrial biomes in the world? a) tundra and chaparral; b) desert and forest; c) taiga and tundra; d) taiga and chaparral; e) desert and chaparral.

9. In what ways was *Silent Spring* important or relevant to the vision and the mission of The Wildlife Society's Wildlife Toxicology Working Group?

10. Which of the following wildlife species is not specifically mentioned in this chapter in relation to wildlife toxicology issues? a) kestrels; b) clapper rails; c) loons; d) ospreys.

11. Name four animal species that can adapt to the climate in a chaparral, and four that can adapt to the climate in a coastal desert.

12. What are the four general analytical components included in ecological risk assessment?

13. Briefly describe the *analysis* phase included as the key stage in a typical ecological risk assessment. And how is it relevant to the *risk characterization* phase?

14. Define the terms *conceptual model*, *stressor*, *receptor*, and *assessment endpoint*, as used in the U.S. EPA framework for ecological risk assessment.

15. Which of the following is regarded as the most comprehensive global environmental agreement on toxic and other wastes? a) Basel Convention; b) Stockholm Convention; c) Vienna Convention; d) Montreal Convention.

16. What are the main differences between the two U.S. hazardous waste pollution legislations *RCRA of 1976* and *CERCLA of 1980*, in terms of their jurisdictions and authorities?

17. Match each example of hazardous waste given in the left column to the specific type in the right column that the waste belongs to, as classified by U.S. EPA.

(1) unused DES (diethylstilbestrol)	(a) the P-list
(2) unused parathion	(b) the U-list
(3) used TCE (trichloroethylene)	(c) universal wastes
(4) acetaldehyde-based distillation bottoms	(d) the F-list
(5) used batteries	(e) the K-list

18. Give the general algorithm for deriving a simple hazard quotient (HQ). And what would be the risk implication if this calculated HQ were close to unity (e.g., 0.95)?

19. Briefly describe the distinction between short-term removal actions and long-term remedial responses as authorized under Superfund.

20. Which of the following was the United Heckathorn toxic site used for in 1981? a) packaging of pesticides; b) bulk shipping facilities; c) bulk storage; d) fishery facilities.

21. Briefly describe the two technical steps used in cleaning up the United Heckathorn Superfund toxic site during the 1990s.

22. Which of the following were used in 2001 or 2008 as test organisms in monitoring the tissue levels of dieldrin and total DDTs at the United Heckathorn Superfund toxic site? a) oysters, fish; b) oysters, mussels; c) clams, shrimp; d) mussels, fish.

23. In which years were the three phases of investigation on release source carried out for the United Heckathorn Superfund toxic site?

24. Which specific location at the United Heckathorn Superfund toxic site had the highest water concentrations of dieldrin and total DDTs detected in 2002?

25. What and where was the highest fish tissue concentration of total DDTs detected around the United Heckathorn Superfund toxic site in 2008?

CHAPTER 23

Environmental Health Risk Assessment

23.1. Introduction

Three decades ago, U.S. National Research Council (NRC, 1983) published a human health-based risk assessment paradigm that now has become a standard framework applied by many regulatory entities. Since the publication of this classic framework, numerous volumes of textbooks, guidance documents, and other reference materials have been written to advocate or extend its application. One volume noteworthy is the training manual *Chemical Risk Assessment* prepared jointly by the United Nations Environment Programme and the International Programme on Chemical Safety (UNEP/IPCS, 1999). This manual represents the joint effort by the two organizations in advancing the three separate frameworks that they have constructed for human risk assessment, environmental risk assessment, and ecological risk assessment.

The UNEP/IPCS framework for *human* risk assessment includes an exposure component focusing on workers, consumers, and the general public exposed to environmental pollutants as the receptors of concern. That framework is largely comparable to those adopted by many other entities for human health-based risk assessment, including the ones by U.S. EPA (1986, 1991, 1996, 1998a, 2005) and by the Australia Department of Health Services (DHAEC, 2002). However, the exposure component in the UNEP/IPCS framework for *environmental* risk assessment has a somewhat confusing theme not easy to follow. That second framework considers not only the exposures of humans and other mammals from drinking water polluted by chemical substances, but also the exposures of aquatic organisms to the same or different pollutants in surface waters. Given that the exposures of people and aquatic organisms to water pollutants can be covered in the human and the ecological risk assessment, respectively, the UNEP/IPCS framework for environmental risk assessment may not have a focus as specific as intended.

Despite the confusion by UNEP/IPCS, environmental health risk assessment is synonymous with human health risk assessment within the realm of environmental toxicology, at least in terms of principle and process. The former is used as this chapter's title and implicit throughout this book simply because it has a nicer ring to environmental toxicology. Nevertheless, to ease the writing in this chapter, much of the time either term has been shortened to *health risk assessment*.

23.1.1. Health Risk Assessment Activities

A reality with health risk assessment is that its framework and activities are not only subject to public concerns and social values. In practice, its activities also tend to be carried out in fragments at some government levels or within some nongovernment organizations, inasmuch as most of these entities have limited resources and special agenda. It is due to this kind of fragmentation that environmental toxicology, environmental epidemiology, and other relevant sciences cannot always play a more significant role in health risk assessment to promote public health.

Yet in spite of these hurdles, many health risk assessment activities continue to expand considerably and are performed in many places every day, particularly by government health agencies in the advanced countries. For simplicity, these health risk assessment activities can be subsumed under four major risk categories as follows.

The first category involves those health risks that rely on either an individual's self-initiative or a medical organization's effort for exposure mitigation, rather than on some government interventions. In the United States, this type is considered mostly by the U.S. Department of Health and Human Services (DHHS), by its National Institutes of Health (NIH), and by its Centers for Disease Control and Prevention (CDC). A familiar case study under this risk category is CDC's health risk assessment for the tampon-toxic shock syndrome and its episode reported in 1980 (Section 3.2).

The second category deals with those health risks subject to regulatory control and mitigation of exposure. This type is mostly associated with environmental pollution and product use. As hinted in Figure 1.1 and noted by Thongsinthusak and Dong (2010), although exposure mitigation is a key component of health risk *management*, the necessity of its implementation is contingent on the outcome of a health risk assessment performed under a structured framework. In the United States, health risks under this category are assessed mostly by U.S. EPA. Other regulatory agencies under this category include FDA (U.S. Food and Drug Administration) and CPSC (U.S. Consumer Product Safety Commission). In terms of health risk assessment activities, CPSC has been less involved in federal efforts to regulate toxic chemicals, in part due to its small size and limited operating budget. Yet owing to the unique provisions contained in the older version of the Federal Hazardous Substances Act, CPSC is among the forefronts in providing criteria for toxicity tests, particularly those on acute toxicity in animals (e.g., the primary irritation assay in rabbits). Otherwise, CPSC obtains much of its health risk assessment information from other sources, including predominately U.S. EPA and FDA.

The third category differs from the second only in that the health risks involved are those due to exposures occurring in a workplace. In the United States, health risks in this category are regulated by OSHA (U.S. Occupational Safety and Health Administration). OSHA's most controversial health and safety standards have been exposure limits for toxicants present in the workplace. In its early years, OSHA rejected the use of health risk assessment for occupational carcinogens and other toxic agents under the presumption that its statute would not permit the use of such a quantitative process. However, one key impetus to the adoption of health risk assessment as a decision-making tool by many U.S. health regulatory agencies today, including OSHA, was the U.S. Supreme Court's decision on the OSHA standard for worker exposure to benzene (NRC, 1994). That court decision argued for some form of health risk assessment as a prelude to the determination whether a health risk is high enough to merit regulatory action.

The fourth category includes all environmental health risks generated or aggravated by (economic) development policies and programs (DPP), particularly in the developing regions. DPP can be broadly subsumed under five subgroups leading to five different sources for potential adverse effects: (1) agricultural growth and food supply; (2) macro-economic growth; (3) energy; (4) housing; and (5) industrialization. Health risk assessment's connection with DPP, unlike with public health, is more subtle and indirect but at times equally relevant and forceful. One general step included in an environmental health impact assessment (EHIA), which is an integral part of most if not all the DPP-associated actions and activities, is the assessment of potential health and environmental impacts. It is for this assessment step that some form of health risk assessment is required to complete an EHIA for many of these development projects.

23.1.2. Subtleties of Health Risk Assessment

The four key components of NRC's initial human health-based risk assessment paradigm, as depicted below in Figure 23.1, are introduced in Chapter 1 without much discussion except for laying out the ground that the principles for environmental toxicology are integral to and revolved around such a scientific (regulatory) framework. In many ways and particularly in concept, the basic process of ecological risk assessment discussed in Section 22.3.3 is similar to the one involved in this health-based risk assessment paradigm. In the present and final chapter, further elaborations are given on each of the four components in an effort to bring the book to a closure, with the intent to integrate as many as practical the concepts and issues presented in the other chapters.

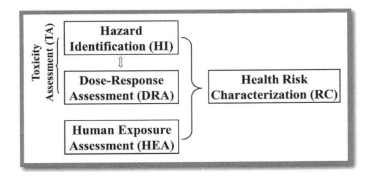

Figure 23.1. Key Components (Phases) of Environmental Health Risk Assessment

As a prelude to the elaborations, one subtlety worth reminding here is that health risk characterization, as reflected in Figure 23.1, is the final phase in the health risk assessment paradigm. Literally, this phase is the final step in which the potential health risk of

concern is *characterized*, utilizing all relevant information gathered from hazard identification, dose-response assessment, and human exposure assessment. Given that a health
risk cannot be characterized until it has been *assessed* at least qualitatively, health risk
assessment as a *quatitation* task or (sub)process, rather than as a framework, construct, or
discipline, can be regarded as a subpart of health risk characterization.

Another subtlety noteworthy here is that nearly two decades ago, NRC (1994) revised
its initial paradigm to combine hazard identification and dose-response assessment into a
single phase termed *toxicity assessment* (Figure 23.1). NRC based its revision on the notion that the data and tasks required for the two uniting phases are practically inseparable.

23.2. Toxicity Assessment

Unlike ecological risk assessment (Section 22.3.3), health risk assessment generally
does not start with *problem formulation* as the formal first step. Instead, it generally
starts with hazard identification (HI), the phase that involves the determination of potential adverse health effects from a biological, physical, or chemical agent of concern.
Problem formulation is almost not needed in performing health risk assessment because
the action plan, the justification, and the conceptual model involved are relatively more
straightforward. Many (toxic) substances under health risk assessment either are active
ingredients in products that are subject to safety evaluation before they may be registered
or re-registered for use, or are those suspected to cause environmental health hazard. In
practice, the main task of HI is to first characterize all potential *toxic* endpoints identified
and then to determine the one(s) *of critical concern*, usually in terms of severity, toxic effect, or both. In contrast, the output of the problem formulation phase will include a set
of *assessment* endpoints that, while reflecting the ecosystem, are determined to be both
measurable and affected by the ecological stressor(s) in question.

More specifically, an assessment endpoint in ecological risk assessment is defined as
an explicit expression of the ecological value to be protected or upheld (Section 22.3.3;
U.S. EPA, 1998b). The ecological attributes for the value to be protected and thereby to
be assessed can be as broad as maintaining a balanced indigenous population in waters
receiving radioactive plumes from a nuclear power plant, as stipulated by Section 316(b)
of the U.S. Clean Water Act. In contrast, when performing the health risk assessment for
a particular toxic agent, the practice in the HI phase has been to let the available toxicity
tests define the toxic endpoints (Suter and Barnthouse, 1993).

23.2.1. Hazard Identification

Conceptually, the HI (hazard identification) task need not be initiated with the use of
chemical-specific animal or human toxicity data. Yet for health risk assessment purposes,
the use of well-conducted chemical-specific animal toxicity studies is not only encour-
aged but in most cases also warranted. This is because strong evidence is needed to ensure that the toxic effect is caused by the suspect agent or activity involved. More so than

ecological risk assessment, health risk assessment needs such strong evidence because there is more at stake with the suspect agent's use and the activity involved.

Naturally, the most convincing evidence for a causal relationship is a well-conducted epidemiological study in which a positive association between exposure and adverse effect in human subjects has been observed, since human data offer evidence that is more direct. Yet well-conducted epidemiological studies are hard to come by, as it is unethical to deliberately subject humans to doses sufficient to cause them bodily harm. The use of animal data from well-designed experiments thereby becomes a crucial part of the HI component. At the least, the dose given to the test animals is more controllable, compared to human exposure. Regardless, as expected, the main problem with utilizing animal toxicity results is that the test agent could have a different effect in animals than in humans. After all, the rodent and human bodies are anatomically very different.

Other types of studies used in HI include short-term tests ranging from bacterial mutation assays performed entirely *in vitro* to more elaborate short-term bioassays such as skin-painting studies. A test agent's physicochemical properties also play a key role in providing crucial information on its toxicity.

23.2.2. Animal Toxicity Studies

The assessment of a toxic agent's adverse effects in animals normally examines most, if not all, of the eight general toxicity categories listed in Table 23.1 for one or more of the three common routes of exposure: oral (by ingestion); inhalation; and dermal (by absorption through the skin). For illustration purposes, also included in the table are select test guidelines published by U.S. EPA for the eight toxicity categories listed.

Table 23.1. General Categories of Health Effects and Their Select Test Guidelines as Considered (by U.S. EPA) in a Typical Health Risk Assessment

Category of Health Effects	Select Guidelines Published by U.S. EPA
Acute toxicity	Acute Oral Toxicity (2002)
Subchronic toxicity	Ninety-Day Inhalation (1998c)
Chronic toxicity	Chronic Toxicity (1998d)
Genetic toxicity	Bacterial Reverse Mutation (1998e)
Neurotoxicity	Neurotoxicity Screening Battery (1998f)
Carcinogenicity	Carcinogenicity (1998g)
Immunotoxicity	Immunotoxicity (1998h)
Reproductive/Developmental	Reproduction/Developmental Screening (2000a)

The health effects test guidelines published by U.S. EPA total to about 50. This is not the only set available for the public to use as study protocols in testing the safety of pesticides, food additives, industrial chemicals, and pharmaceuticals. Comparable guidelines have been made available by other organizations, including prominently the Organization for Economic Cooperation and Development (OECD) and the International Conference on Harmonization (ICH). The OECD guidelines represent a collection of about 100 most relevant testing protocols used by government, industry, and independent laboratories to identify and characterize potential hazards of new and existing chemical substances in all categories. These OECD guidelines, which are now accessible online at the organization's website, are regularly updated with the assistance of thousands of experts from its 30 or so member countries (e.g., Australia, Chile, France, Italy, Japan, Korea, Mexico, Norway, Spain, United Kingdom, United States). The ICH guidelines, which are currently available online on the FDA website, are intended for pharmaceuticals only. They represent the joint effort of the six ICH founding members from the United States, the European Union, and Japan, with one regulatory authority and one industry trade association serving for each jurisdiction. As expected, FDA is the regulatory authority representing the United States. At the present moment, Canada, the European Free Trade Association, and World Health Organization (WHO) are the observer members of ICH.

At times, the potential health effects of a toxic agent may also be conveniently categorized into the following three groups or six subgroups: acute *vs*. chronic effects; local *vs*. systemic effects; and reversible *vs*. irreversible effects (as defined in Table 9.1). Regardless of the categorization scheme used, in practice the toxic endpoints of concern are quantified primarily in terms of NOAEL (no observed *adverse* effect level) or NOEL (no observed effect level) for (almost) all types of health effects subject to health risk analysis, except for acute toxicity and cancer. Acute toxicity is one that manifests shortly after a single exposure and is typically expressed as LD_{50} or LC_{50}, which is the dose or concentration (respectively) required to kill half of the study population. For cancer, the effect unit of concern generally is the so-called cancer potency factor (CPF), which is the slope of the dose-response curve generated for the toxic agent at issue. The rationale for the application of CPF is discussed in the next (sub)section on dose-response assessment, which is concerned with how health effects can be quantified and reassured.

23.2.3. Dose-Response Assessment

Once the toxic endpoints of concern are identified, the next crucial step is to determine the highest dose at which biologically and statistically no significant adverse effect is expected to occur relative to the control group. This highest dose is referred to as NOEL or NOAEL, the dose ideally *just* below the lowest observed [adverse] effect level (LO[A]EL) which ideally *just* begins to show significant increase in the observed effect. The difference between NOEL and NOAEL rests on the definition of *adverse* effect (NRC, 1994). As noted in Section 23.1.2, most toxicity studies are conducted not only for HI purposes, but also for dose-response assessment (DRA). It is for this reason that NRC (1994) made an effort to revise its initial health risk assessment paradigm to combine HI and DRA into a single phase termed *toxicity assessment*.

One crucial function of DRA is to ascertain the reasonable lowest dose to be used as the LO[A]EL, or the reasonable highest dose used as the NO[A]EL. Oftentimes there are merely three or four dose levels and a very limited number of animals used per level in a toxicity study, largely because any type of animal toxicity studies is expensive to conduct costing between $10,000 and $500,000 or more each (e.g., Klaassen and Eaton, 1991). The resultant LO[A]EL or NO[A]EL thus generally turns out to be less appreciable' particularly when a dose-response curve cannot be constructed from the very few responses observed. As a point for argument, if the intermediate dose of a threesome yielded the highest response (e.g., that having most test animals with the effects), the lower or negative response from the lowest dose tested could be construed as an artifact, or due to chance. In any case, if a dose-response curve could indeed be constructed showing a very steep slope, then the response would be regarded as highly sensitive to dose level, suggesting that the NO[A]EL is very close to the LO[A]EL. Conversely, if the slope were less steep, the response would be treated as less dose-sensitive (Figure 23.2). The use of NO[A]EL or LO[A]EL in health risk assessment is based on the notion that the exposure has to reach a threshold before any (non-cancer) adverse health effects can occur.

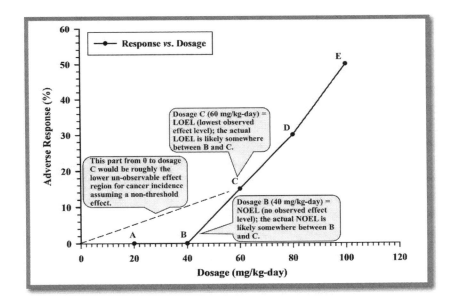

Figure 23.2. Dose-Response Curve (Relationship) from a Hypothetical Study
Having Five Dosage Points (A, B, C, D, E)

DRA plays a relatively more prominent role where the adverse health effect is cancer, for which usually no threshold is assumed. Because human doses are typically lower than the experimental LO[A]EL derived from animal studies, there are many uncertainties and interests about how a human dose behaves biologically in the *unobservable* region below the experimental LO[A]EL, particularly when a no threshold effect is assumed. The practice has been to extrapolate from responses at the experimental doses down to the region below the LO[A]EL (as illustrated in Figure 23.2) by means of a theorized mechanistic model such as a linearized multistage or a low-dose linear model (e.g., U.S. EPA, 2005). This type of extrapolation is part of the DRA task.

The slope extrapolated from these theorized models is known as cancer slope factor (CSF) or CPF (cancer potency factor), typically expressed in units of $(mg/kg\text{-}day)^{-1}$. This slope is basically a rate constant implicating that the magnitude (or level) of the response is linearly proportional to the exposure level (typically in units of mg carcinogen per kg body weight per day). As hinted earlier, the steeper the slope, the more potent each dosage is implicated for cancer risk since it takes less exposure to induce the same level of cancer response (risk). As further elaborated in Section 23.4.1, excess lifetime cancer risk can be quantified by multiplying an estimated dose of concern by the associated CPF.

23.3. Human Exposure Assessment

In this key phase of the health risk assessment, those assessors responsible for the task will often face chemical, physical, or biological contaminants that are less concrete than desired. The perspectives that follow explain why scientists with sufficient knowledge in epidemiology tend to have a better edge in assessing human exposure to environmental toxicants than many of those in other disciplines would. The exposure media and pathways in Figure 23.3 are provided to reflect the complexity as well as the general scheme involved in performing this difficult task known as human exposure assessment.

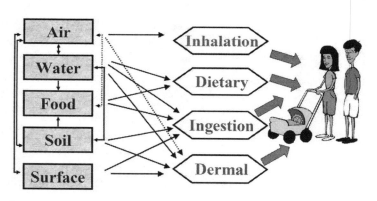

Figure 23.3. Simplified Complexity of Human Exposure Assessment

In essence, human exposures to environmental toxicants can occur via dermal contact, ingestion, dietary intake, and inhalation. Figure 23.3 also suggests that in addition to the common environmental media such as air, soils, foods, and drinking water, the contaminant may be present on foliar or structural surfaces. For some environmental toxicants, certain exposure routes and media play a more prominent role than others do. For example, compared to dermal contact, inhalation generally is a route more crucial for soil fumigants due to their high volatility. Throughout the book, ingestion and dietary intake are considered different although in both cases the route of exposure is oral. Dietary intake involves the exposure from daily food consumption, frequently including drinking water. In contrast, ingestion refers to any other oral intake, such as from hand-to-mouth by a toddler after crawling on a carpet treated with a flea killer fogger.

23.3.1. Past and Current Perspectives

Several definitions have been given for human exposure assessment. To some scholars, there may be a necessary distinction between the terms *human exposure measurement* and *human exposure assessment*. The former generally is limited to the quantification of human exposure, whereas the latter extends to considering the implication or impact of the human exposure level that has been measured. In this section, however, the term *exposure analysis* is used most of the time for no reasons other than to avoid such a distinction as well as to ease the writing somewhat.

Exposure analysis rests on the widely accepted toxicological concept that the magnitude, the frequency, and the route of dosing all have a significant impact on the nature, the severity, and the potential that an adverse effect is exerted. Oftentimes, repeated exposures at a lower dosage are assumed to have the same (or at least similar) toxic effects induced by a single exposure at a higher dosage (*see*, e.g., Section 10.2.2.A).

As pointed out in the guidelines published by U.S. EPA (1992), exposure analysis in various forms dates back at least to the early 20th century, particularly in the field of epidemiology and those dealing with occupational exposure. U.S. EPA defines exposure as the contact between an agent and a human body's outer boundary (e.g., the skin, lungs, gastrointestinal tract). In contrast, applied dose refers to the amount of a substance placed at or around one or more of these outer boundaries which act as absorption barriers. The term *dosage* differs from *dose* only in the former referring to an amount that is relative to a physiological parameter (e.g., per kg of body weight) or to a time interval (e.g., per day). Another closely related term is internal dose, which is the amount of a substance that has been absorbed via all body barriers plus the portion produced in the body, if any; it is simply the total amount available for biological interaction with receptors located in any body tissue. (These distinctions are introduced in Section 1.2.1).

Despite the supposition that exposure analysis is important to toxicologists engaging in health risk assessment, documentation of this subject matter in toxicology textbooks is incomplete and fragmented. To this date, most toxicology textbooks have offered at most only a few sections on exposure analysis, usually as part of a chapter on some form of health risk assessment. Many toxicologists do not find exposure analysis appealing in part because they are better trained to use animal models or bioassays as investigation tools. Another reason is that health risk assessment, of which exposure analysis is a key part, is still a young field. There are undoubtedly toxicologists measuring exposure levels for pathological examination, forensic investigation, and the kind. Yet measurements of such are on single individuals without the intent of protecting public health.

In any event, it is somewhat a relief to find that these days more toxicologists have been willingly and constantly working with epidemiologists and other health scientists in performing exposure analysis. For instance, toxicologists have been conducting animal (and at times human) studies to determine the dermal or inhalation absorption of chemicals. These studies would enable exposure assessors to estimate the internal dose from dermal or inhalation exposure to the chemical (i.e., using the animal value as a surrogate). Food toxicologists and nutritional epidemiologists are also frequently seen working together in assessing dietary intakes. Overall, nowadays, environmental toxicologists generally have acquired a fair amount of knowledge about the air, water, and soil concentrations of certain contaminants in various parts of a country or the world.

For somewhat different objectives, exposure analysis is covered more fully and more frequently in epidemiology textbooks. Despite such coverage or efforts, there are still reasons why some epidemiologists too may find exposure analysis not appealing. First, the efforts by many epidemiologists to associate human exposures to health outcomes are primarily for etiology testing, not for health risk assessment. Second, exposure analyses are conducted primarily for chemical, physical, or biological contaminants present in the environment. Yet epidemiologists outside of the environmental or occupational health discipline frequently face different issues or agenda whenever they assess human exposures to or for intrinsic factors. Third, as noted earlier, health risk assessment as a scientific discipline is in its adolescence, if not still in its infancy.

Epidemiologists who are less concerned with exposure analysis are those dealing with either intangible exposures or exposures of more concrete levels. For instance, when conducting a clinical trial, most epidemiologists already have a good idea on the dose or treatment levels at which the patients are being exposed. And for psychosocial epidemiologists or the kind, they tend to work with personal trait, lifestyle, or socioeconomic status as the risk factors. These factors are intangible; their measurements thereby often rely on the use of more quantifiable but less relevant determinants as surrogates, such as through work histories, observed behaviors, and surveys.

23.3.2. Direct and Indirect Measurements

There are essentially two approaches to estimating (daily) human exposures to an environmental toxicant. One approach is to first identify the major exposure sources or media involved (e.g., inhalation, dermal, dietary, ingestion, onsite). The exposures from, to, or with these components are then assess separately and indirectly. In most cases, indirect exposure measurements are performed by means of the toxicant's concentrations in one or more appropriate media (e.g., air, water, foods, foliage).

Most, if not all, indirect measurement methods available to these days are still built on the well received, yet not fully validated, simple algorithm presented below in Box 23.1:

Box 23.1. Basic Algorithm for Calculation of Human Environmental Exposure

Human Exposure = [Environmental Concentration of Toxicant] x [Human Contact]

It is intuitive that the reverse implication of the premise in Box 23.1 is always true. That is, no human exposure would occur if there were no human contact with the toxicant whether directly or indirectly. Nor would there be any human exposure to the toxicant if the toxicant is not available in the person's environment.

Another approach to measuring human exposure is to estimate the (daily) dosage of the person directly through biomonitoring *(as defined in Section 20.3.2)*. Biomonitoring of human exposure generally involves the measurement of an internal dose. Yet in reality, the biomonitoring approach does not truly offer a direct measurement method. This is because the dose so measured technically is still through some form of indirect estimation. In practice, the internal dose so derived is almost always based on the amounts of the toxicant measured in a couple of biological media such as blood, expired air, or urine. More specifically, the amounts estimated for other body tissues need to be inferred or accounted for indirectly. If a metabolite were monitored instead, which is often the case, then additional correction or back-calculation would be needed to account for the portion of the parent compound that had been biotransformed to the metabolite, so that the total amount of human exposure to the parent compound (which is often the chemical species of regulatory concern per risk assessment) could be fully determined.

For a comprehensive exposure analysis, the calculations of *aggregate* and *cumulative* doses are often warranted. Aggregate dose is defined as that level accumulated from multiple exposure pathways and media, whereas cumulative dose refers to an aggregate dose that accounts for the additional exposures to (all) relevant chemicals sharing a common mechanism of toxicity. The advantage of using biomonitoring data to estimate exposure is thus manifold. Because biomonitoring integrates the exposures by all routes of entry, this type of exposure monitoring reduces the concern with exposure events that may occur concurrently. In addition, the use of aggregate or cumulative dose derived from well-designed biomonitoring studies would reduce the uncertainties inherent in animal dermal absorption or other types of extrapolation (Dong and Ross, 2001; Ross *et al.*, 2000).

The limitations of using biomonitoring data are likewise enormous, unfortunately. The total body burden derived from this type of data is not route-specific, unless further efforts are made such as collecting air samples on the side to separate the dose from inhalation exposure. Regardless, for risk mitigation purposes, it is important to know which route of entry is the principal exposure pathway. For instance, if exposure via dermal route turns out to be much more crucial than from inhalation, then the workers will be required to wear adequate protective clothing, not an approved respirator.

In human exposure assessment, the indirect measurement method currently is much more popular compared to biomonitoring. This is because the indirect approach currently is still more practical and economical. Another reason is that knowledge of a substance's toxicokinetics is a prerequisite for the interpretation and application of the human monitoring data obtained on the substance; yet quite frequently, such knowledge is not available or attainable. Furthermore, collection of body fluids, including urine, from human subjects is considered as an invasive ordeal to many people.

23.3.3. Aggregate and Cumulative Exposures

The exposure scenario depicted below in Figure 23.4 may serve to illustrate the complexity involved in measuring aggregate exposure (and, to some extent, cumulative exposure as well) with the indirect method. This example scenario involves the multiple exposure pathways via multiple media for children spending some time at a playground in which the playset was treated with a wood preservative of concern such as chromated copper arsenate (CCA). For an extensive assessment of the children's daily exposure to the CCA residues, of which one or more metallic ingredients are presumed to be ubiquitous in the local environment, it is necessary to consider at least the four common routes of exposure conceptualized graphically below in Figure 23.4.

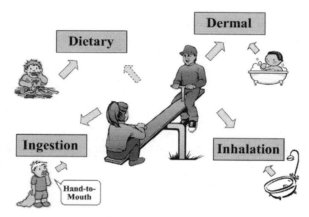

Figure 23.4. Potential Routes for Aggregate Exposure of Children to Wood Preservative Residues *(e.g., to Residues in Pressure-Treated Wood Used in Playground Structures)*

In reality, it is possible for a young child to be exposed to the CCA residues from dermal contact with the contaminated soil around the playset. The child's skin and clothing could also come in contact with the residues (long) left on the treated playset structure, or potentially even with indoor surface residues that had been translocated from the playground through contaminated outdoor air or other means. Another source of dermal uptake could be through contaminated bath or shower water. The child could additionally inhale the residues in the bath or shower water contaminated from the same or other sources. Both the indoor and the outdoor ambient air could be sources for inhalation exposure. In addition to foods and drinking water, the child could ingest the residues on the playset structures or the soil through hand-to-mouth exposure.

Note that in performing the exposure analysis as part of a health risk assessment, the background level from sources other than the treated site is also critical. This is because the adverse effect, if any, is induced by the *total* effective amount of the substance in or on the body. Furthermore, if and when one or more relevant chemicals share a common mechanism of toxicity at issue and are present in the child's local environment at a significant level, the child's daily exposures from many of the aforesaid pathways should be estimated also for these other chemicals in the same manner as for the target chemical, and then to be added to the total exposure for the day, the month, or the year.

Both the consideration and the estimation of aggregate or cumulative exposure for the above or similar scenarios are complex. Many presumptions and assumptions are needed to deal with the exposure nature and duration range for each of the pathways involved. The concentration range for each of the exposure media is required as well. All of these parameters are subject to challenge by the stakeholders, the scientific community, and the higher (or other) regulatory entities. With cumulative exposure, there is an additional need for defending the decision made that the target chemical shares a common mechanism of toxicity with the other relevant chemical(s). U.S. EPA (2003, 2007b) has published a resource guide and a framework document that together provide the much needed concepts, methods, and data sources to assist in the conduct of multi-exposure, multi-chemical, and population-focused cumulative risk assessments.

23.4. Health Risk Characterization

According to U.S. EPA's *Risk Characterization Handbook* (2000b), health risk characterization (henceforth risk characterization) is *"The final, integrative step of risk assessment"* that *"conveys the risk assessor's judgment as to the nature and existence (or the lack) of human health or ecological risks."* That handbook reiterates NRC's paradigm, asserting that HI (hazard identification), DRA (dose-response assessment), HEA (human exposure analysis), and RC (risk characterization) are the key steps in the assessment of health risk. In that sense, risk characterization can be regarded as a major part of the newly emerging discipline called (environmental) health risk assessment.

In a narrower context, risk characterization can be treated, however, as a simple (quantitative) process *comparing* one or more estimated human exposure levels of concern *to* a benchmark (i.e., safe) exposure level predetermined as insignificant by regulatory standards. The health risk is assumed to be proportionally greater if the human exposure is increased farther (within a reasonable range) beyond the safe level. In many instances, the benchmark level used is expressed as or derived from one of the health risk measures described in the next (sub)section.

23.4.1. Health Risk Measures

Over the years, there have been a dozen or so quantitative measures used to account for, directly or indirectly, the significance of a health risk assessed. These health risk measures, often known more by their acronyms, include ADI, RfD, RfC, CPF, ECR, PEL, TLV, STEL, BMD, BMC, NO[A]E, LO[A]EL, and MCL. Among these, the first three (ADI, RfD, RfC) have their values built in with a safety margin. Closely related to these dozen measures are the likewise commonly utilized MOE and HQ.

ADI (*acceptable daily intake*) is the predetermined daily dosage (e.g., mg per kg body weight) of a chemical substance (e.g., pesticide, food additive, metal) that presumably may be *ingested* daily by people over their entire lifetime without causing any significant adverse health effect. This dosage is determined by dividing the NO[A]EL by a set of safety factors (SFs), usually of multiples of 10, to account for *intra*species sensitivity, *inter*species variation, and other uncertainties of concern (e.g. low quality of toxicity data used). The definitions of NO[A]EL and LO[A]EL are given in Section 23.2.3 above. The term *ADI* was first used by the United Nations Food and Agriculture Organization/World Health Organization Expert Committee on Food Additives in 1961. Now it is also used extensively by FDA in the United States.

RfD (*reference dose*), used by many programs within U.S. EPA, is derived similarly. The potential difference between RfD and ADI is the possibly different SFs and toxicity studies used by the different agencies. RfC (*reference concentration*) is likewise determined and used similarly by U.S. EPA. It differs from RfD only in that air, water, or soil *concentration*, instead of the actual exposure (dose), is used.

PEL (*permissible exposure limit*) and the kind, such as TLV (*threshold limit value*) and TLV-STEL (TLV *short-term exposure limit*), are the maximum environmental concentrations of a toxicant that workers (or sometimes a community) presumably can be exposed to within a given period without causing any significant adverse health effect (Chapter 20). In the United States, exposure limits of this type are utilized mainly by OSHA. As used mostly by U.S. EPA, MCL is the *maximum contaminant level* of a substance in a (public) water system that is considered as harmless to consumers.

BMD (*benchmark dose*) can be determined and used to represent a lower confidence limit on a dose that produces an acceptable small percentage (e.g., 5%) increase in a particular adverse effect. It is thereby a more accurately quantified as well as a more realistic LO[A]EL. BMC (*benchmark concentration*) differs from BMD in that it deals with the toxicant's concentration to be exposed to, instead of its dose received.

For carcinogenicity, excess lifetime risk is generally calculated by multiplying an estimated dose of concern by the associated CPF (cancer potency factor). This product represents an upper bound on the probability of having *excess cancer risk* (ECR) from lifetime or long-term exposure to a carcinogen. The probability is expressed as a population risk, such as 1×10^{-6} meaning that 1 in 1 million exposed persons is estimated to have the cancer. As ECR = dose x CPF, it follows that dose = ECR ÷ CPF. Therefore, the exposure *dose* considered as safe for the cancer risk at issue can be estimated in terms of CPF alone, as long as an acceptable level of ECR has been predetermined.

Those measures used to characterize health risk *indirectly* include ADI, RfD, RfC, PEL, CPF, and the kind. They are treated as *indirect* health risk measures because their values must be checked against the exposure at issue before their risk implications can be appreciated. For example, a higher ADI value for toxicant A might turn out to implicate a higher health risk than a lower ADI value would for toxicant B, if the same person were exposed to a much higher level of toxicant A than of toxicant B.

ECR is considered a *direct* health risk measure in that no further comparison with any estimated dose is required. For noncarcinogenic adverse effects, the direct risk measures commonly used by regulatory agencies are margin of exposure (MOE), HQ (hazard quotient), and some variants of the two.

Until recently, MOE was used interchangeably with margin of safety (MOS). It is determined by dividing the NO[A]EL by the estimated dose of concern. HQ is the ratio of the exposure dose to a pre-established RfC, RfD, or a similar effect concentration or dose (Box 22.1). The main difference between MOE and HQ is that the latter can be used as is, since one or more SFs have been incorporated to derive the RfD or RfC. Accordingly, an HQ value much less than 1 is considered to have a low ecological or health risk. In contrast, an acceptable MOE (or the so-called benchmark MOE) is typically 100 or greater to account for at least an uncertainty factor of 10 for interspecies variation and another 10 for intraspecies sensitivity. Given that MOE = (NO[A]EL ÷ dose) x SF_{MOE}, HQ = dose ÷ RfD, and RfD = NO[A]EL ÷ SF_{HQ}, it follows that MOE ≅ (SF_{MOE} x SF_{HQ}) ÷ HQ.

23.4.2. Uncertainty and Safety Factors

From the discussion given thus far in this chapter, it is clear that health risk assessment is inadequate without at least some consideration of how the uncertainty or safety factors are determined and used. Their impacts on health risk implication are substantial, given that they are deliberately incorporated into some health risk measures (e.g., RfD, RfC, ADI). It is intuitive that here the uncertainties of concern can be broadly subsumed under the two key assessment components with which they tend to associate: (1) toxicity assessment; and (2) human exposure assessment. Despite such triviality, any fair account of the uncertainties involved in most any health risk assessment would require volumes of discussion, for which this chapter as well as this book is not the appropriate place. In this (sub)section, only certain uncertainties that are deemed to have the most impacts on health risk assessment are highlighted, all in an effort to illustrate the complexity and dynamics involved. It is of note that in many cases, it is due to the difficult, lengthy process of resolving many of the uncertainties involved that a full-scale health risk assessment for any toxic substance can take years to finalize.

One of the major uncertainty issues frequently encountered is that many toxicants can each be found to cause more than one type of adverse health effects, depending on the species tested and on the route, the amount, as well as the duration of dosing used. Where two or more types of effects were observed, they might not have been caused by exposure(s) at the same level or via the same route. It is therefore important for the risk assessor to analyze and determine which observed adverse effect(s) should be treated as the toxic endpoint(s) *of (critical) concern*, supposedly by following the strength- and weight-of-evidence principles. The health effects test guidelines such as those listed in Table 23.1 are provided with the intent to help minimize this type of uncertainties.

In particular, the main problems with HI (hazard identification) are the interpretation of toxicity data and the concerns with strength- and weight-of-evidence. For instance, the toxic effect could show up in a study with dogs, but not with rats. Does this mean that the dog is more sensitive to the toxicant? Or that only the dog study was conducted properly?

Concrete examples can be found in Chapter 10 concerning species and other biological traits as cofactors that can seriously affect toxicity.

The various types of adverse health effects listed in Table 23.1 are also problematic in terms of their actual application. For example, *acute* toxicity involves an adverse effect that by definition manifests within a short time interval following dosing. However, the upper end of this interval is not always well defined or agreed upon; that is, should it be 1, 24, or 72 hours (in the animal)? Another issue is that much implication of mutagenesis for carcinogenesis has not been fully resolved. Still another issue is that irritation scores given in a skin sensitization test are based on some degree of subjective evaluation. This type of evaluation can make skin sensitization less accepted as a primary adverse effect even when compared to decrease in body weight gain. This is not so much that the former effect is treated as less detrimental, but because it is less quantifiable.

Another limitation with toxicity assessment is that the toxic endpoint with the lowest NO[A]EL observed among studies may not always be the best candidate, as such a more health protective endpoint is credible only if it is derived from convincing data. Moreover, the adverse effects observed via different exposure routes may not be the same. Many times the toxic endpoints of regulatory concern do not represent the most severe effects, but are those with a low enough NO[A]EL to call for exposure mitigation. Here the notion is that if the *lower* critical exposure required for inducing the (often less severe) adverse effect under regulatory concern were adequately mitigated, so would the *higher* critical exposures required for inducing other (more severe) toxic effects.

The uncertainty with animal-to-human extrapolation is one of the most concerning issues in toxicity assessment. Yet contrary to general brief, when an adverse effect is observed in an animal study, the first thing that will come to the health risk assessor's mind is not always the question whether or not the same health effect would occur in humans. Oftentimes, the question is whether the same effect would occur in other strains of the test species or in another animal species. This is because knowing that human data are hard to come by, the strength- and the weight-of-evidence would have to rest on animal data alone, and would increase if the same health effect could be reproduced in another strain or in another animal species. Rats are commonly used as a test model mainly because they are relatively inexpensive and inbred to reduce variability (Ross *et al.*, 2000). However, certain chemicals or drugs, such as the notorious teratogen thalidomide, are highly species-specific or fairly sensitive to exposure time .

The uncertainty issues associated with exposure analysis (i.e., with human exposure assessment) are likewise tremendous and in many situations even more overwhelming. Exposure analysis is often thought to be more dynamic and more complicated than toxicity assessment. Such a notion is based on the general observation that overall, both the framework and the process for toxicity assessment are more solid and controllable compared to those for exposure analysis. To put it another way, relatively fewer assumptions and presumptions are needed in toxicity assessment while at the same time animal toxicity studies in general are better designed compared to exposure monitoring studies.

Human contact, being a behavioral as well as a physiological variable, is often more difficult to define and quantify. For example, inhalation exposure is a function of a person's respiration rate and of the toxicant's air concentration in that person's breathing zone. Yet respiration rate is not only gender- and age-specific, but also a function of human activity which cannot be quantified easily. And the toxicant's concentrations in the air are not only a source-dependent but also a temporal as well as a spatial variable. It is fair to say that the toxicant's actual concentration in a specific space and time period at best can only be approximated with some level of uncertainty.

Another important uncertainty with exposure analysis is how to determine duration and frequency for chronic exposure. It is not easy to give a fair account of all the human exposure events for an average day or month. It is even harder to determine the number of times a person is exposed to a toxicant in a year or a season. The uncertainty with the determination of exposure duration or frequency may be better appreciated using the following analogies or challenges: Would the (health) effect on a person be the same between the person taking 1 pill a day for a year and the same person taking 3 pills a day for 122 days (i.e., 1 year ≈ 122 days x 3)? Or would the effect be the same between the person taking 3 pills a day for 122 *consecutive* days and the same person taking 3 pills a day *intermittently* for 122 days over the year? If the effects from these various dosage schemes cannot be the same, then how should they be normalized or weighed?

Also, values used for the exposure parameters are generally based on policy defaults, professional judgment, or preferably empirical data. It is important to realize, however, that nearly all of such empirical data available to date were derived from small, unrepresentative spot or grab samples. By spot samples, it means that the sample size is less than adequate and, more critical, the measurements are less than complete or representative. Grab samples are those in which the test subjects or observation units were not randomly selected or assigned. These are simply opportunistic samples. Therefore, any conclusion or assertion that spot or grab samples would give a fair account about the target population's exposure-related activities or routines is an intention at best.

For instance, the Nationwide Food Consumption Survey conducted every ten years by the U.S. Department of Agriculture covers all ages, genders, and regions in the United States. Yet even with a survey so complexly large, there is still a missing link between people living in regions with known food residue levels and their consumption rates. That is, there is still a lack of correlation between where a contaminant concentrates and what the dietary patterns are for the residents living in that contaminated region.

There can also be uncertainties with the default values used as exposure factors, such as for soil ingestion by children in recreational areas where playground structures were treated with a wood preservative (e.g., Figure 23.4). Two- or three-year-olds might not stay and play in the sandbox for longer time than older children would. The hand-to-mouth movements of the younger children could be more or less frequent. And how well or how frequent their hands would be cleaned during playtime or shortly afterwards depends much on how health conscious these children and their parents are. The *Exposure*

Factors Handbook published by U.S. EPA (2011) provides the percentiles and other statistics of soil ingestion rate, body weight, and many other factors by age and gender intended for the *general* population. It is debatable whether or not these default values should be used to represent the distributions of soil ingestion rate, body weight, and the kind for the children under assessment whose physical build might be different.

To this date, most regulatory agencies still apply an uncertainty factor (UF) of 10 for interspecies extrapolation, thinking that humans can be up to 10 times more susceptible than the test species used in an animal study. Yet there is no sound justification for the adequacy of this UF of 10, other than perhaps the account by Dourson and Stara (1983). Before such an uncertainty can be truly accounted for, the equivalence of animal to human dose must be resolved first. For example, would 1 unit of dose given to a test animal exactly equal to 1 unit of dose received by a human, even after normalization for body weight? Is it not possible that the test animal (e.g., the rat) would detoxify or bioactivate the same amount of the chemical faster or slower than a human would?

Another UF commonly applied in health risk assessment is the 10-fold factor for intraspecies sensitivity which also has a direct impact on the derivation of RfD or ADI. Where the human exposure was calculated for populations other than workers, should this UF be greater than 10 to account for the lack of healthy worker effect? Or should this UF be less than 10 when worker exposure is considered? By healthy worker effect (*see*, e.g., Li and Sung, 1999), it means that workers on the whole are healthier and thus likely less susceptible to toxic insults compared to those of the same age group that are disabled or too ill to work. In essence, there seems to be always the uncertainty about the way in which or the extent to which the factor of 10 should be applied for intraspecies variation.

23.4.3. Health Risk Perception

As noted in Section 23.1.1, health risk assessment activities are bound by social values and public concerns. Such constraints imply that health risk perception plays a key role in having a health risk assessment done with a certain level of success, as evident from the tampon-toxic shock story discussed briefly in Section 3.2. The society's risk perception has much to do with how health risk assessment or characterization is actually performed. Health risk perception on this level may later be translated into practice through health regulations and will eventually complicate the health risk assessment or characterization process. For example, through the U.S. Food Quality Protection Act of 1996, the federal government now mandates the consideration of cumulative as well as aggregate exposure assessment for children's health (as defined in Section 23.3.3).

The centerpiece of risk perception is subjective or perceived risk which can be defined as the *sum* of objective risk (or hazard) *and* outrage (Beecher *et al.*, 2005; Covello and Sandman, 2001; Sandman, 1987). As stated in Section 22.3.3, (health) risk can be technically defined as the probability of an adverse effect on the receptor. More broadly, it is the likelihood that a dangerous event would occur. Yet the outrage of a stakeholder (i.e., one having an interest in the issue) is influenced by a number of perception factors, including dread, control, nature of the hazard (e.g., natural or anthropogenic), familiarity, trust, and more (Covello and Sandman, 2001; U.S. EPA, 2007a). Moreover, according to U. S. EPA (2007a), although a subjective risk takes much more into account, with the proper perspective it is just as manageable as an objective risk.

Any appreciation of health risk assessment thereby should rest on the public's risk and health perceptions of the hazard at issue. Risk and health perceptions each have a strong impact on the populace's choices of health agenda and are basic elements to health risk assessment movement. They rest on the two key human behavioral factors *(un)controllability* and *(un)familiarity* with the hazard. Stakeholders tend to accept greater risks linked to voluntary activities than to those imposed on them without their consent. On the other hand, shock, fear, and horror to people tend to multiply when the event is unexpected or sudden, or when the nature of the risk is complex.

The public reacts differently to most misfortunes, as do many organizations and professional groups including regulatory toxicologists. By definition, health risk perception starts with health effects that people perceive. Inasmuch as health effects may be determined by various types of toxicity tests, interpretations of test outcomes are not always consistent among regulatory agencies. Such differences in health risk perception explain in part why FDA, U.S. EPA, and some other entities in and outside of the United States apply different terminology to safe human dose for exposure hazards in their health risk analysis. As noted in Section 23.4.1, U.S. EPA prefers to use RfD for benchmark human exposure level in their analysis. In contrast, FDA opts to use ADI instead. ADI values are also used by WHO to define lifetime allowable daily intake of pesticide and food additive residues. Differences between RfD and ADI rest on the way in which the NO[A]EL and the uncertainty factors are treated, and often on the choice of toxicity data as well.

23.4.4. Health Risk Communication

In all cases, health risk assessment should never end with just the completion of a risk characterization. Risk assessment as a process is merely a regulatory or scientific tool, not an end in itself. The entity that has performed the human health (or ecological) risk assessment is obligated to relate the outcomes to its stakeholders and other audiences. In the past (or in some cases even now), the conventional way in which many government agencies dealt with the public on regulatory decisions is the *decide-announce-defend* or *"DAD"* approach (e.g., Beecher *et al.*, 2005; Scherer and Juanillo, 2003). This classic approach is built on the notion that the decisions that the experts make are fair and sound, and defend their decisions only when they are challenged. However, in recent years, many public sectors are seen to increasingly challenge government decisions and demand active involvement in the decision-making process, especially those decisions involving health risks. Nowadays, the experts are also perceived as ones not always capable of accurately assessing health risks.

In response to this new trend for greater participation by the public sectors, many regulatory agencies begin to appreciate the need for taking (health) risk communication into fuller consideration in their health risk assessment processes. As NRC (1989) puts it, the risk characterization process can be regarded as successful only if it *"satisfies those involved that they are adequately informed within the limits of available knowledge."* The U.S. Agency for Toxic Substances and Disease Registry (ATSDR, 1994) further contends that *"Merely disseminating the outcome information without regard for communicating the complexities and uncertainties of risk does not ensure necessarily effective risk communication."* It is therefore important that any productive risk characterization must rest on how health risk assessors can treat the uncertainties involved professionally and then address them effectively to stakeholders and other audiences.

According to NRC (1989), *"(Health) risk communication is an interactive process of exchange of information and opinions among individuals, groups, and institutions. It often involves multiple messages about the nature of the risk or expressing concerns, opinions, or reactions to risk messages or to the legal and institutional arrangements for risk management."* U.S. EPA (2007a) refines this concept to suggest that any ideal risk communication process would put a risk into proper perspective, would make contrasts with other risks, and would advocate a fruitful dialogue between those that deliver and those that receive the risk assessment outcome. In that same document, U.S. EPA reiterates its seven cardinal rules (Covello and Allen, 1988) for the practice of (health) risk communication. Those cardinal rules are reproduced below in Box 23.2.

Box 23.2. Cardinal Rules for Risk Communication (Covello and Allen, 1988)

- Accept and involve the public as a partner.
- Listen to the public's specific concerns.
- Be honest, frank, and open.
- Work with other credible sources.
- Meet the needs of the media.
- Speak clearly and with compassion.
- Plan carefully and evaluate the communication effort.

In addition to the seven cardinal rules, U.S. EPA (2007a) references the following four theories for a sound risk communication practice: (1) the trust determination theory; (2) the negative dominance theory; (3) the mental noise theory; and (4) the risk perception theory. In essence, the trust determination theory hypothesizes that when people are upset or under stress, they easily do not trust that other people are listening, caring, competent, empathetic, or committed. The negative dominance theory suggests that when people are upset or under stress, they focus more on the negative than on the positive aspects of a situation. The mental noise theory contends that when people are upset or under stress, they have difficulty listening, understanding, and remembering relevant information. The risk perception theory postulates that when people are upset or under stress, their concerns and perceptions of threat differ from those of experts. Overall, these risk communication theories all revolve around the message receiver's state of mind, and together lend strong support for the cardinal rules listed in Box 23.2.

In closing, it is important to note that public sectors are not the only audiences to a health (or ecological) risk assessment. At the professional or legal end, risk assessors and risk managers must realize that concerns with adverse health effects vary considerably among health statutes and hence among regulatory agencies. Such variations need to become explicit in the risk characterization document, so that the variations in health risk perceptions and risk prevention goals can be kept to a minimum among stakeholders and other audiences. As a case in point, the U.S. Clean Water Act requires *best available technology*, whereas the U.S. Clean Air Act promulgates *risk-based standards*. The risk-based approach requires that the ambient air quality be upheld in terms of a set of air quality standards, such as the U.S. National Ambient Air Quality Standards (Chapter 11). In contrast, the best available technology approach limits discharges of (water) contaminants by applying technologically feasible abatement principles and strategies. Similar terms for the best available technology approach include *best available techniques*, *best practicable means*, and *best practicable environmental option*. In all cases, such regulatory requirements need to be effectively communicated in the risk characterization report not only to the peer reviewers and the public, but also to all other audiences.

References

ATSDR (U.S. Agency for Toxic Substances and Disease Registry), 1994. A Primer on Health Risk Communication Principles and Practices. U.S. Department of Health and Human Services, Atlanta, Georgia, USA.

Beecher N, Harrison E, Goldstein N, McDaniel M, Field P, Susskind L, 2005. Risk Perception, Risk Communication, and Stakeholder Involvement for Biosolids Management and Research. *J. Environ. Qual.* 34:122-128.

Covello V, Allen F, 1988. Seven Cardinal Rules of Risk Communication. OPA-87-020 (leaflet). Office of Policy Analysis, Washington DC, USA.

Covello VT, Sandman PM, 2001. Risk Communication: Evolution and Revolutions. In *Solutions to an Environment in Peril* (Wolbarst AB, Ed.). Baltimore, Maryland, USA: John Hopkins University Press, Chapter 15.

Dong MH, Ross JH, 2001. Coping with Aggregate Pesticide Exposure Assessment: An Integration Approach. In *Hayes' Handbook of Pesticide Toxicology* (Krieger R, Ed.), Second Edition. San Diego, California, USA: Academic Press, Chapter 19.

Dourson ML, Stara JF, 1983. Regulatory History and Experimental Support of Uncertainty (Safety) Factors. *Regul. Toxicol. Pharmacol.* 3:224-238.

Klaassen CD, Eaton DL, 1991. Principles of Toxicology. In *Casarett and Doull's Toxicology: The Basic Science of Poisons* (Amdur MO, Doull J, Klaassen CD, Eds.), Fourth Edition. New York, New York, USA: Pergamon Press, Chapter 2.

Li CY, Sung FC, 1999. A Review of the Healthy Worker Effect in Occupational Epidemiology. *Occup. Med. (Lond.)* 49:225-229.

NRC (U.S. National Research Council), 1983. *Risk Assessment in the Federal Government: Managing the Process*. Washington DC, USA: National Academic Press.

NRC (U.S. National Research Council), 1989. *Improving Risk Communication*. Washington DC, USA: National Academy Press.

NRC (U.S. National Research Council), 1994. *Science and Judgment in Risk Assessment*. Committee on Risk Assessment of Hazardous Air Pollutants, Board on Environmental Studies and Technology, Commission on Life Science. Washington DC, USA: National Academy Press.

Ross JH, Dong MH, Krieger RI, 2000. Conservatism in Pesticide Exposure Assessment. *Regul. Toxicol. Pharmacol.* 31:53-58.

Sandman PM, 1987. Communicating Risk: Some Basics. *Health Environ. Digest* 1:3-4.

Scherer CW, Juanillo NK Jr, 2003. The Continuing Challenge of Community Health Risk Management and Communication. In *Handbook of Health Communication* (Thompson TL, Dorsey AM, Miller KL, Parrott R, Eds.). Mahwah, New Jersey, USA: Lawrence Erlbaum Associate, Chapter 11.

Suter GW II, Barnthouse LW, 1993. Assessment Concepts. In *Ecological Risk Assessment* (Suter GW II, Ed.). Boca Raton, Florida, USA: CRC Press, Chapter 2.

Thongsinthusak T, Dong MH, 2010. Mitigation Measures for Exposure to Pesticides. In *Hayes' Handbook of Pesticide Toxicology* (Krieger R, Ed.), Third Edition. San Diego, California, USA: Academic Press, Chapter 54.

UNEP/IPCS (United Nations Environment Programme/International Programme on Chemical Safety), 1999. *Training Module No. 3 – Chemical Risk Assessment: Human Risk Assessment, Environmental Risk Assessment and Ecological Risk Assessment*. WHO/PCS/99.2. World Health Organization, Geneva, Switzerland.

U.S. EPA (U.S. Environmental Protection Agency), 1986. Guidelines for Mutagenicity Risk Assessment. *Federal Register* 51:34006-34012.

U.S. EPA (U.S. Environmental Protection Agency), 1991. Guidelines for Developmental Toxicity Risk Assessment. *Federal Register* 56:63798-63826.

U.S. EPA (U.S. Environmental Protection Agency), 1992. Guidelines for Exposure Assessment. *Federal Register* 57:22888-22938.

U.S. EPA (U.S. Environmental Protection Agency), 1996. Guidelines for Reproductive Toxicity Risk Assessment. *Federal Register* 61:56274-56322.

U.S. EPA (U.S. Environmental Protection Agency), 1998a. Guidelines for Neurotoxicity Risk Assessment. *Federal Register* 63:26926-26954.

U.S. EPA (U.S. Environmental Protection Agency), 1998b. Guidelines for Ecological Risk Assessment. *Federal Register* 63:26846-26924.

U.S. EPA (U.S. Environmental Protection Agency), 1998c. Health Effects Test Guidelines: OPPTS 870.3465 – 90-Day Inhalation Toxicity. EPA 712-C-98-204. Office of Prevention, Pesticides, and Toxic Substances, Washington DC, USA.

U.S. EPA (U.S. Environmental Protection Agency), 1998d. Health Effects Test Guidelines: OPPTS 870.4100 – Chronic Toxicity. EPA 712-C-98-210. Office of Prevention, Pesticides, and Toxic Substances, Washington DC, USA.

U.S. EPA (U.S. Environmental Protection Agency), 1998e. Health Effects Test Guidelines: OPPTS 870.5100 – Bacterial Reverse Mutation Test. EPA 712-C-98-247. Office of Prevention, Pesticides, and Toxic Substances, Washington DC, USA.

U.S. EPA (U.S. Environmental Protection Agency), 1998f. Health Effects Test Guidelines: OPPTS 870.6200 – Neurotoxicity Screening Battery. EPA 712-C-98-238. Office of Prevention, Pesticides, and Toxic Substances, Washington DC, USA.

U.S. EPA (U.S. Environmental Protection Agency), 1998g. Health Effects Test Guidelines: OPPTS 870.4200 – Carcinogenicity. EPA 712-C-98-211. Office of Prevention, Pesticides, and Toxic Substances, Washington DC, USA.

U.S. EPA (U.S. Environmental Protection Agency), 1998h. Health Effects Test Guidelines: OPPTS 870.7800 – Immunotoxicity. EPA 712-C-98-351. Office of Prevention, Pesticides, and Toxic Substances, Washington DC, USA.

U.S. EPA (U.S. Environmental Protection Agency), 2000a. Health Effects Test Guidelines: OPPTS 870.3550 – Reproduction/Developmental Toxicity Screening Test. EPA 712-C-00-367. Office of Prevention, Pesticides, and Toxic Substances, Washington DC, USA.

U.S. EPA (U.S. Environmental Protection Agency), 2000b. *Risk Characterization Handbook*. EPA 100-B-00-002. Science Policy Council, Washington, DC, USA.

U.S. EPA (U.S. Environmental Protection Agency), 2002. Health Effects Test Guidelines: OPPTS 870.1100 – Acute Oral Toxicity. EPA 712-C-02-190. Office of Prevention, Pesticides, and Toxic Substances, Washington DC, USA.

U.S. EPA (U.S. Environmental Protection Agency), 2003. Framework for Cumulative Risk. EPA/630/P-02/001F. Risk Assessment Forum, Washington DC, USA.

U.S. EPA (U.S. Environmental Protection Agency), 2005. Guidelines for Carcinogen Risk Assessment. EPA/630/P-03/001F. Risk Assessment Forum, Washington DC, USA.

U.S. EPA (U.S. Environmental Protection Agency), 2007a. Risk Communication in Action: The Risk Communication Workbook. EPA/625/R-025/003. Office Research and Development, Cincinnati, Ohio, USA.

U.S. EPA (U.S. Environmental Protection Agency), 2007b. Concepts, Methods, and Data Sources for Cumulative Health Risk Assessment of Multiple Chemicals, Exposures and Effects: A Resource Document. EPA/600/013F. Office Research and Development, Cincinnati, Ohio, USA.

U.S. EPA (U.S. Environmental Protection Agency), 2011. Exposure Factors Handbook 2011 Edition (Final). EPA/600/R-09/052F. National Center for Environmental Assessment, Washington DC, USA.

Review Questions

1. What are the four key components or steps of human health-based risk assessment?

2. What are the main differences between the hazard identification phase in health risk assessment and the problem formulation phase in ecological risk assessment?

3. What is the main task of hazard identification, and its overall task?

4. List the types of adverse health effects commonly considered in a health risk assessment.

5. Name three organizations that help harmonize the health effects test guidelines used by government agencies and the industry.

6. What is the crucial function (task) of dose-response assessment in health risk analysis?

7. What is the implication for effect response when the dose-response slope is very steep?

8. What does the term *toxicity assessment* refer to?

9. What are the (subtle) differences among exposure, applied dose, dosage, and internal dose?

10. Briefly explain why compared to environmental toxicologists, environmental epidemiologists tend to be more ready to assess human exposure to environmental toxicants.

11. What is the widely received, yet not fully validated, simple algorithm for the determination of human exposure?

12. Briefly distinguish the direct and indirect measurement methods generally used for human exposure assessment.

13. In their simplest terms, what are aggregate and cumulative exposure assessments?

14. In their simplest terms, what are health risk characterization and health risk assessment?

15. Why does it become a crucial uncertainty issue when the upper end of the exposure interval is not well defined for an acute toxicity test?

16. When an untoward health effect is observed in an animal study, what is likely the first thing that will come to the health risk assessor's mind in performing the toxicity assessment?

17. Match each of the health risk measures in the left column to its definition, characteristics, or application in the right column.

    (1) PEL   (a) [NOEL in concentration] ÷ [Safety Factor]
    (2) RfC   (b) direct risk measure for carcinogenic effects
    (3) BMD   (c) direct risk measure for non-cancer effects
    (4) MOE   (d) likely a more accurately quantified LO[A]EL
    (5) CPF   (e) cancer slope factor
    (6) ECR   (f) primarily used by FDA for intake of food additives
    (7) ADI   (g) primarily used by OSHA

18. Match each of the U.S. federal agencies (left column) to the type of health risk assessment activities that it engages in (right column).

    (1) OSHA   (a) replying on self for exposure mitigation
    (2) CDC   (b) relying on regulation for exposure mitigation
    (3) U.S. EPA   (c) involving health risks in a workplace

19. What is the basic definition of perceived (subjective) risk?

20. With the proper perspective, subjective risks are as manageable as objective risks.

    (A) TRUE   (B) FALSE

21. What appears to be the major problem with using the empirical data available to date to set values for the exposure parameters used in human exposure analysis?

22. Briefly explain why health risk assessors might need to take into account the healthy worker effect when applying the safety factor for intraspecies variation.

23. Which of the following was the classic "*DAD*" approach that many government agencies used in the past in dealing with the public on regulatory decisions? a) define-announce-decide; b) decide-announce-defend; c) define-announce-defend; d) define-anticipate-defend.

24. List the seven cardinal rules for (health) risk communication. And briefly explain how they are related to the risk communication theories mentioned in this chapter.

25. Briefly describe the main differences between the risk-based approach and the best practical means approach in regulating environmental health hazards.

INDEX

γ

γ-GABA. *See gamma*-aminobutyric acid (γ-GABA)

γ-HCH (γ-hexachlorocyclohexane). *See* lindane (γ-HCH)

1

1,2-dibromo-3-chloropropane, 143, 364

1,3-dimethylol-5,5-dimethylhydantoin as formaldehyde-releasing ingredient, 399

1,4-dioxane, 399

2

2,3,7,8-TCDD, 55, 71, 73, 81, 83, 134, 145, 269, 295, 296, 297, 298, 341, 357

2,3,7,8-tetrachlorodibenzo-*p*-dioxin. *See* 2,3,7,8-TCDD

2,4,5-T, 269, 270, 294

2,4,5-trichlorophenoxyacetic acid. *See* 2,4,5-T

2,4-D, 269, 270, 294, 378

2,4-dichlorophenoxyacetic acid. *See* 2,4-D

7

7-ethoxyresorufin *o*-deethylase (EROD), 120, 121

A

abiotic transformation. *See* transformation: chemical

acceptable daily intake (ADI), 391, 393, 394, 445, 446, 447, 450, 451

acephate, 265

acetaminophen, 401

acetyl CoA, 115, 241

acetylation, 115

acetylcholinesterase (AChE), 115, 138, 161, 263, 320, 376, 378

ACGIH. *See* American Conference of Industrial Hygienists (ACGIH)

AChE. *See* acetylcholinesterase (AChE)

Acid Deposition Act, U.S., 177

acid rain
    formation, 67

active transport. *See* toxicant(s): mechanisms of entry

acute beryllium disease, 242

acute respiratory distress syndrome, 274

acyl-CoA amino acid:*N*-acyltransferase, 119

additivity. *See* interaction, chemical: additivity

ADI. *See* acceptable daily intake (ADI)

aerodynamic diameter
    definition, 193

aerosol(s)
    atmospheric, 191
    forms, 191

aflatoxicol, 312

aflatoxin(s), 25, 57, 144, 145, 312, 396
    B_1, 25, 116, 134, 158, 312, 334, 335
    B_2, 312
    G_1, 312
    G_2, 312
    M_1, 312
    M_2, 312

Agent Orange, 269, 270

aggregate dose. *See also* aggregate exposure
    definition, 443

aggregate exposure, iv, 155, 444

Ah hydroxylase, 295

AhR. *See* aryl hydrocarbon receptor (AhR)

AIDS (acquired immune deficiency syndrome), 306, 307, 308

air pollutant(s)
    direct deposition. *See* air pollutant(s): dry deposition or wet deposition
    dry deposition, 65, 206
    fate, 63, 64, 65, 66, 67
    indirect deposition, 65
    transport, 63, 64, 65, 66, 67
    wet deposition, 65, 177, 206, 240

air pollution, v, 17, 30, 31, 36, 38, 58, 62, 63, 131, 151, 173, 178, 181, 183, 191, 198, 199, 202, 204, 205, 397, 423
    definition, 17

air toxics. *See* hazardous air pollutants

airborne microbes, 200, 201, 202

ALAD (δ-ALAD). *See delta*-aminolevulinic acid dehydratase (δ-ALAD)

alanycarb, 266

aldehyde oxidase, 160

aldicarb, 266, 425

aldrin, 27, 58, 87, 260, 261, 283

alkaloid(s), 316
    batrachotoxins, 321
    epibatidines, 321
    from toads, 321

histrionicotoxins, 321
indolizidine, 317
pumiliotoxins, 321
pyrrolizidine, 316
taxine, 317
alkylphenols, 283
allergic response, 135, 141
histamine, 135
allura red AC. *See* FD&C red No. 40: food colorant
alpha (α) particle (α radiation), 248, 249
alpha cells, 354
alpha$_{2\mu}$-globulin nephropathy, 163, 164
Alternaria, 55
aluminum (Al), 195, 206, 239, 240, 248, 392, 425
Alzheimer's disease, 85, 139, 205, 240, 247, 392
American Conference of Industrial Hygienists (ACGIH), 375, 376, 377, 378, 383
American Lung Association, 24
American Public Health Association, 415
American Society for Testing and Materials, 415
Ames test, 335
amino acid conjugation, 115
ammonia (NH$_3$), 173, 216, 400
amygdalin, 316
An Inconvenient Truth, 37
anabolism. *See* toxicant(s): metabolism
androgen(s), 354, 355
adrenal, 354
anesthetic effects. *See* toxicant(s): toxicodynamics
aneuploidy. *See* chromosome aberration: aneuploidy
aniline, 115, 219
ankylosing spondylitis, 249
antagonism. *See* interaction, chemical: antagonism
anticoagulant(s), 137, 258, 271, 272
poisoning, 272
antioxidant enzyme(s), 118, 121
antioxidant(s), 26, 57, 115, 119, 120, 122, 132, 164, 335, 390, 394
apoptosis, 142, 274, 311, 336, 337
aquatic environment, 413, 414
aquatic toxicity tests, 411, 414, 415
early-life stage, 416
aquatic toxicology, 411, 412, 413, 414, 415, 416
relevance, 411
Aroclor, 292, *See also* polychlorinated biphenyl(s) [PCB(s)]
aromatase, 271

arsenic (As), 3, 6, 52, 56, 68, 122, 144, 145, 151, 232, 233, 240, 241, 380
arsenate reductase, 240
arsenate(s), 52, 240, 241
arsenide(s), 240
arsenite(s), 240, 241
arsenobetaine, 240
arsine, 145, 241
glutaredoxin. *See* arsenic (As): arsenate reductase
lead arsenate, 240
monosodium methyl arsenate, 240
pentoxide, 240
the Borgias family, 241
trioxide, 162
aryl hydrocarbon receptor (AhR), 120, 133, 134, 292, 294, 357
asbestos, 24, 54, 161, 172, 333, 373, 381, 382, 383
actinolite, 54
anthophyllite, 54
chrysotile, 382
crocidolite, 54, 382
mesothelioma, 54
tremolite, 54
Aspergillus, 55, 307, 312, 335
Aspergillus flavus, 57, 312, 313, 396
Aspergillus parasiticus, 312, 313, 396
asphyxiation. *See* toxicant(s): toxicodynamics
assessment endpoint(s), 421, 422
asthma triggers, 56
atrazine, 75, 271, 358
atropine, 263, 314
ATSDR. *See* U.S. Agency for Toxic Substances and Disease Registry (ATSDR)
attention deficit hyperactivity disorder (ADHD), 265
Aum Shinrikyo cult, 265
Australia Department of Health Services (ADHS), 433
autosomal dominant disorders
definition, 331
azinphos-methyl, 265

B

BAL. *See* British anti-Lewisite (BAL)
Bangkok Fashion City Area, Thailand, 201
base excision repair (BER). See DNA (deoxyribonucleic acid): repair
Basel Convention, 41, 284, 423
Basel Convention on the Control of

Transboundary Movements of Hazardous Wastes and Their Disposal. See Basel Convention

BCF. *See* bioconcentration factor (BCF)

beauvericin, 312, 313

bee sting(s), 319

Beijing, 18, 198, 199

BEIs. *See* biological exposure indices (BEIs)

benchmark concentration (BMC), 445, 446

benchmark dose (BMD), 445, 446

benzaldehyde
   direct food additive, 393

benzene, 52, 56, 57, 59, 113, 145, 184, 213, 214, 215, 217, 218, 219, 220, 221, 223, 260, 262, 269, 270, 285, 293, 294, 380, 394, 402, 417
   exposures and toxic effects, 218, 219, 220
   sources and use, 218

benzo[α]pyrene (BαP), 116, 334, 335

berylliosis, 242, 378

beryllium (Be), 239, 241, 242, 379, 380

best available technology, 453

beta (ß) particle (ß radiation), 248

beta cells, 354

beta-bungarotoxin (ß-bungarotoxin), 320

beta-glucosidase, 316

BHA. *See* butylated hydroxyanisole (BHA)

BHT. *See* butylated hydroxytoluene (BHT)

bioaccumulation, 63, 78, 79, 80, 82, 83, 87, 88, 90, 155, 235, 280, 281, 282, 286, 415
   dynamic equilibrium effect, 89, 90
   environmental mobility, 88, 89
   influencing factors, 87, 88, 89, 90
   lipophilicity and bioavailability, 88
   metabolic potential, 88
   real cases, 83, 84

bioavailability, 88

bioconcentration, 63, 78, 80, 82, 87, 281

bioconcentration factor (BCF), 80, 81, 82, 281

biological agents, 22

biological exposure indices (BEIs), 376, 377
   as biomarkers, 376

biological transformation, 62, 68

biomagnification, 63, 78, 82, 84, 155
   real cases, 83, 84

biomembrane(s), 95, 96, 100, 111
   glycolipids, 96
   integral proteins, 96
   peripheral proteins, 96
   sphingolipids, 96
   structure, 95, 96

biomonitoring (biological monitoring), 220, 376, 377, 443

Bioterrorism Act, U.S., 39, 41

biotransport, 63, 89

birth defect(s), 6, 21, 23, 26, 58, 142, 269, 347, 348, 361, 362, 363, 397
   average annualnational prevalence, U.S., 362
   definition, 23, 348
   impacts and causes, 348
   major structural types, 362
   metabolic diseases, 23

bisphenol A, 48, 49, 360, 394

Blastomyces dermatitidis, 308

bloodborne pathogens (BBP) standard. *See* U.S. Occupational Safety and Health Administration (OSHA): bloodborne pathogens (BBP) standard

blood-brain barrier, 144, 163

bone disease
   industrial disease, 22

botulinum, 2, 57, 310, 311
   toxin, 136

botulism, 305, 310, 311

bovine spongiform encephalopathy (BSE), 11, 12, 305

Brazilian Institute of Environmental and Renewable Natural Resources (IBAMA), 42, 43

brevetoxin, 19, 309, 315

brilliant blue. *See* FD&C blue No. 1: food colorant

British anti-Lewisite (BAL), 241

brominated flame retardants (BFRs), 290

brompheniramine
   antihistamine, 401

Brown Cloud, 206

Brownian diffusional force, 193, 194

BSE. *See* bovine spongiform encephalopathy (BSE)

BTEX, 402

Burkitt's lymphoma, 333

Bush, George W (former U.S. President), 283

butylated hydroxyanisole (BHA), 57, 360, 393

butylated hydroxytoluene (BHT), 57, 393

C

cadmium (Cd), 19, 26, 51, 52, 68, 137, 139, 151, 195, 196, 233, 239, 380, 396
   cigarette (tobacco) smoke, 237
   heavy metal, 236, 237, 238
   itai-itai, 237, 238

calcitonin, 354

calcium (Ca), 133, 137, 159, 162, 177, 233, 243,

354, 391, 392
California Environmental Protection Agency
    (Cal/EPA), 35
California newt, 321
Campylobacter, 305
Canadian Environmental Protection Act (CEPA),
    281
cancer
    characteristics, 330, 331
    childhood type, 21
    definition, 23
    metastatic (secondary), 339
    of the bladder, 116, 241
    of the bone, 249
    of the breast, 24, 359
    of the cervix, 143
    of the colorectum, 399
    of the gastrointestinal tract, 295
    of the head, 249
    of the liver, 55, 116, 144, 241, 261, 312, 316
    of the lung, 24, 54, 122, 144, 153, 154, 161,
        183, 238, 241, 242, 245, 249, 250, 378,
        382
    of the nasal passage (the nose), 216, 249, 378
    of the prostate, 364
    of the respiratory tract, 295
    of the scrotum, 9, 22, 369
    of the skin, 145
    of the testicle, 24, 271
    of the vascular system, 265
    risk, 247
    vaginal clear cell carcinoma, 349
cancer potency factor (CPF), 438, 440
cancer slope factor (CSF). *See* cancer potency
    factor (CPF)
Candida, 307
capsaicin, 401
carbamate(s) [CB(s)], 138, 144, 265, 273
carbaryl, 265
carbofuran, 266
carbon dioxide (CO_2), 17, 19, 52, 65, 67, 105,
    172, 174, 182, 185, 221, 391, 399
carbon disulfide, 145
carbon monoxide (CO), 18, 52, 53, 117, 130, 134,
    142, 143, 145, 156, 162, 172, 173, 181, 182,
    183, 184, 185, 186, 198, 223, 323
    characteristics, 184, 185
    effects on humans and animals, 185, 186
    effects on plants, 186
    poisoning, 156, 162, 223
    sources of pollution, 184
    toxic effects and advisories, 186

carbon tetrachloride, 116, 132, 161, 213, 394
carbonyl reductase, 118
carbosulfan, 266
carboxylesterase, 118
carcinogen(s)
    definition, 328
carcinogenesis, 26, 57, 116, 142, 328, 337, 342,
    448
    concepts, 337
    in relation to cell cycle, 336
    mechanism, 116, 264, 337, 338, 339
carcinogenic effects. *See* toxicant(s):
    toxicodynamics
carcinogenicity
    definition, 328
    potential for humans, 340
cardiac glycosides. *See* glycoside(s): cardiac
Carson, Rachel, 8, 21, 30, 33, 34, 35, 255, 417
catabolism. *See* toxicant(s): metabolism
catalase (CAT), 112, 119, 120
catalytic converter requirement, 184
cataract, 145
cell cycle, 336, 337, 342
    checkpoints, 336, 342
    interphase, 336
cell differentiation. *See* developmental-
    reproductive process: cell differentiation
cell migration. *See* developmental-reproductive
    process: cell migration
cell proliferation, 142, 337, *See also*
    developmental-reproductive process: cell
    proliferation
CEQ. *See* U.S. Council of Environmental
    Quality (CEQ)
cervical stenosis, 143
cetirizine
    antihistamine, 401
chaparral. *See* wildlife environment: chaparral
Charcot-Marie-Tooth neuropathy. *See*
    chromosome aberration: Charcot-Marie-
    Tooth neuropathy
chelation, 135, 136
    therapy, 136, 247
chemical persistence, 280, 281
chemical pneumonitis, 242
Chemical Risk Assessment, 433
chemical transformation, 62, 68
Chernobyl nuclear explosion, 322
chloracne, 55, 145, 269, 296
chlordane, 27, 58, 260, 261, 283
chlordecone. *See* kepone
chlorobenzene, 380

chlorobenzilate, 259
chlorofluorocarbons, 17, 66, 380
chlorosis, of plants, 94, 131
chlorpyrifos, 265
cholestasis, 144
chromated copper arsenate (CCA), 52, 240, 444
chromium (Cr), 18, 26, 52, 53, 57, 160, 233, 243, 244, 247, 380, 395
chromosome aberration, 331, 332, 333
    aneuploidy, 332
    Charcot-Marie-Tooth neuropathy, 333
    clastogenicity, 332
    cri du chat syndrome, 333
    deletion, 332
    Down syndrome, 332, 361, 362
    duplication, 333
    inversion, 333
    Pick complex diseases, 333
    translocation, 333
    Turner syndrome, 332
chromosome deletion. *See* chromosome aberration: deletion
chromosome duplication. *See* chromosome aberration: duplication
chromosome inversion. *See* chromosome aberration: inversion
chromosome translocation. *See* chromosome aberration: translocation
chromosome(s), 330
    autosomes, 329
    chromatids, 330
    chromatin, 329
    definition, 329
chronic glomerulonephritis, 381
chronic obstructive pulmonary disease (COPD), 24, 203
chrysotile. *See* asbestos: chrysotile
cigarette (tobacco) smoke, 20, 23, 24, 116, 118, 143, 144, 178, 192, 205, 215, 217, 218, 335, 338, 364
cigarette (tobacco) smoking, 54, 161, 245, 250
cigarette consumption
    in Japan, 153
ciguatera, 315
ciguatoxin, 25, 304, 315, 396
    Gambierdiscus toxicus, 315
cilantro, 136
cisplatin, 343
citric acid cycle. *See* Krebs cycle
Cladosporium, 55
clastogenicity. *See* chromosome aberration: clastogenicity

cleft lip, 23, 361, 362
cleft palate, 361, 362
Clostridium, 310, 396
Clostridium botulinum, 2
coagulation. *See* ultrafine particles: coagulation
cobalt (Co), 160, 200, 243, 380
cocamide DEA, 397, 398
cocamide diethanolamine. *See* cocamide DEA
Coccidioides immitis, 308
Coccidioides posadasii, 308
codon(s)
    definition, 329
coenzyme(s). *See* enzyme(s): coenzymes
cofactor(s). *See* enzyme(s): cofactors
colony collapse disorder, 273
Commission for Environmental Cooperation (CEC), 42
complexation. *See* chelation
Compound 1080. *See* sodium (mono)fluoroacetate (Compound 1080)
Comprehensive Environmental Response, Compensation, & Liability Act, U.S. (CERCLA), 36, 39, 40, 41, 51, 423, 425, 426, 427, 428
Conventional Reduced Risk Program, 273
COPD. *See* chronic obstructive pulmonary disease (COPD)
copper (Cu), 1, 52, 58, 119, 124, 145, 159, 163, 173, 174, 175, 177, 195, 200, 233, 238, 240, 241, 243, 244, 246, 247, 256, 380, 444
    IUDs (intrauterine devices), 247
    oral contraceptives, 247
corrosive effects. *See* toxicant(s): toxicodynamics
corticosteroids, 354
Corynebacteria, 318
Cosmetic Ingredient Review, 398
coumarin(s), 271, 272
    3,4-coumarin epoxide, 272
CPSC. *See* U.S. Consumer Product Safety Commission (CPSC)
Creutzfeldt-Jakob disease (CJD), 11
cri du chat syndrome. *See* chromosome aberration: *cri du chat* syndrome
Crigler-Nijar syndrome, 118
criteria air pollutants, 53, 58, 172, 191, 234
Criteria Documents, 374
crocidolite. *See* asbestos: crocidolite
Cryptosporidium, 308
CS syndrome, 266
cumulative dose. *See also* cumulative exposure
    definition, 443

cumulative exposure, 155, 161, 255, 444, 445, 450, *See also* health risk assessment: cumulative exposure

cumulative risk, 161

cumulative risk assessment
for atrazine, simazine, and propazine, 270

cyanuric acid, 49

cyclodienes, 261, 262, 266

CYP1A1, 118, 120, 123, 159

CYP1A2, 123, 159

CYP2D6, 121, 123, 164

CYP2E1, 123, 158, 159

CYP3A4, 117, 123, 159, 163

cytochrome 450, 114, 115, 116, 117, 118, 121, 123, 158, 159, 160, 163, 164
activities and locations, 117, 118
characteristics, 117, 118
families, 117

cytochrome *c* oxidase, 134

cytokinesis
definition, 336

D

DBCP. *See* 1,2-dibromo-3-chloropropane

DDD (dichlorodiphenyldichloroethane), 259

DDE (dichlorodiphenyldichloroethylene), 83, 260, 359

DDT (dichlorodiphenyltrichloroethane), 27, 34, 51, 58, 81, 83, 84, 85, 86, 87, 89, 103, 259, 260, 266, 283, 341, 360, 364, 378, 426, 427, 428, 429
analogues, 359

*deca*brominated biphenyl (*deca*BB), 289

*deca*brominated diphenyl ether (*deca*BDE), 56, 290, 292

decide-announce-defend (DAD) approach, 451

Deepwater Horizon BP Oil Spill of 2010, 417

deforestation, 16, 17, 19, 20
source of carbon dioxide, 52

degradation half-life, 80, 280

delayed neuropathy, 264

Delhi, India, 206, 256

delta-aminolevulinic acid dehydratase (δ-ALAD), 139, 235

dengue fever, 317

dermophyte, 307

desert. *See* wildlife environment: desert

development policies and programs (DPP), 435

developmental toxicant(s)
definition, 359

developmental-reproductive cycle, 350, 351, *See*

also developmental-reproductive process

developmental-reproductive effects, 359, 361, 362, 363, 364, 366

developmental-reproductive process, 347
cell differentiation, 350
cell migration, 350
cell proliferation, 350
organogenesis, 350, 351
predifferential period, 350, 351

dextromethorphan (DXM), 135

diabetes (mellitus), 13, 54, 145, 354, 365

dialkylpiperidine hemolytic factors, 319

diazinon, 264, 265, 420

dibromochloropropane, 24

dichlorodiphenyldichloroethane. *See* DDD (dichlorodiphenyldichloroethane)

dichlorodiphenyldichloroethylene. *See* DDE (dichlorodiphenyldichloroethylene)

dichlorodiphenyltrichloroethane. *See* DDT (dichlorodiphenyltrichloroethane)

dichloromethane (DCM). *See* methylene chloride (MC)

dichlorvos, 265

dicofol, 259

Dieffenbachia. See dumb cane (*Dieffenbachia*)

dieldrin, 25, 27, 58, 87, 260, 261, 283, 359, 360, 378, 429

diesel fuel, 56

diesel particulate matter, 205

dietary supplement, 393
definition, 392

Dietary Supplement Health and Education Act, U.S. (DSHHA), 392

diethylstilbestrol (DES), 23, 57, 341, 349, 355, 358, 362, 363, 425

Digitalis purpurea, 316

dioxin(s). *See* polychlorinated dibenzo-*p*-dioxin(s) [PCDD(s)]

direct chemical reversal. *See* DNA (deoxyribonucleic acid): repair

DNA (deoxyribonucleic acid)
damage, 130, 336, 338, 340, 342, 343, 344
definition, 328
hotspots on, 331
repair, 336, 337, 340, 343, 344

DNA adduct(s), 116, 134, 334

DNA AP endonuclease. *See* DNA (deoxyribonucleic acid): repair

DNA damage tolerance mechanism. *See* DNA (deoxyribonucleic acid): repair

DNA glycosylase. *See* DNA (deoxyribonucleic acid): repair

DNA ligase. *See* DNA (deoxyribonucleic acid): repair

DNA polymerase. *See* DNA (deoxyribonucleic acid): repair

DNA repair mechanism. *See* DNA (deoxyribonucleic acid): repair

DNA TLS (translesion synthesis) polymerases. *See* DNA (deoxyribonucleic acid): repair

DNA topoisomerases. *See* DNA (deoxyribonucleic acid): repair

DNA translesion synthesis. *See* DNA (deoxyribonucleic acid): repair

domoic acid, 309, 315, 396

Donora, Pennsylvania, 131, 173, 202

dose-response assessment. *See* health risk assessment: dose-response assessment

dose-response relationship, 140, 150, 151

DOT. *See* U.S. Department of Transportation (DOT)

double-stranded RNA (dsRNA), 309

Down syndrome. *See* chromosome aberration: Down syndrome

doxylamine
    antihistamine, 401

drinking water contaminants, 47, 56

drug (chemical) interaction, 389, 393, 402

dry deposition. *See* air pollutant(s): dry deposition

dumb cane (*Dieffenbachia*), 316, 317

dust storms
    in Beijing, 199
    in Sydney, 199

dysplastic phase. *See* carcinogenesis: mechanism

E

Eastern red-spotted newt, 321

ecological risk assessment, v, vi, 78, 79, 80, 420, 421, 422, 423, 433, 435, 436, 437
    assessment endpoint(s), 436
    effects analysis, 422
    exposure analysis, 421, 422
    framework, 7, 421
    problem formulation, 421, 436
    risk characterization, 421, 422

ecotoxicology
    definition, 8
    human health aspects, 411
    vs. environmental toxicology, 8, 94

EDCs. *See* endocrine-disrupting chemicals (EDCs)

edetate disodium. *See* EDTA

(ethylenediaminetetraacetate)

EDTA (ethylenediaminetetraacetate), 136

EEDs. *See* environmental endocrine disruptors (EEDs)

electronic waste. *See* e-waste

elimination rate constant. *See* toxicant(s): toxicokinetics

emphysema, 24, 183, 237

Employee Right-To-Know Act, U.S., 383

employee right-to-know laws, 322

encephalitis, 306, 307
    Japanese, 307
    rabies, 307
    St. Louis, 307
    Venezuelan equine, 348

Endangered Species Act, U.S., 417

endocrinal effects
    examples, 360

endocrine disruption, iv, 129, 347, 349, 355, 357, 358, 359, 405
    concepts, 349
    modes, 357, 358

endocrine disruptors
    types, 359

endocrine system (endocrine network), 58, 347, 351, 352, 353, 354, 355, 357

endocrine-disrupting chemicals (EDCs), 347, 349, 357, 358, 359
    examples, 360
    types, 358

endocrine-reproductive system, 347, 350

endocytosis. *See* toxicant(s): mechanisms of entry

endosulfan, 260, 283

endotoxins, 136, 310

endrin, 27, 157, 260, 283

Entamoeba histolytica, 308

Enterobius follicularis, 309

enterohepatic circulation, 101, 105

Environment Canada (EC), 42

environmental carcinogenesis, 336, 337, 338, 339, 340

environmental carcinogens, 340

environmental change(s), 15, 16, 17, 19, 30

environmental contaminants
    definition, 47
    grouping, 47

environmental disease(s)
    concerns, 15, 16, 21, 22
    costs, 11, 21
    definition, 20
    grouping, 23, 26

incidence and spectrum, 11, 17, 20
environmental endocrine disruptors (EEDs), 47, 56, 57, 347
environmental estrogen(s), 362, 363
environmental health, iv, 9, 11, 16, 33, 37, 38, 39, 41, 42, 46, 47, 144, 150, 163, 193, 198, 212, 213, 233, 243, 282, 303, 322, 357, 423, 435, 436
    definition, 37
environmental health (science)
    definition, 15
environmental health impact assessment (EHIA), 435
environmental health laws, 37
    in the United States, 39, 40
    international, 41
    outside of the United States, 41, 42, 43
environmental health risk assessment. *See* health risk assessment
environmental justice
    definition, 35
environmental movement, 33, 35, 36, 370, 397
environmental mutagen(s), 333, 335
    examples, 334
environmental mutagenesis, 331, 335
environmental persistence, 280, 281, 282, 283
environmental pollution, v, 9, 11, 13, 15, 31, 35, 42, 261, 323, 389, 397, 434
    concerns, 33, 35, 412
    costs in China, 32
    definition, 30, 33
    impacts, 31, 36
    U.S. EPA's responsibility, 35
environmental reproductive toxicant(s), 363
environmental risk assessment, 433
environmental sciences
    definition, 15
environmental teratogen(s), 361
environmental toxicant(s)
    concerns, 51
    transport of
        advection, 62
        diffusion, 62
environmental toxicology, 31, 149, 150, 304, 418, 433
    ally with epidemiology, 9
    definition, 3, 11
    importance, 11, 17, 21
    knowledge for. *See* environmental toxicology: principles for
    principles for, 3, 5, 6, 7
    scope, 1

vs. ecotoxicology, 8, 94
    with pesticide residues, 255
enzymatic activities
    disruption, 136, 138, 139
enzyme(s)
    characteristics, 112
    coenzymes, 112, 113, 115, 121, 124, 137, 159
        inhibition, 137
    cofactors, 112, 121, 124, 137, 159
        inhibition, 137
    inducers, 122, 123
    inhibitors, 122, 123, 139, 318
ephedrine
    decongestant, 402
epidemiology
    analytical, 9
    definition, 9
    descriptive, 9
    environmental, 10
    human exposure assessment, 10, *See also* health risk assessment: exposure analysis
    occupational, 10
epigenetic carcinogen(s)
    definition, 338
epinephrine, 225, 226, 354, 356, 357
epoxide hydrolase, 118
EPSP synthase, 274
erectile dysfunction (ED), 348, 360, 365
ergotism, 313
Erin Brockovich, 18, 26, 244
Escherichia coli (E. coli), 57, 305, 311
estradiol, 355, 356, 358, 365
estrogen(s), 23, 24, 49, 271, 294, 349, 354, 355, 357, 358, 359
    functions, 355
ethiofencarb, 266
ethion, 265
ethylan, 259
ethylene dibromide, 24
ethylene glycol, 6
ethylene oxide, 364, 399
ethylenediaminetetraacetate. *See* EDTA (ethylenediaminetetraacetate)
European Commission (EC), 281
European Environmental Agency (EEA), 42
European Union (EU), 42, 213, 217, 270, 292, 370
    Framework Directive, 371
eutrophication, 180
e-waste, v, 16, 19, 48, 51, 289, 290, 291, 292
excess cancer risk (ECR), 440, 446
excess lifetime cancer risk. *See* excess cancer

risk (ECR)
exotoxins, 136, 310, 396
Exposure Factors Handbook, 450
Exxon Valdez
   oil pollution incident, 39

F

facilitated diffusion. *See* toxicant(s):
   mechanisms of entry
FAO. *See* United Nations Food and Agriculture
   Organization (FAO)
FD&C blue No. 1
   food colorant, 393
FD&C red No. 40
   food colorant, 393
FD&C yellow No. 5
   food colorant, 393
FDA. *See* U.S. Food and Drug Administration
   (FDA)
fecal excretion. *See* toxicant(s): excretion
Federal Employers Liability Act, U.S. (FELA),
   370
Federal Environment(al) Agency, Germany
   (UBA), 42, 43
Federal Food, Drug, and Cosmetic Act, U.S.
   (FD&C Act), 255, 388, 389
Federal Hazardous Substances Act, U.S. (FHSA),
   39, 40, 434
Federal Insecticide, Fungicide, and Rodenticide
   Act, U.S. (FIFRA), 35, 36, 39, 40, 255, 406
fenthion, 265
Fenton reaction, 131, 132
FHSA. *See* Federal Hazardous Substances Act,
   U.S.
fiberglass. *See* synthetic mineral fibers (SMFs)
fibrogenic dust, 382
Fick's law of diffusion, 97
FIFRA. *See* Federal Insecticide, Fungicide, and
   Rodenticide Act, U.S. (FIFRA)
filtration. *See* toxicant(s): mechanisms of entry
fine particles. *See* $PM_{0.1-2.5}$
fine soot particles, 202
flow-through test. *See* aquatic toxicity tests
fluorocitrate, 138, 275
fluorosis
   dental, 392
   skeletal, 392
follicle-stimulating hormone (FSH), 352, 354
fonofos, 265
food additive
   definition, 388

function, 57
food allergies, 391
food chain(s), 3, 12, 26, 63, 78, 79, 80, 82, 242,
   245, 396
   trophic level, 79
food infection
   definition, 396
food intoxication
   definition, 396
food poisoning, 236, 305, 306, 311, 314, 389,
   396, 406
   melamine, v, *See also* melamine: poisoning
   scombrotoxic, 315
   Staphylococcal, 310
food product(s)
   toxic substances, 390, 391, 392, 393, 394, 395,
     397
Food Quality Protection Act, U.S. (FQPA), 39,
   155, 161, 255, 270, 389
food toxicant(s), 6, 7, 16, 38, 57, 239, 393, 394
   additives, 57
   concerns, 388
   contaminants, 57, 388, 389, 390, 396, 397
   direct additives, 57, 388, 389, 390, 391, 392,
     393
     anticaking agents, 391
     antioxidants, 391, 393
     colorants, 391
     dietary supplement, 392
     emulsifiers, 391, 392
     flavoring agents, 391, 393
     leavening agents, 393
     preservatives, 391, 393
     spices, 391
     stabilizers, 391
     tickeners, 391
     vitamins and minerals, 391
   indirect additives, 388, 389, 390, 393, 394,
     395, 396
     agrochemicals, 395, 396
   learning lessons, 403, 404, 405, 406
   mitigation and prevention, 405, 406
   persistent toxic substances in seafood, 403
   pesticides, 397
   source categories, 390
   toxic metals, 396, 397
   toxins, 396
food web. *See* food chain(s)
foodborne diseases
   statistics, 388
forests. *See* wildlife environment: forests
   environmental importance, 20

formaldehyde, 52, 53, 56, 213, 214, 215, 216, 217, 399, 401, 425
   exposures and toxic effects, 216, 217
   sources and use, 215, 216
FQPA. *See* Food Quality Protection Act, U.S. (FQPA)
fragrance
   sick building syndrome, 399
   toxic household products, 399
frameshift mutation, 332
Framework for Ecological Risk Assessment, 420, 421
free radicals, 25, 56, 57, 119, 130, 131
freshwater biome, 414
   lentic, 414
   lotic, 414
   wetlands, 414
FSH. *See* follicle-stimulating hormone (FSH)
Fukushima nuclear crisis, v, 322
fumonisin(s), 312, 313
   B_1, 312
   B_2, 312

G

gametogenesis, 350
gamma (γ) particle (γ radiation), 248
gamma-aminobutyric acid (γ-GABA), 260, 261, 266
   neurotransmitter, 260, 262
   receptor, 261, 262
gastrointestinal absorption. *See* toxicant(s): uptake of: by humans
gene mutation. *See* point mutation or intragenic mutation
gene(s)
   definition, 329
   DNA repair gene, 337
   oncogene, 329, 330
   proto-oncogene, 329, 330, 337
   tumor suppressor gene, 337
General Industry Air Contaminants Standard, U.S., 374
generally recognized as safe (GRAS), 390, 391
genetic polymorphism, 117, 121, 122
genome
   definition, 329
genotoxic carcinogen(s)
   definition. *See* ultimate carcinogen(s): definition
germinal stage (germinal period). *See* developmental-reproductive process:

   predifferentiation period
Giardia lamblia, 308
Gilbert's syndrome, 118
ginger Jake paralysis, 264
global cooling effect, 192
global warming, 17, 37, 53, 66
glomerular filtration, 103
glucagon(s), 354, 356
glucuronidation, 113, 115, 117
glutathione conjugation, 115
glutathione peroxidase (GPx), 119, 120, 121
glutathione S-transferase (GST), 115, 122, 160
glycol ether, 24
glycoside(s), 316
   cardiac, 316
   cyanogenic, 316
glycosylphosphatidylinositol. *See* malaria: toxin
glyphosate, 273, 274
Gore, Al (former U.S. Vice-President), 37, 349
GRAS. See generally recognized as safe (GRAS)
grasshopper effect, 64, 282
Great Lakes basin, U.S., 282
greenhouse effect, 17, 53, 65, 66
greenhouse gas(es), 17, 66
Guidelines for Ecological Risk Assessment, 420
guinea worm (*Dracunculus medinensis*), 303, 308
Gulf War Oil Spill of 1991, 417
Guyana
   health concerns, 20

H

H1N1 (virus), v, 11, 12, 13, 33, 46, 201
HAB (harmful algal bloom). *See* red tide pollution
Haber's law, 154
Haemophilus influenzae, 305
Harbin, China
   chemical explosion, 219
harmful physical agents. *See* physical hazards
Hazard Communication Standard, 383, 397
hazard identification. *See* health risk assessment: hazard identification
hazard quotient (HQ), 422, 447
   computation and interpretation, 423
hazardous air pollutants, 172, 173
hazardous waste pollution, 411, 417, 423, 424, 425, 426, 427, 428, 429
   relevance, 412, 413
hazardous waste(s), 18, 40, 41, 51, 213, 239, 242, 244, 411, 412, 423, 424, 425, 426

characteristics waste factors, 424
characteristics wastes, 424, 425
definition, 423
F-list, 424
K-list, 425
listed wastes, 424, 425
P-list, 425
U-list, 425
universal wastes, 425
health effects tests
categories, 437
guidelines, 437
health risk
definition, 422, 450
health risk assessment, v, 3, 10, 31, 78, 80, 140,
150, 160, 304, 391, 433, 434, 435, 436, 438,
439, 440, 441, 442, 444, 445, 447, 450, 451,
452
activities, 433, 434, 435, 450
aggregate exposure, 450
animal toxicity studies, 437, 438
assessment endpoints, 436
components, 435
cumulative exposure, 450
dose-response assessment, 7, 436, 438, 439,
440
exposure analysis, 7, 78, 436, 440, 441, 442,
443, 444, 445, 447, 448, 449
aggregate and cumulative exposures, 443,
444, 445
basic algorithm, 442
direct and indirect measurements, 442
past and current perspectives, 441, 442
framework, 7, 433
hazard identification, 7, 10, 436, 437
health risk characterization, 3, 7, 436, 445,
446, 447, 448, 449, 450, 451, 452, 453
health risk communication, 451, 452, 453
health risk measures, 445, 446, 447
health risk perception, 32, 450, 451, 453
role of epidemiology, 10
subtleties, 435
toxicity assessment, 412, 422, 436, 437, 438,
439, 440, 445, 447, 448
uncertainty and safety factors, 446, 447, 448,
449, 450, 451
health risk characterization, 452, 453, *See also*
health risk assessment: health risk
characterization
health risk communication. *See* health risk
assessment: health risk communication
health risk measures. *See* health risk assessment:
health risk measures
health risk perception, vi, 450, 451, 453, *See also*
health risk assessment: health risk perception
definition, 451
healthy worker effect, 450
heavy metal(s)
definition, 233
Henle-Koch postulates, 305
hepatic excretion. *See* toxicant(s): excretion
heptachlor, 27, 71, 260, 261, 283, 360
*hexa*brominated biphenyl (*hexa*BB), 283, 289,
290
hexachlorobenzene (HCB), 27, 86, 262, 283
hexachlorocyclohexane (HCH), 157, 158, 262,
360
Himalayan rhubarb, 316
histones, 329
Histoplasma capsulatum, 308
HIV (human immunodeficiency virus), 122, 123,
145, 305, 306, 341
holoenzyme(s), 124
honey bee depopulation syndrome. *See* colony
collapse disorder
hormone(s), 145, 347, 352
amine, 355
peptide, 355
receptor, 355
steroid, 132, 355, 358
hornet sting(s), 319
household chemicals, toxic, 57, *See also* toxic
household product(s)
Human and Ecological Risk Assessment, 422
human exposure assessment. *See* health risk
assessment: exposure analysis
human herpesviruses (HHVs), 307
human papilloma virus, 143
human risk assessment, 433
humidity
effects, 156
hyaluronidases, 320, 321
hydrogen cyanide (HCN), 134
hydrogen fluoride (HF), 94, 131, 173, 174
hydrogen sulfide (H_2S), 173, 174
hydroxyl radical (HO•), 26, 66, 67, 131, 132, 175,
179, 182, 222, 224, 226
Hypericum, 317
Hypericum perforatum (H. perforatum), 317
hyperplastic phase. *See* carcinogenesis:
mechanism
hypersensitivity. *See* toxicant(s): toxicodynamics
hypervitaminosis A, 26

I

IARC. *See* International Agency for Research on Cancer (IARC)
imidacloprid, 273
imidazolidinyl urea
    as formaldehyde-releasing ingredient, 399
incidence
    definition, 9
indandione(s), 271, 272
indoxacarb, 266
industrial disease(s)
    classic, 369
Industrial Revolution Period, 369
industrialization, 17, 20, 30, 294, 435
infection
    definition, 304
    vs. infectious disease, 304
infectious disease
    definition, 304
    vs. infection, 304
infertility, vi, 143, 313, 314, 348, 360, 361
inhalable coarse particles. *See* $PM_{2.5-10}$
initiation phase. *See* carcinogenesis: mechanism
insulin, 354, 355, 356
integral proteins. *See* biomembrane(s)
interaction, chemical
    additivity, 6, 140, 160, 161, 298
    antagonism, 6, 140, 160, 162, 183
    potentiation, 6, 140, 160, 161
    synergism, 6, 140, 160, 161
Intergovernmental Panel on Climate Change (IPCC), 17, 36, 37
International Agency for Research on Cancer (IARC), 216, 219, 223, 225, 227, 235, 236, 238, 241, 242, 244, 245, 247, 249, 250, 260, 261, 262, 263, 266, 268, 269, 271, 274, 289, 291, 295
    classification of carcinogenicity potential, 340
    examples of human carcinogenicity potential, 341
    objectives, 340
International Conference on Harmonization (ICH), 438
International Programme on Chemical Safety (IPCS), 292, 298
International Standardization Organization, 415
International Union of Pure and Applied Chemistry (IUPAC), 223, 225
INTER-NOISE Congresses, 323, 324
interphase, 336, *See also* cell cycle: interphase
interstrand crosslink. *See* DNA

(deoxyribonucleic acid): damage
intestinal excretion. *See* toxicant(s): excretion
intragenic mutation, 331, 332
intrastrand crosslink. *See* DNA
    (deoxyribonucleic acid): damage
ionophores, 395
iron (Fe), 24, 119, 134, 136, 159, 164, 174, 175, 195, 200, 233, 243, 244, 245, 246, 247, 424, 425
irritation. *See* toxicant(s): toxicodynamics
islets of Langerhans, 354
itai-itai (byo), 52, *See also* cadmium (Cd): *itai-itai*
IUPAC. *See* International Union of Pure and Applied Chemistry (IUPAC)

J

Jack Lewis
    The Birth of EPA, 35
James River pollution, 262
Jinzu river basin, Japan, 237

K

kepone, 24, 122, 123, 260, 261, 283, 360, 425
Krebs cycle, 138, 241, 275

L

lactic acidosis, 393
LC_{50} (median lethal concentration), 2, 152, 154, 156, 422, 438
LD_{50} (median lethal dose), 2, 155, 164, 422, 424, 438
lead (Pb), 1, 3, 18, 19, 48, 51, 52, 103, 139, 162, 233, 234, 235, 239, 240, 242, 364, 380, 403, 404, 425
    acetate, 235
    acute poisoning, 234
    biological exposure index, 376
    children's jewelry and toys, 155, 234, 404
    classic industrial disease, 369
    compounds, 24, 173, 195, 234, 235, 364
    criteria air pollutant, 172
    glazes
        classic industrial disease, 22
    heavy metal, 234, 235
    on toys, 48
    phosphate, 235
    poisoning (plumbism), 21, 235, 369, 403, 405
    pollution, 139
    reproductive effects, 235

spent lead shot, 416, 417
systemic poison, 234
tetraethyl, 218
leaf
structure, 98
lecithin, 391, 392
lectins, 316
Legionella pneumophila, 369, 384
legionellosis, 201, 369, 384
Norway incidence, 384
Philadelphia (Pennsylvania) incidence, 369, 384
Legionnaire's disease. *See* legionellosis
leukemia, 145, 162, 217, 219, 225, 269, 330, 363, 381
chronic myeloid, 122
lily of the valley (*Convallaria majalis*), 316
lindane (γ-HCH), 25, 58, 262, 283, 358
linoleic acid, 159
lipid peroxidation, 116, 131, 159
lipophilicity, 68, 78, 90, 158, 259, 380, 405
lizard(s)
Gila monster (*Heloderma suspectum*), 321
Iguana genus, 321
Komodo dragons, 321
Mexican beaded (*Heloderma horridum*), 321
Monitor species, 321
LO[A]EL. *See* lowest observed [adverse] effect level (LO[A]EL)
London, 151, 173, 178, 198, 202, 369
London fog of 1952, v, 16, 17, 131, 151
long-range transport (LRT), 26, 88, 181, 282, 286
loratadine
antihistamine, 401
Los Angeles, 18, 183, 198, 205
Love Canal, 16, 18, 36, 41, 51, 413, 425
lowest observed [adverse] effect level (LO[A]EL), 5, 438, 439, 445, 446
luteinizing hormone (LH), 352, 354, 365

M

mad-cow disease. *See* bovine spongiform encephalopathy (BSE)
magnesium (Mg), 159, 233, 243, 289
magnesium oxide, 289, 380
malaria, 20, 34, 303, 308, 309, 317
toxin, 309
malathion, 25, 264, 420
malnutrition, 157, 158
manganese (Mn), 119, 195, 243, 245, 374, 380

man-made mineral fibers (MMMFs). *See* synthetic mineral fibers (SMFs)
Mantle cell lymphoma, 333
margin of exposure (MOE), 445, 447
margin of safety (MOS). *See* margin of exposure (MOE)
marine biome, 413, 414
mastitis, 306
Material Safety Data Sheet (MSDS), 155, 397, 398, 399
maximum allowable concentration (MAC), 375
maximum contaminant level (MCL), 271, 445, 446
mechanism(s) of (toxic) action. *See* toxicant(s): mechanism(s) of (toxic) action
median lethal concentration. *See* LC$_{50}$ (median lethal concentration)
median lethal dose. *See* LD$_{50}$ (median lethal dose)
medications
side effects, 135
meiosis
definition, 336
melamine, 49, 215
poisoning, v, 49
melatonin, 157, 353, 356
Menkes syndrome, 246
Merck Veterinary Manual, 22
mercury (Hg), 2, 3, 19, 49, 50, 52, 53, 64, 68, 74, 78, 136, 139, 233, 235, 236, 237, 239, 256, 303, 363, 380, 396, 417, 418, 425
biological exposure index, 376
heavy metal, 235, 236
methylmercury, 78, 235, 236, 362
Minamata syndrome, 54, 236
poisoning (mercurialism), 236
MERS (Middle East respiratory syndrome), v, 12, 13
mesothelioma. *See* asbestos: mesothelioma
MeT. *See* *methyltransferase (MeT)*
metabolism. *See* toxicant(s): metabolism
metal fume fever, 380
metal(s)
definition, 232
environmental health concerns, 233
heavy metals, 233, 234, 235, 236, 237, 238
periodic table, 232
radioactive metals, 247, 249, 250
secondary heavy metals, 238, 239, 240, 241, 242
toxic trace metals, 243, 244, 245, 246, 247
metalloid(s), 52, 232, 240, 241

definition, 232
metallothionein (MT), 238
  Cd-MT binding, 238
metastasis, 331, *See also* carcinogenesis:
  mechanism
methane, 17, 66, 215, 216
methemoglobin, 145
methlochlor, 259
methomyl, 266
methoxychlor, 122, 123, 259, 401
methyl bromide, 172, 256
methyl *tert*-butyl ether (MTBE), 213, 220, 221
  exposures and toxic effects, 221
  sources and use, 221
methylation, 113, 115
methylene chloride (MC), 213, 214, 215, 222,
  223, 225, 226, 380, 394, 402
  exposures and toxic effects, 222, 223
  sources and use, 222
methylmercury. *See* mercury (Hg):
  methylmercury
methyltransferase (MeT), 115, 119
MGK-264, 267
microbic (microbial) invasion, 135, 136, 304
microcephaly, 362, 363, 404
Middle East respiratory syndrome. *See* MERS
  (Middle East respiratory syndrome)
Minamata syndrome. *See* mercury (Hg):
  Minamata syndrome
Mine Safety and Health Act, U.S. (MSH Act),
  374
mineral wool. *See* synthetic mineral fibers
  (SMFs)
mineral(s)
  definition, 233
Ministry of Environmental Protection, China
  (CMEP), 42, 43
Ministry of the Environment, Japan (JMOE), 42,
  43
mirex, 27, 58, 89, 118, 122, 123, 260, 261, 283
mismatch repair. *See* DNA (deoxyribonucleic
  acid): repair
mitosis
  definition, 336
mobility, of toxicants. *See* toxicant(s): mobility
molybdenum (Mo), 160, 243
monosodium glutamate (MSG)
  direct food additive, 393
Montevideo (Latin America)
  PM$_{10}$ levels, 199
Montreal Protocol, 41, 256
Montreal Protocol on Substances That Deplete

the Ozone Layer. See Montreal Protocol
MSDS. *See* Material Safety Data Sheet (MSDS)
MT. *See* metallothionein (MT)
MTBE. *See* methyl *tert*-butyl ether (MTBE)
Mumbai, India, 198
mushroom poisoning (mycetism), 310
mutagen(s)
  definition, 328
mutagenesis, 142, 328, 340, 448
  concepts, 331
mutagenicity
  definition, 328
mycetism. *See* mushroom poisoning (mycetism)
Mycobacterium tuberculosis, 305
mycotoxin*s*, 25, 57, 145, 310, 312, 314, 396
  major groups, 313

N

NAAQS. *See* National Ambient Air Quality
  Standard, U.S. (NAAQS)
N-acetyltransferase (NAT), 115, 119
nanoparticles. *See* PM$_{0.1}$
narcotic effects. *See* toxicant(s): toxicodynamics
NAT. *See* *N*-acetyltransferase (NAT)
National Ambient Air Quality Standard, U.S.
  (NAAQS), 172, 175, 179, 182, 185, 196, 197,
  200
National Environmental Policy Act, U.S.
  (NEPA), 34, 38, 40
National Health and Nutrition Examination
  Survey, U.S. (NHANES), 21, 291
National Pollutant Discharge Elimination System,
  U.S. (NPDES), 416
National Priorities List, U.S. (NPL), 426
National Research Council. *See* U.S. National
  Research Council (NRC)
Nationwide Food Consumption Survey, U.S.
  (NFCS), 34, 449
necrosis, of plants, 94, 131
neonicotinoid(s), 273
neoplasm. *See* cancer
nephron, 103
  distal (convoluted) tubule, 103
  glomerulus, 103, 104
  proximal (convoluted) tubule, 103
  the functional unit, 104
nervous system
  functions, 351, 352
neurological diseases (neurological disorders), 22,
  24, 25, 333, 369
neurotoxic esterase (NTE), 264

neurotoxins, 25, 310, 317, 389

New York, 18, 36, 184, 198, 202, 205, 213, 413

NHANES. *See* National Health and Nutrition Examination Survey, U.S. (NHANES)

nickel (Ni), 52, 119, 195, 243, 244, 245, 247, 380

nickel carbonyl, 245, 246, 380

nickel carbonyl poisoning. *See* nickel carbonyl

nicotine, 58, 258, 273, 358

NIH. *See* U.S. National Institutes of Health (NIH)

NIOSH. *See* U.S. National Institute for Occupational Safety and Health (NIOSH)

nitric acid (HNO_3), 67, 179, 192, 195

nitric oxide (NO), 177

nitrobenzene, 115, 219, 401

nitrogen dioxide (NO_2), 55, 63, 94, 131, 177, 178, 179, 180, 216

    characteristics, 178, 179

    effects on humans and animals, 179, 180

    effects on plants, 180

    sources of pollution, 178

    toxic effects and advisories, 179

nitrogen fixation, 178

nitrogen mustard(s), 334, 335, 343, 358

nitrogen oxides (NO_x), 54, 55, 56, 172, 177, 178, 179, 192, 195, 198, 323

nitrous oxide (N_2O), 17, 66

Nixon, Richard (former U.S. President), 34, 370, 371

no observed [adverse] effect level (NO[A]EL), 3, 391, 438, 445, 446, 447, 448

NO[A]EL. *See* no observed [adverse] effect level (NO[A]EL)

Noise Control Act, U.S., 324

noise pollution, 31, 47, 322, 323, 324

non-inhalable coarse particles. *See* PM_{10+}

North American Agreement on Environmental Cooperation, 42

novel and specialty pesticides, 272, 274, 275

NPDES. *See* National Pollutant Discharge Elimination System, U.S. (NPDES)

NRC. *See* U.S. National Research Council (NRC)

nucleation. *See* ultrafine particles: nucleation

nucleotide excision repair. *See* DNA (deoxyribonucleic acid): repair

nuisance dust, 383

nutrient(s), 157, 158

    definition, 392

    macronutrients, 112, 158, 159, 392

    micronutrients, 158, 159, 160

nutrition

    definition, 157

nutritional status

    anorexia nervosa, 157

    fasting, 157

    malnutrition, 157

    nutritional disorders, 157

    obesity, 157

    starvation, 157

nutritional toxicology

    definition, 157

O

Occupational Disease Control Act, China, 370

occupational disease(s)

    definition, 369

occupational health, 370

    laws, 370, 371

    legislation for, 371, 372, 373, 374, 375

Occupational Health and Safety Act, South Africa, 370

Occupational Health, Safety and Welfare Act, South Australia, 370

Occupational Safety and Health Act, U.S. (OSH Act), 371, 372, 373, 374

occupational toxicant(s), 377, 379, 380, 381, 382, 383, 384, 385

    biological agents. *See* workplace biological hazards

    examples, 378

    fibers/dusts, 377, 378, 381, 382, 383

    metals, 377, 378, 379, 380

    metalworking fluids, 383

    organic solvents, 377, 378, 380, 381

    pesticides, 377, 378, 379

        acute poisoning, 377

    physical agents. *See* workplace physical hazards

occupational toxicology, 8, 370, 372

    basic principles of, 370, 375, 376, 377

ocean regions, 413

*octa*brominated diphenyl ether (*octa*BDE), 56, 283, 290

OH-PCBs. *See* polychlorinated biphenyl(s) [PCB(s)]: OH-PCBs

Oil Pollution Act, U.S. (OPA), 39, 40, 417

oil spills, 31

    concerns, 22

omega-3 fatty acids, 85

    ALA (alpha-linolenic acid), 85

    DHA (docosahexaenoic acid), 85

    DPA (docosapentaenoic acid), 85

    EPA (eicosapentaenoic acid), 85

one-compartment model. *See* toxicant(s):

toxicokinetics
oogenesis, 350
OPA. *See* Oil Pollution Act, U.S. (OPA)
OPIDN. *See* organophosphate-induced delayed
    neuropathy (OPIDN)
Orfila, Mathieu, 1
organic matter, 75, 192, 246
organic solvents, 217, 220, 222, 223, 225, 376,
    402
Organization for Economic Cooperation and
    Development (OECD), 415, 438
    Test Guidelines 305, 82
organochlorine (OC) pesticides, 27, 64, 258, 259,
    260, 261, 263
    chlorinated cyclodiene-related, 259, 260, 262
    chlorinated cyclohexane-related, 259, 262
    dichlorodiphenylethane-related, 259, 260
organogenesis. *See* developmental-reproductive
    process: organogenesis
organophosphate (OP) poisoning, 263
organophosphate pesticides. *See*
    organophosphate(s) [OP(s)]
organophosphate(s) [OP(s)], 25, 47, 100, 115,
    138, 144, 161, 258, 263, 264, 265
    acetylcholinesterase inhibitors, 264, 265
    delayed neurotoxic agents, 264
    SLUDGE, 264
organophosphate-induced delayed neuropathy
    (OPIDN), 264
organotin compounds, 283
OSHA. *See* U.S. Occupational Safety and Health
    Administration (OSHA)
Our Stolen Future, 349
OurStolenFuture.org, 359
ovarian cysts, 24, 348, 365
over-the-counter (OTC) medicines, 50, *See also*
    toxic household product(s): over-the-counter
    (OTC) medicines
    health concerns, 389
oxalates, 316
oxidative phosphorylation, 145, 272
oxidative stress, 26, 94, 119, 120, 131, 164
oxygen free radicals. *See* reactive oxygen
    species (ROS)
ozone (O_3), 17, 41, 52, 63, 66, 67, 94, 131, 172,
    177, 179, 181, 182, 198, 212
    characteristics, 181, 182
    effects on humans and animals, 182, 183
    effects on plants, 183
    sources of pollution, 181
    stratospheric, 256
    toxic effects and advisories, 182, 183

P

p53 (protein), 336
PAHs. *See* polycyclic aromatic hydrocarbons
    (PAHs)
PAN. *See* peroxyacetylnitrate (PAN)
Paracelsus (Phillip von Hohenheim), 1, 150
Paracoccidioides brasiliensis, 308
paraquat, 145, 273, 274
parathion, 25, 263, 264, 376, 425
parathyroid hormone, 354
Paris Basin, France, 199
particulate matter (PM), 56, 58, 63, 89, 144, 172,
    179, 191, 205, 212, 239
    characteristics, 192
    composition, 191, 192
    definition, 191
    effects on cardiovascular system, 205
    effects on respiratory tract, 203, 204
    effects on the environment, 206
    motions of, 193, 194
    other serious health effects, 205
    secondary organic matter, 212
    sizes of regulatory importance, 192, 193, 194,
        195, 196, 197
    toxic effects, 202, 203, 204, 205, 206
        mechanisms and trends, 203
passive diffusion. *See* toxicant(s): mechanisms
    of entry
pathogenic (microbial) agent(s), 304
    bacteria, 305, 306
    fungi, 307, 308
    parasites, 308, 309
        helminthes, 308, 309
        protozoa, 308
    viruses, 306, 307
PBB(s). *See* polybrominated biphenyl(s) [PBB(s)]
PBDE(s). *See* polybrominated diphenyl ether(s)
    [PBDE(s)]
PB-PK (physiologically-based pharmacokinetics)
    model, 106
    modeling
        for TCE, PCE, 227
PB-TK (physiologically-based toxicokinetics)
    model. *See* PB-PK (physiologically-based
    pharmacokinetics): model
PBTs. *See* persistent toxic substance(s) [PTS]
PCB(s). *See* polychlorinated biphenyl(s)
    [PCB(s)]
PCDD(s). *See* polychlorinated dibenzo-*p*-dioxins
    (PCDDs)]
PCDE(s). *See* polychlorinated diphenyl ether(s)

[PCDE(s)]
PCDF(s). *See* polychlorinated dibenzofuran(s)
[PCDF(s)]
PCE (PERC). *See* tetrachloroethylene (PCE)
Pearl River Delta Urban Agglomeration, China, 202
Penicillium, 55
*penta*brominated diphenyl ether (*penta*BDE), 56, 290
pentachlorobenzene, 283
pentachlorophenol (PCP), 71, 73, 395
perfluorooctane sulfonate (PFOS), 283, 284, 285, 286, 287, 360
   environmental health concerns, 286, 287
   use and pollution sources, 286
perfluorooctanoic acid (PFOA), 286
peripheral proteins. *See* biomembrane(s): peripheral proteins
permethrin, 25, 267
permissible exposure limit (PEL), 213, 372, 374, 375, 446
peroxyacetylnitrate (PAN), 66, 67, 177, 179, 181
persistence criteria, 281
persistent organic pollutants (POPs), v, 26, 36, 41, 46, 58, 82, 89, 282, 283, 284, 285, 286, 287, 290, 291, 292
   the dirty dozen, 26, 41, 283
persistent organochlorine compounds (POCs), 27, 47, 54, 55, 58, 68, 69, 70, 71, 72, 73, 79, 80, 81, 82, 83, 85, 87, 88, 89, 90, 396, 403, 406
   bioaccumulation in seafood, 85, 87
   fate and transport in water, 68
      physicochemical and environmental variables, 69
persistent toxic substance(s) [PTS], 80, 281, 282, 403
pesticide residues, 18, 39, 47, 57, 94
   as pollutants, 256
   definition, 255
pesticide(s)
   definition, 255
   health impacts and concerns, 255, 256
   use and classification, 256, 257, 258
PFOA. *See* perfluorooctanoic acid (PFOA)
PFOS. *See* perfluorooctane sulfonate (PFOS)
phagocytosis. *See* toxicant(s): mechanisms of entry
pharmaceutical wastes, 50
Phase I enzymatic reactions, 112, 114, 116
Phase I enzyme(s). *See* cytochrome 450 and Phase I enzymatic reactions
Phase I hydrolysis. *See* Phase I enzymatic reactions

Phase I oxidation. *See* Phase I enzymatic reactions
Phase I reduction. *See* Phase I enzymatic reactions
Phase II enzymatic reactions, 113, 114, 115, 116
Phase II enzyme(s), 113
phase-transfer
   (ad)sorption, 68, 70, 71, 75
   dissolution, 68, 69, 70, 71
   volatilization, 63, 68, 70, 71, 73, 74
phenol, 58, 113, 215, 218
phenoxy pesticide(s), 268, 270
phenylketonuria (PKU), 361, 363
phosphodiesterases, 320
phospholipases, 320, 321
phospholipases-A_2, 320
phossy jaw
   classic industrial disease, 22, 369
photochemical reaction, 66, 216
photochemical smog reaction, 175, 177
photodecomposition. *See* photochemical reaction
photodissociation. *See* photochemical reaction
photosynthesis, 53, 67, 72, 98, 131, 180, 186, 203, 206, 270, 274, 414
phthalates, 283, 394, 395
physical agents, 22, *See also* physical hazards
physical hazards, 322, 323, 324
physiological toxicology, 141
physiologically-based pharmacokinetics model. *See* PB-PK (physiologically-based pharmacokinetics): model
phytochemicals
   antioxidants, 119
   enzyme inhibitors, 122
phytoremediation, 99
Pick complex diseases. *See* chromosome aberration: Pick complex diseases
picrotoxin, 262
pinocytosis. *See* toxicant(s): mechanisms of entry
piperonyl butoxide, 267
pirimicarb, 266
PKU. *See* phenylketonuria (PKU)
plant toxicants, 58
Plasmodium falciparum, 309, 317
plastic marine pollution, v, 50
plastics (polymers), 50, 52, 56, 394
   high-density polyethylene, 395
   low-density polyethylene, 395
   polypropylene, 395
   polystyrene, 218, 290, 395

$PM_{0.1}$, 193, 194, 195, 197, 200
$PM_{0.1-2.5}$, 196, 197
PM_{10}, 193, 194, 196, 197, 198, 199, 201, 202, 203, 204, 205
PM_{10+}, 193, 194, 196
$PM_{2.5}$, 193, 194, 195, 196, 197, 198, 200, 202, 203, 204, 205
$PM_{2.5-10}$, 196, 205
pneumoconiosis, 24, 369, 374, 383
Pocket Guide to Chemical Hazards, 374
POCs. *See* persistent organochlorine compounds (POCs)
point mutation, 331, 332, 343
poison dart frogs, 321
poison ivy, 25, 317
poison oak, 25
poison sumac, 25, 317
poisonous plants, 314
polybrominated biphenyl(s) [PBB(s)], 283, 287, 288, 289, 290, 292, 294, 360
    contamination incident in Michigan, 214, 289, 298
    environmental health concerns, 289, 290
    use and pollution sources, 287, 289
polybrominated diphenyl ether(s) [PBDE(s)], 51, 54, 56, 57, 283, 288, 290, 291, 292, 294, 360, 418
    environmental health concerns, 291, 292
    use and pollution sources, 290, 291
polybromobiphenyl(s). *See* polybrominated biphenyl(s) [PBB(s)]
polychlorinated biphenyl(s) [PCB(s)], 19, 24, 27, 51, 55, 57, 64, 72, 79, 83, 84, 85, 86, 87, 88, 89, 102, 120, 133, 145, 152, 154, 218, 282, 283, 288, 292, 293, 294, 296, 297, 341, 359, 364, 403
    Aroclor compounds, 152
    dioxin-like, 83, 84, 161, 292, 293, 294, 296, 298
    environmental health concerns, 293, 294
    OH-PCBs, 83, 294
    use and pollution sources, 292, 293
polychlorinated dibenzofuran(s) [PCDF(s)], 55, 87, 283, 294, 295, 296, 297
    environmental health concerns, 295, 296
    use and pollution sources, 294, 295
polychlorinated dibenzo-*p*-dioxin(s) [PCDD(s)], 55, 57, 64, 72, 83, 84, 87, 102, 120, 283, 292, 294, 295, 296, 297, 298
    environmental health concerns, 295, 296
    use and pollution sources, 294, 295
polychlorinated diphenyl ether(s) [PCDE(s)], 84

polycyclic aromatic hydrocarbons (PAHs), 120, 133, 399, 418
polyethylene glycol (PEG), 395, 399
polyethylene terephthalate, 394
polyhalogenated aromatic hydrocarbons (PHAHs), 285
polymers. *See* plastics (polymers)
polynuclear aromatic hydrocarbons. *See* polycyclic aromatic hydrocarbons (PAHs)
polystyrene. *See* plastics (polymers): polystyrene
polytetrafluoroethylene (PTFE), 395
POPs. *See* persistent organic pollutants (POPs)
porphyria cutanea tarda, 262
portal venous system, 101
potentiation. *See* interaction, chemical: potentiation
potter's disease. *See* lead (Pb): classic industrial disease
pralidoxime, 263
prevalence
    definition, 9
prion(s), 11, 305
procarcinogen(s)
    definition, 338
progesterone, 354, 355, 356, 358, 360, 365
    functions, 355
progestogen(s), 355
progression phase. *See* carcinogenesis: mechanism
promotion phase. *See* carcinogenesis: mechanism
Prop 65. *See* Proposition 65
propargite, 25, 94, 145
propargyl bromide, 74
propazine, 271
Proposition 65, 21
propoxur, 266
propyl gallate, 360, 393
propylene glycol (PG), 399
proteases, 320
protozoa, 304, 308
pseudoephedrine
    decongestant, 402
Pseudomonas, 305
psoralen, 343
PTS. *See* persistent toxic substance(s) [PTS]
pulmonary excretion. *See* toxicant(s): excretion
pyrethrin and pyrethroid pesticides, 267, 268
pyrethrin(s), 266, 267
    allergic contact dermatitis, 268
Pyrethrins I, 266
Pyrethrins II, 266

pyrethroid(s), 25, 161, 267, 268, 273
  paresthesia, 268
  Type I, 266
  Type II, 266
pyrethrum, 58, 266
pyruvate dehydrogenase, 241

Q

Quieting the World's Cities, 323

R

radiation
  absorption and release, 65
radioactive wastes, 56, 58
radium (Ra), 248, 249
radon (Rn), 52, 57, 192, 200, 248, 249, 250
raphides. *See* oxalates
rate of diffusion. *See* toxicant(s): mechanisms of
  entry
rBST. *See* recombinant bovine somatotropin
  (rBST)
RCRA. *See* Resource Conservation & Recovery
  Act, U.S. (RCRA)
reactive oxygen species (ROS), 26, 57, 130, 164,
  247, 342
receptor(s), 112, 120, 130, 132, 133, 134, 136,
  142, 145, 294, 352, 358, 396, 422, 433, 441
  estrogen, 357
  hormone, 357, 358
re-circulation test. *See* aquatic toxicity tests
recombinant bovine somatotropin (rBST), 396,
  397
recommended exposure limit (REL), 374, 375,
  376
red tide pollution, 19, 37
  Solutions to Avoid Red Tide (START), 37
reference concentration (RfC), 445, 446, 447
reference dose (RfD), 422, 445, 446, 447, 450,
  451
refractory ceramic fibers. *See* synthetic mineral
  fibers (SMFs)
renal excretion. *See* toxicant(s): excretion
renewal test. *See* aquatic toxicity tests
reproductive damage (reproductive disorders)
  concerns, 348, 349
  definition, 23
  fertility, 23
reproductive system
  human female, 366
  human male, 365
reproductive toxicant(s)

definition, 359
sources of exposure, 359
Resource Conservation & Recovery Act, U.S.
  (RCRA), 40, 417, 423, 424, 425, 426
  definition and implications, 424, 425
respiratory diseases
  definition, 24
respiratory uptake. *See* toxicants: uptake of: by
  humans
retro-transposons, 331
RfC. *See* reference concentration (RfC)
RfD. *See* reference dose (RfD)
Rhamnus purshiana, 316
Rhus, 317
Richmond (Inner) Harbor. *See* United
  Heckathorn (Superfund toxic site)
ricin, 316
ringworm, 307
Risk Characterization Handbook, 445
risk communication
  cardinal rules, 452, 453
  mental noise theory, 452
  negative dominance theory, 452
  risk perception theory, 452
  theories, 452, 453
  trust determination theory, 452
risk perception
  definition, 450
risk-based standards, 453
RNA (ribonucleic acid)
  definition, 328
rodenticide(s)
  bromethalin, 272
  DDT, 272
  red squill, 272
  strychnine, 272
  thallium sulfate, 272
  zinc phosphide, 272
ROS. *See* reactive oxygen species (ROS)
Rotterdam Convention, 270
*Rotterdam Convention on the Prior Informed
  Consent Procedure for Certain Hazardous
  Chemicals and Pesticides in International
  Trade. See* Rotterdam Convention
Roundup. *See* glyphosate

S

safety factors. *See* health risk assessment:
  uncertainty and safety factors
Salmonella, 305, 306, 311, 328, 335, 396
  typhimurium, 335

Salmonella assay. *See* Ames test
sarin, 265
SARS (severe acute respiratory syndrome), v, 12,
    13, 201, 385
saxitoxin, 309, 315, 396
scombrotoxin, 315
scorpion(s)
    chlorotoxin, 319
    deathstalker, 319
seasonal affective disorder, 353
selenium (Se), 26, 119, 160, 243
Sentinel Event Notification System for
    Occupational Risks (SENSOR)-Pesticides
    program, 379
serotonin syndrome, 135
SETAC. *See* Society of Environmental
    Toxicology and Chemistry (SETAC)
severe acute respiratory syndrome. *See* SARS
    (severe acute respiratory syndrome)
Seveso dioxin, 296, *See also* 2,3,7,8-TCDD
Sevin. *See* carbaryl
shellfish poisoning, 309, 314
sick building syndrome, 399
sickle-cell anemia, 331, 332
Silent Spring, 8, 21, 33, 34, 35, 255, 397, 417
silicosis, 383
    classic industrial disease, 22, 369
simazine, 75, 270, 271
site of (toxic) action
    definition, 129
skin disorders (skin diseases), 25, 145
skin penetration. *See* toxicant(s): uptake of: by
    humans
SMFs. *See* synthetic mineral fibers (SMFs)
snake(s), 320, 321
    elapid venoms, 320
    Elapidae family, 320
    Viperidae family, 320
Society of Environmental Toxicology and
    Chemistry (SETAC), 15
sodium (mono)fluoroacetate (Compound 1080),
    273, 274
sodium laureth sulfate (SLES), 399
sodium lauryl sulfate (SLS), 398, 399
sodium nitrate
    direct food additive, 393
sodium nitrite
    direct food additive, 393
soil contaminant(s), 98, 99, 224
    degradation, 74
    erosion and runoff, 74
    fate, 73, 74, 75

leaching, 75
    transport, 73, 74, 75
    volatilization, 73, 74
soil contamination, 18
Solanum nigrum L., 151
Solid Waste Disposal Act, U.S. (SWDA), 424
soman, 265
soot pollution, 205
sorbitan monostearate
    stabilizer, 391
sorbitan tristearate
    stabilizer, 391
spermatogenesis, 350
sphingomyelinase D, 318
spider(s)
    black widow spiders (*Latrodectus*), 318
    brown recluse spiders (*Loxosceles*), 318
    jumping species (*Phidippus*), 318
    wolf species (*Pardosa*), 318
    yellow sac species (*Chiranthium*), 318
squill (*Scilla maritima*), 316
St. Anthony's Fire. *See* ergotism
St. John's wort. *See* H. perforatum
Standards Completion Program, 374
Staphylococcus(ci), 305, 396
    aureus, 306, 311
        methicillin-resistant (MRSA), 306
State Environmental Protection Administration,
    China (SEPA), 43
static test. *See* aquatic toxicity tests
steatosis, 144
Stockholm Convention, 26, 27, 36, 41, 282, 283,
    284, 285, 287, 290, 292
    aims and actions, 283, 284
    persistent pollutants of concern, 282, 283
*Stockholm Convention on Persistent Organic
    Compounds (POPs)*, 41
stoma(ta), 176
    functions, 99
strength-of-evidence, 447, 448
Streptococcus(ci), 305
    aureus, 33
Strychnos nux vomica, 272
sudden infant death syndrome (SIDS), 180, 202,
    205
sulfanilamide, 388
sulfation, 113, 115, 117
sulfhemoglobin, 145
sulfhydryl group, 139, 233, 235, 238, 241
sulfite oxidase, 160
sulfosate, 274
sulfotransferase (SULT), 115, 119

sulfur dioxide (SO$_2$), 56, 63, 94, 131, 151, 157, 172, 173, 174, 175, 176, 177, 195, 198
    characteristics, 174, 175
    effects of acid rain, 177
    effects on humans and animals, 176
    effects on plants, 176, 177
    sources of pollution, 173, 174
    toxic effects and advisories, 175
sulfur oxides (SO$_x$), 18, 54, 56, 173, 192
sulfur trioxide (SO$_3$), 67, 173, 175
sulfuric acid (H$_2$SO$_4$), 56, 67, 157, 173, 175, 177, 185, 192
SULT. See sulfotransferase (SULT)
superoxide dismutase (SOD), 119, 120, 121, 122
superoxide radical(s), 26, 131
Swainsonine. *See* alkaloid(s): indolizidine
synergism. *See* interaction, chemical: synergism
synergistic effect
    among NO$_2$, O$_3$, SO$_2$, 180, 183
synthetic mineral fibers (SMFs), 381, 382

T

T syndrome, 266
tabun, 265
taiga. *See* wildlife environment: taiga
tampon-toxic shock scare, 32, 33, 450
tartrazine. *See* FD&C yellow No. 5: food colorant
taxol, 317
Tay-Sachs disease (TSD), 361
TCE. *See* trichloroethylene (TCE)
TDE. *See* DDD (dichlorodiphenyldichloroethane)
TEF. *See* toxic equivalency factor (TEF)
Teflon®. *See* polytetrafluoroethylene (PTFE)
Tegucigalpa (Latin America)
    PM$_{10}$ levels, 199
TEPP. *See* tetraethyl pyrophosphate (TEPP)
TEQ. *See* toxic equivalency (TEQ)
teratogen(s)
    definition, 142, 347
    effects, 142, 223, 350, 351, 359, 362
    environmental, 47, 347
    examples, 363
    ionizing radiation, 23
teratogenic effects. *See* toxicant(s): toxicodynamics
terbufos, 265
testosterone, 117, 271, 354, 355, 356, 358, 360, 365
    functions, 354
tetani, 310, 311

tetanus, 305, 310
tetrachloroethylene (PCE), 213, 214, 215, 223, 225, 400, 424
    exposures and toxic effects, 224, 225
    sources and use, 224
tetraethyl pyrophosphate (TEPP), 264
tetrodotoxin, 25, 304, 315, 321, 396
thalidomide, 6, 23, 448
The Endocrine Society, 349
The Safe Drinking Water and Toxic Enforcement Act of 1986 (California). See Proposition 65
The Wildlife Society, 417
thiol group. *See* sulfhydryl group
thiourea, 164
thorium (Th), 248, 249
threshold limit value(s) [TLV(s)], 375, 376, 377, 446
Threshold of Regulation program, 394
thyroxine, 353, 354, 356, 357
TLV(s). *See* threshold limit value(s) [TLV(s)]
TLV-C. *See* threshold limit value(s) [TLV(s)]
TLV-STEL. *See* threshold limit value(s) [TLV(s)]
TLV-TWA. *See* threshold limit value(s) [TLV(s)]
TMDL. *See* Total Maximum Daily Load, U.S. (TMDL)
TNF. *See* tumor necrosis factor (TNF)
TOCP. *See* tri-*ortho*-cresyl phosphate (TOCP)
Tokyo, 198, 265
toluene, 143, 213, 218, 395, 402
Total Maximum Daily Load, U.S. (TMDL), 416
total suspended particles (TSP), 194, 196, 197, 200, 202
toxaphene, 27, 58, 260, 283
toxic consumer products
    learning lessons, 403, 404, 405, 406
    mitigation and prevention, 405, 406
toxic effects
    on target organs and systems. *See* toxicant(s): toxicodynamics
toxic equivalency (TEQ), 83, 293, 296, 298
toxic equivalency factor (TEF), 83, 161, 293, 296, 297, 298
toxic household product(s), 397
    cleaning agents, 400, 401
    concerns, 389
    gasoline, 402
    lead on children's jewelry and toys, 404
    mitigation and prevention, 405, 406
    other organic compounds, 402
    over-the-counter (OTC) medicines, 401, 402
        antihistamines, 401

cold medicines, 402
  decongestants, 402
  pain relievers, 401
  side effects, 401, 402
personal care products, 398, 399, 400
pesticide products, 402
poisoning statistics, 388
source categories, 398
toxic substances, 397, 398, 399, 400, 401, 402
triclosan in antibacterial products, 405
toxic response
  definition, 129
toxic shock syndrome, 33, 311
Toxic Substances Control Act, U.S. (TSCA), 423
toxicant clearance. *See* toxicant(s):
  toxicokinetics
toxicant(s), v, 2
  bioactivation, 116
  biotransformation, 111, 112, 113, 115, 116,
    118, 121, 122, 124, 129, 158, 160, 163,
    164, 413
    affecting factors, 121, 122, 123, 124
    general processes, 113
  detoxification, 116, 117, 119, 129, 158, 181
  disposition, 94
  distribution, 102, 103, 104, 105
  excretion, 102, 103, 104, 105
  internal organ, 94
  mechanism(s) of (toxic) action, 129, 130, 131,
    294
    adverse indirect actions, 135, 136
    adverse secondary actions, 135, 136
    definition, 129
    disruption of enzymatic activities, 137,
      138, 139
    mediated toxic actions, 131, 132, 133, 134
    primary toxic actions, 131, 132, 133, 134
  mechanisms of entry, 95, 96, 97
  metabolism, 5, 88, 89, 95, 103, 111, 121, 144,
    164
  metabolism *vs.* biotransformation, 111, 112
  mobility, 88
  systemic, 94
  toxicodynamics, 139, 140, 141, 142, 143, 145,
    411
    basic types of toxic effects, 139, 141
    definition, 130, 139
    mechanism-based adverse effects, 141,
      142, 143, 144, 145
  toxicokinetics, 106, 107, 108
    area under the curve, 108
    definition, 106, 139

    elimination rate constant, 108
    mathematical principles, 107, 108
    numerical example, 108
    toxicant clearance, 107, 108
    volume of distribution, 107
  uptake and absorption of, 97, 99, 101
  uptake of
    by humans, 99
    by plants, 97, 98, 99
toxicity
  definition, 149
toxicity affecting factors
  biological factors, 162, 163, 164
  environmental factors, 149, 150, 151, 152,
    153, 154, 155, 156
  extrinsic factors, 149
  intrinsic factors, 149, 150
  nutritional factors, 149, 157, 158, 159, 160
  physicochemical factors, 149, 160, 161, 162
toxicity assessment. *See* health risk assessment:
  toxicity assessment
toxicodynamics. *See* toxicant(s): toxicodynamics
toxicokinetics. *See* toxicant(s): toxicokinetics
toxicologists
  activities for, 7
toxicology
  definition, 1
  historical development, 1
  terminology, 2, 3
toxin K1, 309
toxin K2, 309
toxin K28, 309
toxin(s), v, 2, 389
  from bacteria, 57, 310, 311
  from fishes, 314, 315
  from fungi, 310, 312, 314
  from microorganisms, 309, 310, 311, 312,
    314
  from mushrooms, 310
  from plants, 314, 316, 317
  from viruses. *See* viral toxin
Toxoplasma gondii, 308
traffic congestion, 47, 178, 184, 303, 322, 323
trans fats, 46, 50
transformation
  biological, 71
  chemical, 71
transposons, 331
triazine pesticides, 270, 271
trichloroethylene (TCE), 213, 214, 215, 223, 224,
  225, 226, 227, 380, 394, 424
  exposures and toxic effects, 226, 227

sources and use, 225, 226
trichloromethyl free radical, 116, 132
trichothecene(s), 312, 313
triclosan, 48, 403, 405, *See also* toxic household
    products: triclosan in antibacterial products
triiodothyronine, 353, 354, 356, 357
tri-*ortho*-cresyl phosphate (TOCP), 264
triphenylmethyl radical, 26
trophic level. *See* food chain(s)
TSP. *See* total suspended particles (TSP)
tubular reabsorption, 103
tumor. *See* cancer
tumor necrosis factor (TNF), 309
tumorigenesis. *See* carcinogenesis
tundra. *See* wildlife environment: tundra
Turner syndrome. *See* chromosome aberration:
    Turner syndrome
two-compartment model. *See* toxicant(s):
    toxicokinetics
Type I hypersensitivity. *See* toxicant(s):
    toxicodynamics
Type II hypersensitivity. *See* toxicant(s):
    toxicodynamics
Type III hypersensitivity. *See* toxicant(s):
    toxicodynamics
Type IV hypersensitivity. *See* toxicant(s):
    toxicodynamics

U

U.K. Department for Environmental, Food, and
    Rural Affairs (U.K. DEFRA), 281
U.S. Agency for Toxic Substances and Disease
    Registry (ATSDR), 41, 47, 51, 176, 214, 219,
    221, 224, 245, 249, 452
    creation of, 41
U.S. Bureau of Mines (USBM), 370
U.S. Centers for Disease Control and Prevention
    (CDC), 12, 23, 33, 361, 371, 388
    health risk assessment activities, 434
U.S. Clean Air Act (USCA Act), 36, 172, 453
U.S. Clean Water Act (USCW Act), 36, 39, 415,
    416, 436, 453
U.S. Coast Guard (USCG)
    areas of regulatory concern, 40
U.S. Code of Federal Regulations, 371, 394, 395,
    424, 425
U.S. Consumer Product Safety Act (CPS Act), 38
U.S. Consumer Product Safety Commission
    (CPSC), 7, 39, 42, 58
    areas of regulatory concern, 40
    functions, 38

health risk assessment activities, 434
lead poisoning, 404
toxic household products, 388, 389, 405
U.S. Council of Environmental Quality (CEQ),
    34, 35
U.S. Department of Agriculture (USDA), 422,
    449
U.S. Department of Health and Human Services
    (DHHS), 38, 371, 434
U.S. Department of Transportation (DOT), 38,
    40
    areas of regulatory concern, 40
    functions, 39
U.S. Environmental Protection Agency (U.S.
    EPA), 7, 35, 36, 38, 39, 41, 43, 49, 51, 56, 64,
    81, 86, 155, 175, 179, 193, 194, 205, 212, 217,
    219, 221, 235, 238, 241, 242, 244, 245, 247,
    255, 257, 258, 265, 266, 268, 270, 271, 273,
    274, 281, 295, 340, 379, 397, 406, 451
    air pollutants, 172
    air toxics, 172
    aquatic toxicity tests, 415
    areas of regulatory concern, 40
    cumulative risk assessment, 445
    early efforts, 35
    ecological risk assessment, 420, 421
    endocrine disruptors, 360
    Exposure Factor Handbook, 450
    functions, 38
    health risk assessment activities, 433, 434
    health risk communication, 452
    health risk perception, 451
    maximum contaminant level (MCL), 213, 446
    National Priorities List (NPL), 426
    NPDES, water quality, 416
    oil spills, 417
    persistence criteria, 281
    RCRA, toxic wastes, 424
    reference dose (RfD), 446, 451
    risk characterization, 445
    screening values, 85, 86, 403
    Superfund cleanup, 425, 426, 427, 428, 429
    The Birth of, 35
    TMDL, water quality, 416
    toxic wastes, 424
    toxicity testing, 434, 437
    water quality criteria (WQC), 415
U.S. EPA. *See* U.S. Environmental Protection
    Agency (U.S. EPA)
U.S. Federal Emergency Management Agency
    (FEMA), 217
U.S. Food and Drug Administration (FDA), 7, 39,

42, 49
acceptable daily intake (ADI), 446, 451
areas of regulatory concern, 40
food toxicants, 388, 390, 394
functions, 38
health risk assessment activities, 434, 451
toxic household products, 399
toxicity testing, 438
U.S. Food, Drug, and Cosmetic Act (FD&C Act), 39, 40
U.S. Geological Survey (USGS), 50, 418
U.S. Mine Safety and Health Administration (MSHA), 194, 374, 382
U.S. National Institute for Occupational Safety and Health (NIOSH), 57, 371, 373, 374, 375, 379, 381
U.S. National Institute on Deafness and Other Communication Disorders (NIDCD), 323
U.S. National Institutes of Health (NIH), 2, 434
U.S. National Research Council (NRC), 7, 395, 433
U.S. Occupational Safety and Health Act (OSH Act), 39, 40, 370
U.S. Occupational Safety and Health Administration (OSHA), iv, 7, 38, 42, 194, 213, 219, 371, 372, 373, 374, 375
areas of regulatory concern, 40
bloodborne pathogens (BBP) standard, 373, 385
functions, 39
Hazard Communication Standard, 383
health risk assessment activities, 434, 446
organic solvents, 380
permissible exposure limit, 375
right-to-know standard, 373
synthetic mineral fibers (SMFs), 381, 382
U.S. Personal Care Products Council (U.S. PCPC), 398
UDP-glucuronosyltransferase (UGT), 113, 115, 118, 123
UGT. *See* UDP-glucuronosyltransferase (UGT)
ultimate carcinogen(s)
definition, 338
ultrafine particles, 193, 196, 197, *See also* $PM_{0.1}$
coagulation, 196
nucleation, 196, 197
uncertainty and safety factors, 422, 447, *See also* health risk assessment: uncertainty and safety factors
uncertainty factors. *See* health risk assessment: uncertainty and safety factors
UNEP. *See* United Nations Environment

Programme (UNEP)
United Heckathorn (Superfund toxic site), 51, 426, 427, 428
United Nations Economic Commission for Europe (UNECE), 281
United Nations Environment Programme (UNEP), 42, 89, 281, 283, 433
United Nations Food and Agriculture Organization (FAO), 20, 85
Universal Waste Rule, U.S., 50
uptake of toxicants. *See* toxicant(s): uptake and absorption of
uranium (U), 54, 248, 249, 333, 334, 384
urban particulate pollution, 197, 198, 199, 200, 201, 202
airborne microbes, 200, 201, 202
episodes, 198, 199
lignite mining operations, 199
monitoring issues, 199, 200
urbanization, 17, 19, 30
Urginea maritima, 272

V

vapor migration (vapor intrusion), 226
venom(s), 303
from amphibians, 320, 321, *See also* various species or orders (frogs, newts, toads, etc.) separately
from arachnids, 318, 319
from arthropods, 317, 318, 319
from insects, 319, *See also* bee, hornet, or wasp sting(s) separately
from lizards, 321
from reptiles, 319, 321, *See also* snake(s) or lizard(s) separately
from scorpions, 318, *See also* scorpion(s)
from spiders, 318, *See also* spider(s)
vinyl chloride, 144, 213, 224, 334
viral gastroenteritis, 234, 306, 404
viral toxin, 309
virions, 136, 306
viroids, 305
virus L-A, 309
vitamin A, 26, 119, 359, 363, 391, 392
vitamin B_1 (thiamine), 159
vitamin B_{12} (cobalamin), 160
vitamin C (ascorbic acid), 26, 119, 121, 124, 159, 162, 392
vitamin D, 159, 391, 392
vitamin E, 119, 121, 392
vitamin K, 137, 159

vitellogenin (VTG), 294
    gene, 294
VOCs. *See* volatile organic compounds (VOCs)
volatile organic compounds (VOCs), 18, 47, 52,
    56, 59, 172, 181, 192, 198, 212, 213, 214, 223,
    394
    environmental concerns, 213, 214, 215
    precursors of ozone, 212
    precursors of particulate matter, 212
    sources of pollution, 213
    use standards, 213, 214, 215
volume of distribution. *See* toxicant(s):
    toxicokinetics
VX, 265

W

warfarin, 137, 163, 272
wasp sting(s), 319
water contaminant(s)
    fate, 68, 69, 70, 71, 72, 73
    transport, 68, 69, 70, 71, 72, 73
water pollution, 17, 22, 31, 38, 74, 75, 412, 416,
    423
    definition, 18
water quality
    criteria (WQC), 415
    regulatory efforts for, 416
weight-of-evidence, 447, 448
wet deposition. *See* air pollutant(s): wet
    deposition
WHO (World Health Organization), 3, 11, 12, 16,
    17, 37, 41, 42, 83, 150, 161, 163, 175, 176,
    179, 182, 185, 195, 196, 197, 198, 199, 202,
    204, 214, 222, 223, 224, 225, 226, 227, 255,
    266, 296, 297, 298, 335, 383, 385, 388, 422,
    438, 451
    carcinogenicity potential, 340
wildlife environment, 418, 419, 420
    chaparral, 419
    desert, 419

    forests, 419, 420
    taiga, 419
    tundra, 419
Wildlife Exposure Factors Handbook, 421
wildlife toxicology, 411, 412, 416, 417, 418, 419,
    420, 421, 422
    relevance, 412
    scope and history, 417, 418
Wildlife Toxicology Working Group, 417
Wilson's disease, 247
Wingspread Conference Center, Wisconsin, U.S.
    endocrine disruption, 349
workplace biological hazards, 383
    infectious agents, 384, 385
workplace exposure limit (WEL), 375
workplace physical hazards, 383
    cold, 384
    heat, 384
    ionizing radiation, 384
    noise, 384
    non-ionizing radiation, 384
    vibration, 384
workplace right-to-know movement, 383
World Health Day, 11
World Health Organization. *See* WHO (World
    Health Organization)

X

xanthine oxidase, 160
xenobiotics. *See* toxicology: terminology
xylene(s), 213, 218, 380, 402

Z

zearalenone(s), 312, 313, 314
zinc (Zn), 26, 119, 136, 159, 185, 195, 233, 237,
    238, 243, 244, 246, 247, 380, 392, 425
zinc oxide, 380
zygocin, 309

Made in the USA
Charleston, SC
11 December 2015